Clinical Pharmacology
During Pregnancy

Clinical Pharmacology During Pregnancy

Second Edition

Edited by

Donald Mattison

University of South Carolina,
Arnold School of Public Health,
Columbia, SC, United States

Risk Sciences International, Ottawa, ON, Canada

School of Epidemiology and Public Health,
University of Ottawa, Ottawa, ON, Canada

Lee-Ann Halbert

Associate Professor of Nursing
University of South Carolina
Beaufort, Bluffton
SC, United States

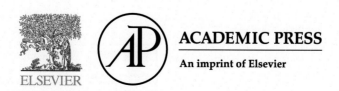

ELSEVIER

ACADEMIC PRESS
An imprint of Elsevier

Library of Congress Cataloging-in-Publication Data
A catalog record for this book is available from the Library of Congress

British Library Cataloguing-in-Publication Data
A catalogue record for this book is available from the British Library

ISBN: 978-0-12-818902-3

For information on all Academic Press publications visit our website at https://www.elsevier.com/books-and-journals

Publisher: Andre Gerhard Wolff
Acquisitions Editor: Erin Hill-Parks
Editorial Project Manager: Tracy I. Tufaga
Production Project Manager: Stalin Viswanathan
Cover Designer: Victoria Pearson

Typeset by TNQ Technologies

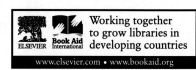

This book is dedicated to all the individuals who have added to and benefit from the collective knowledge and wisdom presented within this book. The chapter authors share their insights with the express goal of helping health care practitioners and their clients make the best clinical decisions when it comes to the use of medications in pregnancy.

Contents

CHAPTER 6   Treating the placenta: an evolving therapeutic concept...79

Michael D. Reed and Donald R. Mattison

CHAPTER 7   Conducting randomized controlled pharmaceutical trials in the pregnant population: challenges and solutions......................93

Isabelle Hardy and William D. Fraser

CHAPTER 15   Diabetes in pregnancy...................................251
Kimberly K. Trout and Cara D. Dolin

CHAPTER 16   Cardiovascular medications in pregnancy...........271
Andrew Youmans

CHAPTER 19   Antenatal thyroid disease and pharmacotherapy in pregnancy...........339
Shannon M. Clark and Luis A. Monsivais

CHAPTER 20   Management of dermatological conditions in pregnancy 357
Carmen V. Harrison

CHAPTER 24   **Challenges in predicting the pharmacokinetics of drugs in premature and mature newborns: example with piperacillin and tazobactam**

Jeffrey W. Fisher, Darshan Mehta, Miao Li and Xiaoxia Yang

Contributors

Mahmoud Abdelwahab
Ohio State University, Columbus, OH, United States

Mahmoud S. Ahmed
Department of Obstetrics & Gynecology, University of Texas Medical Branch, Galveston, TX, United States

Sarah Armstrong
Frimley Park Hospital, Surrey, United Kingdom

Cheston M. Berlin, Jr.
Department of Pediatrics/Division of Academic General Pediatrics, Penn State College of Medicine, Penn Statae Children's Hospital, Hershey, PA, United States

Brookie M. Best
University of California, Skaggs School of Pharmacy and Pharmaceutical Sciences, San Diego, CA, United States

Carolyn Bottone-Post
University of Northern Colorado, Greeley, CO, United States

Shannon M. Clark
Department of ObGyn, Division of Maternal-Fetal Medicine, University of Texas Medical Branch-Galveston, Galveston, TX, United States

Maged M. Costantine
Ohio State University, Columbus, OH, United States

Kala R. Crobarger
Tanner Health System School of Nursing, University of West Georgia, Carrollton, GA, United States

Cara D. Dolin
Department of Obstetrics and Gynecology, University of Pennsylvania, Perelman School of Medicine, Philadelphia, PA, United States

Jeffrey W. Fisher
Division of Biochemical Toxicology, National Center for Toxicological Research, Food and Drug Administration, Jefferson, AR, United States; ScitoVation, LLC, Durham, NC, United States

David A. Flockhart
Indiana University School of Medicine, Indianapolis, IN, United States

Jeffrey S. Fouche-Camargo
School of Health Sciences, Georgia Gwinnett College, Lawrenceville, GA, United States

William D. Fraser
Department of Obstetrics and Gynecology, Université de Sherbrooke, Sherbrooke, QC, Canada

Jennifer L. Grasch
Indiana University School of Medicine, Indianapolis, IN, United States

David M. Haas
Indiana University School of Medicine, Indianapolis, IN, United States

Lee-Ann Halbert
University of South Carolina Beaufort, Bluffton, SC, United States

Isabelle Hardy
Department of Obstetrics and Gynecology, Université de Sherbrooke, Sherbrooke, QC, Canada

Carmen V. Harrison
School of Nursing, Simmons University, Boston, MA, United States

Mary F. Hebert
Departments of Pharmacy and Obstetrics & Gynecology, University of Washington, Seattle, WA, United States

Henry M. Hess
Emeritus Professor of Obstetrics and Gynecology, University of Rochester School of Medicine, Rochester, NY

Janelle Komorowski
Department of Nurse-midwifery, Frontier Nursing University, Versailles, KY, United States

Miao Li
Division of Biochemical Toxicology, National Center for Toxicological Research, Food and Drug Administration, Jefferson, AR, United States

Megan Lutz
University of Wisconsin School of Medicine and Public Health, Department of Medicine, Madison, WI, United States

Donald R. Mattison
University of South Carolina, Arnold School of Public Health, Columbia, SC, United States; Risk Sciences International, Ottawa, ON, Canada; School of Epidemiology and Public Health, University of Ottawa, Ottawa, ON, Canada

Darshan Mehta
Division of Biochemical Toxicology, National Center for Toxicological Research, Food and Drug Administration, Jefferson, AR, United States

Jeremiah D. Momper
University of California, Skaggs School of Pharmacy and Pharmaceutical Sciences, San Diego, CA, United States

Luis A. Monsivais
Department of ObGyn, Division of Maternal-Fetal Medicine, University of Texas Medical Branch-Galveston, Galveston, TX, United States

Jennifer A. Namazy
Scripps Clinic, San Diego, CA, United States

Luis Pacheco
University of Texas Medical Branch, Galveston, TX, United States

Maria P. Ramirez-Cruz
Department of Obstetrics and Gynecology, University of New Mexico School of Medicine, Albuquerque, NM, United States

William F. Rayburn
Obstetrics and Gynecology, University of New Mexico School of Medicine, Albuquerque, NM, United States

Michael D. Reed
Professor Emeritus of Pediatrics, Department of Pediatrics, School of Medicine, Case Western Reserve University, Cleveland, United States

Sharon E. Robertson
Department of Obstetrics and Gynecology, Indiana University School of Medicine, Indianapolis, IN, United States

Erik Rytting
Department of Obstetrics & Gynecology, University of Texas Medical Branch, Galveston, TX, United States

Rachel Ryu
Department of Pharmacy, University of Washington, Seattle, WA, United States

Sumona Saha
University of Wisconsin School of Medicine and Public Health, Department of Medicine, Madison, WI, United States

Michael Schatz
Kaiser Permanente, San Diego, CA, United States

Jeanne M. Schilder
Department of Obstetrics and Gynecology, Indiana University School of Medicine, Indianapolis, IN, United States

Steven A. Seifert
Department of Emergency Medicine, University of New Mexico School of Medicine, Albuquerque, NM, United States; Medical, New Mexico Poison and Drug Information Center, Clinical Toxicology, Albuquerque, NM, United States

Harry Soljak
Frimley Park Hospital, Surrey, United Kingdom

Kimberly K. Trout
Department of Family and Community Health, University of Pennsylvania, School of Nursing, Philadelphia, PA, United States

Jennifer Waltz
School of Medicine, University of Texas Medical Branch, Galveston, TX, United States

Xiaoxia Yang
Division of Infectious Disease Pharmacology, Center for Drug Evaluation and Research, Food and Drug Administration, Silver Spring, MD, United States

Andrew Youmans
University of Michigan School of Nursing, MI, United States

Acknowledgment

Although each chapter author is acknowledged by having his/her/their name associated with the chapters, the timing of this book necessitates an additional thank you to each author. Research and writing for this book started before anyone was aware that a pandemic would change the world and raise concerns about therapeutic interventions during pregnancy.

As the authors became involved with the challenges of working in healthcare, a world turned upside down—long hours in uncertain times, isolation, trying to understand and predict the impact of coronavirus on pregnancy, shortages of equipment and staff, and countless other trials of the times—the authors continued their research and writing for these chapters.

Under normal times, completing a book chapter takes dedication and commitment, and during pandemic, it goes beyond measure. For this, we are appreciative.

Introduction

Donald R. Mattison[1,2,3], Lee-Ann Halbert[4]

[1]University of South Carolina, Arnold School of Public Health, Columbia, SC, United States;
[2]Risk Sciences International, Ottawa, ON, Canada; [3]School of Epidemiology and Public Health,
University of Ottawa, Ottawa, ON, Canada; [4]University of South Carolina Beaufort, Bluffton,
SC, United States

Over the past decade, attention to clinical therapeutics during pregnancy has grown substantially [1−3]. Examples of these advances are summarized in many different chapters in this edition Despite these advances, there is increasing concern that discovery and development of new drugs for these important populations is lagging [4−9]. For example, while there are many advances in treating depression and mood disorders, we are still struggling with questions concerning whether these diseases should be treated during pregnancy [Chapter 14]. Clearly, select populations are excluded from drug development, especially women and children [5,10−12]. One consequence of this failure to develop drugs for maternal and child health is to dissociate therapeutic opportunities for women and children from the drugs and treatments currently available. This distancing of women and children from drug development and therapeutic knowledge produces a host of clinical challenges for the concerned practitioner. In the absence of sufficient therapeutic knowledge, appropriate dosing is not known [[13−17], see Chapter 26]. Without the understanding of appropriate dosing, the clinician does not know if the dose recommended on the product label will produce the desired drug concentration at the site of action, or if the concentration produced will be above or below the needed concentration, producing toxicity or inadequate response, respectively. Similarly, without thoughtful therapeutic development in women and children, it is not known if differences in pharmacodynamics will produce different treatment goals and needs for monitoring effectiveness and safety [14,18−21].

A consequence of the failure to develop drugs for use in pregnancy is that most drugs are not tested for use during pregnancy [4,22]; consequently, labeling, which may include extensive information about fetal safety [10,23], includes nothing about dosing, appropriate treatment, efficacy, or maternal safety [3−5,10,11,22,23]. Yet, these are concerns of health care providers considering treatment during pregnancy. Therefore, the practitioner treats the pregnant woman with the same dose recommended for use in adults (typically men) or may decide not to treat the disease at all. However, is the choice of not treating a woman during pregnancy better than dealing with the challenges which accompany treatment? Clearly, treatment of

Clinical Pharmacology During Pregnancy. https://doi.org/10.1016/B978-0-12-818902-3.00012-9

depression poses risks for both mother and fetus, as does stopping treatment [24–26]. This is also the case with respect to influenza during pregnancy [13,27,28]. All combined, the state of therapeutics during pregnancy underscores the continued tension that exists between maternal–placental–fetal health and maternal quality of life during pregnancy and the lack of critical study of "gestational therapeutics." This book hopes to address many of these imbalances.

A second and equally important aspect of this edition is the focus on collaborative practice. Physicians and their students, nurses (advanced practice and generalist) and their students, and physician assistants (and their students) are all involved in the care of the pregnant woman. The American College of Nurse-Midwives and the American College of Obstetricians and Gynecologists formalized support of the collaborative practice between midwives and physicians in statements dating back to 2011 [29]. The American College of Obstetricians and Gynecologists 2016 Executive Summary on collaborative practice extends interdisciplinary practice support to include not only physicians and nurses but also pharmacists and physician assistants [30]. This edition reflects this goal of collaborative practice, with an editorial team comprised of a physician and certified nurse-midwife.

Medical and health care providers caring for women during pregnancy have many excellent resources describing the safety of medications for the fetus [10,23]. However, none of these references provide information on appropriate dosing as well as the efficacy of the various medications used during pregnancy for maternal/placental therapeutics. We are all familiar with the potential/actual costs, financial and psychosocial, of having treatments which produce developmental toxicity; however, how many of us ever think critically about the costs of having inadequate therapeutic options to treat the major diseases of pregnancy, growth restriction, pregnancy loss, and preeclampsia/eclampsia? Where we have effective treatments for maternal diseases, infection, depression, diabetes, and hypertension, we are recognizing that continuation of treatment during pregnancy carries benefit for mother, placenta, and baby. In the end what is important for the mother, baby, and family is the appropriate balancing of benefit and risk—as indeed is the important balancing for all clinical therapeutics [11,12]. This book provides medical and health professionals involved in the care of pregnant women with contemporary information on clinical pharmacology for pregnancy. It covers an overview of the impact of pregnancy on drug disposition, summarizing current research about the changes of pharmacokinetics and pharmacodynamics during pregnancy. This is followed by specific sections on the treatment, dosing, and clinical effectiveness of medications during pregnancy, providing health care providers with an essential reference on how to appropriately treat women with medications during pregnancy. At one level, the question is simple: how to treat, how to monitor for benefit and risk, or how to know if treatment is successful? This book was developed to explore that question for women during pregnancy. The book is meant to be a guide to clinicians who care for women during pregnancy. We hope the busy clinician and student of obstetrics will find this a useful guide.

References

[1] Zajicek A, Giacoia GP. Obstetric clinical pharmacology: coming of age. Clin Pharmacol Ther 2007;81(4):481–2.

[2] Schwartz JB. The current state of knowledge on age, sex, and their interactions on clinical pharmacology. Clin Pharmacol Ther 2007;82(1):87–96.

[3] Kearns GL, Ritschel WA, Wilson JT, Spielberg SP. Clinical pharmacology: a discipline called to action for maternal and child health. Clin Pharmacol Ther 2007;81(4):463–8.

[4] Malek A, Mattison DR. Drug development for use during pregnancy: impact of the placenta. Expet Rev Obstet Gynecol 2010;5(4):437–54.

[5] Thornton JG. Drug development and obstetrics: where are we right now? J Matern Fetal Neonatal Med 2009;22(Suppl. 2):46–9.

[6] Woodcock J, Woosley R. The FDA critical path initiative and its influence on new drug development. Annu Rev Med 2008;59:1–2.

[7] The PME. Drug development for maternal health cannot be left to the whims of the market. PLoS Med 2008;5(6):e140.

[8] Hawcutt DB, Smyth RL. Drug development for children: how is pharma tackling an unmet need? IDrugs 2008;11(7):502–7.

[9] Adams CP, Brantner VV. Estimating the cost of new drug development: is it really $802 million? Health Aff 2006;25(2):420–8.

[10] Lo WY, Friedman JM. Teratogenicity of recently introduced medications in human pregnancy. Obstet Gynecol 2002;100(3):465–73.

[11] Fisk NM, Atun R. Market failure and the poverty of new drugs in maternal health. PLoS Med 2008;5(1):e22.

[12] Thornton J. The drugs we deserve. BJOG 2003;110(11):969–70.

[13] Beigi RH, Han K, Venkataramanan R, Hankins GD, Clark S, Hebert MF, et al. Pharmacokinetics of oseltamivir among pregnant and nonpregnant women. Am J Obstet Gynecol 2011;204(6 Suppl. 1):S84–8.

[14] Rothberger S, Carr D, Brateng D, Hebert M, Easterling TR. Pharmacodynamics of clonidine therapy in pregnancy: a heterogeneous maternal response impacts fetal growth. Am J Hypertens 2010;23(11):1234–40.

[15] Eyal S, Easterling TR, Carr D, Umans JG, Miodovnik M, Hankins GD, et al. Pharmacokinetics of metformin during pregnancy. Drug Metab Dispos 2010;38(5):833–40.

[16] Hebert MF, Ma X, Naraharisetti SB, Krudys KM, Umans JG, Hankins GD, et al. Are we optimizing gestational diabetes treatment with glyburide? The pharmacologic basis for better clinical practice. Clin Pharmacol Ther 2009;85(6):607–14.

[17] Andrew MA, Easterling TR, Carr DB, Shen D, Buchanan ML, Rutherford T, et al. Amoxicillin pharmacokinetics in pregnant women: modeling and simulations of dosage strategies. Clin Pharmacol Ther 2007;81(4):547–56.

[18] Na-Bangchang K, Manyando C, Ruengweerayut R, Kioy D, Mulenga M, Miller GB, et al. The pharmacokinetics and pharmacodynamics of atovaquone and proguanil for the treatment of uncomplicated falciparum malaria in third-trimester pregnant women. Eur J Clin Pharmacol 2005;61(8):573–82.

[19] Hebert MF, Carr DB, Anderson GD, Blough D, Green GE, Brateng DA, et al. Pharmacokinetics and pharmacodynamics of atenolol during pregnancy and postpartum. J Clin Pharmacol 2005;45(1):25–33.

[20] Meibohm B, Derendorf H. Pharmacokinetic/pharmacodynamic studies in drug product development. J Pharmacol Sci 2002;91(1):18—31.

[21] Lu J, Pfister M, Ferrari P, Chen G, Sheiner L. Pharmacokinetic-pharmacodynamic modelling of magnesium plasma concentration and blood pressure in preeclamptic women. Clin Pharmacokinet 2002;41(13):1105—13.

[22] Feghali MN, Mattison DR. Clinical therapeutics in pregnancy. J Biomed Biotechnol 2011;2011:783528.

[23] Adam MP, Polifka JE, Friedman JM. Evolving knowledge of the teratogenicity of medications in human pregnancy. Am J Med Genet C Semin Med Genet 2011;157(3): 175—82.

[24] Markus EM, Miller LJ. The other side of the risk equation: exploring risks of untreated depression and anxiety in pregnancy. J Clin Psychiatr 2009;70(9):1314—5.

[25] Marcus SM, Heringhausen JE. Depression in childbearing women: when depression complicates pregnancy. Prim Care 2009;36(1):151—65 [ix].

[26] Marcus SM. Depression during pregnancy: rates, risks and consequences — Motherisk Update 2008. Can J Clin Pharmacol 2009;16(1):e15—22.

[27] Mirochnick M, Clarke D. Oseltamivir pharmacokinetics in pregnancy: a commentary. Am J Obstet Gynecol 2011;204(6 Suppl. 1):S94—5.

[28] Greer LG, Leff RD, Rogers VL, Roberts SW, McCracken Jr GH, Wendel Jr GD, et al. Pharmacokinetics of oseltamivir according to trimester of pregnancy. Am J Obstet Gynecol 2011;204(6 Suppl. 1):S89—93.

[29] Statement of policy: joint statement of practice relations between obstetrician-gynecologists and certified nurse-midwives/certified midwives, vol. 129; 2017. p. e117—e122.

[30] Executive summary: collaboration in practice: implementing team-based care. Obstet Gynecol 2016;127:612—7.

Physiologic changes during pregnancy

Mahmoud Abdelwahab[1], Maged M. Costantine[1], Luis Pacheco[2]

[1]*Ohio State University, Columbus, OH, United States;* [2]*University of Texas Medical Branch, Galveston, TX, United States*

2.1 Physiologic changes during pregnancy

Human pregnancy is characterized by profound anatomic and physiologic changes that affect virtually all systems and organs in the body. Many of these changes begin in early gestation. Understanding of the various physiologic adaptations in pregnancy is vital to the clinician and the pharmacologist as many of these alterations will have a significant impact on pharmacokinetics and pharmacodynamics of different therapeutic agents. A typical example involves the increase in glomerular filtration rate (GFR) during pregnancy leading to increased clearance of heparins, thus requiring the use of higher doses during pregnancy. This chapter discusses the most relevant physiologic changes that occur during human gestation.

2.2 Cardiovascular system

Profound changes in the cardiovascular system characterize human pregnancy and are likely to affect the pharmacokinetics of different pharmaceutical agents. Table 2.1 summarizes the main cardiovascular changes during pregnancy.

Cardiac output (CO) increases by 30%–50% during pregnancy, secondary to an increase in both heart rate and stroke volume; the increase in CO in early pregnancy is thought to be mainly mediated by an increase in stroke volume, whereas later in gestation the increase is attributed to elevated heart rate [1]. Most of the increase in CO occurs early in pregnancy such that by the end of the first trimester 75% of the increase has already occurred. In addition, CO is expected to be 15% more in a twin pregnancy compared to a singleton [2]. CO plateau at 28–32 weeks and afterward remains relatively stable until delivery. At 32 weeks, CO increased to about 7.21 l/min vs 4.88 l/min prior to conception [3].

As CO increases, pregnant women experience a significant decrease in both systemic and pulmonary vascular resistances [4]. Systemic vascular resistance decreases in early pregnancy, reaching a nadir (5–10 mm below baseline) at 14–24 weeks. Subsequently, vascular resistance starts rising, progressively approaching the prepregnancy value at term [4]. Blood pressure tends to fall toward the end of the

Table 2.1 Summary of cardiovascular changes during pregnancy.

Variable	Change
Mean arterial pressure	No significant change
Central venous pressure	No change
Pulmonary arterial occlusion pressure	No change
Systemic vascular resistance	Decreased by 21% (nadir at 14–24 weeks)
Pulmonary vascular resistance	Decreased by 34%
Heart rate	Increased by 10–20 bpm maximum in third trimester
Stroke volume	Increases to a maximum of 85 mL at 20 weeks of gestation
Colloid osmotic pressure	Decreased by 14% (associated with a decrease in serum osmolarity noticed as early as the first trimester of pregnancy)
Hemoglobin concentration	Decreased (maximum hemodilution is achieved at 30–32 weeks)

first trimester and then rises again in the third trimester to prepregnancy levels [5]. Physiologic hypotension may be present between weeks 14 and 24, likely due to the decrease in the systemic vascular resistance observed during pregnancy.

Maternal blood volume increases in pregnancy by 40%–50%, reaching maximum values at 32 weeks [6]. Despite the increase in blood volume, central filling pressures like the central venous and pulmonary occlusion pressures remain unchanged secondary to an increase in compliance of the right and left ventricles [7]. The precise etiology of the increase in blood volume is not clearly understood. However, increased mineralocorticoid activity with water and sodium retention does occur [8]. Production of arginine vasopressin (resulting in increased water absorption in the distal nephron) is also increased during pregnancy and thought to further contribute to hypervolemia. Secondary hemodilutional anemia and a decrease in serum colloid osmotic pressure (due to a drop in albumin levels) are observed.

Finally, left ventricular wall thickness and left ventricular mass increase by 28% and 52% above pregnancy values [9]. Despite the multiple changes in cardiovascular parameters, left ventricular ejection fraction does not appear to change during pregnancy [10].

The latter physiological changes could have theoretical implications on the pharmacokinetics of drugs in pregnancy. The increase in blood volume, increased capillary hydrostatic pressure, and decrease in albumin concentrations would be expected to increase significantly the volume of distribution of hydrophilic substances. In addition, highly protein-bound compounds may display higher free levels due to decreased protein binding availability.

2.3 **Respiratory system**

The respiratory system undergoes both mechanical and functional changes during pregnancy. Table 2.2 summarizes these changes.

The sharp increase in estrogen concentrations during pregnancy leads to hypervascularity and edema of the upper respiratory mucosa [11]. These changes result in an increased prevalence of rhinitis and epistaxis in pregnant individuals. Theoretically, inhaled medications such as steroids used in the treatment of asthma could be more readily absorbed in the pregnant patient. Despite this theoretical concern, however, there is no evidence of increased toxicity with the use of these agents during pregnancy.

Progesterone acts centrally to increase the sensitivity of respiratory center to carbon dioxide [12]. This drives an increase in minute ventilation by 30%−50% secondary to an increase in tidal volume. As a result of in the increase in ventilation, there in an increase in the arterial partial pressure of oxygen to 101−105 mmHg and a diminished arterial partial pressure of carbon dioxide ($PaCO_2$), with normal values of $PaCO_2$ of the range 28−31 mmHg during pregnancy. This decrement allows for a gradient to exist between the $PaCO_2$ of the fetus and the mother so that carbon dioxide can diffuse freely from the fetus into the mother through the placenta and then be eliminated through the maternal lungs. Of note, maternal respiratory rate remains unchanged during pregnancy [13].

The normal maternal arterial blood pH in pregnancy is between 7.4 and 7.45, consistent with a mild respiratory alkalosis. The latter is partially corrected by an

Table 2.2 Summary of respiratory changes during pregnancy.

Variable	Change
Tidal volume	Increased by 30%−50% (increase starts as early as the first trimester)
Respiratory rate	No change
Minute ventilation	Increased by 30%−50% (increase starts as early as the first trimester)
Partial pressure of oxygen	Increased (increase starts as early as the first trimester)
Partial pressure of carbon dioxide	Decreased (decrease starts as early as the first trimester)
Arterial pH	Slightly increased (increase starts as early as the first trimester)
Vital capacity	No change
Functional residual capacity	Decreased by 10%−20% (predisposes pregnant patients to hypoxemia during induction of general anesthesia)
Total lung capacity	Decreased by 4%−5% (maximum diaphragmatic elevation happens during the third trimester of pregnancy)

increased renal excretion of bicarbonate to allow for a normal serum bicarbonate between 18 and 21 meq/L during gestation [14]. As pregnancy progresses, the increased intraabdominal pressure (likely secondary to uterine enlargement, bowel dilation, and third-spacing of fluids into the peritoneal cavity secondary to decreased colloid osmotic pressure) displaces the diaphragm upward by 4–5 cm leading to alveolar collapse in the bases of the lungs. Bibasilar atelectasis results in a 10%–20% decrease in the functional residual capacity and increased right to left vascular shunt [15,16]. The decrease in expiratory reserve volume is coupled with an increase in inspiratory reserve volume. As a result, no change is seen in the vital capacity [15].

An increase in the transverse diameter of the rib cage occurs to accommodate the upward shit of the diaphragm due to the enlarging gravid uterus and upward displacement of intraabdominal contents, in order to allow space for the lung and preserve total lung capacity. The average subcostal angle of the ribs at the xiphoidal level increases from 68.5 degrees at the beginning of pregnancy to 103.5 degrees at term [17].

Changes in respiratory physiology may impact the pharmacokinetics of certain drugs. Topical drugs administered into the nasopharynx and upper airway could be more readily available to the circulation as local vascularity and permeability of the mucosa are increased. As discussed earlier, the latter assumption is theoretical, and no evidence of increased toxicity from inhaled or topical agents during pregnancy has been demonstrated.

2.4 Renal system

Numerous physiologic changes occur in the renal system during pregnancy. These changes are summarized in Table 2.3.

The relaxing effect of progesterone on smooth muscle and mechanical effects of the enlarging uterus leads to dilation of the urinary tract with subsequent urinary stasis. It is estimated that the dilated collecting system seen in pregnancy can hold 200–300 mL of urine [18]. Hydronephrosis affects 43%–100% of pregnant women and is more prevalent with advancing gestation. However, studies have shown that exogenous administration of progesterone in nonpregnant women fails to cause hydronephrosis. The changes observed in the urinary tract predispose pregnant women to infectious complications, most notably urinary tract infections [19].

The 50% increase in renal blood flow during early pregnancy leads to a parallel increase in the GFR of approximately 50%. This massive elevation in GFR is present as early as 14 weeks of pregnancy [20]. As a direct consequence of increased GFR, creatinine clearance increases and serum values of creatinine and blood urea nitrogen decrease. In fact, a serum creatinine above 0.8 mg/dL may be indicative of underlying renal dysfunction during pregnancy.

Besides detoxification, one of the most important functions of the kidney is to regulate sodium and water metabolism. Progesterone favors natriuresis, while

Table 2.3 Summary of renal changes during pregnancy.

Variable	Change
Renal blood flow	Increased by 50%. Increase noticed as early as 14 weeks of gestation
Glomerular filtration rate	Increased by 50%. Increase noticed as early as 14 weeks of gestation
Serum creatinine	Decreased (normal value is 0.5—0.8 mg/dL during pregnancy)
Renin—angiotensin—aldosterone system	Increased function leading to sodium and water retention noticed from early in the first trimester of pregnancy
Total body water	Increased by up to 8 L. 6 L gained in the extracellular space and 2 L in the intracellular space
Ureter—bladder muscle tone	Decreased secondary to increases in progesterone. Smooth muscle relaxation leads to urine stasis with increased risk for urinary tract infections
Urinary protein excretion	Increased secondary to elevated filtration rate. Values up to 260 mg of protein in 24 h are considered normal in pregnancy
Serum bicarbonate	Decreased by 4—5 meq/L. Normal value in pregnancy is 18—22 meq/L (24 meq/L in nonpregnant individuals)

estrogen favors sodium retention [21]. Although the increase in GFR leads to more sodium wasting, it is counterbalanced by an elevated level of aldosterone which reabsorbs sodium in the distal nephron [21]. Relaxin may also play a role in water retention since it stimulates ADH production in animal studies and is normally elevated in pregnancy [22]. The net effect during pregnancy is a state of avid water and sodium retention leading to a significant increase in total body water with up to 6 L of fluid gained in the extracellular space and 2 L in the intracellular space. This "dilutional effect" leads to a mild decrease in both serum sodium (concentration of 135—138 meq/L) and serum osmolarity (normal value in pregnancy $\sim$280 mOsm/L) [23]. In comparison, in the nonpregnant state, normal serum osmolarity is 286—289 mOsm/L with a concomitant normal serum sodium concentration of 135—145 meq/L.

Changes in renal physiology have profound repercussions on drug pharmacokinetics. Agents cleared renally are expected to have shorter half-lives, and fluid retention is expected to increase the volume of distribution of hydrophilic agents. A typical example involves lithium. Lithium is mainly cleared by the kidney, and during the third trimester of pregnancy, clearance is doubled compared to the nonpregnant state [24]. However, not all renally cleared medications undergo such dramatic increases in excretion rates. For example, digoxin clearance is only increased by 30% during the third trimester of pregnancy.

2.5 Gastrointestinal system

The gastrointestinal tract is significantly affected during pregnancy secondary to progesterone-mediated inhibition of smooth muscle motility [25]. Table 2.4 summarizes these changes.

Gastric emptying and small bowel transit time are considerably prolonged during pregnancy. The increase in intragastric pressure (secondary to delayed emptying and external compression from the gravid uterus) together with a decrease in resting muscle tone of the lower esophageal sphincter favors gastroesophageal regurgitation. Of note, studies have shown that gastric acid secretion is not affected during pregnancy [26]. However, overall gastric acidity might be increased due to increased serum levels of gastrin [27]. Finally, constipation commonly affects pregnant women and is multifactorial in nature. The combination of increased bowel transit time, mechanical obstruction by gravid uterus, decreased maternal activity, decreased motilin, increased colonic water and sodium absorption, and routine iron supplementation all contribute to constipation in pregnancy [28].

Conflicting data exist regarding liver blood flow during pregnancy. Recently, with the use of Doppler ultrasonography, investigators found that blood flow in the hepatic artery does not change during pregnancy, but portal venous return to the liver was increased [29].

Most of the liver function tests are not altered. Specifically, serum transaminases, bilirubin, lactate dehydrogenase, and gamma-glutamyl transferase are all unaffected by pregnancy. Serum alkaline phosphatase is elevated secondary to production from the placenta and levels two to four times higher than that of nonpregnant individuals may be seen [30]. Other liver products that are normally elevated include serum cholesterol, fibrinogen, and most of the clotting factors, ceruloplasmin,

Table 2.4 Summary of gastrointestinal changes during pregnancy.

Variable	Change
Gastric emptying time	Prolonged, increasing the risk of aspiration in pregnant women. Intragastric pressure is also increased
Gastric acid secretion	Unchanged
Liver blood flow	Unchanged in the hepatic artery; however, more venous return in the portal vein has been documented with ultrasound Doppler studies
Liver function tests	No change during pregnancy except for alkaline phosphatase (increases in pregnancy secondary to placental contribution)
Bowel/gallbladder motility	Decreased, likely secondary to smooth muscle relaxation induced by progesterone
Pancreatic function enzymes (amylase and lipase)	Unchanged

thyroid-binding globulin, and cortisol-binding globulin (CBG). The observed increase in all of these proteins is likely estrogen mediated [30]. Progesterone, on the other hand, decreases gallbladder motility rendering the pregnant woman at increased risk for cholelithiasis.

These observed physiologic changes can clearly affect pharmacokinetics of orally administered agents, with delayed absorption and onset of action resulting. For example, the pharmacokinetics of antimalarial agents undergo significant changes at the gastrointestinal level during pregnancy that could decrease their therapeutic efficacy [31].

2.6 Hematologic and coagulation systems

Pregnancy is associated with an increased white cell count, mainly consisting of an increase in neutrophils. On the contrary, lymphocyte count decreases during the first and second trimesters with return to baseline in the third trimester. The rise in white cell count is thought to be related to increased bone marrow granulopoiesis and may make a diagnosis of infection difficult at times. However, it is usually not associated with significant elevations in immature forms like bands. There is also an absolute monocytosis and increase in the monocyte-to-lymphocyte ratio, which is thought to aid in preventing fetal allograft rejection by infiltrating decidual tissue at 7—20 weeks of gestation [32].

An increase in red cell mass by 30% during pregnancy is likely secondary to an increase in renal erythropoietin production. Placental lactogen may also enhance the effect of erythropoietin on erythropoiesis [32]. This occurs simultaneously with a much higher (around 45%) increase in plasma volume leading to what is referred to as "physiologic anemia" of pregnancy which peaks early in the third trimester (30—32 weeks) [33,34]. This hemodilution is thought to confer maternal and fetal survival advantage as the patient will lose more dilute blood during delivery. In addition, the decreased blood viscosity improves uterine perfusion, while the increase in red cell mass serves to optimize oxygen transport to the fetus. As an example, patients with preeclampsia, despite having fluid retention, suffer from reduced intravascular volume (secondary to diffuse endothelial injury and resultant third-spacing), which makes them less tolerant to peripartum blood loss [35,36].

Pregnancy is also associated with changes in the coagulation and fibrinolytic pathways that favor a hypercoagulable state. Plasma levels of fibrinogen, clotting factors (VII, VIII, IX, X, and XII), and von Willebrand factor increase during pregnancy leading to a hypercoagulable state. Factor XI decreases and levels of prothrombin and factor V remain the same. Protein C is usually unchanged, but protein S is decreased in pregnancy. There is no change in the levels of antithrombin III. The fibrinolytic system is suppressed during pregnancy as a result of increased levels of plasminogen activator inhibitor (PAI-1) and reduced plasminogen activator levels. Platelet function remains normal in pregnancy. Routine coagulation screen panel will show values around normal.

Table 2.5 Hemoglobin values during pregnancy.

Gestational age	Mean hemoglobin value (g/dL)
12 weeks	12.2
28 weeks	11.8
40 weeks	12.9

Table 2.6 Summary of hematological changes during pregnancy.

Variable	Change
Fibrinogen level	Increased (elevation starts in the first trimester of pregnancy and peaks during the third trimester)
Factors VII, VIII, and X	Increased
Von Willebrand factor	Increased
Factors II, IX, and V	No change
Clotting times (prothrombin and activated partial thromboplastin times)	No change
Protein C, antithrombin III	No change
Protein S	Decreased. Free antigen levels above 30% in the second trimester and 24% in the third trimester are considered normal during pregnancy
Plasminogen activator inhibitor	Levels increase 2–3 times leading to a decrease in fibrinolytic activity
White blood cell count	Elevated. This increase results in a "left shift" with granulocytosis. Increased peaks at 30 weeks of gestation. May see values of 20,000–30,000/mm^3 during labor
Platelet count	No change

This hypercoagulable state predisposes the pregnant patient to a higher risk of thromboembolism. However, it is also thought to offer survival advantage in minimizing blood loss after delivery [37]. Tables 2.5 and 2.6 summarize some of the most relevant changes discussed previously.

2.7 Endocrine system

Pregnancy is defined as a "diabetogenic" state. Increased insulin resistance is due to elevated levels of human placental lactogen, progesterone, estrogen, and cortisol. Carbohydrate intolerance that occurs only during pregnancy is known as gestational diabetes. Most gestational diabetes patients are managed solely with a modified diet. Approximately 10% of patients will require pharmacological treatment, mainly in the form of insulin, glyburide, or even metformin. Available literature suggests that glyburide and metformin may be as effective as insulin for the treatment of gestational diabetes.

Pregnancy is also associated with higher glucose levels following a carbohydrate load. In contrast, maternal fasting is characterized by accelerated starvation, increased lipolysis, and faster depletion of liver glycogen storage [38]. This is thought to be related to the increased insulin resistance state of pregnancy induced by placental hormones such as human placental lactogen. Pancreatic β-cells undergo hyperplasia during pregnancy resulting in increased insulin production leading to fasting hypoglycemia and postprandial hyperglycemia. All of these changes facilitate placental glucose transfer, as the fetus is primarily dependent on maternal glucose for its fuel requirements [39].

Leptin is a hormone primarily secreted by adipose tissues. Maternal serum levels of leptin increase during pregnancy and peak during the second trimester. Leptin in pregnancy is also produced by the placenta.

When considering changes in certain endocrine glands during pregnancy, the thyroid gland faces a particular challenge. Due to the hyperestrogenic milieu, thyroid-binding globulin (the major thyroid hormone (TH)−binding protein in serum) increases by almost 150% from a prepregnancy concentration of 15−16 mg/L to 30−40 mg/L in mid-gestation. This forces the thyroid gland to increase its production of THs to keep their free fraction in the serum constant [40,41]. The increase in THs production occurs mostly in the first half of gestation and plateaus around 20 weeks until term.

Other factors that influence THs in pregnancy include a minor thyrotropic action of human chorionic gonadotropin hormone (hCG), higher maternal metabolic rate as pregnancy progresses, in addition to increase in transplacental transport of TH to the fetus early in pregnancy, inactivity of placental type III monodeiodinase (which converts T4 to reverse T3), and in maternal renal iodine excretion.

Although the free fraction of T4 and T3 concentrations declines somewhat during pregnancy (but remains within normal values), these patients remain clinically euthyroid [40,41]. Thyroid-stimulating hormone (TSH) decreases during the first half of pregnancy secondary to a negative feedback from peripheral THs secondary to thyroid gland stimulation by hCG. During the first half of pregnancy, the upper limit of normal value of TSH is 2.5 mIU/L (as compared to 5 mIU/L in the nonpregnant state).

Serum cortisol levels are increased during pregnancy. Most of this elevation is secondary to increased synthesis of CBG by the liver. Free cortisol levels are also increased by 30% during gestation.

Serum parathyroid hormone and 1, 25 dihydroxy vitamin D increase to favor an environment of calcium accumulation in the fetus. The placenta forms a calcium

Table 2.7 Summary of endocrine changes during pregnancy.

Variable	Change
Leptin	Increases
Free T4 and T3 levels	Unchanged
Total T4 and T3 levels	Increased secondary to increased levels of thyroid-binding globulin (TBG) induced by estrogen. This elevation begins as early as 6 weeks and plateaus at 18 weeks of pregnancy
Thyroid-stimulating hormone (TSH)	Decreases in the first half of pregnancy and returns to normal in the second half of gestation. During the first 20 weeks of pregnancy, a normal value is between 0.5 and 2.5 mIU/L
Parathyroid hormone	Increases to favor calcium accumulation in the fetus (PTH) and 1, 25 dihydroxy vitamin D
Total calcium	Decreases
Ionized calcium	Unchanged
Prolactin	Increases
Total cortisol levels	Increased, mainly driven by increased liver synthesis of cortisol-binding globulin (CBG)
Free serum cortisol	Increased by 30% in pregnancy

pump in which a gradient of calcium and phosphorus is established which favors the fetus. The total level of calcium decreases, but ionized calcium remains the same [42].

Finally, the anterior pituitary enlarges 2—3-fold in pregnancy primarily due to hyperplasia and hypertrophy of lactotrophs, which causes increase in serum prolactin as pregnancy progress. The increase in pituitary size is thought to cause hypophyseal artery compression and predisposes the pituitary to infarction in cases of hypotension secondary to postpartum (i.e., Sheehan syndrome) [43]. The endocrine changes during pregnancy are summarized in Table 2.7.

2.8 Summary

Pregnancy is associated with profound changes in human physiology. Virtually every organ in the body is affected and the clinical consequences of these changes are significant. Unfortunately, our knowledge of how these changes affect the pharmacokinetics and pharmacodynamics of therapeutic agents is still very limited. Future research involving pharmacokinetics of specific agents during pregnancy is desperately needed.

References

[1] Sanghavi M, Rutherford JD. Cardiovascular physiology of pregnancy. Circulation 2014; 130(12):1003—8.

[2] Hunter S, Robson S. Adaptation of the maternal heart in pregnancy. Br Heart J 1992; 68(6):540—3.

[3] Robson SC, Hunter S, Boys RJ, et al. Serial study of factors influencing changes in cardiac output during human pregnancy. Am J Physiol 1989;256:H1060—5.

[4] Clark SL, Cotton DB, Lee W, et al. Central hemodynamic assessment of normal term pregnancy. Am J Obstet Gynecol 1989;161:1439—42.

[5] Seely EW, Ecker J. Chronic hypertension in pregnancy. N Engl J Med 2011;365(5): 439—46.

[6] Hytten FE, Paintin DB. Increase in plasma volume during normal pregnancy. J Obstet Gynaecol Br Commonw 1963;70:402—7.

[7] Bader RA, Bader MG, Rose DJ, et al. Hemodynamics at rest and during exercise in normal pregnancy as studied by cardiac catheterization. J Clin Invest 1955;34: 1524—36.

[8] Winkel CA, Milewich L, Parker CR, et al. Conversion of plasma progesterone to desoxycorticosterone in men, non pregnant, and pregnant women, and adrenalectomized subjects. J Clin Invest 1980;66:803—12.

[9] Robson S, Dunlop W, Hunter S. Haemodynamic changes during the early puerperium. Br Med J 1987:294.

[10] Ducas RA, Elliott JE, Melnyk SF, Premecz S, daSilva M, Cleverley K, Wtorek P, Mackenzie GS, Helewa ME, Jassal DS. Cardiovascular magnetic resonance in pregnancy: insights from the cardiac hemodynamic imaging and remodeling in pregnancy (CHIRP) study. J Cardiovasc Magn Reson 2014;16:1.

[11] Taylor M. An experimental study of the influence of the endocrine system on the nasal respiratory mucosa. J Laryngol Otol 1961;75:972—7.

[12] Lyons HA, Antonio R. The sensitivity of the respiratory center in pregnancy and after administration of progesterone. Trans Assoc Am Phys 1959;72:173—80.

[13] McAuliffe F, Kametas N, Costello J, et al. Respiratory function in singleton and twin pregnancy. BJOG 2002;109:765—8.

[14] Elkus R, Popovich J. Respiratory physiology in pregnancy. Clin Chest Med 1992;13: 555—65.

[15] Baldwin GR, Moorthi DS, Whelton JA, et al. New lung functions in pregnancy. Am J Obstet Gynecol 1977;127:235—9.

[16] Hankins GD, Harvey CJ, Clark SL, et al. The effects of maternal position and cardiac output on intrapulmonary shunt in normal third-trimester pregnancy. Obstet Gynecol 1996;88(3):327—30.

[17] LoMauro A, Aliverti A. Respiratory physiology of pregnancy. Breathe 2015;11(4): 297—301.

[18] Cheung KL, Lafayette RA. Renal physiology of pregnancy. Adv Chronic Kidney Dis 2013;20(3):209—14. https://doi.org/10.1053/j.ackd.2013.01.012.

[19] Schneider DH, Eichner E, Gordon MB. An attempt at production of hydronephrosis of pregnancy, artificially induced. Am J Obstet Gynecol 1953;65(3):660—5.

[20] Davison JM, Dunlop W. Changes in renal hemodynamics and tubular function induced by normal human pregnancy. Semin Nephrol 1984;4:198—207.

[21] Barron WM, Lindheimer MD. Renal sodium and water handling in pregnancy. Obstet Gynecol Annu 1984;13:35—69.

[22] Thornton SM1, Fitzsimons JT. The effects of centrally administered porcine relaxin on drinking behaviour in male and female rats. J Neuroendocrinol 1995;7(3):165—9.

[23] Davison JM, Vallotton MB, Lindheimer MD. Plasma osmolality and urinary concentration and dilution during and after pregnancy. BJOG 1981;88:472—9.

[24] Schou M, Amdisen A, Steenstrup OR. Lithium and pregnancy: hazards to women given lithium during pregnancy and delivery. Br Med J 1973;2(5859):137—8.

[25] Parry E, Shields R, Turnbull AC. Transit time in the small intestine in pregnancy. J Obstet Gynaecol Br Commonw 1970;77:900—1.

[26] Cappell M, Garcia A. Gastric and duodenal ulcers during pregnancy. Gastroenterol Clin North Am 1998;27:169—95.

[27] Milev N, Todorov G, Pumpalov A, Ignatov A. The serum gastrin level in pregnancy running a normal course. Probl Rentgenol Radiobiol 1982;3:106—11.

[28] Singer AJ1, Brandt LJ. Pathophysiology of the gastrointestinal tract during pregnancy. Am J Gastroenterol 1991;86(12):1695—712.

[29] Nakai A, Sekiya I, Oya A, et al. Assessment of the hepatic arterial and portal venous blood flows during pregnancy with Doppler ultrasonography. Arch Obstet Gynecol 2002;266(1):25—9.

[30] Lockitch G. Clinical biochemistry of pregnancy. Crit Rev Clin Lab Sci 1997;34:67—139.

[31] Wilby KJ, Ensom MH. Pharmacokinetics of antimalarials in pregnancy: a systematic review. Clin Pharmacokinet 2011;50(11):705—23.

[32] Chandra S, Tripathi A, Mishra A, Amzarul M, Vaish A. Physiological changes in hematological parameters during pregnancy. Indian J Hematol Blood Transfus 2012;28(3):144—6.

[33] Pritchard JA. Changes in the blood volume during pregnancy and delivery. Anesthesiology 1965;26:393—9.

[34] Peck TM, Arias F. Hematologic changes associated with pregnancy. Clin Obstet Gynecol 1979;22:785—98.

[35] Letsky EA. Erythropoiesis in pregnancy. J Perinat Med 1995;23:39—45.

[36] Koller O. The clinical significance of hemodilution during pregnancy. Obstet Gynecol Surv 1982;37:649—52.

[37] Hehhgren M. Hemostasis during pregnancy and puerperium. Hemostasis 1996;26:244—7.

[38] Boden G. Fuel metabolism in pregnancy and in gestational diabetes mellitus. Obstet Gynecol Clin North Am 1996;23:1—10.

[39] Phelps R, Metzger B, Freinkel N. Carbohydrate metabolism in pregnancy. XVII. Diurnal profiles of plasma glucose, insulin, free fatty acids, triglycerides, cholesterol, and individual amino acids in late normal pregnancy. Am J Obstet Gynecol 1981;140:730—6.

[40] Glinoer D. The regulation of thyroid function in pregnancy: pathways of endocrine adaptation from physiology to pathology. Endocr Rev 1997;18:404—33.

[41] Glinoer D. What happens to the normal thyroid during pregnancy? Thyroid 1999;9(7): 631−5.

[42] Tal R, Taylor HS, Burney RO, Mooney SB, Giudice LC. Endocrinology of pregnancy. 2021.

[43] Laway B, Mir A. Pregnancy and pituitary disorders: challenges in diagnosis and management. Indian J Endocrinol Metab 2013;17(6):996−1004.

Impact of pregnancy on maternal pharmacokinetics of medications

3

Rachel Ryu[1], Mary F. Hebert[2]

[1]*Department of Pharmacy, University of Washington, Seattle, WA, United States;* [2]*Departments of Pharmacy and Obstetrics & Gynecology, University of Washington, Seattle, WA, United States*

3.1 Introduction

Variability in drug efficacy and safety is multifactorial. Both the pharmacokinetics (how the body handles the drug) and the pharmacodynamics (how the body responds to the drug) play significant roles in drug efficacy and safety. This chapter will discuss the effects of pregnancy on medication pharmacokinetics.

The physiologic changes that occur during pregnancy result in marked changes in the pharmacokinetics for some medications. Whether or not the physiologic changes will result in clinically significant pharmacokinetic changes for an individual medication depends on many factors. The discussion of these factors will be the focus of this chapter. Generally speaking, pharmacokinetic changes are most important clinically for medications with narrow therapeutic ranges. The therapeutic range includes all the concentrations above the minimum effective concentration, but less than the maximum tolerated concentration (Fig. 3.1A and B). Medications such as cyclosporine, tacrolimus, lithium, warfarin, carbamazepine, valproic acid, phenytoin, digoxin, vancomycin, and the aminoglycosides are examples of narrow therapeutic range drugs. These are medications for which the concentrations needed for therapeutic benefit are very close to those that result in toxicity. For these agents, small changes in drug concentrations can lead to inefficacy if the concentrations decrease or intolerable toxicity if the concentrations increase. Typically, when drug interactions, disease states or conditions alter the concentration-time profile for a medication, if no changes have occurred in the pharmacodynamics, the patient's dosage is adjusted to keep the concentrations similar to those prior to the altered state or similar to those for the population in which the drug has been approved. This dosage adjustment is done to maintain concentrations within the therapeutic range. For narrow therapeutic range medications, even a 25% change in drug concentration can be considered clinically significant. In contrast, for most medications, which have wide therapeutic ranges, small changes in

Clinical Pharmacology During Pregnancy. https://doi.org/10.1016/B978-0-12-818902-3.00015-4

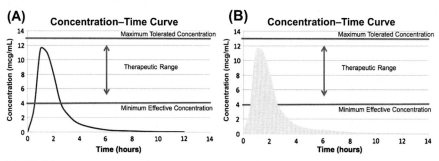

FIGURE 3.1

(A) is a stereotypic oral concentration-time curve. The *upper horizontal solid line* represents the maximum tolerated concentration, and the *lower horizontal solid line* represents the minimum effective concentration. The therapeutic range for this drug, represented by the *vertical double-sided arrow*, includes all the concentrations between the minimum effective concentration and the maximum tolerated concentration.
(B) illustrates a stereotypic oral concentration-time curve with the shaded area depicting the area under the concentration-time curve, which is a measure of total drug exposure.

pharmacokinetics have little to no clinical effect. However, given the magnitude of some of the pharmacokinetic changes that occur during pregnancy in which there can be 2–6-fold changes in drug exposure (Fig. 3.2A), even medications that have wide therapeutic ranges can be clinically affected.

3.2 Effects of pregnancy on pharmacokinetic parameters

A change in pharmacokinetics for a medication can result in the need to change dosage. As described above, altered concentrations during pregnancy can result in the need for higher (Fig. 3.2A) or lower (Fig. 3.2B) drug dosage to maintain concentrations within the therapeutic range. The changes in medication pharmacokinetics during pregnancy in some cases are so great that altered medication selection should be considered. For example, oral metoprolol concentrations are 2–4-fold lower during pregnancy than in the nonpregnant state [1,2]. Given the magnitude and variability in metoprolol concentrations during pregnancy, for those patients that require a beta blocker (e.g., cardiac rate control), selecting another agent such as atenolol, which is renally eliminated, should be considered. Even with the changes in renal function that are expected during pregnancy, atenolol will give much more consistent and reliable drug concentrations in pregnant patients than metoprolol [1–3]. Although there are fetal risks with the utilization of beta blockers during pregnancy, such as intrauterine growth restriction, if a beta blocker is required during pregnancy, selecting an agent that will consistently and reliably achieve the desirable therapeutic effect requires consideration of pharmacokinetic changes in medication selection.

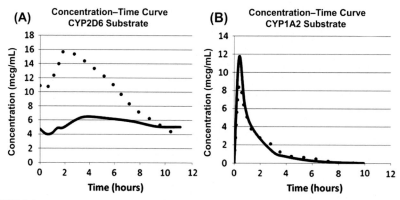

FIGURE 3.2

(A) depicts concentration-time curves for a CYP2D6 substrate during pregnancy represented by the *solid line* and in the same subject three months postpartum represented by the *dotted line*. The increase in metabolism that occurs during pregnancy results in 2–6-fold lower area under the concentration-time curve (AUC) for CYP2D6 substrates during pregnancy than in the nonpregnant state in patients given the same dose. (B) depicts concentration-time curves for a CYP1A2 substrate during pregnancy represented by the *solid line* and in the same subject 10 days postpartum represented by the *dotted line*. The inhibition of metabolism that occurs during pregnancy results in a higher AUC for CYP1A2 substrates during pregnancy than in the nonpregnant state.

The following sections will discuss the commonly estimated pharmacokinetic parameters, their application, and how they might be altered during pregnancy. The actual calculation of these parameters will not be discussed in this chapter. However, the reader is referred to the many publications that discuss in detail the mathematical equations used to determine the pharmacokinetic parameters [4,5].

3.2.1 Extraction ratio

Extraction ratio (ER) is the fraction of drug that is removed from the blood or plasma as it crosses the eliminating organ (e.g., liver or kidney). Knowing whether a drug has a high (ER > 0.7; e.g., morphine, metoprolol, verapamil), intermediate (ER 0.3–0.7; e.g., codeine, midazolam, nifedipine, metformin, cimetidine), or low (ER < 0.3; e.g., phenytoin, indomethacin, cyclosporine, amoxicillin, digoxin, atenolol) ER is important in predicting which factors such as intrinsic clearance, protein binding, and/or blood flow will alter the pharmacokinetic parameters for the drug.

3.2.2 Area under the concentration-time curve

The area under the concentration-time curve is a measure of the overall systemic drug exposure (Fig. 3.1B). Since we rarely can measure the drug concentration at the site of action (e.g., brain, lung, or heart); blood, plasma, or serum concentrations are typically used to determine systemic drug exposure. The area under the concentration-time curve (AUC) is dependent on the dose, clearance, and bioavailability of the drug. For some medications, AUC is the key determinant of medication efficacy and safety; while for other medications, either the maximum concentration and/or minimum concentration are better correlated with outcomes. For low ER drugs (both oral and intravenous administration), an increase in enzyme activity and/or a decrease in plasma protein binding will lead to a lower total drug AUC with changes in blood flow having no effect. For high hepatic ER, intravenously administered drugs, a decrease in blood flow will increase the total AUC; whereas, enzyme activity and protein binding have no effect on the total AUC. For high hepatic ER, orally administered drugs, the decrease in clearance caused by a decrease in blood flow is equal to the decrease in bioavailability such that changes in blood flow have no effect on oral AUC. However, increased enzyme activity or decreased plasma protein binding will decrease the total AUC through their effect on oral bioavailability.

3.2.3 Bioavailability

Bioavailability is the fraction of the dose administered that reaches the systemic circulation unchanged. Sometimes, the bioavailability term is used to encompass both the rate and extent of absorption from the site of administration to the systemic circulation. For orally administered drugs, the bioavailability is affected by the amount of drug that is absorbed from the gut as well as first pass metabolism as the drug crosses the intestine and liver on it's way to the systemic circulation. An increase or decrease in bioavailability directly impacts the oral AUC or total drug exposure. For low hepatic ER drugs, bioavailability is not affected by enzyme activity, hepatic blood flow, or protein binding. In contrast, for high hepatic ER drugs, bioavailability is decreased by an increase in enzyme activity, decreased hepatic blood flow, and/or a decrease in plasma protein binding. In addition to the above-described changes in enzyme activity, protein binding and blood flow which can alter medication pharmacokinetics, other physiologic changes that occur during pregnancy which might influence the bioavailability of drugs include: gastric acidity, gastrointestinal transit time, and hypertrophy of duodenal villi, which can alter drug absorption [6−9].

3.2.4 Clearance

Clearance is a parameter used to describe how well the body can metabolize or eliminate drugs. The clearance directly affects total drug exposure as well as average steady state drug concentrations and is utilized to determine maintenance dosage. There are three major determinants of hepatic drug clearance: hepatic blood flow, protein binding, and the intrinsic activity of hepatic drug metabolizing enzymes. Hepatic blood flow plays an important role in determining the hepatic clearance of drugs, particularly those with high ERs. Physiologic, pathologic, and drug-induced changes in hepatic blood flow can alter the systemic clearance and oral bioavailability of many important therapeutic agents, resulting in changes in patient response. For high hepatic ER drugs, clearance is directly affected by hepatic blood flow such that an increase in blood flow will increase clearance. The rate-limiting step for metabolism of high hepatic ER drugs is the delivery of the drug to the liver. Visualizing this process in which everything that is delivered to the eliminating organ, such as the liver, will be cleared from the body can be helpful. This process will proceed so that the faster the drug is delivered to the eliminating organ, the faster the drug is eliminated from the body.

In contrast, for low ER drugs, the rate-limiting step is not blood flow; therefore, a change in organ blood flow does not alter clearance. Instead, clearance is affected by the enzyme activity and protein binding, such that an increase in enzyme activity or a decrease in protein binding will increase the drugs total clearance. For intermediate ER drugs, clearance will be dependent on changes in enzyme activity, protein binding, and organ blood flow.

3.2.5 Protein binding

As described above, plasma protein binding can affect the pharmacokinetics of medications. There are multiple issues to consider with regards to protein binding of medications. Some of the plasma proteins are known to be altered both in normal pregnancy as well as pathologic conditions [10]. In normal pregnancy, albumin concentrations decrease by approximately 1% at 8 weeks, 10% at 20 weeks, and 13% at 32 weeks [11]. In pregnant patients with pathologic conditions, albumin concentrations can be substantially lower. Changes in albumin concentrations are important for many medications (e.g., phenytoin, valproic acid, carbamazepine). Other plasma proteins such as α-1-acid glycoprotein are involved in binding of drugs like betamethasone, bupivacaine, lopinavir, and lidocaine. Plasma α-1-acid glycoprotein has been reported to be 52% lower in late pregnancy (30−36 weeks gestation) than postpartum (2−13 weeks) [12]. In addition, some agents (e.g., cyclosporine, tacrolimus) concentrate within the red blood cells. For these agents, binding might be altered as a result of anemia during pregnancy. Hematocrits are known to fall during normal pregnancy by 2% at 8 weeks and 4% at 20−32 weeks [11]. For some medications, disease states or conditions during pregnancy can lead to severe anemia, which would be expected to have a much greater effect on binding of these medications. In contrast, there are plasma proteins which increase during pregnancy. For example, corticosteroid-binding globulin (CBG or transcortin) binds glucocorticoids such as cortisol and progesterone in the plasma/serum [13] and is increased by 2−3-fold during pregnancy [14]. The increase in CBG impacts the binding of drugs such as prednisone and prednisolone.

Drug binding is important for many reasons. The first reason is that the unbound drug is in equilibrium with the site of action and is therefore considered the active moiety as well as being able to cross membranes including the placenta. Unbound drug not only will cause beneficial effects but also potentially toxic effects.

For drugs that are highly bound to albumin such as phenytoin, changes in albumin concentrations during pregnancy can be associated with alterations in protein binding. Yerby et al. reported a significant increase in the percent of unbound phenytoin during the second and third trimesters of pregnancy as well as labor and delivery as compared to the prepregnancy state [15]. This is particularly important clinically because phenytoin is a highly protein bound drug with a narrow therapeutic range. The second reason is that understanding protein binding is critical in the interpretation of total drug concentrations. For phenytoin, when interpreting total drug concentrations, knowing whether protein binding has been altered is important. Changes in phenytoin protein binding would require either measuring unbound phenytoin concentrations or accounting for protein binding changes in the interpretation of total phenytoin concentrations.

Fig. 3.3A illustrates the total concentration for the drug in plasma measured to be 10, and the unbound concentration measured to be 1. In contrast, in Fig. 3.3B, the total drug concentration is 5, but the unbound concentration is still 1. In this example, although the total concentration is reduced in half, since the unbound concentration is still the same, no dosage adjustment should be made clinically because the active form of the drug (unbound) is the same. This would be expected to occur if there was a change in protein binding and no change in enzyme activity, leading to a change in total clearance, but no change in unbound clearance.

For prednisone and prednisolone, both are highly bound to albumin and CBG. The protein binding of prednisone and prednisolone has been shown to increase with the increase in CBG during pregnancy [16]. The total prednisolone clearance

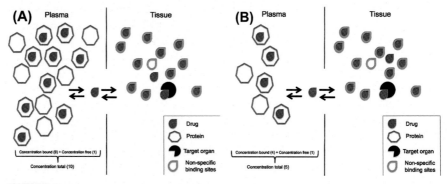

FIGURE 3.3

(A) illustrates a drug with a total plasma concentration of 10, unbound concentration of 1 and bound concentration of 9. It is the unbound drug that is in equilibrium with the bound drug and is available to cross membranes and get to the site of action. (B) illustrates a drug with a total plasma concentration of 5, unbound concentration of 1 and bound concentration of 4. Although the total drug concentrations are 50% in (B) compared to the example in (A), in both cases, the unbound or active form of the drug is the same.

(A) and (B) are adapted with permission from figures included in Beringer P, Winter's Basic Clinical Pharmacokinetics, 6th Ed. Wolters Kluwer, 2017.

is lower during pregnancy compared to postpartum; however, unbound prednisolone clearance did not change [16]. Since there is no change in unbound prednisolone concentrations, then no dosage adjustment is required based on pharmacokinetics alone. However, this does not take into account changes in immune response during pregnancy. Prednisone and prednisolone binding is a saturable process both during pregnancy and in the nonpregnant state resulting in increased fraction unbound at higher concentrations along with increased variability [16].

An alternate situation could occur in which there is no change in total concentrations, but a change in protein binding, leading to an increase in unbound drug concentration and toxicity. It is essential that in the case of a highly bound drug with a narrow therapeutic range to either measure the unbound concentration or to mathematically account for the changes in protein binding when total concentrations are measured, such as in pregnant patients with low-albumin concentrations. Tacrolimus binds to red blood cells, albumin, and α1-acid glycoprotein, all of which significantly decrease during pregnancy [17,18]. Mean tacrolimus oral clearance was 39% higher during mid- and late-pregnancy compared to postpartum [17]. Since tacrolimus has a narrow therapeutic index and dosage is adjusted based on whole blood trough concentrations, the increase in oral clearance might suggest a need for a dosage increase. However, the estimated unbound tacrolimus oral clearance did not change, and the unbound percent of tacrolimus in plasma was reported to be approximately two-fold higher in mid- and late-pregnancy compared to postpartum [17]. If drug binding is not accounted for and the total drug concentration is measured in a patient with an increase in fraction unbound and no change in unbound clearance, the total concentration will be lower, but the dosage should not be adjusted. If the clinician does not account for the altered binding and increases the dosage, the patient might develop drug toxicity.

The physiologic changes that occur during pregnancy can translate into changes in multiple pharmacokinetic parameters that can alter the interpretation of drug concentrations. For example, you often have changes in both protein binding and unbound clearance during pregnancy, as is the case with phenytoin. These patients require consideration of both factors in interpreting total phenytoin concentrations. It is important to note that not all highly protein bound drugs have increased percent unbound during pregnancy. Some highly protein bound drugs such as midazolam and glyburide have little to no change in protein binding during pregnancy, but significant changes in their clearances [10,19].

3.2.6 Organ blood flow

Changes in hepatic and renal blood flows can alter drug clearance. As described above, changes in organ blood flow are particularly important for high ER drugs. During pregnancy, cardiac output is markedly increased. On average, during normal pregnancy, cardiac output has been reported to be 35% higher in the second trimester and 40% higher in the third trimester as compared to postpartum [20]. In nonseptic critically ill patients, there is a good correlation ($r = 0.92$) between cardiac output and effective hepatic blood flow [21]. In an animal model of reduced cardiac output, there was an associated decrease in portal venous flow [22]. Unfortunately, there is limited information available evaluating the effects of pregnancy on hepatic blood flow. Nakai et al. [23] studied the effects of pregnancy on hepatic arterial and portal venous blood flows during the first trimester of pregnancy (n = 13), second trimester (n = 25), third trimester (n = 29), and in nonpregnant women (n = 22). They found an increase in total liver blood flow (2.98 ± 1.13 L/min, $P < .05$) and portal vein blood flow (1.92 ± 0.83 L/min, $P < .05$) during the third trimester of pregnancy as compared to the nonpregnant women (1.82 ± 0.63 L/min and 1.25 ± 0.46 L/min respectively). Rudolf et al. [24] reported indocyanine-green clearance in 16 women with hyperemesis gravidarum with all but one subject within the upper limit of normal. Robson et al. [25] found no change in hepatic blood flow in 12 women 12−14 weeks, 24−26 weeks, and 36−38 weeks gestation as compared to 10−12 weeks after delivery. Probst et al. [26] conducted a study in seven healthy pregnant women during labor and delivery and compared them to nonpregnant controls. They found that hepatic blood flow was decreased to 70% of the control value during labor. In a cross-sectional study of 210 pregnant women between 6 and 40 weeks gestation and 40 healthy nonpregnant women, Doppler resistance indices [hepatic artery pulsatility (PI) and resistive index (RI)] were measured to evaluate hepatic liver blood flow [27]. Mandic-Markovic et al. [27] found PI and RI in hepatic artery was decreased during the third trimester compared to nonpregnant state and the first two trimesters. This is likely a result of systemic arterial vasodilation during the third trimester of pregnancy [27]. All of the studies were underpowered and in most cases did not have the pregnant women serve as their own control. At this point, it is unclear whether hepatic blood flow is increased or unchanged during pregnancy.

Pregnancy is associated with increased renal filtration, increased creatinine clearance, and increased renal clearance of drugs [3,10,28,29]. During normal pregnancy, effective renal plasma flow increases on average 50%−85%, with a corresponding 50% increase in glomerular filtration rate [30,31]. Because the estimated tubular ER for metformin is moderately high, the gestational changes in the metformin's renal clearance and net secretory clearance can in part be explained by enhanced renal plasma flow [32].

3.2.7 Intrinsic clearance

The intrinsic clearance generally refers to the liver's inherent ability to metabolize drug. It is a term used to describe enzyme activity and is independent of protein binding and hepatic blood flow.

3.2.8 Metabolism

Drug metabolism is the conversion of one chemical structure to another. The formation of metabolites often occurs via drug metabolizing enzymes. There are many drug metabolizing enzymes involved in both phase I [e.g., CYP3A4, CYP3A5,

CYP2D6, CYP1A1, CYP1A2, CYP2C8 CYP2C9, CYP2C19, CYP2E1, CYP2A6, CYP2B6, esterases, epoxide hydrolase, dihydropyrimidine dehydrogenase, alcohol dehydrogenase (ADH), carbonyl reductase 1 (CBR1)] and phase II (e.g., uridine diphosphate glucuronyltransferase (UGT), sulfotransferase, methyltransferase, N-acetyltransferase, catechol-O-methyl transferase, thiopurine S-methyltransferase, histamine methyltransferase, glutathione S-transferase) metabolism. Phase I metabolism usually precedes phase II metabolism, but not always. Phase I reactions typically include: oxidation, reduction, hydrolysis, cyclization, and decyclization reactions. Phase II reactions involve conjugation with glucuronic acid, sulfate, glutathione, or amino acids. Occasionally, there is back conversion of metabolites to the parent compound. For some medications that are administered as inactive compounds (prodrugs), metabolism is necessary to convert the drug to active compound.

As described above, many different drug metabolizing enzymes exist. The enzyme involved in the metabolism of a drug is dependent on the chemical structure of the agent. For some medications, only one enzyme is involved in the metabolism. For other drugs, multiple enzymes with differing affinities are involved in the formation of the metabolites. One method that has been used to evaluate the effects of pregnancy on drug metabolizing enzymes is to use probe substrates as markers for enzyme activity. A probe substrate is a drug that is primarily metabolized by a single enzyme. The drug is administered and a pharmacokinetic study is completed. From this, drug clearance, urinary excretion of metabolite, metabolite formation clearance, area under the concentration-time curve, or metabolite to parent concentration ratio are used as surrogate markers for enzyme activity. The discussion below will describe the effects of pregnancy on key drug metabolizing enzyme activities (Table 3.1).

3.2.8.1 CYP3A

CYP3A is responsible for the metabolism of more drugs than any other P450 enzyme. Examples of CYP3A substrates can be found in Table 3.2. Midazolam is one of the "gold standard" probes for CYP3A activity. We conducted a study evaluating the effect of pregnancy on CYP3A activity utilizing midazolam as the probe drug. Mean midazolam area under the concentration time curve and maximum concentration were markedly lower during pregnancy than postpartum. This corresponded to an average of 108% increase in midazolam apparent oral clearance and 123% increase in 1'-hydroxymidazolam formation clearance during pregnancy as compared to postpartum. Apparent oral unbound midazolam clearance and unbound 1'-hydroxymidazolam formation clearance were on average 86% and 99% higher, respectively, in pregnancy than postpartum [10]. Other CYP3A substrates (dextromethorphan N-demethylation, nelfinavir, indinavir, rilpivirine, nifedipine, atazanavir, darunavir, elvitegravir) have also been studied during pregnancy. N-demethylation of oral dextromethorphan was increased by 35%−38% during pregnancy [33]. Similarly, nelfinavir was reported to have a 25%−33% increase in apparent oral clearance in pregnancy [34,35]. Indinavir has an approximately threefold lower average AUC in pregnancy than postpartum [36]. Rilpivirine AUC

Table 3.1 The effects of pregnancy on enzymes and renal transporters.

	Pregnancy effect	Substrates
Enzymes		
ADH	Unchanged (83)	Abacavir
CBR1	Decreased (87)	Doxorubicin
CYP1A2	Decreased (33, 56)	Caffeine, dacarbazine
CYP2B6	Unchanged (63), increased (62)	Efavirenz
CYP2C9	Increased (19, 60)	Glyburide, phenytoin
CYP2C19	Unchanged (58), decreased (54,57)	Proguanil, etravirine
CYP2D6	Increased (1, 2, 43)	Metoprolol, clonidine
CYP2E1	Increased (55, 64)	Acetaminophen, caffeine, theophylline
CYP3A4	Increased (10, 33–38)	Dextromethorphan, indinavir, nelfinavir, midazolam, rilpivirine
UGT1A1	Increased (75)	Labetalol
UGT1A4	Increased (71)	Lamotrigine
UGT2B7	Unchanged (78), increased (79)	Morphine, zidovudine
Renal transporters		
OATP	Increased (10)	Digoxin
OAT1	Increased (97)	Amoxicillin
OCT2	Increased (32)	Metformin
P-gp	Increased (10)	Digoxin

ADH, *alcohol dehydrogenase;* CBR1, *carbonyl reductase;* CYP, *cytochrome P450;* OAT1, *organic anion transporter 1;* OATPs, *organic anion transporter polypeptides;* OCT2, *organic cation transporter 2;* P-gp, *P-glycoprotein;* UGT, *uridine diphosphate-glucuronosyltransferase.*

was also decreased by 23% during the second trimester [37] and 45% during the third trimester of pregnancy compared to postpartum [38]. These data are consistent with increased CYP3A activity during pregnancy as compared to the nonpregnant state.

Because CYP3A is involved in the metabolism of many medications, this finding has clinical implications for medication dosages during pregnancy. In particular, CYP3A substrates with narrow therapeutic ranges may fall below effective concentrations during pregnancy if dosage adjustments are not made. Many antiretroviral medications are CYP3A substrates, in which therapeutic concentrations are critical in providing adequate viral suppression and minimizing risk of HIV resistance and transmission to the infant [38]. Such medications might need their dosage increased during pregnancy to achieve adequate plasma concentrations. When CYP3A substrates are initiated during pregnancy and titrated to response, subsequent dosage reductions might be needed postpartum to avoid toxicity.

Table 3.2 Cytochrome P450 substrate examples.

CYP3A	CYP2D6	CYP2C9	CYP2C19	CYP1A2	CYP2B6
Alfentanil	Alprenolol	Diclofenac	Citalopram	Caffeine	Bupropion
Alprazolam	Amitriptyline	Flubiprofen	Clopidogrel	Clozapine	Efavirenzy
Amlodipine	Clomipramine	Glipizide	Escitalopram	Duloxetine	Methadone
Amprenavir	Codeine	Glyburide	Esomeprazole	Lidocaine	Propofol
Buspirone	Debrisoquine	Ibuprofen	Etravirine	Melatonin	
Chlorpheniramine	Dextromethorphan	Losartan	Lansoprazole	Ondansetron	
Citalopram	Doxepin	Naproxen	Mephenytoin	Ramelteon	
Cyclosporine	Flecainide	Omeprazole	Omeprazole	Ropivacaine	
Dapsone	Fluoxetine	Phenytoin	Pantoprazole	Theophylline	
Diltiazem	Fluvoxamine	Piroxicam	Proguanil	Triamterene	
Erythromycin	Haloperidol	Sulfamethoxazole	Rabeprazole		
Felodipine	Hydrocodone	Tolbutamide	Sertraline		
Fentanyl	Imipramine	Voriconazole			
Indinavir	Metoprolol	Warfarin			
Isradipine	Mexiletine				
Itraconazole	Nortriptyline				
Lidocaine	Paroxetine				
Loratidine	Promethazine				
Methadone	Propafenone				
Midazolam	Propranolol				
Nelfinavir	Resperidone				
Nicardipine	Thioridazine				
Nifedipine	Tolterodine				
Oxycodone	Venlafaxine				
Simvastatin					
Sirolimus					
Tacrolimus					
Zolpidem					

3.2.8.2 CYP2D6

CYP2D6 is responsible for the metabolism of the second highest number of drugs metabolized by P450 enzymes. Substrates for CYP2D6 can be found in Table 3.2. CYP2D6 is a particularly challenging enzyme to understand and study because of its genetic polymorphism. Genetic variation for this enzyme can result in some patients having no enzyme, some having a low amount of enzyme activity with only one active allele, some having two active alleles, and some having duplicate genes. Clinically, these genetic differences result in poor, intermediate, normal (extensive), and ultrarapid metabolizers of CYP2D6 substrates. Historically, CYP2D6 was thought to be a noninducible enzyme by classic pathways for enzyme induction. However, more recently, data suggest that changes in transcription regulation play a role in CYP2D6 induction during pregnancy [39,40].

Metoprolol is the "gold standard" probe for CYP2D6 activity. In a small study, oral metoprolol AUC was reported to be 2−4-fold lower during pregnancy than in the nonpregnant population [1,2]. In a recent study, metoprolol apparent oral clearance was higher during mid- and late-pregnancy compared to postpartum in intermediate and extensive metabolizers [41]. Other CYP2D6 substrates have been studied during pregnancy. For example, dextromethorphan is primarily a CYP2D6 substrate (although its N-demethylation occurs via CYP3A as described above). Utilizing dextromethorphan as a CYP2D6 probe, Tracy et al. [33] reported an increase in CYP2D6 activity by ~25% at 14−18 weeks gestation, ~35% at 24−28 weeks gestation, and ~50% at 36−40 weeks gestation. In addition, we have found clonidine to primarily be a CYP2D6 substrate [42]. The mean apparent oral clearance of clonidine is approximately 80% higher in pregnant women compared with the nonpregnant population. Of note, in the nonpregnant population, clonidine is primarily renally eliminated. However, only 36% of the clonidine was excreted unchanged in the urine in pregnant women compared with 59% in the nonpregnant population [43−46]. Interestingly, the increase in CYP2D6 activity during pregnancy is so great that the major pathway for elimination for clonidine switched from primarily renal to primarily metabolic.

3.2.8.3 CYP2C9

CYP2C9 is involved in the elimination of approximately 10% of the metabolized drugs from the list of top 100 drugs by US sales. Substrates for CYP2C9 can be found in Table 3.2. CYP2C9 is the primary metabolic pathway for phenytoin elimination. Because of the high-protein binding for phenytoin, when considering phenytoin as a probe for CYP2C9, utilizing free phenytoin clearance is important given the known changes in phenytoin protein binding during pregnancy. CYP2C9 activity as measured by free phenytoin clearance is increased ~1.5-fold during all three trimesters of pregnancy as compare to the prepregnant state [15].

Glyburide is another agent that is metabolized by CYP2C9, although CYP3A and CYP2C19 are also involved in its metabolism in vitro [47−49]. In vivo, glyburide appears to be a CYP2C9 substrate in the nonpregnant population [50−53]. At equivalent doses, glyburide plasma concentrations were ~50% lower in pregnant women compared to nonpregnant women [19]. The large gestational increase in unbound glyburide CL/F and unbound formation clearance of the primary metabolite 4-trans OH-glyburide (>two-fold increase) suggest that higher dosages might be needed during pregnancy. The gestational increase in unbound glyburide CL/F most likely reflects induction of CYP2C9 and CYP3A, since these activities have been previously shown to be increased (and CYP2C19 activity decreased) during pregnancy [10,15,54].

3.2.8.4 CYP1A2

CYP1A2 is involved in the metabolism of fewer drugs than the enzymes previously discussed. However, some agents that are substrates for CYP1A2 are being used more and more frequently during pregnancy, such as ondansetron (Table 3.2). A commonly used probe substrate for CYP1A2 activity is caffeine. The activity of CYP1A2 as determined by caffeine clearance is reported to be decreased by approximately 30% at 14−18 weeks gestation, 50% at 24−28 weeks gestation, and 70% at 36−40 weeks gestation [33]. Dose normalized caffeine serum and urine concentrations were significantly increased between first and third trimesters of pregnancy [55]. Caffeine's metabolite theophylline concentrations increased over the course of pregnancy, primarily during the third trimester [55]. CYP1A2 is also involved in the metabolism of dacarbazine. In a case report, a subject who received the prodrug dacarbazine was found to have a 7% increase in dacarbazine AUC during pregnancy compared to postpartum, whereas the active metabolite of dacarbazine, 5-[3-hydroxy-methyl-3-methyl-triazen-1-yl]-imidazole-4-carboxamide, AUC was 27% lower compared to postpartum [56]. The apparent decrease in CYP1A2 activity potentially could result in increased toxicity for CYP1A2 substrates. This is in contrast to the effect seen with CYP3A, CYP2D6, and CYP2C9, which all have markedly increased activities during pregnancy and potentially will result in decreased drug efficacy.

3.2.8.5 CYP2C19

Substrates for CYP2C19 can be found in Table 3.2. Medications that are metabolized by CYP2C19 include omeprazole, pantoprazole, citalopram, sertraline, and etravirine. CYP2C19 is a polymorphic enzyme leading to extensive and poor metabolizers. Similar to CYP1A2, CYP2C19 activity appears to be inhibited during pregnancy in extensive metabolizers [54]. The ratio of proguanil to cycloguanil has been utilized as a probe for CYP2C19 activity. Although no significant changes are seen in CYP2C19 activity during pregnancy in poor metabolizers, in extensive metabolizers there is a doubling in the plasma ratio of proguanil to cycloguanil 6 h after dosing when comparing women in their third trimester of pregnancy to women two months postpartum, suggesting a decrease in CYP2C19 activity in late pregnancy [54]. Etravirine, a second generation nonnucleoside reverse transcriptase inhibitor, is primarily metabolized by CYP2C19 [57]. It is also metabolized by CYP2C9 and CYP3A4 to minor metabolites [57]. Studies have shown mixed results on the pharmacokinetics of etravirine in pregnancy. When compared to nonpregnant adults, etravirine pharmacokinetics during late pregnancy were not significantly different [58]. However, a recent study found a 52% lower etravirine apparent oral clearance and 36%−39% higher plasma concentrations during late pregnancy compared to postpartum [59], which is consistent with the reported decrease in CYP2C19 activity during pregnancy [60]. Despite the higher etravirine concentrations seen during pregnancy, there has not been an increase in the reported frequency or severity of adverse events in this population [61]. In light of these data, monitoring for medication toxicity and in some cases consideration of altered dosage might be warranted.

3.2.8.6 CYP2B6

CYP2B6 is involved in metabolism of drugs such as efavirenz, bupropion, methadone, and propofol. Efavirenz is a non-nucleoside reverse transcriptase inhibitor used for the treatment of HIV/AIDS. CYP2B6 is responsible for metabolizing 90% of efavirenz [62]. CYP2B6 genotype contributes to efavirenz pharmacokinetic variability [62]. In one study, pregnancy appeared to have the greatest effect on efavirenz apparent oral clearance in women with CYP2B6 516GG genotype. This study reported a doubling of efavirenz apparent oral clearance during pregnancy in women with CYP2B6 516GG genotype and no significant change in efavirenz apparent oral clearance in women with CYP2B6 516GT and CYP2B6 516TT genotypes [62]. In another study that did not include genotyping for CYP2B6, the apparent oral clearance of efavirenz during pregnancy, although reported to be significantly higher than postpartum, was only slightly higher and not sufficient to warrant dosage adjustment [63]. Future studies are needed to determine if alternate dosage strategies are needed and the role of CYP2B6 genotype in this determination.

3.2.8.7 CYP2E1

CYP2E1 metabolizes endogenous and exogenous substrates, but is better known to be involved in metabolizing toxins and procarcinogens. CYP2E1 metabolizes a relatively small number of medications with acetaminophen (paracetamol) being one of the most important. In pregnant mice, placental lactogen induced CYP2E1 expression in human hepatocytes [64]. Acetaminophen is primarily metabolized by glucuronidation and sulfation, but is also metabolized by CYP2E1 producing 3-hydroxy-paracetamol and a reactive metabolite, N-acetyl-p-benzoquinone imine (NAPQI) [65]. Miners et al. reported acetaminophen apparent oral clearance was 58% higher in pregnancy compared to nonpregnant women [66]. In another study, acetaminophen clearance was 1.8-fold higher at the time of delivery compared to nonpregnant adults [67]. Although decreased exposure to acetaminophen is likely in pregnancy, dose adjustments are not advised since there is potential for increased NAPQI formation that may lead to hepatotoxicity [67]. More studies are needed to determine how pregnancy affects the toxicodynamics of NAPQI. The implications of increased CYP2E1 activity in pregnancy remain to be determined.

3.2.8.8 Uridine diphosphate glucuronyltransferase

UGT is a non-P450 enzyme involved in phase 2 metabolism. UGT metabolizes agents to glucuronide conjugates. There are two families found in humans, UGT1 and UGT2, where UGT1A and UGT2B subfamilies are primarily involved in hepatic glucuronidation [68]. There are many substrates for UGT1A4 such as amitriptyline, doxepin, imipramine, lamotrigine, and promethazine [69,70]. The increase in UGT1A4 activity starts in the first trimester of pregnancy and is reported to return to prepregnancy baseline by two–three weeks postpartum. The clearance of lamotrigine has been reported to increase by 65% during pregnancy [71]. While the initial decrease in lamotrigine concentrations during early pregnancy may largely be attributed to the increased blood flow, estradiol's induction of glucuronidation appears to have a greater impact during the remainder of pregnancy. A strong correlation between increased estradiol serum concentrations and increased lamotrigine- N2-glucuronide/lamotrigine ratio has been reported [72]. This suggests that increased estradiol, a UGT inducer, during pregnancy may contribute to the decreased lamotrigine serum concentrations and potentially decreased efficacy [72]. Consistent with this, an increase in seizure frequency during pregnancy along with a decrease in lamotrigine concentration to dose ratio by $\sim 50\%$ between 11 weeks gestation and term has been reported [73].

UGT1A1 and UGT2B7 were found to be the major enzymes that metabolize labetalol to glucuronides [74]. In vitro, progesterone enhanced UGT1A1 activity mediated by pregnane X receptor [74]. Considering that labetalol oral clearance is increased during the second and third trimesters of pregnancy compared to postpartum women, induction of UGT1A1 may largely be responsible for the increased clearance [75]. Protein binding and oral absorptions are not likely the cause, since protein binding of labetalol does not change during pregnancy [76] and labetalol show complete oral absorption. Acetaminophen is another common medication used during pregnancy that is metabolized by UGT1A1 and CYP2E1. Acetaminophen also undergoes faster elimination in pregnant women and has a 20% shorter half-life in the first trimester of pregnancy compared to nonpregnant adults [77]. Mixed results have been reported on the effects of pregnancy on UGT2B7 activity. UGT2B7 metabolizes medications such as zidovudine and morphine. In one study, zidovudine pharmacokinetics were not altered during pregnancy compared to nonpregnant adults [78]. In contrast, morphine plasma clearance was increased by 70% in pregnant women compared to nonpregnant adults [79]. More research is needed to assess the effects of pregnancy on UGT2B7 activity.

3.2.8.9 Alcohol dehydrogenase

ADH is a polymorphic enzyme which metabolizes variety of substances such as ethanol, vitamin A, simple alcohols, and hydroxysteroids [80]. ADH is predominantly present in the liver, but also in many other tissues in lower amounts [81]. In pregnant rats, alcohol clearance was higher compared to weight matched nonpregnant rats. Interestingly, liver ADH activity did not change during pregnancy; however, gastric ADH activity was 177% greater in pregnant rats compared to the nonpregnant group [80]. Abacavir, a nucleoside analog reverse transcriptase inhibitor, is metabolized in the liver to inactive metabolites by ADH and UGT [82]. Abacavir is used as one of the first line combination agent to treat HIV/AIDs in pregnancy [83]. In a study of 14 pregnant women, abacavir AUC, $T_{1/2}$, and C_{max} were not different between the third trimester of pregnancy and two−six weeks postpartum [83]. Therefore, dosage adjustments do not appear to be needed.

3.2.8.10 Carbonyl reductase 1

Oxidative drug metabolism pathways of cytochrome P450 enzymes have been extensively studied; however, information on reductive pathways of drug metabolism is still limited. CBR1 is a class of short-chain dehydrogenases/reductases primarily expressed in the intestine, liver, and kidney [84]. However, its ubiquitous distribution in other human tissues makes it particularly challenging to predict hepatic clearance through in vitro studies [85]. In preclinical studies, CBR1 has been shown to decrease protein expression in presence of 17β-estradiol [86], and its activity was reported to decrease during pregnancy [87]. CBR1 metabolizes medications such as doxorubicin, daunorubicin, dolasteron, nabumetone, haloperidol, loxoprofen, and bupropion [88,89]. In pregnancy, doxorubicin appears to have 30%−39% decrease in clearance during pregnancy [90].

3.2.9 Renal

Almost one-third of the medication in the top 100 drugs list by US sales is primarily eliminated by the kidneys. During normal pregnancy, creatinine clearance increases by 45% at nine weeks gestation, and peaks in the mid-second trimester at 150% −160% of nonpregnant values. In some women, clearances will decline over the last six weeks of pregnancy. Occasionally, creatinine clearance will return to the nonpregnant state over the last three weeks of pregnancy [28,29]. Pregnancy has been reported to increase tubular secretion of endogenous compounds such as glucose and amino acids [30]. Understanding and accounting for changes in kidney function during pregnancy is important for optimizing dosage for renally eliminated medications.

3.2.9.1 Filtration

Changes in renal filtration as measured by creatinine clearance during pregnancy have been associated with changes in the renal clearance of many medications [3,10,32,91]. In some, but not all cases, these changes will require dosage adjustments during pregnancy. For example, changes in digoxin concentrations during pregnancy often require dosage adjustments to maintain therapeutic concentrations. On average, digoxin renal clearance increases 61% during pregnancy compared to 6−10 weeks postpartum [10]. There is a good correlation (r = 0.8) between creatinine clearance and digoxin renal clearance [10]. Even though digoxin also has an active transport component to its renal elimination, the change in creatinine clearance appears to be a good surrogate marker for the expected change in digoxin renal clearance during pregnancy due to the large fraction of digoxin renal clearance accounted for by filtration compared to net secretion [10].

Metformin is eliminated almost entirely unchanged in the urine. In mid- and late-pregnancy, metformin renal clearance increases on average by 49% and 29%, respectively, compared to three—four months postpartum. The change in renal clearance parallels the 29% and 21% increase in creatinine clearance during mid- and late-pregnancy reported in the same study [32]. There are currently not enough data to determine if dosage increases for metformin are needed during pregnancy.

Atenolol is another drug that is primarily eliminated unchanged in the urine. Pregnancy as compared to three months postpartum results in significant increases in creatinine clearance, 42% and 50% in the second and third trimesters, respectively, and in atenolol renal clearance, 38% and 36% in the second and third trimesters, respectively. There is a very good correlation (r = 0.7) between creatinine clearance and atenolol renal clearance [3]. However, changes in atenolol renal clearance during pregnancy do not translate into clinically significant changes in apparent oral clearance, and therefore dosage adjustments are not necessary based on pharmacokinetic changes. However, changes in hemodynamics and pharmacodynamics over the course of gestation might result in the need for dosage adjustments for atenolol during pregnancy.

3.2.9.2 Secretion/reabsorption

3.2.9.2.1 P-glycoprotein and organic anion transporter polypeptides

Examples of renal transporters can be found in Table 3.3. Digoxin has been considered the "gold standard" probe for p-glycoprotein activity because it mediates secretion of digoxin across the apical membrane of the renal tubular epithelium [92,93]. However, other renal transporters are also involved in the net secretion of digoxin. There is evidence that digoxin is a substrate for organic anion transporter

Table 3.3 Active renal transporters examples.

OATP	OAT1	OCT2	P-gp
Atorvastatin	Acyclovir	Amantadine	Amlodipine
Enalapril	Adefovir	Amiloride	Amprenavir
Caspofungin	Amoxicillin	Cimetidine	Atazanavir
Digoxin	Cidofovir	Cisplastin	Budesonide
Fexofenadine	Didanosine	D-Tubocurarine	Carvedilol
Levofloxacin	Lamivudine	Debrisoquine	Cetirizine
	Stavudine	Guanidine	Clopidogrel
	Tenofovir	Metformin	Cyclosporine
	Zalcitabine	Oxaliplatin	Digoxin
	Zidovudine	Pindolol	Diltiazem
		Procainamide	Erythromycin
		Ranitidine	Fexofenadine, Loperamide, Sirolimus, Tacrolimus, Quinidine

OAT1, organic anion transporter 1; OATPs, organic anion transporter polypeptides; OCT2, organic cation transporter 2; P-gp, P-glycoprotein.

polypeptides (OATPs) [94,95]. Human OATP4C1 (SLCO4C1) plays a primary role in the transport of digoxin on the basolateral membrane of the kidney [96]. Thus, digoxin renal tubular secretion appears to be a serial transport process mediated by p-glycoprotein and OATP. Although, glomerular filtration rate increases during pregnancy, this increase does not completely explain the increased renal clearance of digoxin. Digoxin net secretion clearance was 120% higher during pregnancy as compared to postpartum. Unbound digoxin net secretion clearance was higher (on average 107%) during pregnancy than postpartum [10]. The doubling of digoxin net renal secretion clearance is consistent with an increase in renal p-glycoprotein activity, but might also be explained by an increase in renal OATP activity during pregnancy.

3.2.9.2.2 Organic anion transporter, oligopeptide transporters

The transporters involved in renal transport of amoxicillin are still being worked out. In vivo studies with amoxicillin and probenecid (inhibitor of the renal organic anion transport system) have shown that the renal clearance of amoxicillin is significantly reduced by probenecid, suggesting that amoxicillin is a substrate for an organic anion transporter [97]. The oligopeptide transporters, hPepT1 and hPepT2, are located on the apical membrane of the proximal tubule and are involved in reabsorption of endogenous peptides [98]. Amoxicillin is an inhibitor and substrate for hPepT2 transport with a lower affinity for hPepT1 [99]. In both the second and third trimesters of pregnancy, the renal clearance and net renal secretion of amoxicillin are increased by more than 60% and 50%, respectively [91]. Renal secretion makes up more than half of the renal clearance for amoxicillin. The change in net renal secretion clearance may be a result of increased renal secretion, inhibition of reabsorption, or both.

3.2.9.2.3 Organic cation transporters, multidrug and extrusion transporters, and plasma monoamine transporter

Metformin is a substrate for OCTs, including OCT1, OCT2, the multidrug and toxin extrusion (MATE) transporters [100], and the plasma membrane monoamine transporter [101]. In humans, OCT2 plays an important role in metformin renal clearance [102−104]. Several studies in vitro and in animal species suggest that OCT2 expression and activity in the kidney can be regulated by the steroid hormones [105−107]. Metformin net secretion clearance was on average 45% and 38% higher in mid- and late-pregnancy than postpartum [32]. Metformin renal clearance correlates well with creatinine clearance ($r = 0.8$), but even better with its net tubular secretion clearance ($r = 0.97$), which is not surprising given metformin's high secretory clearance [32]. The increase in metformin net secretory clearance could in part be a result of upregulation in the renal tubular transport (i.e., OCT2 activity). N1-methylnicotinamide (1-NMN), an endogenous probe for OCT2 and MATE (specifically MATE1 and MATE2-K), was found to have increased renal clearance and net renal secretion during both mid- and late-pregnancy compared to postpartum [108]. 1-NMN renal clearance was positively correlated with metformin renal clearance [108]. Increased glomerular filtration and increased OCT2, MATE1, and MATE2-K activities during pregnancy are likely the reasons for the increase in renal clearance of 1-NMN and metformin. Further research is necessary to determine the mechanism underlying these changes.

3.2.9.2.4 pH-dependent changes in secretion and reabsorption

The tendency is to assume that all drugs that are predominantly eliminated by the kidneys in the nonpregnant population will remain as such in the pregnant population. However, this is not always the case. For example, clonidine is a drug that is ~65% eliminated unchanged in the urine in the nonpregnant population with dosage adjustment recommendations for patients with renal disease. Therefore, it is reasonable to assume that the increase in creatinine clearance expected during pregnancy would increase the renal clearance of clonidine. However, even though the patients in our study had an increase in creatinine clearance during pregnancy, there was no change in clonidine renal clearance and a poor correlation ($r = 0.26$) between clonidine renal clearance and creatinine clearance. In fact, the primary pathway for elimination of clonidine during pregnancy switches from renal to metabolic. The explanation for the discrepancy between changes in creatinine clearance being observed, but no change in clonidine renal clearance during pregnancy is related to the chemical properties of clonidine. Clonidine's pKa is 8.05, which resulted in a strong correlation ($r = 0.82$, $P < .001$) between clonidine renal clearance, corrected for GFR, and urine pH (range 5.8−7.5) [43]. This example is a reminder that it is difficult to predict the effects of pregnancy on the pharmacokinetics of medications.

3.2.10 Volume of distribution

Volume of distribution is not a physical space, but rather an apparent one. Volume of distribution is the apparent volume needed to account for the total amount of drug in the body if the drug was evenly distributed throughout the body and in the same concentration as the site of sample collection such as peripheral venous plasma. Some drugs (e.g., tolbutamide, phenytoin, gentamicin, warfarin) are known to have small volumes of distribution (0.1−1 L/kg) while others (e.g., meperidine, propranolol, digoxin) are known to have large volumes of distribution (1−10 L/kg). The volume of distribution for a drug affects the difference between peak and trough concentrations at steady state or maximum concentrations for single intravenous bolus dosing. The volume of distribution can be used to determine the loading dose needed to achieve a certain concentration.

There are many physiologic changes that occur during pregnancy that can result in altered volume of distribution for medications. For example, the recommended total weight gain during a singleton pregnancy depends on the BMI and stature of the pregnant woman, but ranges from 6 to 18 kg. Despite the recommendations, many women will exceed these weight gain guidelines. Of the weight gained, approximately 62% will be water, 30% will be fat, and 8% will be protein. Blood volume typically increases 30%−45% and peaks between 28 and 34 weeks gestation. Total body water increases 6−8 L during pregnancy and peaks at term [109]. Increases in the volume of distribution for a medication will not alter the average steady state concentration, but will result in lower peak and higher trough concentrations. Apparent volume of distribution is dependent on the drug's lipid or water solubility, plasma protein binding as well as tissue binding. Metformin has a larger apparent oral volume of distribution during pregnancy than in women three−four months postpartum [32].

3.2.11 Half-life

Half-life is the time it takes for the drug concentration to be reduced in half and is useful in determining dosing frequency. Half-life is dependent on both clearance and volume of distribution, such that a decrease in clearance, as might be seen with a CYP1A2 or CYP2C19 substrate, or an increase in volume of distribution will prolong the half-life and lead to a longer dosage interval. For medications with increased clearance (e.g., CYP3A, CYP2D6, or CYP2C9 substrates or those eliminated by the kidneys) or decreased volume of distribution will have shorter half-lives and require more frequent dosing. Since half-life is dependent on both clearance and volume of distribution, if there is a similar increase in both clearance and volume, there will be no change in the half-life for the drug as is the case for midazolam and metoprolol [1,2,10]. Although the changes in renal function during pregnancy are small relative to the magnitude of changes seen with some of the hepatic enzymes, altered renal function can change the pharmacokinetics of some medications. We found that both renally eliminated drugs, atenolol and amoxicillin, have shorter half-lives during the second and third trimesters of pregnancy compared to the same women three months postpartum, although these changes were relatively small [3,91]. In contrast, metformin, which is also eliminated by the kidneys, has a longer half-life in the second trimester of pregnancy than women three−four months postpartum, reflecting the increase in volume of distribution seen during pregnancy [32].

3.3 Summary

There is a tremendous amount of variability in patient response to medications during pregnancy. In part, this variability can be explained by changes in pharmacokinetics. The medication's chemical and pharmacokinetic characteristics influence the type of effect pregnancy can have on drug handling and response. Changes in protein binding are most important for highly protein bound drugs and should be taken into account when interpreting total drug concentrations. Changes in hepatic blood flow during pregnancy might affect the hepatic clearance of high ER drugs. Medications that are eliminated by the kidneys as well as those metabolized by CYP3A, CYP2D6, CYP2C9, CYP2E1, and UGT1A4 are likely to undergo increased clearance during pregnancy. Those metabolized by CYP1A2, CYP2C19, and CBR1 might have decreased clearance during pregnancy. For those medications that are metabolized by CYP2B6, changes in clearance might be genotype dependent. Lastly, ADH does not appear to change during gestation. Most medications that are cleared renally will undergo increased clearance as renal filtration increases during gestation. For some medications, the physiologic changes that occur during pregnancy have a significant impact on pharmacokinetics and dosage. For medications with unpredictable pharmacokinetic changes during pregnancy, altered medication selection should be considered. Taking into account the pharmacokinetic changes that occur during pregnancy will help to minimize the variability in patient response. This approach is particularly important for medications with narrow therapeutic ranges. Pharmacokinetics should be considered to be only one component in determining optimum medication selection and dosage.

References

[1] Högstedt S, Lindberg B, Peng DR, Regårdh CG, Rane A. Pregnancy-induced increase in metoprolol metabolism. Clin Pharmacol Ther 1985;37:688−92.

[2] Högstedt S, Lindberg B, Rane A. Increased oral clearance of metoprolol in pregnancy. Eur J Clin Pharmacol 1983;24:217−20.

[3] Hebert MF, Carr DB, Anderson GD, Blough D, Green GE, Brateng DA, Kantor E, Benedetti TJ, Easterling TR. Pharmacokinetics and pharmacodynamics of atenolol during pregnancy and postpartum. J Clin Pharmacol 2005;45:25−33.

[4] Beringer PM. Winter's basic clinical pharmacokinetics. 6th ed. Philadelphia: Walters Kluwer; 2018.

[5] Rowland M, Tozer TN. Clinical pharmacokinetics and pharmacodynamics concepts and applications. 4th ed. Philadelphia: Lippincott Williams & Wilkins; 2011.

[6] Everson GT. Gastrointestinal motility in pregnancy. Gastroenterol Clin N Am 1992;21: 751−76.

[7] Kelly TF, Savides TJ. Gastrointestinal disease in pregnancy. In: Creasy RK, Resnik R, Iams JD, editors. Maternal-fetal medicine: principles and practices. 6th ed. Philadelphia: Saunders; 2009. p. 1041−58.

[8] Steinlauf AF, Chang PK, Traube M. Gastrointestinal complications. In: Burrow GN, Duffy TP, Copel JA, editors. Medical complications during pregnancy. 6th ed. Philadelphia: Saunders; 2004. p. 259−78.

[9] Van Thiel DH, Schade RR. Pregnancy: its physiologic course, nutrient cost, and effects on gastrointestinal function. In: Rustgi VK, Cooper JN, editors. Gastrointestinal and hepatic complications in pregnancy. New York: John Wiley & Sons; 1986. p. 1−292.

[10] Hebert MF, Easterling TR, Kirby B, Carr DB, Buchanan ML, Rutherford T, Thummel KE, Fishbein DP, Unadkat JD. Effects of pregnancy on CYP3A and P-glycoprotein activities as measured by disposition of midazolam and digoxin: a University of Washington specialized center of research study. Clin Pharmacol Ther 2008;84:248−53.

[11] Murphy MM, Scott JM, McParlin JM, Fernandez-Ballart JD. The pregnancy-related decrease in fasting plasma homocysteine is not explained by folic acid supplementation, hemodilution, or a decrease in albumin in a longitudinal study. Am J Clin Nutr 2002;76:614−9.

[12] Aweeka FT, Stek A, Best BM, Hu C, Holland D, Hermes A, Burchett SK, Read J, Mirochnick M, Capparelli EV, International Maternal Pediatric Adolescent AIDS Clinical Trials Group (IMPAACT) P1026s Protocol Team. Lopinavir protein binding in HIV-1-infected pregnant women. HIV Med 2010;11:232−8.

[13] Gardill BR, Vogl MR, Lin HY, Hammond GL, Muller YA. Corticosteroid-binding globulin: structure-function implications from species differences. PLoS One 2012; 7(12):e52759.

[14] Potter JM, Mueller UW, Hickman PE, Michael CA. Corticosteroid binding globulin in normotensive and hypertensive human pregnancy. Clin Sci 1987;72:725−35.

[15] Yerby MS, Friel PN, McCormick K, Koerner M, Van Allen M, Leavitt AM, Sells CJ, Yerby JA. Pharmacokinetics of anticonvulsants in pregnancy: alterations in plasma protein binding. Epilepsy Res 1990;5:223−8.

[16] Ryu RJ, Easterling TR, Caritis SN, Venkataramanan R, Umans JG, Ahmed MS, Clark S, Kantrowitz-Gordon I, Hays K, Bennett B, Honaker MT, Thummel KE, Shen DD, Hebert MF. Prednisone pharmacokinetics during pregnancy and lactation. J Clin Pharmacol 2018;58(9):1223−32.

[17] Zheng S, Easterling TR, Umans JG, Miodovnik M, Calamia JC, Thummel KE, Shen DD, Davis CL, Hebert MF. Pharmacokinetics of tacrolimus during pregnancy. Ther Drug Monit 2012;34(6):660−70.

[18] Feghali MN, Mattison DR. Clinical therapeutics in pregnancy. J Biomed Biotechnol 2011;2011:783528.

[19] Hebert MF, Ma X, Naraharisetti SB, Krudys KM, Umans JG, Hankins GD, Caritis SN, Miodovnik M, Mattison DR, Unadkat JD, Kelly EJ, Blough D, Cobelli C, Ahmed MS, Snodgrass WR, Carr DB, Easterling TR, Vicini P, Obstetric-Fetal Pharmacology Research Unit Network. Are we optimizing gestational diabetes treatment with glyburide? The pharmacologic basis for better clinical practice. Clin Pharmacol Ther 2009; 85:607−14.

[20] Easterling TR, Benedetti TJ, Schmucker BC, Millard SP. Maternal hemodynamics in normal and preeclamptic pregnancies: a longitudinal study. Obstet Gynecol 1990;76: 1061−9.

[21] Mizushima Y, Tohira H, Mizobata Y, Matsuoka T, Yokota J. Assessment of effective hepatic blood flow in critically ill patients by noninvasive pulse dye-densitometry. Surg Today 2003;33:101−5.

[22] Bracht H, Takala J, Tenhunen JJ, Brander L, Knuesel R, Merasto-Minkkinen M, Jakob SM. Hepatosplanchnic blood flow control and oxygen extraction are modified by the underlying mechanism of impaired perfusion. Crit Care Med 2005;33:645−53.

[23] Nakai A, Sekiya I, Oya A, Koshino T, Araki T. Assessment of the hepatic arterial and portal venous blood flows during pregnancy with Doppler ultrasonography. Arch Gynecol Obstet 2002;266:25−9.

[24] Rudolf VK, Rudolf H, Towe J. Indocyaningrun (Ujoviridin®)-Test bei Patientinnen mit Hyperemesis gravidarum. Zbl Hynakol 1982;104:748−52.

[25] Robson SC, Mutch E, Boys RJ, Woodhouse KW. Apparent liver blood flow during pregnancy: a serial study using indocyanine green clearance. Br J Obstet Gynaecol 1990;97:720−4.

[26] Probst P, Paumgartner G, Caucig H, Frohlich H, Grabner G. Studies on clearance and placental transfer of indocyanine green during labor. Clin Chim Acta 1970;29:157—60.

[27] Mandic-Markovic VD, Mikovic ZM, Djukic MK, Vasiljevic MD, Jankovic GL. Doppler parameters of the maternal hepatic artery blood flow in normal pregnancy: maternal hepatic artery blood flow in normal pregnancy. Eur J Obstet Gynecol Reprod Biol 2014;181:275—9.

[28] Davison JM, Dunlop W, Ezimokhai M. 24-hour creatinine clearance during the third trimester of normal pregnancy. Br J Obstet Gynaecol 1980;87:106—9.

[29] Davison JM, Noble MC. Serial changes in 24 hour creatinine clearance during normal menstrual cycles and the first trimester of pregnancy. Br J Obstet Gynaecol 1981;88: 10—7.

[30] Davison JM, Dunlop W. Renal hemodynamics and tubular function normal human pregnancy. Kidney Int 1980;18:152—61.

[31] Sturgiss SN, Dunlop W, Davison JM. Renal haemodynamics and tubular function in human pregnancy. Baillieres Clin Obstet Gynaecol 1994;8:209—34.

[32] Eyal S, Easterling TR, Carr D, Umans JG, Miodovnik M, Hankins GD, Clark SM, Risler L, Wang J, Kelly EJ, Shen DD, Hebert MF. Pharmacokinetics of metformin during pregnancy. Drug Metab Dispos 2010;38:833—40.

[33] Tracy TS, Venkataramanan R, Glover DD, Caritis SN, National Institute for Child Health and Human Development Network of Maternal-Fetal-Medicine Units. Temporal changes in drug metabolism (CYP1A2, CYP2D6 and CYP3A activity) during pregnancy. Am J Obstet Gynecol 2005;192:633—9.

[34] van Heeswijk RP, Khaliq Y, Gallicano KD, Bourbeau M, Seguin I, Phillips EJ, Cameron DW. The pharmacokinetics of nelfinavir and M8 during pregnancy and post partum. Clin Pharmacol Ther 2004;76(6):588—97.

[35] Hirt D, Treluyer JM, Jullien V, Firtion G, Chappuy H, Rey E, et al. Pregnancy-related effects on nelfinavir-M8 pharmacokinetics: a population study with 133 women. Antimicrob Agents Chemother 2006;50(6):2079—86.

[36] Unadkat JD, Wara DW, Hughes MD, Maathias AA, Holland DT, Paul ME, Connor J, Huang S, Nguyen B-Y, Watts DH, Mofenson LM, Smith E, Deutsch P, Kaiser KA, Tuomala RE. Pharmacokinetics and safety of indinavir in human immunodeficiency virus-infected pregnant women. Antimicrob Agents Chemother 2007;51:783—6.

[37] Tran AH, Best BM, Stek A, Wang J, Capparelli EV, Burchett SK, Kreitchmann R, Rungruengthanakit K, George K, Cressey TR, Chakhtoura N, Smith E, Shapiro DE, Mirochnick M, IMPAACT P1026s Protocol Team. Pharmacokinetics of rilpivirine in HIV-infected pregnant women. J Acquir Immune Defic Syndr 2016;72(3):289—96.

[38] Schalkwijk S, Colbers A, Konopnicki D, Gingelmaier A, Lambert J, van der Ende M, Moltó J, Burger D, Pharmacokinetics of Newly Developed Antiretroviral Agents in HIV-Infected Pregnant Women (PANNA) Network. Lowered rilpivirine exposure during the third trimester of pregnancy in human immunodeficiency virus type 1—infected women. Clin Infect Dis 2017;65(8):1335—41.

[39] Koh KH, Pan X, Shen HW, Arnold SL, Yu AM, Gonzalez FJ, Isoherranen N, Jeong H. Altered expression of small heterodimer partner governs cytochrome P450 (CYP) 2D6 induction during pregnancy in CYP2D6-humanized mice. J Biol Chem 2014;289(6): 3105—13.

[40] Koh KH, Pan X, Zhang W, McLachlan A, Urrutia R, Jeong H. Krüppel-like factor 9 promotes hepatic cytochrome P450 2D6 expression during pregnancy in CYP2D6-humanized mice. Mol Pharmacol 2014;86(6):727—35.

[41] Ryu RJ, Eyal S, Easterling TR, Caritis SN, Venkataraman R, Hankins G, Rytting E, Thummel K, Kelly EJ, Risler L, Phillips B, Honaker MT, Shen DD, Hebert MF. Pharmacokinetics of metoprolol during pregnancy and lactation. J Clin Pharmacol 2016; 56(5):581−9.

[42] Claessens AJ, Risler LJ, Eyal S, Shen DD, Easterling TR, Hebert MF. CYP2D6 mediates 4-hydroxylation of clonidine in vitro: implication for pregnancy-induced changes in clonidine clearance. Drug Metab Dispos 2010;38:1393−6.

[43] Buchanan ML, Easterling TR, Carr DB, Shen DD, Risler LJ, Nelson WL, Mattison DR, Hebert MF. Clonidine pharmacokinetics in pregnancy. Drug Metab Dispos 2009;37:702−5.

[44] Cunningham FE, Baughman VL, Peters J, Laurito CE. Comparative pharmacokinetics of oral versus sublingual clonidine. J Clin Anesth 1994;6:430−3.

[45] Porchet HC, Piletta P, Dayer P. Pharmacokinetic-pharmacodynamic modeling of the effects of clonidine on pain threshold, blood pressure, and salivary flow. Eur J Clin Pharmacol 1992;42:655−62.

[46] Arndts D. New aspects of clinical pharmacology of clonidine. Chest 1983;83: 397−400.

[47] Naritomi Y, Terashita S, Kagayama A. Identification and relative contributions of human cytochrome P450 isoforms involved in the metabolism of glibenclamide and lansoprazole: evaluation of an approach based on the in vitro substrate disappearance rate. Xenobiotica 2004;34:415−7.

[48] Van Giersbergen PL, Treiber A, Clozel M, Bodin F, Dingemanse J. In vivo and in vitro studies exploring the pharmacokinetic interaction between bosentan, a dual endothelin receptor antagonist and glyburide. Clin Pharmacol Ther 2002;71:253−62.

[49] Zhou L, Naraharisetti SB, Liu L, Wang H, Lin YS, Isoherranen N, Unadkat JD, Hebert MF, Mao Q. Contributions of human cytochrome P450 enzymes to glyburide metabolism. Biopharm Drug Dispos 2010;31:228−42.

[50] Kirchheiner J, Brockmöller J, Meineke I, Bauer S, Rohde W, Meisel C, Roots I. Impact of CYP2C9 amino acid polymorphisms on glyburide kinetics and on the insulin and glucose response in healthy volunteers. Clin Pharmacol Ther 2002;71:286−96.

[51] Yin OQ, Tomlinson B, Chow MS. CYP2C9 but not CYP2C19 polymorphisms affect the pharmacokinetics and pharmacodynamics of glyburide in Chinese subjects. Clin Pharmacol Ther 2005;78:370−7.

[52] Niemi M, Cascorbi I, Timm R, Kroemer HK, Neuvonen PJ, Kivisto KT. Glyburide and glimepiride pharmacokinetics in subjects with different CYP2C9 genotypes. Clin Pharmacol Ther 2005;78:90−2.

[53] Zhang YF, Chen XY, Guo YJ, Si DY, Zhou H, Zhong DF. Impact of cytochrome P450 CYP2C9 variant allele CYP2C9*3 on the pharmacokinetics of glibenclamide and lornoxicam in Chinese subjects. Yao Xue Xue Bao 2005;40:796−9.

[54] McGready R, Stepniewska K, Seaton E, Cho T, Cho D, Ginsberg A, Edstein MD, Ashley E, Looareesuwan S, White NJ, Nosten F. Pregnancy and use of oral contraceptives reduces the biotransformation of proguanil to cycloguanil. Eur J Clin Pharmacol 2003;59:553−7.

[55] Yu T, Campbell SC, Stockmann C, Tak C, Schoen K, Clark EA, Varner MW, Spigarelli MG, Sherwin CM. Pregnancy-induced changes in the pharmacokinetics of caffeine and its metabolites. J Clin Pharmacol 2016;56(5):590−6.

[56] Kantrowitz-Gordon I, Hays K, Kayode O, Kumar AR, Kaplan HG, Reid JM, Safgren SL, Ames MM, Easterling TR, Hebert MF. Pharmacokinetics of dacarbazine (DTIC) in pregnancy. Cancer Chemother Pharmacol 2018;81(3):455—60.

[57] Yanakakis LJ, Bumpus NN. Biotransformation of the antiretroviral drug etravirine: metabolite identification, reaction phenotyping, and characterization of autoinduction of cytochrome P450-dependent metabolism. Drug Metab Dispos 2012;40(4):803—14.

[58] Izurieta P, Kakuda TN, Feys C, Witek J. Safety and pharmacokinetics of etravirine in pregnant HIV-1-infected women. HIV Med 2011;12(4):257—8.

[59] Mulligan N, Schalkwijk S, Best BM, Colbers A, Wang J, Capparelli EV, Moltó J, Stek AM, Taylor G, Smith E, Hidalgo Tenorio C, Chakhtoura N, van Kasteren M, Fletcher CV, Mirochnick M, Burger D. Etravirine pharmacokinetics in HIV-infected pregnant women. Front Pharmacol 2016;4(7):239.

[60] Ke AB, Nallani SC, Zhao P, Rostami-Hodjegan A, Unadkat JD. Expansion of a PBPK model to predict disposition in pregnant women of drugs cleared via multiple CYP enzymes, including CYP2B6, CYP2C9 and CYP2C19. Br J Clin Pharmacol 2014;77(3): 554—70.

[61] Montaner J, Yeni P, Clumeck NN, Fätkenheuer G, Gatell J, Hay P, Seminari E, Peeters MP, Schöller-Gyüre M, Simonts M, Woodfall B, TMC125-C203 Study Group. Safety, tolerability, and preliminary efficacy of 48 weeks of etravirine therapy in a phase IIb dose-ranging study involving treatment-experienced patients with HIV-1 infection. Clin Infect Dis 2008;47(7):969—78.

[62] Olagunju A, Bolaji O, Amara A, Else L, Okafor O, Adejuyigbe E, Oyigboja J, Back D, Khoo S, Owen A. Pharmacogenetics of pregnancy-induced changes in efavirenz pharmacokinetics. Clin Pharmacol Ther 2015;97(3):298—306.

[63] Cressey TR, Stek A, Capparelli E, Bowonwatanuwong C, Prommas S, Sirivatanapa P, Yuthavisuthi P, Neungton C, Huo Y, Smith E, Best BM, Mirochnick M, IMPAACT P1026s Team. Efavirenz pharmacokinetics during the third trimester of pregnancy and postpartum. J Acquir Immune Defic Syndr 2012;59:245—52.

[64] Lee JK, Chung HJ, Fischer L, Fischer J, Gonzalez FJ, Jeong H. Human placental lactogen induces CYP2E1 expression via PI 3-kinase pathway in female human hepatocytes. Drug Metab Dispos 2014;42(4):492—9.

[65] Prescott LF. Kinetics and metabolism of paracetamol and phenacetin. Br J Clin Pharmacol 1980;10(Suppl. 2):291S—8S.

[66] Miners JO, Robson RA, Birkett DJ. Paracetamol metabolism in pregnancy. Br J Clin Pharmacol 1986;22(3):359—62.

[67] Kulo A, Peeters MY, Allegaert K, Smits A, de Hoon J, Verbesselt R, Lewi L, van de Velde M, Knibbe CA. Pharmacokinetics of paracetamol and its metabolites in women at delivery and post-partum. Br J Clin Pharmacol 2013;75(3):850—60.

[68] King CD, Rios GR, Green MD, Tephly TR. UDP-glucuronosyltransferases. Curr Drug Metabol 2000;1(2):143—61.

[69] Zhou J, Tracy TS, Remmel RP. Glucuronidation of dihydrotestosterone and trans-androsterone by recombinant UDP-glucuronosyltransferase (UGT) 1A4: evidence for multiple UGT1A4 aglycone binding sites. Drug Metab Dispos 2010;38:431—40.

[70] Green MD, Bishop WP, Tephly TR. Expressed human UGT1.4 protein catalyzes the formation of quaternary ammonium-linked glucuronides. Drug Metab Dispos 1995; 23:299—302.

[71] Tran TA, Leppik IE, Blesi K, Sathanandan ST, Remmel R. Lamotrigine clearance during pregnancy. Neurology 2002;59:251—5.

[72] Reimers A, Helde G, Bråthen G, Brodtkorb E. Lamotrigine and its N2-glucuronide during pregnancy: the significance of renal clearance and estradiol. Epilepsy Res 2011;94(3):198−205.

[73] de Haan GJ, Edelbroek P, Segers J, Engelsman M, Lindhout D, Dévilé-Notschaele M, Augustijn P. Gestation-induced changes in lamotrigine pharmacokinetics: a monotherapy study. Neurology 2004;63:571−3.

[74] Jeong H, Choi S, Song JW, Chen H, Fischer JH. Regulation of UDP-glucuronosyltransferase (UGT) 1A1 by progesterone and its impact on labetalol elimination. Xenobiotica 2008;38(1):62−75.

[75] Hardman J, Endres L, Fischer P, Fischer J. Pharmacokinetics of labetalol in pregnancy. Pharmacotherapy 2005;25(10):1493.

[76] Choi S, Jeong H, Deyo K, Fischer J. Protein binding of labetalol in pregnancy. Clin Pharmacol Therapeut 2007;81(S1):S79.

[77] Beaulac-Baillargeon L, Rocheleau S. Paracetamol pharmacokinetics during the first trimester of human pregnancy. Eur J Clin Pharmacol 1994;46(5):451−4.

[78] O'Sullivan MJ, Boyer PJ, Scott GB, Parks WP, Weller S, Blum MR, Balsley J, Bryson YJ. The pharmacokinetics and safety of zidovudine in the third trimester of pregnancy for women infected with human immunodeficiency virus and their infants: phase I acquired predictions resulted in the lowest $C_{ss,avg}$ in the third trimester (median [interquartile range]: 4.5 [3.8-5.1] mg/L), while C_s immunodeficiency syndrome clinical trials group study (protocol 082). Zidovudine Collaborative Working Group. Am J Obstet Gynecol 1993;168(5):1510−6.

[79] Gerdin E, Salmonson T, Lindberg B, Rane A. Maternal kinetics of morphine during labour. J Perinat Med 1990;18(6):479−87.

[80] Shankar OK, Ronis MJJ, Badger TM. Effects of pregnancy and nutritional status on alcohol metabolism. Alcohol Res Health 2007;30(1):55−9.

[81] Crabb DW, Matsumoto M, Chang D, You M. Overview of the role of alcohol dehydrogenase and aldehyde dehydrogenase and their variants in the genesis of alcohol-related pathology. Proc Nutr Soc 2004;63(1):49−63.

[82] Yuen GJ, Weller S, Pakes GE. A review of the pharmacokinetics of abacavir. Clin Pharmacokinet 2008;47:351−71.

[83] Vannappagari V, Koram N, Albano J, Tilson H, Gee C. Abacavir and lamivudine exposures during pregnancy and non-defect adverse pregnancy outcomes: data from the antiretroviral pregnancy registry. J Acquir Immune Defic Syndr 2015;68(3):359−64.

[84] Hua W, Zhang H, Ryu S, Yang X, Di L. Human Tissue distribution of carbonyl reductase 1 using proteomic approach with LC-MS/MS. J Pharmaceut Sci 2017;106:1405−11.

[85] Shi SM, Di L. The role of carbonyl reductase 1 in drug discovery and development. Expet Opin Drug Metabol Toxicol 2017;13(8):859−70.

[86] Waclawik A, Jabbour HN, Blitek A, Ziecik AJ. Estradiol-17beta, prostaglandin E2 (PGE2), and the PGE2 receptor are involved in PGE2 positive feedback loop in the porcine endometrium. Endocrinology 2009;150(8):3823−32.

[87] Iwata N, Inazu N, Satoh T. Changes and localization of ovarian carbonyl reductase during pseudopregnancy and pregnancy in rats. Biol Reprod 1990;43(3):397−403.

[88] Malatkova P, Wsol V. Carbonyl reduction pathways in drug metabolism. Drug Metab Rev 2014;46:96−123.

[89] Rosemond MJ, Walsh JS. Human carbonyl reduction pathways and a strategy for their study in vitro. Drug Metab Rev 2004;36:335−61.

[90] Ryu RJ, Eyal S, Kaplan HG, Akbarzadeh A, Hays K, Puhl K, Easterling TR, Berg SL, Scorsone KA, Feldman EM, Umans JG, Miodovnik M, Hebert MF. Pharmacokinetics of doxorubicin in pregnant women. Cancer Chemother Pharmacol 2014;73(4): 789–97.

[91] Andrew MA, Easterling TR, Carr DB, Shen D, Buchanan ML, Rutherford T, Bennett R, Vicini P, Hebert MF. Amoxicillin pharmacokinetics in pregnant women: modeling and simulations of dosage strategies. Clin Pharmacol Ther 2007;81:547–56.

[92] Tanigawara Y, Okamura N, Hirai M, Yasuhara M, Ueda K, Kioka N, Komano T, Hori R. Transport of digoxin by human P-glycoprotein expressed in a porcine kidney epithelial cell line (LLC-PK1). J Pharmacol Exp Therapeut 1992;263:840–5.

[93] Ernest S, Rajaraman S, Megyesi J, Bello-Reuss EN. Expression of MDR1 (multidrug resistance) gene and its protein in normal human kidney. Nephron 1997;77:284–9.

[94] Kullak-Ublick GA, Ismair MG, Stieger B, Landmann L, Huber R, Pizzagalli F, Fattinger K, Meier PJ, Hagenbuch B. Organic anion-transporting polypeptide B (OATP-B) and its functional comparison with three other OATPs of human liver. Gastroenterology 2001;120:525–33.

[95] Lau YY, Wu C-Y, Okochi H, Benet LZ. Ex situ inhibition of hepatic uptake and efflux significantly changes metabolism: hepatic enzyme-transporter interplay. J Pharmacol Exp Therapeut 2004;308:1040–5.

[96] Lowes S, Cavet ME, Simmons NL. Evidence for a non-MDR1 component in digoxin secretion by intestinal Caco-2 epithelial layers. Eur J Pharmacol 2003;458:49–56.

[97] Shanson DC, McNabb R, Hijipieris P. The effect of probenecid on serum amoxicillin concentrations up to 18 hours after a single 3 g oral dose of amoxicillin: possible implications for preventing endocarditis. J Antimicrob Chemother 1984;13:629–32.

[98] Daniel H, Kottra G. The proton oligopeptide cotransporter family SLC15 in physiology and pharmacology. Pflueg Arch Eur J Physiol 2004;447:610–8.

[99] Li M, Anderson GD, Phillips BR, Kong W, Shen DD, Wang J. Interactions of amoxicillin and cefaclor with human renal organic anion and peptide transporters. Drug Metab Dispos 2006;34:547–55.

[100] Becker ML, Visser LE, van Schaik RH, Hofman A, Uitterlinden AG, Stricker BH. Genetic variation in the multidrug and toxin extrusion 1 transporter protein influences the glucose-lowering effect of metformin in patients with diabetes: a preliminary study. Diabetes 2009;58:745–9.

[101] Zhou M, Xia L, Wang J. Metformin transport by a newly cloned proton-stimulated organic cation transporter (plasma membrane monoamine transporter) expressed in human intestine. Drug Metab Dispos 2007;35:1956–62.

[102] Song IS, Shin HJ, Shim EJ, Jung IS, Kim WY, Shon JH, Shin JG. Genetic variants of the organic cation transporter 2 influence the disposition of metformin. Clin Pharmacol Ther 2008;84:559–62.

[103] Wang ZJ, Yin OQ, Tomlinson B, Chow MS. OCT2 polymorphisms and in-vivo renal functional consequence: studies with metformin and cimetidine. Pharmacogenetics Genom 2008;18:637–45.

[104] Chen Y, Li S, Brown C, Cheatham S, Castro RA, Leabman MK, Urban TJ, Chen L, Yee SW, Choi JH, Huang Y, Brett CM, Burchard EG, Giacomini KM. Effect of genetic variation in the organic cation transporter 2 on the renal elimination of metformin. Pharmacogenetics Genom 2009;19:497–504.

[105] Urakami Y, Nakamura N, Takahashi K, Okuda M, Saito H, Hashimoto Y, Inui K. Gender differences in expression of organic cation transporter OCT2 in rat kidney. FEBS Lett 1999;461:339−42.

[106] Shu Y, Bello CL, Mangravite LM, Feng B, Giacomini KM. Functional characteristics and steroid hormone-mediated regulation of an organic cation transporter in Madin-Darby canine kidney cells. J Pharmacol Exp Therapeut 2001;299:392−8.

[107] Alnouti Y, Petrick JS, Klaassen CD. Tissue distribution and ontogeny of organic cation transporters in mice. Drug Metab Dispos 2006;34:477−82.

[108] Bergagnini-Kolev MC, Hebert MF, Easterling TR, Lin YS. Pregnancy increases the renal secretion of N1-methylnicotinamide, an endogenous probe for renal cation transporters, in patients prescribed metformin. Drug Metab Dispos 2017;45(3):325−9.

[109] Blackburn ST. Maternal, fetal & neonatal physiology. A clinical perspective. 3rd ed. St Louis: Saunders Elsevier; 2007.

Medications and the breastfeeding mother

4

Cheston M. Berlin, Jr.

Department of Pediatrics/Division of Academic General Pediatrics, Penn State College of Medicine, Penn Statae Children's Hospital, Hershey, PA, United States

4.1 Medication use by the breastfeeding mother

Mothers may need medication both during and after pregnancy. In both cases, it is important not only to protect the infant but also to provide the mother with necessary drug treatment. The infant may be born having been exposed to maternal medication during gestation. It is important to remember, in addition to drug exposure of the infant during breastfeeding, that previous exposure during pregnancy may potentiate any adverse effects during lactation. This would especially be true in the immediate postnatal period, but for some drugs, the window of adverse reactions in the infant may be longer (e.g., antidepressants).

4.2 Clinical pharmacology of drug transfer into breast milk

The determining factors for the transport of drugs from maternal circulation to the alveolar lumen in the mammary cell are as follows [1]: molecular weight [2], binding to maternal plasma proteins [3], lipid solubility, and [4] degree of ionization. Drugs which are transferred most rapidly and/or in the highest amount are those with high lipid solubility, no electrical charge, low molecular weight, and low or no binding to maternal plasma proteins. There are four diffusion mechanisms for drug transfer into the mammary cell alveolar lumen: transcellular, intercellular, passive, and ionophore (transfer of polar compounds bound to carrier proteins) [1]. Transcellular diffusion probably accounts for most drug transfer. The intercellular diffusion route, which avoids the interior of the cell, may account for the appearance in milk of high-molecular weight compounds such as immunoglobulins (from maternal plasma) and monoclonal antibody drugs such as etanercept (Enbrel, molecular weight 52,000). High-molecular weight compounds do appear in milk. Most obvious are antibodies from maternal plasma. Many of the newer pharmacological agents are high-molecular weight entities such as monoclonal antibodies. For drugs like etanercept, the amount appearing in milk is extremely small (2−5 ng/mL) compared to the maternal serum level of 1450−2000 ng/mL [2]. Such a small amount of a protein is most likely pharmacologically inactive both because of the extremely small dose

Clinical Pharmacology During Pregnancy. https://doi.org/10.1016/B978-0-12-818902-3.00004-X

and also because of lack of absorption from the infant's gastrointestinal tract. Because virtually all drugs of a molecular weight below 200 or 300 Da will cross into milk, the dose that the child receives (concentration × volume) is usually pharmacologically insignificant. For most drugs, less than 1%−2% of the maternal dose is potentially available to be excreted into breast milk [3−5].

4.3 During delivery

The obvious concern in this period of time is the type and anesthesia/analgesia that the mother may have received. This drug exposure may delay the onset of lactogenesis, may affect the mother's mentation and ability to nurse, and the infant may show effects from transplacental transfer that interfere with latch and ingestion. An important concept is that regardless of the type of anesthesia and/or analgesia used after delivery, the amount of any agent potentially transferred to the infant would be less than the amount transferred during labor and delivery via the placenta.

4.4 General anesthesia

4.4.1 Volatile anesthetic agents

There are very little data on the concentration of these compounds in human milk. This is due to rapid washout after administration, and by the time the mother wakens to nurse her infant, her plasma levels are very low or absent.

4.4.1.1 Halothane

There are no published reports measuring the amount of halothane in milk after general anesthesia to the mother. It has been reported that patients can exhale measurable amounts of halothane for 11−20 days after anesthesia [6]. A female anesthesiologist had levels of 2 ppm of halothane in her milk after working in an operating room for up to 5 h [7]. Because of this observation, it is reasonable to assume that it would appear in the milk of a mother administered halothane for a cesarean section or any postdelivery complication.

4.4.1.2 Desflurane and sevoflurane

These two inhalation anesthetic agents are highly fluorinated and not very soluble in fat and other peripheral tissues. Thus, induction and recovery are rapid. Although there are no reports of measurement of these two compounds in milk, the levels are very likely to be low or absent because of very low fat solubility.

4.4.2 Intravenous anesthetic agents

4.4.2.1 Ketamine

There are no reports of the measurement of ketamine in the milk of postpartum women. The half-life of ketamine is about 3 h, so that permitting a mother to breastfeed several hours after delivery would expose the infant to extremely small amounts of this drug.

4.4.2.2 Propofol

This drug is a lipid and must be administered to the mother via a lipid emulsion. The half-life of the drug is about 2 h. The amounts found in milks are very low—usually 1 mg/L of milk or less [8]. Such low amounts would be unlikely to be absorbed by the nursing infant.

4.4.2.3 Etomidate

Concentrations of etomidate in milk are very low (less than 1 mg/L) and absent 4 h after administration. Maternal half-life is about 3 h [9].

4.4.2.4 Thiopental

Concentrations of thiopental in milk are usually 2 mg/dL or less depending on the time of sampling after intravenous administration to the mother. Serum concentrations usually decline to less than 1 mg/dL after 4 h from the last dose [9]. One study compared the excretion of thiopental in both breast-fed and nonbreast-fed infants and found no difference in the amount excreted [10]. It is unlikely that the breast-fed infant would receive a significant amount of thiopental by the time lactation is established. This drug has been the subject of much debate because of its use as a component in lethal injection for capital punishment. It has not been manufactured in the United States of America since 2009, and its importation from foreign suppliers is a source of litigation.

4.4.3 A general statement

It is interesting to speculate on whether initial difficulty in breastfeeding (especially poor latch) may be due to residual general anesthetics (either inhalation or intravenous) in breast milk. It is safe for mother (and infant) to start or resume breastfeeding as soon as she emerges from a general anesthetic agent [11–14].

4.5 Epidural anesthesia

The usual anesthetic agents employed in epidural anesthesia are bupivacaine or ropivacaine. The opioid fentanyl is frequently added to the injection fluid. These local anesthetic agents provide rapid onset of pain relief and when used in the usual concentrations do not cause significant loss of muscle power. They are both highly bound to maternal plasma protein and hence transfer to milk is limited. Two recent, prospective, random allocated studies did not show any appreciable difference in breastfeeding between groups receiving epidural anesthesia with a local anesthetic and/or with fentanyl [15,16]. There was a suggestion that women receiving only meperidine did have a lower rate of successful breastfeeding. Chang and Heaman reported on 53 women receiving either ropivacaine or bupivacaine for an average infusion time of 3.5 h. There was no effect on neurobehavior including breastfeeding when compared to a group that received no anesthesia [17]. Both of these local anesthetic agents are poorly, if at all, absorbed from the gastrointestinal tract, so that even if a small amount was present in milk, the infant should not be affected. Rosen and Lawrence studied 83 mother–child pairs and found no difference between breastfed and bottle-fed infants on the ability to feed or initial weight loss [18].

4.6 Galactogogues including dietary supplements (including herbs)

Several drugs and many dietary supplements have been tried to improve lactation both in initiation of milk formation and increase in milk supply. The Dietary Supplement Health and Education Act of 1994 removed dietary supplements from review by the USA FDA. They are not subject to the scrutiny for safety and effectiveness as are drugs. Many dietary supplements may be imported with no guarantee of purity [19]. There are no studies which can confirm that any of these substances are effective [20]. Mothers should be advised not to use dietary supplements as both their purity and efficacy are not established. Adverse reactions to herbal products have been reported and frequently may be associated with impurities including legumes and tree nuts [21]. There is no substitute for lactation support and evaluation by the physician, the hospital, and a lactation consultant [22].

4.7 Immediate postpartum period

During the immediate postpartum period, the major concerns for drug administration to the mother are the following [1]: pain relief [2], resumption of medications for chronic conditions that may have been interrupted by pregnancy, and [3] treatment of newly diagnosed conditions.

4.8 Pain

For immediate postpartum pain relief (cesarean section and episiotomy), acetaminophen or a nonsteroidal antiinflammatory drug (NSAID) may be sufficient if appropriate dosing is used. There have been recent concerns over the use of higher doses of acetaminophen for chronic therapy particularly when associated with the use of alcoholic beverages. Should acetaminophen or NSAIDs provide insufficient pain control, a switch to a narcotic would be appropriate.

4.8.1 Morphine

Regardless of the route of administration to the mother (oral, intravenous, epidural, and intrathecal), the amount of morphine and its active metabolite, morphine-6-glucuronide, transferred in milk is very small and unlikely to cause symptoms in the infant except possibly in the very young term or premature infant. As an example, mothers given 4 mg of morphine epidurally had peak milk levels of 82 mcg/L. If the morphine was given parenterally (5–15 mg), the peak level was 500 mcg/L [23]. The half-life of morphine is about 3 h (adult), so if the mother waited 3 h after any dose of morphine, the level in milk would be quite low and most likely have no clinical effect.

4.8.2 Codeine

The active metabolites of codeine are morphine and the morphine metabolite morphine-6-glucuronide. The enzyme systems responsible for this metabolism are as follows: CYP2D for codeine and UGT2B7 for morphine, codeine-6-glucuronide, and morphine-6-glucuronide. Both of these systems are subject to genetic variation. Some patients are ultrarapid metabolizers of codeine and produce higher levels of morphine and active metabolites in a very short period of time after administration. These increased levels will produce increased side effects, especially drowsiness and central nervous system depression in both the mother and nursing child [24,25]. One death has been reported from morphine poisoning [24]. It would be prudent to avoid using codeine in the immediate postpartum period and perhaps never in breastfeeding mothers regardless of the infant's age. Older infants, especially those receiving solid foods in addition to breast milk, may not have significant symptoms even though their mothers are ultrafast metabolizers [25].

4.8.3 Meperidine

Meperidine does appear in milk and in infant plasma after the administration of the drug for cesarean section and also for postpartum pain management [26,27]. The infant's plasma level was found to be 1.4% of the maternal plasma level [26]. Meperidine given postpartum for pain control does produce decreased alertness in 3- to 4-day-old infants compared to equivalent doses of morphine [27,28]. Hodgkinson et al. using the Early Neonatal Neurobehavioral Scale showed a suppression of most of the 13 items (including alertness, rooting, and sucking) on the first and second postpartum days. The effects were dose related [29]. Morphine appears to be the preferred opioid for intra- and postpartum pain.

4.8.4 Hydrocodone

Hydrocodone is metabolized to the more active metabolite hydromorphone and both are excreted into breast milk. If the daily dosage is limited to 30 mg per day, it is unlikely to affect the established nursing infant [30,31]. The estimated median opiate dose to which the infant might be exposed is 0.7% of the therapeutic dosage for older infants.

There has been much concern expressed over the potential toxicity of opioids delivered to the infant through breastfeeding. Adverse events are usually associated with high maternal dose in very young infants.

4.9 Methadone

Women who have been on methadone during pregnancy for narcotic addiction should be encouraged to breastfeed and continue to take methadone [32]. Babies who nurse from mothers on methadone have both a slower onset and less severe neonatal abstinence syndrome. They also have less need for pharmacological treatment of the abstinence syndrome [33]. Concentrations of methadone are low in breast milk: 21−314 ng/mL [34]. Only about 1%−3% of the maternal dose is excreted into milk [35]. These infants will still require very close observation in the hospital and after discharge to monitor possible withdrawal symptoms.

4.10 Resumption of prepregnancy medications

With the possible exception of psychotropic drugs, almost all medications for acute and chronic maternal conditions are safe for the breastfeeding infant. Adverse reactions in the infant to maternal drug administration are very rare and usually confined to infants under the age of 2 months [36,37]. Anderson et al. found 100 reports of adverse reactions in several database searches from 1966 to 2002 [36]. None were considered definitely related to the drug used, 53 were possibly related, and 47 were probably related. There were 3 deaths among the 100 infants; one was a sudden infant death syndrome. These reports were before the concern about the use of codeine in mothers of very young infants. Only 4% of the reports were in infants older than 6 months of age. Information on over 1000 drugs is on the LactMed website [38] (see below).

4.11 Psycho- and neurotropic drugs

4.11.1 Antidepressants, antipsychotics, anxiolytics, antiepileptics, and drugs for attention deficit hyperactivity disorder

These drugs are grouped together because they target the brain; the pharmacodynamic action of these compounds involves alterations of neurotransmitters within the central nervous system. These alterations may be in the amount of neurotransmitter, sensitivity of the receptor on the neuron, or number of active receptors. These drugs include antidepressants, antipsychotics, tranquilizers, antiepilepsy drugs, and drugs to treat attention deficient hyperactivity disorder. These compounds may be transmitted during both pregnancy and lactation. This group of drugs is perhaps the most significant challenge to the physician caring for the mother; she needs the drug or drugs, but what of the effect or effects on the infant? Since they all act by influencing transmitter function and since central nervous system receptors are developing in the fetus and young infant, will there be permanent effects on neurodevelopment? The evidence is far from complete; long-term studies are not available. Limited information suggests that the effect of these compounds on long-term development may not be significant or at the most difficult to measure because of so many variables such as genetic background and social and economic status [39]. It is impossible to separate drug effect during breastfeeding from effect due to exposure during pregnancy. The important information to be given to the mother is the following [1]: all of these drugs if measured in breast milk do appear [2], the amount in milk is very small and frequently the drug does not appear in infant plasma, and [3] long-term studies (over childhood and adolescence) are not available.

It appears that the sensitive period for exposure and adverse effects may be within the first weeks and months.

The antidepressants are of special interest for obstetricians because of the well-known incidence of depression during pregnancy as well as in the postpartum period, as many as 18%−20% of women may experience depression either during pregnancy or during the first 3 months after delivery [40,41]. Most of the antidepressants currently in use are members of the selective serotonin uptake inhibitors (SSRIs) class. They all have prolonged half-lives of 15−36 h [42]. Several of the SSRIs also have active metabolites (fluoxetine and sertraline) which may extend pharmacological action for a further 4−16 days. There is a neonatal withdrawal syndrome associated with the use of SSRIs. These symptoms can vary from infant to infant and usually consist of difficulty feeding, jitteriness, tremor, sneezing, and sleep difficulties [43]. Symptoms are usually mild and subside within 2 weeks [44].

4.12 Drugs not to give to the nursing mother postpartum

This list is quite small and would include the following:

- drugs of abuse (cocaine and heroin);
- several of the beta-blocking agents such as atenolol and sotalol. These have a high percentage of maternal dose excreted and symptoms have been reported in the nursing infant [45];
- lithium—significant blood levels (from 11% to 56% of maternal levels) reported in nursing infants [46]. 24 infants reported nursed without difficulty; 4 infants reported with symptoms (all under 2 months of age) [47];
- amiodarone—3.5%−45% of the maternal dose may be excreted in milk [48]. This drug contains 39% iodine and may interrupt thyroid function. The half-life in adults is 100 days [49]. Infant serum levels can be 25% of maternal serum levels [50].

4.13 Oral contraceptives

There have been two concerns with the use of oral contraceptives (OCPs) in the breastfeeding woman: quality and quantity of milk produced.

The quality of milk does not seem to vary between mothers not taking OCPs and mothers taking a variety of OCPs. There have been many studies showing decreased milk supply especially with the older high-dose estrogen compounds and especially with starting in the first few weeks after delivery. Progestins seem not to inhibit lactation as much as the estrogen compounds do. A recent study compared immediate postpartum placement of two progestin contraceptives: etonogestrel (ENG, 3-year protection) or levonorgestrel (LNG, 5-year protection). Exclusivity of breastfeeding at 6 months was high for both compounds (71% for ENG and 72% for LNG). Continuation of breastfeeding at 21 months was 100% (ENG) and 93.2% (LNG). There was no difference in exclusivity and continuation between women using the two progestin compounds and the general population of breastfeeding women [51]. The Academy of Breastfeeding Medicine places progestin-only compounds as a second choice for contraception and estrogen contraceptives as the third choice [52]. The first choices are the following: LAM (Lactational Amenorrhea Method), natural family planning, barrier contraception, and intrauterine devices. Mothers wishing to use LAM should be referred to a physician or lactation consultant for advice on how to use LAM. When used correctly, it is 98% effective [53].

4.13.1 Biologics and biopharmaceuticals (e.g., monoclonal antibodies)

A large number of biopharmaceutical drugs have been introduced in to medicine in recent years. They are usually large molecular weight compounds given by injection to the mother in order to modify many diseases. In rheumatology therapy, they are known as Disease Modifying Antirheumatic Drugs. Because they are of high molecular weight, transfer into milk is either low or absent. If transfer does occur, the compounds most likely would be broken down in the infant's intestinal tract. Rarely are detectable levels seen in the infant's plasma [54,55].

4.13.2 Marijuana

With increasing legalization of marijuana for recreational use, its consumption will continue to increase. One study reports 36% of women use it during pregnancy and 18% report using it duration lactation [56]. The cannabis plant is a very complex biological system. There is a field of chemistry called natural product chemistry which has provided several important pharmacology compounds. Some of these compounds may also have with significant capacity for biologic damage of all human organs. Like tobacco, the cannabis plant has over 400 identified compounds [57,58]. The most prominent of the cannabinoids that provide changes in mood and mentation is Δ-9-tetrahydrocannabinol. Another cannabinoid is cannabidiol which has found some efficacy in treatment certain types of seizures. Like coffee and tobacco, there are hundreds of other compounds without significant biological and toxicity studies. The cannabinoid receptor system not only is in the central nervous system but also in peripheral organs. A most important pharmacological property of this class of compounds is the very long half-life in humans (Sharma, Atakan). Because these compounds may affect receptors in the central nervous system, there is concern over possible long-term effects on the infant as discussed above in the section of central nervous system compounds. There is also concern over the exposure to the infant from cannabis smoke in the environment [59–63]. It would be prudent for the nursing mother to avoid the use of cannabis products.

4.14 Summary

Important lessons for any drug that may be transferred in breast milk to the infant are as follows: neonates up to 2 weeks of age are particularly susceptible to toxicity; most adverse reports are in infants less than 2 months of age; there is a dose (maternal) response (infant) relationship; there are significant interindividual variations in drug response; and both maternal and infant pharmacogenetics play a critical response in drug toxicity [64].

Finally, precise analytic methods have identified compounds in such extremely small (e.g., nanograms per liter of milk) amounts that it will be difficult to correlate with biological measures.

4.15 Where to find information

The most up-to-date, comprehensive, and authoritative information is to be found in LactMed [38]. This is a website of the National Library of Medicine, TOXNET (Toxicology Data Network). Over 1000 drugs, including herbal preparations, are referenced; the information is peer reviewed, evidence based, and updated frequently during each year. LactMed can be accessed with a mobile device. The LactMed app for iPhone/iPod Touch and Android can be downloaded at http://toxnet.nlm.nih.gov/help/lactmedapp.htm. Another source is Briggs et al. which also offers detailed information about the use of drugs during pregnancy [65]. In 2015, the US Food and Drug Administration published the Pregnancy and Lactation Labeling Rule. This Rule removed the pregnancy letter categories of A, B, C, D, and X and requires publishing known clinical pharmacology date including risks for any compound used in pregnancy and lactation [66,67].

References

[1] Berlin CM. Neonatal and pediatric pharmacology. In: Yaffe SJ, Aranda JV, editors. Neonatal and pediatric pharmacology: therapeutic principles in practice. 4th ed. Philadelphia: Lippincott Williams & Wilkins; 2011. p. 210–20.
[2] Berthelsen BG, Fjeldsoe-Nielsen H, Nielsen CT, Hellmuth E. Etanercept concentrations in maternal serum, umbilical cord serum, breast milk and child serum during breastfeeding. Rheumatology 2010;49:2225–7.

[3]   Bennett PH, Notarianni LJ. Risk from drugs in breast milk; an analysis by relative dose. Br J Clin Pharmacol 1996;42:673—4.

[4]   Anderson PO. Drugs in lactation. Pharm Res 2018;35:1—13. https://doi.org/10.1007/s11095-017-2287-z.

[5]   Anderson PO, Sauberan JB. Modeling drug passage into human milk. Clin Pharmacol Ther 2016;100:42—52.

[6]   Corbett TH, Ball GL. Respiratory excretion of halothane after clinical and occupational exposure. Anesthesiology 1973;39:342—5.

[7]   Cote CJ, Kenepp NB, Reed SB, Strobel GE. Trace concentrations of halothane in human breast milk. Br J Anaesth 1976;48:541—3.

[8]   http://toxnet.nlm.nih.gov/cgi-bin/sis/search/f?/temp/~SrnBRA:1 [propofol].

[9]   Esener Z, Sarihasan B, Guven H, Ustun E. Thiopentone and etomidate concentrations in maternal and umbilical plasma, and in colostrum. Br J Anaesth 1992;69:586—8.

[10] Morgan DJ, Beamiss CG, Blackman GL, Paull JD. Urinary excretion of placentally transferred thiopentone by the human neonate. Dev Pharmacol Ther 1982;5:136—42.

[11] Hale TW. Anesthetic medications in breastfeeding mothers. J Hum Lactat 1999;15:185—94.

[12] Montgomery A, Hale TW, Academy of Breastfeeding Medicine Protocol Committee. ABM Clinical Protocol #15: analgesia and anesthesia for the breastfeeding mother. Breastfeed Med 2006;1:271—7.

[13] Dalal PG, Bosak J, Berlin CM. Safety of the breast-feeding infant after maternal anesthesia. Paediatr Anaesth 2014;24:359—71.

[14] Martin E, Vickers B, Landau R, Reece-Stremtan S, Academy of Breastfeeding Medicine. ABM clinical protocol #28. Peripart Analges Anaesthes Breastfeed Mother 2018;13:164—71.

[15] Beilin Y, Bodian CA, Weiser J, Hossain S, Arnold I, Feierman DE, et al. Effect of labor epidural analgesia with and without fentanyl on infant breast- feeding: a prospective, randomized, double-blind study. Anesthesiology 2005;103:1211—7.

[16] Wilson MJ, MacArthur C, Cooper GM, Bick D, Moore PA, Shennan A, et al. Epidural analgesia and breastfeeding: a randomised controlled trial of epidural techniques with and without fentanyl and a non-epidural comparison group. Anaesthesia 2010;65:145—53.

[17] Chang ZM, Heaman MI. Epidural analgesia during labor and delivery: effects on the initiation and continuation of effective breastfeeding. J Hum Lactat 2005;21:305—14.

[18] Rosen AR, Lawrence RA. The effect of epidural anesthesia on infant feeding. J Univ Roch Med Ctr 1994;6:3—7.

[19] Anderson PO. Herbal use during breastfeeding. Breastfeed Med 2017;12:507—9.

[20] Anderson PO, Valdes V. A critical review of pharmaceutical galactagogues. Breastfeed Med 2007;2:229—42.

[21] Posadzki P, Watson L, Ernst E. Contamination and adulteration of herbal medicinal products (HMPs): an overview of systemic reviews. Eur I Clin Pharmacol 2013;69:295—307.

[22] Academy of Breastfeeding Medicine Protocol Committee. ABM Clinical Protocol #9: use of galactogogues in initiating or augmenting maternal milk production. Breastfeed Med 2018;13:307—14 [second revision 2018].

[23] Feilberg VL, Rosenborg D, Broen Christensen C, Mogensen JV. Excretion of morphine in human breast milk. Acta Anaesthesiol Scand 1989;33:426—8.

[24] Koren G, Cairns J, Chitayat D, Gaedigk A, Leeder SJ. Pharmacogenetics of morphine poisoning in a breastfed neonate of a codeine-prescribed mother. Lancet 2006;368: 33–5.

[25] Madadi P, Ross CJD, Hayden MR, Carleton BC, Gaedigk A, Leeder SJ, et al. Pharmacogenetics of neonatal opioid toxicity following maternal use of codeine during breastfeeding: a case–control study. Clin Pharmacol Ther 2009;85:31–5.

[26] Al-Tamimi Y, Ilett KF, Paech MJ, O'Halloran SJ, Hartman PE. Estimation of infant dose and exposure to pethidine and norpethidine via breast milk following patient-controlled epidural pethidine for analgesia post caesarean delivery. Int J Obstet Anesth 2011;20:28–34.

[27] Wittels B, Scott DT, Sinatra RS. Exogenous opioids in human breast milk and acute neonatal neurobehavior: a preliminary study. Anesthesiology 1990;73:864–9.

[28] Wittels B, Glosten BT, Faure EA, Moawad AH, Ismail M, Hibbard J, et al. Postcesarean analgesia with both epidural morphine and intravenous patient-controlled analgesia: neurobehavioral outcomes among nursing neonates. Anesth Analg 1997;85:600–6.

[29] Hodgkinson R, Bhatt M, Wang CN. Double-blind comparison of the neurobehavior of neonates following the administration of different doses of meperidine to the mother. Can Anaesth Soc J 1978;25:405–41.

[30] Sauberan JB, Anderson PO, Lane JR, Rafie S, Nguyen N, Rossi SS, et al. Breast milk hydrocodone and hydromorphone levels in mothers using hydrocodone for postpartum pain. Obstet Gynecol 2011;117:611–7.

[31] Anderson PO, Sauberan JB, Lane JR, Rossi SS. Hydrocodone excretion into breast milk: the first two reported cases. Breastfeed Med 2007;2:10–4.

[32] Academy of Breastfeeding Medicine Protocol Committee. ABM Clinical Protocol #21: guidelines for breastfeeding and the drug-dependent woman. Breastfeed Med 2009;4: 225–8.

[33] Abdel-Latif ME, Pinner J, Clews S, Cooke F, Lui K, Oei J. Effects of breast milk on the severity and outcome of neonatal abstinence syndrome among infants of drug-dependent mothers. Pediatrics 2007;117:e1163–9.

[34] Jansson LM, Choo R, Harrow C, Velez M, Schroeder JR, Lowe R, et al. Methadone maintenance and long-term lactation. J Hum Lactat 2007;23:184–90.

[35] http://toxnet.nlm.nih.gov/cgi-bin/sis/search/f?/temp/~nMXQon:1 [methadone].

[36] Anderson PO, Pochop SL, Manoguerra AS. Adverse drug reactions in breastfed infants: less than imagined. Clin Pediatr 2003;42:325–40.

[37] Ito S, Blajchman A, Stephenson M, Eliopoulos C, Koren G. Prospective follow-up of adverse reactions in breastfed infants exposed to maternal medication. Am J Obstet Gynecol 1993;168:1393–9.

[38] LactMed (drugs and lactation database). http://toxnet.nlm.nih.gov/cgi-bin/sis/htmlgen? LACT.

[39] Nulman I, Rovet J, Stewart DE, Wolpin J, Pace-Asciak P, Shuhaiber S, et al. Child development following exposure to tricyclic antidepressants or fluoxetine throughout fetal life: a prospective, controlled study. Am J Psychiatr 2002;159:1889–95.

[40] Marcus SM. Depression during pregnancy: rates, risks, and consequences – motherisk update 2008. Can J Clin Pharmacol 2009;16:e15–22.

[41] Gavin NI, Gaynes BN, Lohr KN, Meltzer-Brody S, Gartlehner G, Swinson T. Perinatal depression: a systematic review of prevalence and incidence. Obstet Gynecol 2005;106: 1071–83.

[42] Davanzo R, Copertino M, De Cunto A, Minen F, Amaddeo A. Antidepressant drugs and breastfeeding: a review of the literature. Breastfeed Med 2011;6:89—98.

[43] Monk C, Fitelson EM, Werner E. Mood disorders and their pharmacological treatment during pregnancy: is the future child affected? Pediatr Res 2011;69:3R—10R.

[44] Moses-Kolko EL, Bogen D, Bregar A, Uhl K, Levin B, Wisner KL. Neonatal signs after late in utero exposure to serotonin reuptake inhibitors: literature review and implications for clinical applications. J Am Med Assoc 2005;293:2372—83.

[45] Atkinson H, Begg EJ. Concentrations of beta-blocking drugs in human milk. J Pediatr 1990;116:156.

[46] Viguera AC, Newport DJ, Ritchie J, Stowe Z, Whitfield T, Mogielnicki J, et al. Lithium in breast milk and nursing infants: clinical implications. Am J Psychiatr 2007;164: 342—5.

[47] http://toxnet.nlm.nih.gov/cgi-bin/sis/search/f?/temp/~r7lQ4W:1 [lithium].

[48] http://toxnet.nlm.nih.gov/cgi-bin/sis/search/f?/temp/~yGm4ch:1 [amiodarone].

[49] Basaria S, Cooper DS. Amiodarone and the thyroid. Am J Med 2005;118:706—14.

[50] McKenna WJ, Harris L, Rowland E, Storey G, Holt D. Amiodarone therapy during pregnancy. Am J Cardiol 1983;51:1231—3.

[51] Krashin JW, Lemani C, Nkambule J, Talama G, Chiunula L, Flax VL, Stuebe AM, Tang JH. A comparison of breastfeeding exclusivity and duration rates between immediate postpartum levonorgestrel versus etonogestrel implant users: a prospective cohort study. Breastfeed Med 2019;14:69—76.

[52] Academy of Breastfeeding Medicine Protocol Committee. ABM Clinical Protocol #13: contraception during breastfeeding. Breastfeed Med 2006;1:43—50.

[53] Labbok MH, Hight-Laukaran V, Peterson AE, Fletcher V, von Hertzen H, Van Look PFA. Multicultural study of the lactational amenorrhea method (LAM): I. efficacy, duration, and implications for clinical application. Contraception 1997;55: 327—36.

[54] Krause ML, Amin S, Makol A. Use of DMARDS and biologics during pregnancy and lactation in rheumatoid arthritis: what the rheumatologist needs to know. Ther Adv Musculoskelet Dis 2014;6:169—84.

[55] Witzel SJ. Lactation and the use of biologic immunosuppressive medications. Breastfeed Med 2014:543—6.

[56] Wang GS. Pediatric concerns due to expanded cannabis use: unintended consequences of legalization. J Med Toxicol 2017;13:99—105.

[57] Sharma P, Murthy P, Bharath MMS. Chemistry, metabolism and toxicology of cannabis: clinical implications. Iran J Psychiatry 2012;7:149—56.

[58] Atakan Z. Cannabis: a complex plant: different compounds and different effects on individuals. Ther Adv Psychopharmacol 2012;2:241—54. https://doi.org/10.1177/2045125312457586.

[59] Ryan S. A modern conundrum for the paediatrician: the safety of breast milk and the cannabis-using mother. Pediatrics 2018;142:21—2. e20181921.

[60] Ryan SA, Ammerman SD, O'Connor ME. Committee of Substance Use and Prevention, Section on Breastfeeding. Marijuana use during pregnancy and breastfeeding: implications for neonatal and childhood outcomes. Pediatrics 2018;142:117—31. e20181889.

[61] Bertrand KA, Hanan NJ, Honerkamp-Smith G, Best BM, Chambers CD. Marijuana use by breastfeeding mothers and cannabinoid concentrations in breast milk. Pediatrics 2018;142:1—8. e20181076.

[62] Mourh J, Rowe H. Marijuana and breastfeeding: applicability of the current literature to clinical practice. Breastfeed Med 2017;12:582–96.

[63] Anderson PO. Cannabis and breastfeeding. Breastfeed Med 2017;12:580–1.

[64] Berlin Jr CM, Paul IM, Vesell ES. Safety issues of maternal drug therapy during breastfeeding. Clin Pharmacol Ther 2009;85:20–2.

[65] Briggs GG, Freeman RK, Yaffe SJ. Drugs in pregnancy and lactation. 9th ed. Philadelphia: Wolters Kluwer/Lippincott Williams & Wilkins; 2011.

[66] Sahin L, Nallani SC, Tassinari MS. Medical Use in pregnancy and the pregnancy and lactation labeling rule. Clin Pharmacol Ther 2016;100:23–5.

[67] Anderson PO. Medication information sources for breastfeeding mothers. Breastfeed Med 2017;12:396–7.

Fetal drug therapy

5

Erik Rytting[1], Jennifer Waltz[2], Mahmoud S. Ahmed[1]

[1]*Department of Obstetrics & Gynecology, University of Texas Medical Branch, Galveston, TX, United States;* [2]*School of Medicine, University of Texas Medical Branch, Galveston, TX, United States*

5.1 Introduction

The intention of most drugs prescribed during pregnancy is to treat a condition affecting maternal health. Careful attention is placed on the appropriate selection of the medication and its dose that would reduce transplacental drug transport and minimize consequences of fetal drug exposure. However, this chapter will focus on the administration of drugs intended to treat medical conditions afflicting the fetus, rather than the mother. In order to achieve therapeutic drug concentrations in the fetus, efforts are made to circumvent the placenta's function as a barrier. In this case, it is imperative to reduce maternal exposure to a medication that she does not need and consequently might adversely affect her well-being.

The first section of this chapter will discuss a number of medical indications for which fetal drug therapy might be warranted. As the focus is on pharmacological therapy, the reader is referred to other sources for details regarding fetal medical interventions such as prenatal repair of myelomeningocele [1], blood transfusions to treat fetal anemia [2], and others [3].

The second part of this chapter will describe strategies for fetal drug delivery, including transplacental transfer following maternal administration, direct fetal injection, gene therapy, stem cell transplantation, and nanomedicine. This chapter will conclude with a brief discussion of the ethics associated with this challenging subject (see also Chapter 8 which discusses the ethics of clinical pharmacology in pregnancy).

5.2 Indications for fetal therapy

Table 5.1 lists some common indications for fetal therapy and details regarding these conditions are provided below (see also Table 5.2). Nevertheless, as this table is not comprehensive, this section will identify a number of additional settings where fetal drug therapy may be beneficial.

Clinical Pharmacology During Pregnancy. https://doi.org/10.1016/B978-0-12-818902-3.00007-5

Table 5.1 Examples of indications for fetal drug therapy and medications used.

Indication for fetal drug therapy	Medications
Cardiac arrhythmias	Digoxin, flecainide, and sotalol
Endocrinological disorders	
Congenital adrenal hyperplasia	Dexamethasone
Fetal thyroid disorders	Levothyroxine
Hematological disorders	
Alloimmune thrombocytopenia	Gamma globulin
Erythrocyte alloimmunization	anti-D immunoglobulin
Lung maturation	Dexamethasone, betamethasone
Neuroprotection	Magnesium sulfate

Please note that this is not a comprehensive list of indications or medications.

Table 5.2 Pharmacokinetic considerations for some medications used in fetal drug therapy (see Table 5.1).

Drug	Typical dosing	Notes	References
Digoxin	0.5 mg bid for 2 days, then 0.25–0.75 mg/day	Therapeutic concentration 1.0–2.5 ng/mL; fetal/maternal ratio: 0.3–1.3; hydrops reduces placental transfer; and substrate for P-glycoprotein	[4–12]
Flecainide	100 mg tid or qid	Therapeutic concentration 0.2–1.0 µg/mL; fetal/maternal ratio: 0.5–1.0; and crosses placenta even in the presence of hydrops	[4,11,13–17]
Sotalol	80–160 mg bid or tid	Therapeutic concentration 2–7 µg/mL (atrial flutter); fetal/maternal ratio 1.0 ± 0.5	[4,16,18–25]
Dexamethasone (for lung maturation)	6 mg, four intramuscular doses, 12 h apart	Fetal/maternal ratio ranged from 0.20 (50 min after dose) to 0.44 (after 265 min); a fraction is metabolized in the placenta to the inactive 11-ketosteroid	[26–30]

Table 5.2 Pharmacokinetic considerations for some medications used in fetal drug therapy (see Table 5.1).—*cont'd*

Drug	Typical dosing	Notes	References
Betamethasone	12 mg, two intramuscular doses, 24 h apart	Fetal/maternal ratio: 0.28 ± 0.04; a fraction is metabolized in the placenta to the inactive 11-ketosteroid	[31—35]
Levothyroxine	Case studies report intraamniotic doses ranging from 50 to 800 μg (median dose 250 μg), every 1 —4 weeks	Concurrent dose reduction of maternal antithyroid drugs may be necessary; it may be advisable to start with a low dose (150 μg), then increase if necessary; and cordocentesis should be limited	[36—40]
Gamma globulin	1—2 g/kg/week i.v., depending on risk	Prednisone is often used in combination	[41]
Anti-D immunoglobulin	1500 IU as a single intramuscular injection at 28 weeks of gestation	A two-dose regimen consisting of either 500 or 1250 IU each at 28 and 34 weeks may be more effective in maintaining sufficient anti-D levels at term	[42—44]
Dexamethasone (for congenital adrenal hyperplasia)	20 μg/kg/day based on prepregnancy body weight, divided in three doses	See notes on dexamethasone above	[45]
Magnesium sulfate	4 g over 20 min, then 1 g/h for a maximum of 24 h	Fetal/maternal ratio: 0.94 ± 0.15; maternal and fetal concentrations are dependent on maternal BMI	[46—48]

Among the most common pharmacological interventions for fetal therapy is the administration of antenatal corticosteroids in anticipation of preterm delivery to promote *fetal lung maturation*. Dexamethasone and betamethasone are the most common drugs prescribed for this purpose and have demonstrated clinically significant reductions in respiratory distress syndrome, neonatal mortality, cerebroventricular hemorrhage, necrotizing enterocolitis, intensive care admission, and systemic infections in the first 48 h of life [49,50].

Magnesium sulfate is commonly used in obstetric practice for seizure prophylaxis in preeclampsia, but growing evidence supports its role of *neuroprotection* in low birth weight children [46]. Randomized placebo-controlled trials of antenatal administration of magnesium sulfate have consistently demonstrated a decreased risk of cerebral palsy and severe motor dysfunction in preterm infants [51–53]. Long-term cognitive, behavioral, growth, and functional advantages were not observed at school age [54].

Fetal cardiac arrhythmias affect at least 2% of low-risk pregnancies and as much as 16.6% of high-risk pregnancies [55,56]. Although intermittent extrasystoles can be common and may not require treatment, sustained fetal arrhythmias demand vigorous attention because this can lead to hydrops within 48 h, a condition with poor prognosis [57–60]. Hydrops can impair transplacental transport, thereby necessitating fetal injection of a medication [60]. The most common fetal arrhythmias are supraventricular tachycardia, atrial flutter, and severe bradyarrhythmia associated with complete heart block [58]. Drugs used to treat fetal tachycardia include digoxin, flecainide, sotalol, procainamide, propranolol, amiodarone, and adenosine; questions remain regarding the use of steroids and sympathomimetics for bradycardia caused by heart block [58]. Attentive monitoring of response to most antiarrhythmic drugs is needed due to narrow therapeutic margins, and certain drug–drug interactions, as in the case of verapamil and digoxin, could lead to significant maternal toxicity and even fetal death [61,62]. Maternal side effects to fetal antiarrhythmic therapy include palpitations, second-degree atrioventricular block, Wenckebach phenomenon, and hypotension [61].

Congenital adrenal hyperplasia is most often due to a 21-hydroxylase deficiency (CYP21A2) [59]. Decreased cortisol production results in excess androgen synthesis, which causes virilization of female genitalia. In the future, genetic testing could play a stronger role in the prenatal counseling of this condition, as the extent of virilization may be linked to fetal genotype [63]. *In utero* treatment with dexamethasone reduces the abnormal levels of androgens, and this therapy prevents the devastating consequences of wrong sex assignment in affected females. Differentiation of external genitalia occurs between 7 and 12 weeks of gestation, so therapy in at-risk pregnancies must begin earlier, preferably by the fifth week [45]. Cell-free DNA testing can provide noninvasive determination of fetal sex at as early as 5 weeks of gestation, thereby enabling rapid discontinuation of dexamethasone for male fetuses [64,65]. Chorionic villus sampling (CVS) can be performed at 10–12 weeks, at which point therapy can be halted for unaffected females [45]. Dexamethasone treatment (three times daily) will continue throughout pregnancy for an affected female fetus. Maternal side effects of fetal dexamethasone therapy include edema, striae, excess weight gain, Cushingoid facial features, facial hair, glucose intolerance, hypertension, gastrointestinal problems, and emotional irritability [45,59,66].

Congenital hypothyroidism, which affects approximately 1 out of every 4500 pregnancies, is usually a secondary condition caused by treatment of maternal hyperthyroidism, such as Graves' disease [59]. Fetal goiter can interfere with fetal swallowing and lead to polyhydramnios and premature rupture of membranes. Furthermore, fetal goiter can cause tracheal compression and asphyxia at birth

[36,59]. Fetal hypothyroidism can be successfully treated with levothyroxine. Levothyroxine is administered via intraamniotic injection due to its low transplacental transfer [36,59].

Fetal hematological disorders that can be treated include alloimmune thrombocytopenia and erythrocyte alloimmunization. *Fetal and neonatal alloimmune thrombocytopenia* (FNAIT) has an incidence rate of 1 in 1500 and is caused by a maternal antibody-mediated response against a fetal platelet—specific antigen; this may lead to in utero intracranial hemorrhage [67]. Women at risk for a pregnancy with FNAIT are usually only identified after having a previous child with the disorder, but maternal administration of intravenous gamma globulin can successfully increase fetal platelet counts [59,67]. *Erythrocyte alloimmunization*—the reaction of maternal antibodies with fetal erythrocyte antigens—can lead to hemolysis, fetal anemia, and hydrops fetalis [59]. Antepartum anti-D immunoglobulin given to Rh-negative women carrying an Rh-positive fetus reduced the incidence of Rh immunization during pregnancy from 1.8 to 0.14% [68]. Intravenous immunoglobulin treatment in pregnant women with a fetus at risk for hemolytic disease may lower the demand for intrauterine transfusions [69]. It should be noted that there are other types of red-cell alloimmunization besides anti-RhD without prophylactic immune globulins yet available [70].

In addition to the aforementioned indications, there are a number of fetal conditions for which experimental therapeutics are in various stages of testing. *Polyhydramnios* (excess amniotic fluid) affects approximately 1% of pregnancies, of which 55% are idiopathic and 25% are related to fetal diabetes [57,71]. Amnioreduction and betamethasone are used in the management of severe polyhydramnios [72]. Although indomethacin likely decreases fetal urine production in mothers with severe refractory symptoms, it is not recommended for reducing amniotic fluid because of its associated neonatal risks [72,73]. Randomized controlled trials are essential to evaluate the safety and efficacy of novel treatments. For example, preliminary studies had suggested some advantages of sildenafil as an option for *intrauterine growth restriction* [74], but larger trials failed to show improved outcomes and the studies were terminated early due to increased mortality in the treatment arm [75]. On the other hand, it is clear that smoking cessation lowers rates of low birth weight and preterm birth [76]. Injection of picibanil into the pleural cavity for pleurodesis appears promising for the treatment of early second trimester, non-hydropic *fetal chylothorax* [77,78]. Digoxin and furosemide have been injected into fetal intravascular space to treat idiopathic *nonimmune hydrops fetalis* [79], and infection-induced nonimmune hydrops fetalis has been treated with transplacental antiviral or antibiotic therapy [80]. *Fetal malignancies* are rarely diagnosed in utero [81], but this may represent a future area of potential fetal chemotherapy. There are also several examples of maternal prescriptions with direct or indirect fetal benefit, including tocolytics preventing preterm birth, penicillin to treat syphilis [57], spiramycin for toxoplasmosis [57], antibiotics before delivery to reduce neonatal sepsis [82], and the reduction of maternal—fetal HIV transmission rates by the use of highly active antiretroviral therapy [83].

5.3 Strategies to achieve fetal drug therapy

5.3.1 Transplacental drug transfer

Many medications intended for the fetus are administered to the mother, with a portion of the dose crossing the placenta and reaching the fetal circulation. Although this method of drug delivery can cause maternal side effects, it is often preferred over the invasiveness and risks associated with direct fetal injection. To understand this process, it is important to provide a brief introduction to the role of human placenta as a functional barrier (see Fig. 5.1).

Human placenta is a tissue of fetal origin localized at the interface between the maternal and fetal circulations. During gestation, placental functions include those of several organs in the newborn/adult. For example, the placenta is responsible for exchange of gases, uptake of nutrients from the maternal circulation, elimination of waste products, and the biosynthesis of specific hormones (steroids and proteins) that regulate autocrine and/or paracrine functions. Taken together, placental functions begin by ensuring implantation, supporting normal fetal organogenesis and development, and maintaining a healthy pregnancy until parturition.

In the early 20th century, the human placenta had been viewed as a barrier similar to the blood—brain barrier but with the role to "protect" the fetus from exposure to xenobiotics and environmental toxins. The thalidomide-induced birth defects of the 1960s shattered that concept and provided evidence for differences in transplacental transfer of compounds between placentas of human and other mammals. Currently, it is assumed that small molecules (<1000 Da, which includes most current medications) can freely cross the placenta between the maternal and fetal circulations by simple diffusion. However, the bidirectional transfer of compounds between the maternal and fetal circulations across the placenta by simple diffusion does not preclude the simultaneous involvement of two other transport processes, namely facilitated diffusion and active transport [91,92]. Endocytosis is another transport mechanism relevant to fetal drug therapy with the use of drug-loaded nanoparticles designed to alter the transplacental passage of therapeutics [93].

The transfer of a drug by both facilitated diffusion and active transport is mediated by proteins that are usually selective for a particular compound or group of compounds. Facilitated diffusion does not require metabolic energy because the transfer of the compound occurs down a concentration gradient until steady state equilibrium is reached. Active transport is unidirectional, requires metabolic energy, and can transport compounds against a concentration gradient. For example, uptake transporters in the apical membrane are responsible for the transfer of many nutrients from the maternal to fetal circulation [94]. On the other hand, efflux transporters (such as P-glycoprotein, breast cancer resistance protein, and multidrug resistance—associated proteins) are responsible for the extrusion of compounds from the fetal to maternal circulation [95]. Efflux transporters are crucial for decreasing fetal exposure to xenobiotics and each one of them is responsible for the extrusion of a diverse number of drugs. For example, dexamethasone and digoxin, two of the medications listed in Table 5.2, are both susceptible to reduced passage due to P-glycoprotein [93,96].

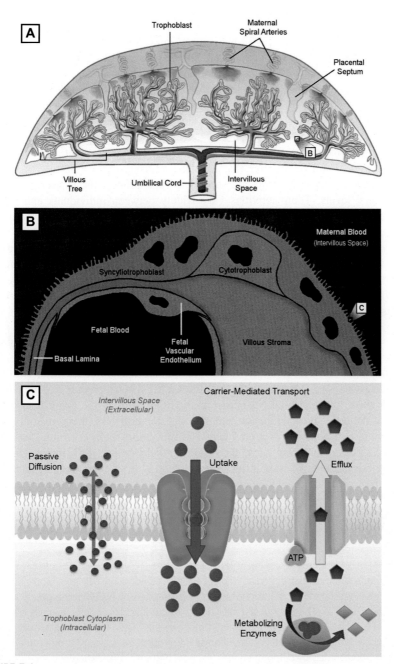

FIGURE 5.1

Mechanisms of maternal–fetal transfer: (A) Overview of human placental morphology showing fetal vessels from the umbilical cord branching into villous trees, which are bathed by maternal blood entering the placenta via spiral arteries. Trophoblast cells on the surface of the villous structures separate the maternal blood in the intervillous space from

Several trophoblast tissue metabolic enzymes are responsible for placental biotransformation of drugs [97,98]. Placental enzymes are occasionally identical to those in the liver, but in most cases, their activity is $\leq 10\%$ of the hepatic enzymes. One placental enzyme, CYP19/aromatase, has a role in steroidogenesis, but is also involved in the placental biotransformation of xenobiotics [98], thus catalyzing reactions which are usually performed by other hepatic enzymes that have not been identified in the placenta, or do not have detectable activity (e.g., CYP3A4) [99,100].

Thus, placental metabolic enzymes and efflux transporters define the human placenta as a functional barrier that regulates transplacental transport of drugs. The activities of these proteins are subject to regulation at the transcription and translational levels. Their activities vary widely between individuals and in the same individual with gestational age [101—104]. In terms of maximizing the transplacental transfer of maternally administered medications intended for fetal drug therapy, substrates of uptake transporters are more likely to reach therapeutic levels in the fetal circulation. Drugs which are substrates for efflux transporters and/or metabolizing enzymes, on the other hand, are more likely to result in maternal side effects, as higher doses will be necessary to reach therapeutic drug levels in the fetal circulation.

5.3.2 Direct fetal injection

Ultrasound-guided injections can be introduced into the umbilical cord, amniotic fluid, intravenously, or into specific fetal tissues [2]. This approach may be advantageous when transplacental transfer is limited due to hydropic conditions or the chemical nature of the therapeutic agent [2,49]. Nevertheless, there are important disadvantages to consider. Not only can fetal movement make the initial injection challenging but it may also cause the needle to dislodge [82,105]. In one extreme example of an attempted fetal intracardiac injection, the needle overshot its target, passed through to the other side of the fetal heart, and resulted in a severe adverse effect for the mother [106]. The weighted procedure-related risk of fetal loss by CVS or amniocentesis is 0.2%—0.3% [107]. Repeated injections will increase the risks of infection or death [2,49].

the fetal circulation, as highlighted in (B). (B) Cellular components of a placental villus, wherein multinucleated syncytiotrophoblast cells are formed by fusion of the precursor cytotrophoblast cells. The trophoblast cells and the fetal vascular endothelial cells are separated by basal lamina. Several transport mechanisms within the trophoblast cell layer are highlighted in (C). (C) Transport mechanisms in trophoblast cells, with different molecules represented by different shapes. Passive diffusion is governed by the concentration gradient of any compound (xenobiotic or intermediary metabolite). Two types of carrier-mediated transport (uptake and efflux) involve transport proteins that span the phospholipid bilayer of the cell membrane. The biotransformation of molecules by metabolizing enzymes is also represented [84—90].

5.3.3 **Gene therapy**

Fetal gene therapy has the potential to benefit severe genetic diseases that lack effective postnatal therapy, including cystic fibrosis, hemophilia, thalassemia, and others [108]. The fetal period may present a unique window of opportunity for gene therapy. Access to an expanding population of stem cells, a higher vector to target cell ratio, the comparative immaturity of the immune system, and the possible induction of immune tolerance in the fetus are all considered advantages to initiating gene therapy during this period [109,110]. Nevertheless, current utility is hampered by the selection of an appropriate vector and a series of unknown risks, such as increased chance of fetal loss upon injection during the first trimester, induction of preterm labor, infection, immune reaction, interference with normal fetal development, insertional mutagenesis, germline integration, and the chance that maternal harm may affect future pregnancies [109,110].

5.3.4 **Stem cell transplantation**

Diseases where in utero stem cell transplantation might prove beneficial include hemoglobinopathies, immunodeficiencies, and inborn errors of metabolism [111]. As proposed for gene therapy, it has been anticipated that a naive fetal immune system would readily accept stem cell transplantation, but to date, such therapy has only been realized in fetuses with immunodeficiencies that might facilitate engraftment [111,112]. The most common sources of stem cells include maternal bone marrow, paternal bone marrow, fetal liver, and amniotic fluid [112,113]. An advantage of using stem cells from amniotic fluid is eliminating the need for a donor source. Intraperitoneal injection of transduced amniotic fluid stem cells appears to be a promising strategy [113,114]. Another strategy gaining attention is generating immune tolerance through fetal stem cell transplantation, followed by repeated postnatal transplantation to achieve phenotypic correction [115].

5.3.5 **Nanoparticles**

Nanoparticles present a number of advantages for drug delivery, including sustained drug release promoting reduced dosing frequency and improved patient compliance, the potential for efficient drug targeting by passive and/or active targeting approaches, protection of therapeutic payload, and improved bioavailability for certain compounds. Besides traditional small-molecule drugs, nanoparticles can also be used to deliver peptides, proteins, genes, siRNA, and vaccines [116]. Examples of nanoparticles developed for drug delivery include liposomes, solid lipid nanoparticles, polymeric nanoparticles, polymeric micelles, and dendrimers. Multifunctional nanoparticles—combining drug delivery and biomedical diagnostic imaging—may have the potential to evaluate toxicity during fetal development in real time, but as yet have not been fully realized [117]. Targeted nanoparticle-based drug delivery systems offer the potential to increase the amount of drug reaching the fetus, thereby reducing the side effects associated with unnecessary maternal drug exposure. *Ex vivo* dual perfusion of the term human placental lobule is a representative model of in vivo placental transport and metabolism. To date, this model has been used with a few sets of nanoparticles to elucidate the effects of particle composition, size, and charge on the placental transfer of nanoparticles [118−121]. These studies have shown that particle size is not the only determinant for transfer. This should not be surprising because macromolecules such as IgG and vitamin B12 can cross the placenta by carrier-mediated mechanisms, but the transport of other macromolecules such as heparin is negligible [120,122]. Some nanoparticles for fetal therapy may take advantage of receptors in the placenta, such as megalin, for receptor-mediated cellular entry [123]. Nanotoxicology is a significant area of research in order to ensure improved drug delivery without adverse effects to the fetus or mother [124,125].

5.4 Special considerations

Maternal drug therapy during pregnancy requires balancing maternal benefit versus fetal risk, and in the case of drug therapy intended for the fetus, we must weigh maternal risks against potential fetal benefits. Despite the potential of a fetal medication causing maternal side effects, transplacental delivery is often preferred to avoid the risks associated with fetal injections.

Although it is anticipated that targeted therapies would require lower doses and potentially lessen the resultant maternal side effects, the appropriate dose will need to be identified. Fetal drug therapy is associated with different pharmacokinetics than would be expected in adults or children. Compared to an adult, the fetus has more extracellular water, less fat, less metabolic enzyme activity, a lower renal secretion rate, less gastrointestinal absorption, and the fetal brain receives a higher percentage of cardiac output [2,61]. Furthermore, drug elimination is altered due to amniotic recycling [2].

5.5 Ethical considerations

Finally, the ethics of fetal drug therapy must be considered. Depending on gestational age, lung maturity, the availability of neonatal facilities, and maternal preference, in some instances, early delivery may be seen as an alternative to fetal therapies carrying high risk [58]. The risks and potential benefits of each disease are unique, and the recommendations of Moaddah et al. serve as excellent guidelines [126]. It is important that the mother can give informed consent, meaning that she understands all the possible outcomes of each intervention. Protocols for fetal drug therapy must be approved by a research ethics committee. Invasive therapy must have a high probability of saving life or preventing disease; risks to fetal health must be minimized; and risks to maternal health must be negligible. Alongside the mother's right to consent is her right to refuse, and supportive counseling should be made available to the family [126]. As if pregnancy and childbirth were not challenging enough, it is inspiring to see the sacrifices of pregnant women participating in clinical trials, enduring undeserved side effects, and undergoing invasive procedures in order to offer their children more hope for a better future.

Acknowledgments

The authors wish to thank Sanaalarab Al-Enazy for her assistance with Fig. 5.1 and Wayne Snodgrass for helpful suggestions. E.R. and M.S.A. are grateful for research support from NIH grants HD083003 and HD047891.

References

[1] Adzick NS, Thom EA, Spong CY, Brock JW, Burrows PK, Johnson MP, et al. A randomized trial of prenatal versus postnatal repair of myelomeningocele. N Engl J Med 2011;364:993−1004.

[2] Miller RK. Fetal drug therapy: principles and issues. Clin Obstet Gynecol 1991;34: 241−50.

[3] Kohl T. Minimally invasive fetoscopic interventions: an overview in 2010. Surg Endosc 2010;24:2056−67.

[4] Jaeggi E, Tulzer G. Pharmacological and interventional fetal cardiovascular treatment. Paediatr Cardiol 2010:199−218.

[5] Nagashima M, Asai T, Suzuki C, Matsushima M, Ogawa A. Intrauterine supraventricular tachyarrhythmias and transplacental digitalisation. Arch Dis Child 1986;61: 996−1000.

[6] Azancot-Benisty A, Jacqz-Aigrain E, Guirgis NM, Decrepy A, Oury JF, Blot P. Clinical and pharmacologic study of fetal supraventricular tachyarrhythmias. J Pediatr 1992;121:608−13.

[7] Younis JS, Granat M. Insufficient transplacental digoxin transfer in severe hydrops fetalis. Am J Obstet Gynecol 1987;157:1268−9.

[8] Weiner CP, Thompson MI. Direct treatment of fetal supraventricular tachycardia after failed transplacental therapy. Am J Obstet Gynecol 1988;158:570−3.

[9] Wiggins Jr JW, Bowes W, Clewell W, Manco-Johnson M, Manchester D, Johnson R, et al. Echocardiographic diagnosis and intravenous digoxin management of fetal tachyarrhythmias and congestive heart failure. Am J Dis Child 1986;140:202−4.

[10] Spinnato JA, Shaver DC, Flinn GS, Sibai BM, Watson DL, Marin-Garcia J. Fetal supraventricular tachycardia: in utero therapy with digoxin and quinidine. Obstet Gynecol 1984;64:730−5.

[11] Kofinas AD, Simon NV, Sagel H, Lyttle E, Smith N, King K. Treatment of fetal supraventricular tachycardia with flecainide acetate after digoxin failure. Am J Obstet Gynecol 1991;165:630−1.

[12] Hunter J, Hirst BH. Intestinal secretion of drugs. The role of P-glycoprotein and related drug efflux systems in limiting oral drug absorption. Adv Drug Deliv Rev 1997;25: 129−57.

[13] Amano K, Harada Y, Shoda T, Nishijima M, Hiraishi S. Successful treatment of supraventricular tachycardia with flecainide acetate: a case report. Fetal Diagn Ther 1997; 12:328−31.

[14] Palmer CM, Norris MC. Placental transfer of flecainide. Am J Dis Child 1990;144:144.

[15] Barjot P, Hamel P, Calmelet P, Maragnes P, Herlicoviez M. Flecainide against fetal supraventricular tachycardia complicated by hydrops fetalis. Acta Obstet Gynecol Scand 1998;77:353−8.

[16] Wagner X, Jouglard J, Moulin M, Miller AM, Petitjean J, Pisapia A. Coadministration of flecainide acetate and sotalol during pregnancy: lack of teratogenic effects, passage across the placenta, and excretion in human breast milk. Am Heart J 1990;119:700−2.

[17] Bourget P, Pons JC, Delouis C, Fermont L, Frydman R. Flecainide distribution, transplacental passage, and accumulation in the amniotic fluid during the third trimester of pregnancy. Ann Pharmacother 1994;28:1031−4.

[18] O'Hare MF, Murnaghan GA, Russell CJ, Leahey WJ, Varma MP, McDevitt DG. Sotalol as a hypotensive agent in pregnancy. Br J Obstet Gynaecol 1980;87:814−20.

[19] Erkkola R, Lammintausta R, Liukko P, Anttila M. Transfer of propranolol and sotalol across the human placenta. Their effect on maternal and fetal plasma renin activity. Acta Obstet Gynecol Scand 1982;61:31−4.

[20] Hackett LP, Wojnar-Horton RE, Dusci LJ, Ilett KF, Roberts MJ. Excretion of sotalol in breast milk. Br J Clin Pharmacol 1990;29:277−8.

[21] Darwiche A, Vanlieferinghen P, Lemery D, Paire M, Lusson JR. Amiodarone and fetal supraventricular tachycardia. Apropos of a case with neonatal hypothyroidism. Arch Fr Pediatr 1992;49:729−31.

[22] Oudijk MA, Ruskamp JM, Ververs FF, Ambachtsheer EB, Stoutenbeek P, Visser GH, et al. Treatment of fetal tachycardia with sotalol: transplacental pharmacokinetics and pharmacodynamics. J Am Coll Cardiol 2003;42:765−70.

[23] Lisowski LA, Verheijen PM, Benatar AA, Soyeur DJ, Stoutenbeek P, Brenner JI, et al. Atrial flutter in the perinatal age group: diagnosis, management and outcome. J Am Coll Cardiol 2000;35:771−7.

[24] Oudijk MA, Michon MM, Kleinman CS, Kapusta L, Stoutenbeek P, Visser GH, et al. Sotalol in the treatment of fetal dysrhythmias. Circulation 2000;101:2721−6.

[25] Oudijk MA, Ruskamp JM, Ambachtsheer BE, Ververs TF, Stoutenbeek P, Visser GH, et al. Drug treatment of fetal tachycardias. Paediatr Drugs 2002;4:49−63.

[26] Ballard PL, Ballard RA. Scientific basis and therapeutic regimens for use of antenatal glucocorticoids. Am J Obstet Gynecol 1995;173:254−62.

[27] Tsuei SE, Petersen MC, Ashley JJ, McBride WG, Moore RG. Disporition of synthetic glucocorticoids. II. Dexamethasone in parturient women. Clin Pharmacol Ther 1980; 28:88−98.

[28] Levitz M, Jansen V, Dancis J. The transfer and metabolism of corticosteroids in the perfused human placenta. Am J Obstet Gynecol 1978;132:363−6.

[29] Dancis J, Jansen V, Levitz M. Placental transfer of steroids: effect of binding to serum albumin and to placenta. Am J Physiol 1980;238:E208−13.

[30] Smith MA, Thomford PJ, Mattison DR, Slikker Jr W. Transport and metabolism of dexamethasone in the dually perfused human placenta. Reprod Toxicol 1988;2:37−43.

[31] Della Torre M, Hibbard JU, Jeong H, Fischer JH. Betamethasone in pregnancy: influence of maternal body weight and multiple gestation on pharmacokinetics. Am J Obstet Gynecol 2010;203. 254e1—12.

[32] Petersen MC, Nation RL, Ashley JJ, McBride WG. The placental transfer of betamethasone. Eur J Clin Pharmacol 1980;18:245—7.

[33] Anderson AB, Gennser G, Jeremy JY, Ohrlander S, Sayers L, Turnbull AC. Placental transfer and metabolism of betamethasone in human pregnancy. Obstet Gynecol 1977; 49:471—4.

[34] Stark MJ, Wright IM, Clifton VL. Sex-specific alterations in placental 11beta-hydroxysteroid dehydrogenase 2 activity and early postnatal clinical course following antenatal betamethasone. Am J Physiol Regul Integr Comp Physiol 2009;297: R510—4.

[35] Murphy VE, Fittock RJ, Zarzycki PK, Delahunty MM, Smith R, Clifton VL. Metabolism of synthetic steroids by the human placenta. Placenta 2007;28:39—46.

[36] Bliddal S, Rasmussen ÅK, Sundberg K, Brocks V, Skovbo P, Feldt-Rasmussen U. Graves' disease in two pregnancies complicated by fetal goitrous hypothyroidism: successful in utero treatment with levothyroxine. Thyroid 2011;21:75—81.

[37] Stoppa-Vaucher S, Van Vliet G, Deladoëy J. Discovery of a fetal goiter on prenatal ultrasound in women treated for Graves' disease: first, do no harm. Thyroid 2011;21:931.

[38] Hashimoto H, Hashimoto K, Suehara N. Successful in utero treatment of fetal goitrous hypothyroidism: case report and review of the literature. Fetal Diagn Ther 2006;21: 360—5.

[39] Miyata I, Abe-Gotyo N, Tajima A, Yoshikawa H, Teramoto S, Seo M, et al. Successful intrauterine therapy for fetal goitrous hypothyroidism during late gestation. Endocr J 2007;54:813—7.

[40] Ribault V, Castanet M, Bertrand AM, Guibourdenche J, Vuillard E, Luton D, et al. Experience with intraamniotic thyroxine treatment in nonimmune fetal goitrous hypothyroidism in 12 cases. J Clin Endocrinol Metab 2009;94:3731—9.

[41] Bussel JB, Berkowitz RL, Hung C, Kolb EA, Wissert M, Primiani A, et al. Intracranial hemorrhage in alloimmune thrombocytopenia: stratified management to prevent recurrence in the subsequent affected fetus. Am J Obstet Gynecol 2010;203. 135e1—14.

[42] Moise Jr KJ. Management of rhesus alloimmunization in pregnancy. Obstet Gynecol 2008;112:164—76.

[43] Davies J, Chant R, Simpson S, Powell R. Routine antenatal anti-D prophylaxis–is the protection adequate? Transfus Med 2011;21:421—6.

[44] Turner RM, Lloyd-Jones M, Anumba DO, Smith GC, Spiegelhalter DJ, Squires H, et al. Routine antenatal anti-D prophylaxis in women who are Rh(D) negative: meta-analyses adjusted for differences in study design and quality. PLoS One 2012; 7:e30711.

[45] Nimkarn S, New MI. Congenital adrenal hyperplasia due to 21-hydroxylase deficiency: a paradigm for prenatal diagnosis and treatment. Ann N Y Acad Sci 2010; 1192:5—11.

[46] Pryde PG, Mittendorf R. Contemporary usage of obstetric magnesium sulfate: indication, contraindication, and relevance of dose. Obstet Gynecol 2009;114:669—73.

[47] Brookfield KF, Su F, Elkomy MH, Drover DR, Lyell DJ, Carvalho B. Pharmacokinetics and placental transfer of magnesium sulfate in pregnant women. Am J Obstet Gynecol 2016;214. 737e1—9.

[48] Vilchez G, Dai J, Lagos M, Sokol RJ. Maternal side effects & fetal neuroprotection according to body mass index after magnesium sulfate in a multicenter randomized controlled trial. J Matern Fetal Neonatal Med 2018;31:178−83.

[49] Evans MI, Pryde PG, Reichler A, Bardicef M, Johnson MP. Fetal drug therapy. West J Med 1993;159:325−32.

[50] Roberts D, Brown J, Medley N, Dalziel SR. Antenatal corticosteroids for accelerating fetal lung maturation for women at risk of preterm birth. Cochrane Database Syst Rev 2017;3:Cd004454.

[51] Crowther CA, Hiller JE, Doyle LW, Haslam RR. Effect of magnesium sulfate given for neuroprotection before preterm birth: a randomized controlled trial. JAMA 2003;290:2669−76.

[52] Rouse DJ, Hirtz DG, Thom E, Varner MW, Spong CY, Mercer BM, et al. A randomized, controlled trial of magnesium sulfate for the prevention of cerebral palsy. N Engl J Med 2008;359:895−905.

[53] Marret S, Marpeau L, Zupan-Simunek V, Eurin D, Lévêque C, Hellot MF, et al. Magnesium sulphate given before very-preterm birth to protect infant brain: the randomised controlled PREMAG trial. BJOG 2007;114:310−8.

[54] Doyle LW, Anderson PJ, Haslam R, Lee KJ, Crowther C. School-age outcomes of very preterm infants after antenatal treatment with magnesium sulfate vs placebo. JAMA 2014;312:1105−13.

[55] Weber R, Stambach D, Jaeggi E. Diagnosis and management of common fetal arrhythmias. J Saudi Heart Assoc 2011;23:61−6.

[56] Silverman NH, Enderlein MA, Stanger P, Teitel DF, Heymann MA, Golbus MS. Recognition of fetal arrhythmias by echocardiography. J Clin Ultrasound 1985;13:255−63.

[57] Rosenberg AA, Galan HL. Fetal drug therapy. Pediatr Clin 1997;44:113−35.

[58] Carvalho JS. Fetal dysrhythmias. Best Pract Res Clin Obstet Gynaecol 2019;58:28−41.

[59] Yankowitz J, Weiner C. Medical fetal therapy. Baillieres Clin Obstet Gynaecol 1995;9:553−70.

[60] Kleinman CS, Nehgme RA. Cardiac arrhythmias in the human fetus. Pediatr Cardiol 2004;25:234−51.

[61] Ward RM. Pharmacology of the maternal-placental-fetal-unit and fetal therapy. Prog Pediatr Cardiol 1996;5:79−89.

[62] Ledwitch KV, Barnes RW, Roberts AG. Unravelling the complex drug-drug interactions of the cardiovascular drugs, verapamil and digoxin, with P-glycoprotein. Biosci Rep 2016;36.

[63] Gurgov S, Bernabé KJ, Stites J, Cunniff CM, Lin-Su K, Felsen D, et al. Linking the degree of virilization in females with congenital adrenal hyperplasia to genotype. Ann N Y Acad Sci 2017;1402:56−63.

[64] Fernández-Martínez FJ, Galindo A, Garcia-Burguillo A, Vargas-Gallego C, Nogués N, Moreno-García M, et al. Noninvasive fetal sex determination in maternal plasma: a prospective feasibility study. Genet Med 2012;14:101−6.

[65] Rijnders RJ, Christiaens GC, Bossers B, van der Smagt JJ, van der Schoot CE, de Haas M. Clinical applications of cell-free fetal DNA from maternal plasma. Obstet Gynecol 2004;103:157−64.

[66] Mercè Fernández-Balsells M, Muthusamy K, Smushkin G, Lampropulos JF, Elamin MB, Abu Elnour NO, et al. Prenatal dexamethasone use for the prevention of virilization in pregnancies at risk for classical congenital adrenal hyperplasia because of 21-hydroxylase (CYP21A2) deficiency: a systematic review and meta-analyses. Clin Endocrinol 2010;73:436−44.

[67] Winkelhorst D, Oepkes D. Foetal and neonatal alloimmune thrombocytopenia. Best Pract Res Clin Obstet Gynaecol 2019;58:15−27.

[68] Bowman JM, Chown B, Lewis M, Pollock JM. Rh isoimmunization during pregnancy: antenatal prophylaxis. Can Med Assoc J 1978;118:623−7.

[69] Zwiers C, van der Bom JG, van Kamp IL, van Geloven N, Lopriore E, Smoleniec J, et al. Postponing Early intrauterine Transfusion with Intravenous immunoglobulin Treatment; the PETIT study on severe hemolytic disease of the fetus and newborn. Am J Obstet Gynecol 2018;219:291e1−9.

[70] Moise KJ. Fetal anemia due to non-Rhesus-D red-cell alloimmunization. Semin Fetal Neonatal Med 2008;13:207−14.

[71] Harman CR. Amniotic fluid abnormalities. Semin Perinatol 2008;32:288−94.

[72] Dashe JS, Pressman EK, Hibbard JU. SMFM consult series #46: evaluation and management of polyhydramnios. Am J Obstet Gynecol 2018;219:B2−b8.

[73] Hammers AL, Sanchez-Ramos L, Kaunitz AM. Antenatal exposure to indomethacin increases the risk of severe intraventricular hemorrhage, necrotizing enterocolitis, and periventricular leukomalacia: a systematic review with metaanalysis. Am J Obstet Gynecol 2015;212. 505e1−13.

[74] Groom KM, David AL. The role of aspirin, heparin, and other interventions in the prevention and treatment of fetal growth restriction. Am J Obstet Gynecol 2018;218: S829−40.

[75] Sharp A, Cornforth C, Jackson R, Harrold J, Turner MA, Kenny L, et al. Mortality in the UK STRIDER trial of sildenafil therapy for the treatment of severe early-onset fetal growth restriction. Lancet Child Adolesc Health 2019;3:e2−3.

[76] Hui L, Challis D. Diagnosis and management of fetal growth restriction: the role of fetal therapy. Best Pract Res Clin Obstet Gynaecol 2008;22:139−58.

[77] Nygaard U, Sundberg K, Nielsen HS, Hertel S, Jørgensen C. New treatment of early fetal chylothorax. Obstet Gynecol 2007;109:1088−92.

[78] Yang YS, Ma GC, Shih JC, Chen CP, Chou CH, Yeh KT, et al. Experimental treatment of bilateral fetal chylothorax using in-utero pleurodesis. Ultrasound Obstet Gynecol 2012;39:56−62.

[79] Anandakumar C, Biswas A, Wong YC, Chia D, Annapoorna V, Arulkumaran S, et al. Management of non-immune hydrops: 8 years' experience. Ultrasound Obstet Gynecol 1996;8:196−200.

[80] Randenberg AL. Nonimmune hydrops fetalis part I: etiology and pathophysiology. Neonatal Network 2010;29:281−95.

[81] Sebire NJ, Jauniaux E. Fetal and placental malignancies: prenatal diagnosis and management. Ultrasound Obstet Gynecol 2009;33:235−44.

[82] Rayburn WF. Fetal drug therapy: an overview of selected conditions. Obstet Gynecol Surv 1992;47:1−9.

[83] Siegfried N, van der Merwe L, Brocklehurst P, Sint TT. Antiretrovirals for reducing the risk of mother-to-child transmission of HIV infection. Cochrane Database Syst Rev 2011:Cd003510.

[84] Sastry BV. Techniques to study human placental transport. Adv Drug Deliv Rev 1999; 38:17−39.

[85] Weiss L. Cell and tissue biology: a textbook of histology. 6th ed., vol. 20. Baltimore: Elsevier Inc; 1989. Urban & Schwartzenberg.

[86] Baergen RN. Overview and microscopic survey of the placenta. In: Baergen RN, editor. Man. Pathol. Hum. Placenta. Boston, MA: Springer US; 2011. p. 85−108.

[87] Ernst LM. Placenta. In: Ernst LM, Ruchelli ED, Huff DS, editors. Color atlas fetal neonatal histol. New York, NY: Springer New York; 2011. p. 363−88.

[88] Huppertz B. The anatomy of the normal placenta. J Clin Pathol 2008;61:1296−302.

[89] Benirschke K, Burton GJ, Baergen RN. Basic structure of the villous trees. Pathol. Hum. Placenta. Berlin, Heidelberg: Springer Berlin Heidelberg; 2012. p. 55−100.

[90] Moe AJ. Placental amino acid transport. Am J Physiol 1995;268:C1321−31.

[91] Vähäkangas K, Myllynen P. Drug transporters in the human blood-placental barrier. Br J Pharmacol 2009;158:665−78.

[92] Prouillac C, Lecoeur S. The role of the placenta in fetal exposure to xenobiotics: importance of membrane transporters and human models for transfer studies. Drug Metab Dispos 2010;38:1623−35.

[93] Albekairi NA, Al-Enazy S, Ali S, Rytting E. Transport of digoxin-loaded polymeric nanoparticles across BeWo cells, an in vitro model of human placental trophoblast. Ther Deliv 2015;6:1325−34.

[94] Ganapathy V, Prasad PD, Ganapathy ME, Leibach FH. Placental transporters relevant to drug distribution across the maternal-fetal interface. J Pharmacol Exp Therapeut 2000;294:413−20.

[95] Young AM, Allen CE, Audus KL. Efflux transporters of the human placenta. Adv Drug Deliv Rev 2003;55:125−32.

[96] Mark PJ, Waddell BJ. P-glycoprotein restricts access of cortisol and dexamethasone to the glucocorticoid receptor in placental BeWo cells. Endocrinology 2006;147: 5147−52.

[97] Pasanen M, Pelkonen O. The expression and environmental regulation of P450 enzymes in human placenta. Crit Rev Toxicol 1994;24:211−29.

[98] Nanovskaya TN, Deshmukh SV, Nekhayeva IA, Zharikova OL, Hankins GD, Ahmed MS. Methadone metabolism by human placenta. Biochem Pharmacol 2004; 68:583−91.

[99] Deshmukh SV, Nanovskaya TN, Hankins GD, Ahmed MS. N-demethylation of levo-alpha-acetylmethadol by human placental aromatase. Biochem Pharmacol 2004;67: 885−92.

[100] Deshmukh SV, Nanovskaya TN, Ahmed MS. Aromatase is the major enzyme metabolizing buprenorphine in human placenta. J Pharmacol Exp Therapeut 2003;306: 1099−105.

[101] Hakkola J, Pasanen M, Hukkanen J, Pelkonen O, Mäenpää J, Edwards RJ, et al. Expression of xenobiotic-metabolizing cytochrome P450 forms in human full-term placenta. Biochem Pharmacol 1996;51:403−11.

[102] Hakkola J, Raunio H, Purkunen R, Pelkonen O, Saarikoski S, Cresteil T, et al. Detection of cytochrome P450 gene expression in human placenta in first trimester of pregnancy. Biochem Pharmacol 1996;52:379−83.

[103] Nanovskaya TN, Nekhayeva IA, Hankins GD, Ahmed MS. Transfer of methadone across the dually perfused preterm human placental lobule. Am J Obstet Gynecol 2008;198. 126e1−4.

[104] Hemauer SJ, Patrikeeva SL, Nanovskaya TN, Hankins GD, Ahmed MS. Opiates inhibit paclitaxel uptake by P-glycoprotein in preparations of human placental inside-out vesicles. Biochem Pharmacol 2009;78:1272−8.

[105] Fan SZ, Susetio L, Tsai MC. Neuromuscular blockade of the fetus with pancuronium or pipecuronium for intra-uterine procedures. Anaesthesia 1994;49:284−6.

[106] Coke GA, Baschat AA, Mighty HE, Malinow AM. Maternal cardiac arrest associated with attempted fetal injection of potassium chloride. Int J Obstet Anesth 2004;13: 287−90.

[107] Salomon LJ, Sotiriadis A, Wulff CB, Odibo A, Akolekar R. Risk of miscarriage following amniocentesis or chorionic villus sampling: systematic review of literature and updated meta-analysis. Ultrasound Obstet Gynecol 2019;54:442−51.

[108] David AL, Waddington SN. Candidate diseases for prenatal gene therapy. In: Coutelle C, Waddington SN, editors. Prenat. Gene ther. Concepts, methods, protoc. Totowa, NJ: Humana Press; 2012. p. 9−39.

[109] David AL, Peebles D. Gene therapy for the fetus: is there a future? Best Pract Res Clin Obstet Gynaecol 2008;22:203−18.

[110] Davey MG, Flake AW. Genetic therapy for the fetus: a once in a lifetime opportunity. Hum Gene Ther 2011;22:383−5.

[111] Pschera H. Current status in intrauterine fetal stem cell therapy. J Obstet Gynaecol Res 1998;24:419−24.

[112] Sagar R, Götherström C, David AL, Westgren M. Fetal stem cell transplantation and gene therapy. Best Pract Res Clin Obstet Gynaecol 2019;58:142−53.

[113] Shaw SW, David AL, De Coppi P. Clinical applications of prenatal and postnatal therapy using stem cells retrieved from amniotic fluid. Curr Opin Obstet Gynecol 2011;23: 109−16.

[114] Mehta V, Abi Nader K, Waddington S, David AL. Organ targeted prenatal gene therapy—how far are we? Prenat Diagn 2011;31:720−34.

[115] Peranteau WH, Hayashi S, Abdulmalik O, Chen Q, Merchant A, Asakura T, et al. Correction of murine hemoglobinopathies by prenatal tolerance induction and postnatal nonmyeloablative allogeneic BM transplants. Blood 2015;126:1245−54.

[116] Rytting E, Nguyen J, Wang X, Kissel T. Biodegradable polymeric nanocarriers for pulmonary drug delivery. Expet Opin Drug Deliv 2008;5:629−39.

[117] Sweeney S, Adamcakova-Dodd A, Thorne PS, Assouline JG. Multifunctional nanoparticles for real-time evaluation of toxicity during fetal development. PLoS One 2018;13:e0192474.

[118] Bajoria R, Fisk NM, Contractor SF. Liposomal thyroxine: a noninvasive model for transplacental fetal therapy. J Clin Endocrinol Metab 1997;82:3271−7.

[119] Myllynen PK, Loughran MJ, Howard CV, Sormunen R, Walsh AA, Vähäkangas KH. Kinetics of gold nanoparticles in the human placenta. Reprod Toxicol 2008;26:130−7.

[120] Menjoge AR, Rinderknecht AL, Navath RS, Faridnia M, Kim CJ, Romero R, et al. Transfer of PAMAM dendrimers across human placenta: prospects of its use as drug carrier during pregnancy. J Control Release 2011;150:326−38.

[121] Wick P, Malek A, Manser P, Meili D, Maeder-Althaus X, Diener L, et al. Barrier capacity of human placenta for nanosized materials. Environ Health Perspect 2010;118: 432−6.

[122] Saunders M. Transplacental transport of nanomaterials. Wiley Interdiscip Rev Nanomed Nanobiotechnol 2009;1:671−84.

[123] Akour AA, Kennedy MJ, Gerk P. Receptor-mediated endocytosis across human placenta: emphasis on megalin. Mol Pharm 2013;10:1269−78.

[124] Keelan JA, Leong JW, Ho D, Iyer KS. Therapeutic and safety considerations of nanoparticle-mediated drug delivery in pregnancy. Nanomedicine 2015;10:2229−47.

[125] Wang R, Song B, Wu J, Zhang Y, Chen A, Shao L. Potential adverse effects of nanoparticles on the reproductive system. Int J Nanomed 2018;13:8487−506.

[126] Moaddab A, Nassr AA, Belfort MA, Shamshirsaz AA. Ethical issues in fetal therapy. Best Pract Res Clin Obstet Gynaecol 2017;43:58−67.

Treating the placenta: an evolving therapeutic concept

6

Michael D. Reed[1], Donald R. Mattison[2,3,4]

[1]*Professor Emeritus of Pediatrics, Department of Pediatrics, School of Medicine, Case Western Reserve University, Cleveland, United States;* [2]*University of South Carolina, Arnold School of Public Health, Columbia, SC, United States;* [3]*Risk Sciences International, Ottawa, ON, Canada;* [4]*School of Epidemiology and Public Health, University of Ottawa, Ottawa, ON, Canada*

6.1 Introduction

Generally, from the perspective of clinical pharmacology, one thinks of the placenta as the route of passage from mother to fetus or the reverse [1–4], with or without metabolism. With few exceptions, it is generally not thought of as the target for therapy. However, we believe that as our understanding of placental function grows and as the science and application of obstetric-based clinical pharmacology broadens, the placenta may become an important therapeutic target for the mother, the fetus, or both [54]. Clinically important diseases where such a strategy is employed today include the prevention of vertical HIV-1 virus transmission from mother to fetus and in the treatment of malaria where the placenta serves as an important reservoir for the malaria parasite. In this chapter, we critically review what is known about placental functions and its modulations throughout gestation and how placental processes can and might be manipulated for therapeutic gain.

Two recent reviews have explored drug development from the perspective of placental dysfunction (Sibley, 2017 #4) or from the perspective of prevention of abnormal fetal brain development from hypoxia [54]. Sibley started his review with the premise that obstetrical challenges (e.g., fetal growth retardation, preeclampsia, preterm labor, preterm premature rupture of membranes, late spontaneous abortion, and placental abruption.) were a consequence of placental dysfunction. From that perspective, he illustrated how a contemporary drug development program could be developed for multiple compounds including sildenafil citrate, adenovirus vector with VEGF, pomegranate juice, tempol, resveratrol, melatonin, sofalcone, proton pump inhibitors, statins, and metformin. Phillips et al. proposed that placental secretions in response to hypoxia might play a role in brain development resulting in adult onset diseases. Using a nanoparticle-bound antioxidant, they demonstrated reduced oxidative stress in the placenta and reduced the reduction in birth weight. The treatment target in the Phillips et al. research was the placenta with an indirect impact on the pup/fetus. Both studies emphasize the potential benefit of treating the placenta.

Clinical Pharmacology During Pregnancy. https://doi.org/10.1016/B978-0-12-818902-3.00023-3

6.2 The placenta as the therapeutic target: the past

An early example of targeting placental function for therapeutic purposes that was both unsuccessful as well as resulting in unexpected tragic consequences is the experience with diethylstilbestrol (DES). The DES experience highlights the importance of the need for a good understanding of the disease process, drug pharmacokinetics and pharmacodynamics, and acute, chronic, and generational toxicity before undertaking widespread drug-based manipulation of the maternal, placental, and/or fetal compartments [5]. DES is a synthetic estrogen structurally similar to estradiol with potent estrogen-like activity that is rarely used today. From the 1940s to ∼1971, DES was commonly used for prevention of spontaneous abortions. An innovative randomized controlled clinical trial conducted at the Chicago Lying-In Hospital demonstrated that DES was unable to prevent pregnancy loss, and may have actually led to missed abortion [6]. Unknown at the time but recently described, DES beneficial clinical effects are most likely a result of the drug's positive effects on placentation and trophoblast stem cell differentiation [7] (see also [54]; Sibley, 2017 #4 for discussion of placental treatments). Unfortunately, maternal use of DES results in a high incidence of developmental toxicity on the reproductive tracts of males and females and the subsequent development of vaginal clear cell adenocarcinoma in women of childbearing age [6–8]. Many environmental chemicals and pollutants either as the intact compound or metabolite can also have similar or unique devastating adverse consequences on the mother, the placenta, and/or the fetus [5] complicating our assessment of individual compounds during pregnancy. These and many other tragic experiences underscore the importance of careful study of mother–fetal benefit–risk profiles of drugs intended to treat the placenta.

6.2.1 Placental function

The placenta provides a link between the mother and fetus, metabolizing and transferring nutrients for growth and development of the fetus as well as for its own growth and development. Metabolic waste products generated in the fetus or placenta are eliminated by transfer into the maternal circulation. A unique function of the placenta is its role as an endocrine organ producing steroid and protein hormones. These characteristics must be considered in thinking about treating the placenta to enhance therapeutic success in placental, fetal, or maternal disease. A detailed description of placental anatomy, physiology, and gestational maturation is addressed in Chapter 5. However, for completeness, we provide a brief overview of those anatomic and physiologic functions important to understanding therapeutic targeting of placental function for maternal and fetal health.

Briefly, fetal and maternal circulations are separated by placental tissue that changes throughout pregnancy; anatomically, the surface area over which maternal–fetal exchange occurs increases and the distance between maternal and fetal blood decreases. Morphologically, the syncytiotrophoblast layer is reduced in thickness and the cytotrophoblast becomes discontinuous as gestation progresses. Changes in the villous structure are also observed, with an increasing number of microvilli facilitating exchange between mother and fetus. These villi and the syncytiotrophoblast layer permit the maternal and fetal circulations to be close to each other, without contact while providing a transport barrier between the two circulations [1,9,10].

In human placenta, the syncytiotrophoblast arises from the fusion of cytotrophoblast, forming a syncytium over the surface of the placenta facing the maternal blood. The plasma membranes of the syncytiotrophoblast are polarized; the brush border membrane is in direct contact with maternal blood and the basal membrane facing the fetal circulation. The brush border membrane possesses a microvillus structure that effectively amplifies the surface area, whereas the basal membrane lacks this structure.

Anatomic differences between species in the number of trophoblast layers and connection between maternal and fetal tissues result in species-specific variation in placental function that influences data gathered during the preclinical stages of drug development. The human placenta is unique in its villous structure. Factors such as diffusion, electrical potential across the placenta, magnitude of maternal and fetal blood flows, and differences in metabolism, transport proteins, and other mechanisms for exchange between maternal and fetal circulations should be considered as the placental transfer and metabolism of drugs varies dramatically among differing species. Discordant results for maternal—fetal drug disposition between humans and many animal species are often noted due to these anatomical differences in placental morphology and function [9—11]. The thalidomide tragedy was the most important event to dispel the erroneous belief that the placenta was a barrier and spawned regulation for controlled, animal-based preclinical teratology studies [11—13]. These anatomical and physiological differences can also lead to false implications for teratogenic effect(s). The widely used drugs diazepam and salicylates were shown to induce teratogenic effects in animals with no increased risk of any such effects in humans.

The previously widely used and therapeutically effective drug Benedictine (doxylamine plus pyridoxine) was shown in animal studies to cause cardiac and limb defects leading to enormous litigation and ultimately withdrawal from the US market though no increase in human teratogenic effects have been described [13], and this drug combination remains the most effective intervention for treating pregnancy-associated nausea and vomiting (see Chapter 12). These misleading and sometimes erroneous findings are directly attributable to the interspecies differences that exist in placental structure and function. Despite these disparities and the need for better mechanisms for screening possible placental toxins or teratogens, animal screening remains the best process today [11], although structure activity analysis is rapidly gaining credence (Wu, 2013 #11).

Drugs for treatment of placental disease should be concentrated within the placenta with little access to, and toxicity for, mother or fetus. Drugs developed for treatment of the mother should have minimal transport to fetal circulation and minimal impact on placental and fetal health. Drugs for treatment of fetal diseases should have unhindered access to the fetal circulation with minimal adverse impact on mother or placenta [1,14].

6.2.2 Placental transport mechanisms

The syncytiotrophoblast, the outermost layer of the human placenta, is the main site of exchange for drugs and metabolites, nutrients, waste products, and gases between the maternal and fetal circulations. Efficient transfer of nutrients, gases, electrolytes, and solutes across the placenta is essential for fetal growth and development. There are several mechanisms by which transfer occurs, and depending on the mechanism of transfer, the direction may be toward the maternal or fetal circulation.

As noted in Chapter 5, the placenta performs a multitude of important, complex, simultaneous functions at a differing functional capacity that changes as gestation progresses. Drugs may transfer from the maternal to fetal compartments via simple passive diffusion, facilitated diffusion, active transport, filtration, or pinocytosis. The physiochemical characteristics of a drug substantially influence its maternal–fetal disposition profile. Structural modifications of a proposed drug's physical and chemical characteristics including molecular weight/size, degree of ionization at physiologic and pathophysiologic pH linked to water/lipid solubility, and affinity for membrane transporters and drug metabolizing enzymes represent just a few of a multitude of targets for drug therapy. Xenobiotics with a molecular weight of <600 Da can usually transfer across the placenta via passive diffusion, whereas compounds of 1000+ daltons, e.g., heparin and insulin, cross very poorly. With a small, highly lipid soluble, low plasma protein-bound drug, its transfer across the placenta will primarily be dependent upon maternal and fetal blood flow combined with involvement, if any, of a membrane transporter. Important to the treatment of placental-based disorders (see below, e.g., malaria), a drug may have high affinity for placental tissue and bind to and/or accumulate within the syncytiotrophoblast [15]. Depending upon the inherent physiochemical characteristics of a drug, it may be released into the fetal circulation or be released back into maternal circulation without reaching the fetal compartment. The rates of these transfer processes can be very different than the individual or combined maternal or fetal clearance rates of the drug [1–5,9,10,15–19].

6.3 The placenta: therapeutic targets

As noted above, the placenta is a multifunctional dynamic organ continuously evolving throughout gestation with the sole purpose of maintaining maternal–fetal homeostasis up to the time of optimal preprogrammed delivery of the newborn infant. The many perturbations that occur with each of these processes during gestation heighten the complexity of effectively targeting one or more functions as a therapeutic target [20]. Nevertheless, as our understanding of maternal–fetal physiology and pathophysiology increases in concert with advances in digital technology fostering more sophisticated patient monitoring and safer anatomical manipulation, therapeutic targeted strategies are a reality now and will continue to expand. With respect to possible therapeutics, enzymes capable of metabolizing (CYPs) or conjugating drugs (transferases) as well as uni- and bidirectional transporters facilitating or preventing drug movement from one location to another are ripe for pharmacologic manipulation to maximize maternal or fetal therapeutics [3,4,16,19−27]. Similarly, a drug development plan focused on an analog's structure−activity relationship linked to specific manipulations of its physiochemical characteristics will foster safer and more effective therapy [1−4,16,18]. Moreover, our increasing understanding of the maternal-fetal environment/communications has advanced the development of increasingly sophisticated physiologically based pharmacokinetic modeling methods fostering more accurate predictions of maternal/fetal drug disposition and action [28].

Tables 6.1−6.3, respectively, outline placental expression of known CYPs, enzymes involved in conjugation, and cellular transporters relative to gestational age that are active in maternal−fetal homeostasis. The overall influence of these placental-based processes on xenobiotic disposition must be considered in total with the functional activity of the mother and the fetus. Changes in the functional capacity and activity of these processes important to drug disposition occur between the mother, placenta, and fetus throughout gestation. In general, fetal tissue activity of these processes increases, whereas placental activity decreases with gestation such that at birth, placental metabolic activity is minimal [4,25−27]. This gestational ontogeny may be the basis for much of the conflicting data regarding placental drug disposition that exist in current literature. For example, the energy-dependent

Table 6.1 Placental expression of cytochrome P450 enzymes involved in drug metabolism.

| Specific enzyme | Placental maturity | | |
	First trimester	Term	Inducible
CYP1A1	A, P, R	A, P, R	Yes
CYP1A2	A, R	A, P	Yes
CYP2C8/9/19	R	P, R	Yes
CYP2D6	R	ND	Yes
CYP2E1	P, R	A, P,[a] R[a]	Yes
CYP3A4-7	P, R	A, P, R	Yes

A, activity; CYP, cytochrome P450 isozyme; ND, no substantive activity/excesses detected; P, protein; R, mRNA.
[a] CYP2E1 has only been detected in the term placenta of heavy ethanol-consuming mothers.
Adapted from Myllynen P, Immonen E, Kummu M, Vahakangas K. Developmental expression of drug metabolizing enzymes and transporter proteins in human placenta and fetal tissues. Expet Opin Drug Metabol Toxicol 2009;5(12):1483−99; Blanco-Castaneda R, Galaviz-Hernandez C, Souto PCS, Lima VV, Giachini FR, et al. The role of xenobiotic-metabolizing enzymes in the placenta: a growing research field. Expet Rev Clin Pharmacol 2020;13:247−63.

Table 6.2 The expression of cellular transporter proteins in human placenta.

	Placenta		
Transporter	**First trimester**	**Second trimester**	**Third trimester**
ABCB1	R, P	R, P	R, P, A
ABCB4	R	NA	R
ABCC1	R	NA	R, P, A
ABCC2	R, P	R, P	R, P
ABCC3	R	NA	R, P, A
ABCC4	NA	NA	R, P
ABCC5	R	R	R, P, A
ABCC6	NA	NA	NA
ABCC10	NA	NA	NA
ABCC11	NA	NA	R
ABCG2	R, P	R, P	R, P, A
NET	NA	NA	R, A
SERT	NA	NA	R, P, A
OCT1	NA	NA	R, A
OCT2	NA	NA	R
OCT3	R	NA	R, P, A
OCTN1	NA	NA	NA
OCTN2	NA	NA	R, P, A
OAT1	NA	NA	NA
OAT4	P	NA	R, P
OATP1A2	R	NA	R
OATP1B1	R	NA	ND
OATP281	P	P	R, P, A
OATP3A1	R	NA	R
OATP4A1	R	NA	R, P

A, activity; NA, data not available; ND, not detected; NET, noradrenalin transporter; OAT, organic anion transporter; OATP, organic anion transporting polypeptide; OCT, organic cation transporter; P, protein; R, mRNA; SERT, 5-HT.

Adapted from Myllynen P, Immonen E, Kummu M, Vahakangas K. Developmental expression of drug metabolizing enzymes and transporter proteins in human placenta and fetal tissues. Expet Opin Drug Metabol Toxicol 2009;5(12):1483–99; Dallman A, Liu XI, Burckart GJ, van den Anker J. Drug transporters expressed in the human placenta and models for studying maternal-fetal drug transfer. J Clin Pharmacol 2019;59(Suppl. 1):S70–81.

efflux (placental) transporter P-glycoprotein (Pgp) is of little importance in term placenta but very important during earlier stages of gestation in preventing xenobiotic access to the fetal compartment. This ontogenic pattern through gestation is very important to the rate and extent of digoxin placental transfer for the treatment of fetal arrhythmias (see Chapter 5) [22].

Table 6.3 Therapeutic agents that are substrates for P-glycoprotein and/or breast cancer resistance protein.

Pgp	BCRP
Azithromycin	
Cyclosporine	Glyburide
Digoxin	Methotrexate
Erythromycin	Sulfated estrogens
Indinavir	Zidovudine
Levofloxacin	
Methylprednisolone	
Morphine	
Phenobarbital	
Phenytoin	
Ritonavir	
Saquinavir	
Verapamil	

BCRP, *breast cancer resistance protein*; Pgp, *P-glycoprotein.*
Adapted from Hutson JR, Koren G, Matthews SG. Placental P-glycoprotein and breast cancer resistance protein: influence of polymorphisms on fetal drug exposure and physiology. Placenta 2010; 31:351—7.

It is conceivable if not inevitable that drugs will be developed that function as a pure antagonist, i.e., high affinity with no intrinsic activity, which occupies a specific placental transporter, enzyme, or other target antagonizing its effects. Such a compound could be used alone or in combination with other therapeutic compounds with the sole purpose of blocking drug transfer into the fetal compartment thus leading to maternal drug accumulation, or conversely, to block back transfer from the fetal compartment to maternal circulation leading to drug accumulation or persistence in the fetal compartment. Such a strategy is employed today with digoxin for fetal arrhythmias where Pgp inhibitors (e.g., verapamil) are coadministered to enhance fetal compartment digoxin concentrations [22]. As noted above, this strategy is of variable success but clearly dependent upon the fetus's gestational age [22].

6.4 The placenta as a therapeutic target today

6.4.1 Diabetes during pregnancy

Poorly or uncontrolled diabetes during pregnancy has been clearly shown to markedly increase maternal and fetal risk for a spectrum of untoward effects, many that are serious and attenuated or prevented with effective therapy [9,29]. However, a major concern in the selection of drug therapy for maternal diabetes is strictly preventing fetal hypoglycemia [9,17,30−32]. The design of drug therapy for optimal treatment of maternal diabetes is a case study for the contemporary targeting of the placenta for successful therapeutics. In this case, the target is exploiting the known influences the placenta has on drug distribution and overall maternal disposition to limit fetal exposure [9,17,30,32] (Sibley, 2017 #4).

The best example of manipulation of maternal and placental function to influence drug disposition for optimal maternal therapeutics is the story of glibenclamide (GBC) (glyburide) [9,17,30,32]. GBC is an oral hypoglycemic drug that stimulates the pancreatic beta cells to secrete insulin and is often used to treat diabetes, including diabetes during pregnancy. This particular drug dosing strategy capitalized on the known influences of drug protein binding, maternal drug clearance rate, and affinity for placental−fetal transporters to achieve the desired therapeutic effect. GBC is highly bound to maternal plasma proteins (primarily albumin) to the extent of 99.8%. This extensive degree of drug binding to circulating maternal plasma protein substantially reduces the amount of free active drug available for placental transfer. Augmenting this effect is the drug's relative short maternal elimination half-life ($t_{1/2}$), minimizing the duration of time the free GBC is present in maternal circulation for transplacental transfer. A third and extremely important characteristic of GBC is the drug's affinity as a substrate for multiple efflux proteins, Pgp, multidrug-resistant protein 1, 2, or 3, and breast cancer resistant protein (BCRP). Very recent data suggest that GBC may be preferentially transported from the fetal to the maternal circulations by BCRP [9,15,18]. When all three of these characteristics are combined, with the latter, probably the most important to limiting drug access to the fetal compartment, highly effective and safe maternal therapeutic regimens can be constructed with easily achieved drug structure−activity relationships targeted at specific maternal and placental function.

6.4.2 Malaria in pregnancy

Malaria during pregnancy is a medical as well as public health concern owing to maternal (anemia, fever, cerebral infection, hypoglycemia, and death), placental, fetal (abortion, stillbirth, and congenital infection), and neonatal (prematurity, growth restriction, infection, and death) effects [14,33,34]. Therapy has been complicated by the emergence and rapid spread of drug resistance, necessitating combination therapy. In addition, malaria and HIV can be found in the same populations and interact to the detriment of the mother, placenta, and fetus [34,35]. Finally, of special relevance are the interactions between malaria and the placenta, as placental malaria may be asymptomatic until adverse pregnancy outcome [36−38].

Drug development for malaria in pregnancy encounters two significant obstacles: malaria is a disease of developing countries and afflicts women during pregnancy [33,34,39,40]. Existing treatments are poorly characterized with respect to pharmacokinetics, pharmacodynamics, safety, and efficacy, yet the tools for studying the existing drugs and new drug development are readily available. Further complicating this scenario is the fact that *Plasmodium falciparum*, the most common human malarial species, manifests differently in pregnant women than in nonpregnant women. In pregnant women *P. falciparum* expresses a different antigen variant to that found in nonpregnant women. Malaria-infected red blood cells possess adhesive proteins on their surface which appear to interact with chondroitin sulfate on the placental surface [37]. These and other cellular perturbations lead to infected erythrocytes preferentially accumulating in the intervillous space of the placenta resulting in a thickening of the trophoblast basement membrane. This later event appears to be an adaptive mechanism in response to the enormous amount of secreted cytokines released in response to the infection. The thickened trophoblast basement membrane damages the syncytiotrophoblastic surface of chorionic villi [38] leading to the negative maternal and fetal consequences associated with this parasitic disease. Thus, an effective therapeutic strategy must not only focus on parasite eradication at the placental and peripheral levels but might concurrently target antagonism of select chemokines and cytokines elevated with placental malaria [38].

6.4.3 **HIV-1 infection in pregnancy**

As noted above, referring to the placenta as a "barrier," the placental barrier has been discouraged for decades and for the most part falsely. This myth has been dispelled for many decades [1,3,12]. For some, however, the placenta does serve as a barrier to fetal transmission of viruses. Cytomegalovirus easily crosses the syncytiotrophoblast to the fetus, whereas the HIV-1 virus crosses very poorly. In untreated HIV-1−infected mothers, more than 90% of their offspring will be HIV-1 negative reflecting the maternal and placental focus of the infection [31]. Mother-to-child transmission of HIV-1 can be reduced to <1% with the use of antiviral drugs during pregnancy and in the neonate. The most common antiretroviral drug used to prevent maternal-to-child HIV-1 transmission is zidovudine (ZDV)—in 1994, maternal ZDV monotherapy was clearly shown to decrease maternal-to-child HIV-1 transmission by two thirds [41]. ZDV is metabolized to its active moiety in the placenta and inhibits HIV-1 replication within placental cells [42].

The exact mechanism(s) of HIV-1 transmission in utero is poorly understood, but the role of the placenta as the primary target is clear. Histological examination of term placentas from HIV-1−positive women revealed HIV-1 infection in syncytiotrophoblast, cytotrophoblast, and villous endothelial cells. Similar histological examination of placenta at 16 weeks revealed syncytiotrophoblast and cytotrophoblast infection, whereas chorionic villi were rarely involved [42]. All these data combined underscore the importance of the placenta as the primary therapeutic target for the prevention of mother-to-child transmission of HIV-1 infection. Further supporting this contention are the data showing increased expression of human beta defensins, a natural defense mechanism in the maternal−fetal interface, in HIV-1−seropositive mothers [43].

Like malarial infection during pregnancy, many factors influence the efficacy of maternal HIV therapy in preventing mother-to-child transmission. Understanding and accounting for the changes in drug pharmacokinetics during pregnancy (see Chapter 3) is of paramount importance to the efficacy and safety of maternal and fetal drug therapy. Although the placenta is well perfused, inadequate prevention, the development of HIV-1 drug resistance, or drug-induced toxicity can occur if maternal antiretroviral drug dose regimens do not account for the changes in drug disposition observed throughout gestation. Subtherapeutic antiviral drug tissue and fluid concentrations can lead to inadequate fetal prevention and/or the development of HIV-1 drug resistance, whereas too large doses may increase the risk of maternal and/or fetal toxicity.

6.5 The placenta as a therapeutic target in the future

The ideal drug for maternal therapy would be an agent that neither reaches the fetal compartment nor alters maternal physiology sufficiently to adversely affect placental function. Similarly, the ideal maternally administered drug targeting the fetal compartment would have no negative maternal or placental effects. To our knowledge, this "ideal" drug does not yet exist—but soon "they" will. Furthermore, a drug may be maternally administered to the mother to inhibit or stimulate individual or multiple placental functions to achieve the desired therapeutic goal.

The value of nanosized materials as a method for drug delivery, and more specifically targeting specific anatomic site delivery, is gaining considerable interest. The number of nanoparticle polymer constructs supporting the engineering of compounds with novel physical and chemical characteristics has increased dramatically over the last decade [44]. Based on the ability to manufacture nanosized compounds (e.g., drugs) of specific size, charge, and disintegration characteristics, it is not surprising that the maternal—placental—fetal compartments are specific targets for ongoing research [44—47]. We envision that nanotechnology will foster the development of a number of specific compounds that target specific placental characteristics, i.e., targeting specific maternal sites, specific placental sites, and/or fetal compartment penetration and binding to specific fetal sites [44—46]. However, before these benefits are fully realized, the methodical study of placental nanopharmaceuticals will provide tremendous insight into placental anatomy and physiology [46]. Advances in placental imaging, particularly of transport mechanisms [27,48] and other functions, should augment the rate at which such new therapies are realized.

Lastly, the genomics of placental function will further expand the therapeutic armamentarium for specific placental diseases and functions [49—51]. Genetic technology has impacted greatly on the ability to detect perinatal genetic disorders and their susceptibility at multiple time points during gestation [49]. Pharmacogenomics in reproductive and perinatal medicine is in its infancy [50]. Although a few clinically useful drugs in perinatal medicine contain pharmacogenetic information in their official labeling, the relevance to contemporary perinatal care is extremely limited. Pharmacogenomics of placental receptors, transporters, enzymes, and other functions will be exploited for therapeutic purposes. As such, placental epigenetics are of great interest with respect to the treatment of placental disease as well as possible manipulation of the fetal compartment by using the placenta as the "gateway to the fetus" [51,52]. Much more information serving to define specific therapeutic targets is being described at a faster and faster rate as advances continue to occur in our technical capabilities. A recent example of such advances described differential expression of several human placental proteins between lean and obese pregnant women that could lead to a number of therapeutic strategies targeting many maternal, placental, and fetal perturbations [53]. This is just the beginning.

6.6 Conclusions

The placenta is the most important structure to the health and viability of the mother and the fetus and for fetal development up to delivery. Nevertheless, the majority of therapeutic strategies used during pregnancy today focus on manipulation of the placenta for maternal or fetal therapeutics. Increasing information defines the importance of therapies directed at, or focused on, the placenta for maternal–fetal health. Advances in molecular biology, technology, imaging, and genomics are among just a few avenues that are fostering a much better understanding of placental anatomy, physiology, maturation, and pathophysiology and serving as the foundations for effective treatment of the placenta.

References

[1] Malek A, Mattison DR. Drug development for use during pregnancy: impact of the placenta. Expet Rev Obstet Gynecol 2010;5:437–54.
[2] Myllynen P, Kummu M, Sieppi E. ABCB1 and ABCG2 expression in the pla- centa and fetus: an interspecies comparison. Expet Opin Drug Metabol Toxicol 2010;6:1385–98.
[3] Vahakangas K, Myllynen P. Drug transporters in the human blood–placental barrier. Br J Pharmacol 2009;158:665–78.
[4] Myllynen P, Immonen E, Kummu M, Vahakangas K. Developmental expression of drug metabolizing enzymes and transporter proteins in human placenta and fetal tissues. Expet Opin Drug Metabol Toxicol 2009;5(12):1483–99.
[5] Miller KP, Borgeest C, Greenfeld C, Tomic D, Flaws JA. In utero effects of chemicals on reproductive tissues in females. Toxicol Appl Pharmacol 2004;198:111–31.
[6] Hoover RN, Hyer M, Pfeiffer RM, Adam E, Bond B, Cheville AL, et al. Adverse health outcomes in women exposed in utero to diethylstilbestrol. N Engl J Med 2011;365:14.
[7] Tremblay GB, Kunath T, Bergeron D, Lopointe L, Champigny C, Bader J, et al. Diethylstilbestrol regulates trophoblast stem cell differentiation as a ligand of orphan nuclear receptor ERRB. Genes Dev 2001;15:833–8.

[8] Levine RU, Berkowitz KM. Conservative management and pregnancy out- come in diethylstilbestrol-exposed women with and without gross genital tract abnormalities. Am J Obstet Gynecol 1993;169(5):1125—9.

[9] Pollex EK, Denice SF, Koren G. Oral hypoglycemic therapy: understanding the mechanisms of transplacental transfer. J Matern Fetal Neonatal Med 2010;23:224—8.

[10] Eshkokoli T, Sheiner E, BenZvi Z, Feinstein V, Holcberg G. Drug transport across the placenta. Curr Pharmaceut Biotechnol 2011;12:707—14.

[11] Daston GP. Laboratory models and their role in assessing teratogenesis. Am J Med Genet 2011;157:183—7.

[12] Ito T, Hideki A, Handa H. Teratogenic effects of thalidomide: molecular mechanisms. Cell Mol Life Sci 2011;68:1569—79.

[13] Koren G, Pastuszak A, Ito S. Drugs in pregnancy. N Engl J Med 1998;338:1128—37.

[14] van Hasselt JG, Andrew MA, Hebert MF, Tarning J, Vicini P, Mattison DR. The status of pharmacometrics in pregnancy: highlights from the 3(rd) American Conference on Pharmacometrics. Br J Clin Pharmacol 2012. https://doi.org/10.1111/j.1365-2125.2012.04280.x [Epub ahead of print].

[15] Pollex EK, Hutson JR. Genetic polymorphisms in placental transporters: implications for fetal drug exposure to oral antidiabetic agents. Expet Opin Drug Metabol Toxicol 2011;7(3):325—39.

[16] Syme MR, Paxton JW, Keelan JA. Drug transfer and metabolism by the human placenta. Clin Pharmacokinet 2004;43:487—514.

[17] Gedeon C, Koren G. Designing pregnancy centered medications: drugs which do not cross the human placenta. Placenta 2006;27:861—8.

[18] Hutson JR, Koren G, Matthews SG. Placental P-glycoprotein and breast cancer resistance protein: influence of polymorphisms on fetal drug exposure and physiology. Placenta 2010;31:351—7.

[19] Nanovskaya TN, Patrikeeva S, Hemauer S, Fokina V, Mattison D, Hankins GD, et al. Effect of albumin on transplacental transfer and distribution of rosiglitazone and glyburide. J Matern Fetal Neonatal Med 2008;21(3):197—207.

[20] Evseenko DA, Paxton JW, Keelan JA. Independent regulation of apical and basolateral drug transporter expression and function in placental trophoblasts by cytokines, steroids, and growth factors. Drug Metab Dispos 2007;35:595—601.

[21] Behravan J, Piquette-Miller M. Drug transport across the placenta, role of the ABC drug efflux transporters. Expet Opin Drug Metabol Toxicol 2007;3:819—30.

[22] Holcberg G, Sapir O, Tsadkin M, Huleihel M, Lazer S, Katz M, et al. Lack of interaction of digoxin and P-glycoprotein inhibitors, quinidine, verapamil in human placenta in vitro. Eur J Obstet Gynecol Reprod Biol 2003;109:133—7.

[23] Ceckova-Novotna M, Pavek P, Staud F. P-glycoprotein in the placenta: expression, localization, regulation and function. Reprod Toxicol 2006;22:400—10.

[24] Liu L, Liu X. Contributions of drug transporters to blood-placental barrier. Adv Exp Med Biol 2019;1141:505—48.

[25] Bloise E, Ortiga-Carvalho TM, Reis FM, Lye SJ, Gibb W, Matthews SG. ATP-binding cassette transporters in reproduction: a new frontier. Hum Reprod Update 2016;22:164—81.

[26] Blanco-Castaneda R, Galaviz-Hernandez C, Souto PCS, Lima VV, Giachini FR, et al. The role of xenobiotic-metabolizing enzymes in the placenta: a growing research field. Expet Rev Clin Pharmacol 2020;13:247—63.

[27] Dallman A, Liu XI, Burckart GJ, van den Anker J. Drug transporters expressed in the human placenta and models for studying maternal-fetal drug transfer. J Clin Pharmacol 2019;59(Suppl. 1):S70−81.

[28] Abduljalil K, Jamei M, Johnson TN. Fetal physiologically based pharmacokinetic models: systems information on the growth and composition of fetal organs. Clin Pharmacokinet 2019;58:235−62.

[29] Ballas J, Moore TR, Ramos GA. Management of diabetes in pregnancy. Curr Diabet Rep 2012;12:33−42.

[30] Hebert MF, Ma X, Naraharisetti SB, Krudys KM, Umans JG, Hankins GD, et al. Are we optimizing gestational diabetes treatment with glyburide? The pharmacologic basis for better clinical practice. Clin Pharmacol Ther 2009;85:607−14.

[31] Zharikova OL, Fokina VM, Nanovskaya TN, Hill RA, Mattison DR, Han- kins GD, et al. Identification of the major human hepatic and placental enzymes responsible for the biotransformation of glyburide. Biochem Pharmacol 2009;78:1483−90.

[32] Jain S, Zharikova OL, Ravindran S, Nanovskya TN, Mattison DR, Hankins GDV, et al. Glyburide metabolism by placentas of healthy and gestational diabetics. Am J Perinatol 2008;25(3):169−74.

[33] White NJ, McGready RM, Nosten FH. New medicines for tropical diseases in pregnancy: catch-22. PLoS Med 2008;6(5):e133.

[34] Riijken MJ, McGready R, Boel ME, Poespoprodjo R, Singh N, Syafruddin D, et al. Malaria in pregnancy in the Asia-Pacific region. Lancet Infect Dis 2012;12:75−88.

[35] Flateau C, LeLoup G, Pialoux G. Consequences of HIV infection on malaria and therapeutic implications: a systematic review. Lancet Infect Dis 2011;11:541−56.

[36] Kattenberg JH, Ochodo EA, Boer KR, Schallig HDFH, Mens PF, Leeflang MMG. Systematic review and meta-analysis: rapid diagnostic tests versus placental histology, microscopy and PCR for malaria in pregnant women. Malar J 2011;10:321.

[37] Higgins MK. The structure of chondroitin sulfate-binding domain important in placental malaria. J Biol Chem 2008;28:21842−6.

[38] Mens PF, Bojtor EC, Schallig HDFH. Molecular interactions in the placenta during malaria infection. Eur J Obstet Gynecol Reprod Biol 2010;152:126−32.

[39] The PME. Drug development for maternal health cannot be left to the whims of the market. PLoS Med 2008;6(5):e140.

[40] Fisk NM, Atun R. Market failure and the poverty of new drugs in maternal health. PLoS Med 2008;1(5):e22.

[41] Stek AM. Antiretroviral medications during pregnancy for therapy or prophylaxsis. HIV/AIDS Rep 2009;6:68−76.

[42] Al-husaini AM. Role of placenta in the vertical transmission of human immunodeficiency virus. J Perinatol 2009;29:331−6.

[43] Aguilar-Jimenez W, Zapata W, Rugeles MT. Differential expression of human beta defensins in placenta and detection of allelic variants in the DEFB1 gene from HIV-1 positive mothers. Biomedica 2011;31(1):44−54.

[44] Wick P, Malek A, Manser P, Meili D, Maeder-Althaus X, Diener L, et al. Barrier capacity of human placenta for nanosized materials. Environ Health Perspect 2010;118: 432−6.

[45] Keelan JA. Nanoparticles versus the placenta. Nat Nanotechnol 2011;6:321−8.

[46] Menezes V, Malek A, Keelan JA. Nanoparticulate drug delivery in pregnancy: placental passage and fetal exposure. Curr Pharmaceut Biotechnol 2011;12:731−42.

[47] Zhang B, Liang R, Zheng M, Cai L, Fan X. Surface-functionalized nanoparticles as efficient tools in targeted therapy of pregnancy complications. Int J Med Sci 2019;20:3642.

[48] Solder E, Rohr I, Kremser C, Hutzler P, Debbage PL. Imaging of placental transport mechanisms. Eur J Obstet Gynecol Reprod Biol 2009;144:114−20.

[49] Bodurtha J, Strauss J. Genomics and perinatal care. N Engl J Med 2012;366:64−73.

[50] Alfirevic A, Alfirevic Z, Pirmohamed M. Pharmacogenetics in reproductive and perinatal medicine. Pharmacogenomics 2010;11:65−79.

[51] Gundacker C, Neesen J, Straka E, Ellinger I, Dolznig H, Hengstschlager. Genetics of the human placenta: implications for toxicokinetics. Arch Toxicol 2016;90:2563−81.

[52] Novakovic B, Saffery R. DNA methylation profiling highlights the unique nature of the human placental epigenome. Epigenomics 2010;2:627−38.

[53] Oliva K, Barker G, Riley C, Bailey MJ, Permezel M, Rice GE, Lappas M. The effect of pre-existing maternal obesity on the placental proteome: two dimensional difference gel electrophoresis coupled with mass spectrometry. J Mol Endocrinol 2012;48:139−49.

[54] Phillips TJ, Scott H, Menassa DA, Bignell AL, Sood A, Morton JS, et al. Treating the placenta to prevent adverse effects of gestational hypoxia on fetal brain development. Sci Rep 2017;7(1):9079.

Conducting randomized controlled pharmaceutical trials in the pregnant population: challenges and solutions

Isabelle Hardy, William D. Fraser

Department of Obstetrics and Gynecology, Université de Sherbrooke, Sherbrooke, QC, Canada

7.1 Introduction

The development of a new drug for use in humans classically follows a strict sequence, beginning with in-vitro and animal experiments to identify promising novel molecules, their sites of action, and biological effects. After efficacy and safety in animals is confirmed, three phases of human clinical trials need to be completed prior obtaining approval for use in clinical practice. Phase I studies are conducted with healthy volunteers and serve to establish the safety of the drug, its therapeutic range, and appropriate dosage. Phase II trials involve a limited number of participants and are conducted in precisely defined conditions to demonstrate drug efficacy in a carefully selected population. Phase III trials are large, usually multicenter trials, which include a broader population and serve to establish the effectiveness and safety of drugs, simulating usual clinical use. After commercialization, phase IV trials are used to document drug effectiveness and adverse events at the population level, or to investigate new dosages or indications [1]. The randomized controlled trial (RCT) is the gold standard for the evaluation of a new drug or technology, and is the design usually used for phase II and III trials.

This stepwise process is essential to ensuring the development and approval of new drugs which are both effective and safe. However, this process is difficult to apply to the development of drugs used in pregnant women. Indeed, due to the potential teratogenic effects of new drugs on the fetus, the ethical dilemma of knowing how much evidence is required to justify conducting a clinical trial including pregnant women has often led to the complete exclusion of this population from drug trials. Apart from data available in registries, there is little high-quality evidence on the innocuity and effectiveness of common medications in the pregnant population. Furthermore, few drugs are developed specifically to target obstetrical diseases, and the ones which are tested or repurposed for these indications often fail at the phase III trial level.

Clinical Pharmacology During Pregnancy. https://doi.org/10.1016/B978-0-12-818902-3.00018-X

This chapter will explore the specific considerations and challenges of conducting randomized controlled pharmaceutical trials in pregnant women and provide potential solutions to help safely include this population in future trials.

7.2 Ethical considerations

7.2.1 Maternal and fetal risks in pharmaceutical research

The most sensitive and controversial ethical aspect of pharmaceutical trials in the pregnant population is the risk of harm to the embryo or fetus. Historically, this risk has led to the systematic exclusion of pregnant women from pharmaceutical research [2]. Although the AIDS/HIV epidemic led to the recognition that all groups of the population should be offered inclusion in the studies of new medications which might benefit them [3], pregnant women are still vastly underrepresented in pharmaceutical trials [4]. The ethical considerations of clinical research in the pregnant population are discussed in detail in Chapter 8. A key point to consider in this endeavor is that pregnant women have agency. The National Institute of Health and the American College of Obstetrician and Gynecologists advocate that pregnant women should no longer be considered a vulnerable population, but rather a scientifically and ethically complex one [5,6]. Indeed, women who are pregnant retain their full agency and can decide independently whether or not they wish to take part in research. Furthermore, consent of the male partner is not necessary to the participation of women in a research project [6].

In 2018, the Food and Drug Administration (FDA) published a draft guidance document which may help direct research efforts in the pregnant population. This document outlines that pregnant women should be included in pharmaceutical trials of any medication that might benefit them, as long as there is sufficient evidence derived from animal studies and nonpregnant women to provide an estimate of the potential risks to the mother and fetus. Research in the pregnant population is deemed acceptable if: "The risk to the fetus is caused solely by interventions or procedures that hold out the prospect of direct benefit for the woman or the fetus; or, if there is no such prospect of benefit, the risk to the fetus is not greater than minimal and the purpose of the research is the development of important biomedical knowledge which cannot be obtained by any other means" [7].

The evolution of ethical considerations concerning the integration of pregnant women in research calls for their broader inclusion in pharmaceutical trials. Recent recommendations by the FDA provide a key impetus to both industry and the academic community to pursue clinical trials involving pregnant women.

7.2.2 Equipoise

Equipoise is an ethical standard that needs to be met to justify the conduct of any clinical trial. A more precise definition of equipoise has been proposed as "a state of genuine agnosticism or conflict in the expert medical community about the net preferred medically established procedure for the condition under study" [8]. A trial is warranted when there is "equipoise," that is when there is a reasonable uncertainty concerning the benefit of an experimental treatment over placebo or an existing treatment. This is a delicate balance between the presence of insufficient evidence to justify a trial (in which case more preliminary/elementary research is needed) and a state of overabundance where an additional trial would not be ethically acceptable. Physician-researchers and members of institutional review boards (IRBs) have the task of determining whether a trial will help resolve equipoise [8]. Different IRBs can disagree markedly on the same protocol as to their opinion on the presence or absence of equipoise [9]. This may reflect variations in the expertise of the members on the IRB, as well as the absence of guidelines regarding what is evidence of sufficient quality to justify a trial.

7.2.3 What is sufficient evidence to conduct a trial?

7.2.3.1 General considerations

In fact, the evidence required to justify the decision to conduct a phase III RCT in the area of maternal-fetal medicine has not been adequately defined. The hypothesis for a trial is normally based on an understanding of the impact of a drug on a specific disease process. The hypothesis should be supported both by in-vitro and animal studies [10]. There must be sufficient preliminary evidence from phase II trials to indicate that the treatment under investigation might improve patient outcomes in a clinically significant way, and that it is not harmful [11]. A phase III clinical trial is "warranted if there is sufficient but not definitive evidence that the intervention to be assessed would have a favorable risk-benefit ratio in the population to be enrolled" [9].

To determine this, the available evidence needs to be reviewed and assessed, usually through a systematic review. The proposed RCT must add to the existing knowledge base; thus, it is important to establish what information is missing from the current knowledge base so that the trial can be designed to fill these knowledge gaps. A thorough understanding of the available evidence is key to formulating the appropriate research question, in defining the target population, in estimating the effect size, and in assessing feasibility.

> *If available evidence is reliable and already provides a definitive answer, there is no need for a study, although there may be a need for a study in a specific target group or a larger study to refine therapeutic strategies or define optimal dosage* [12].

A methodological question arises as to what constitutes sufficient evidence to consider that a treatment is efficacious. If the effect estimate derived from a number of small trials shows statistical evidence of an effect, what conclusion should be drawn? Is an additional large RCT justified? This question is even more difficult to address given that studies have underlined the discrepancy between the findings of meta-analyses and the largest trials of the same therapy [13,14]. One important factor to consider when examining the results of a systematic review is the potential for publication bias. Indeed, clinical trials with significant findings are more likely to be published and are published faster than negative trials [15], and phase I and II trials are more likely to suffer from publication bias than phase III and IV trials [16]. This has the potential to lead to an overestimation of the effect of an intervention in meta-analyses of small randomized clinical trials. Therefore, when the efficacy of a treatment is established based on several small randomized clinical trials, a robust phase III RCT may still be warranted to confirm the treatment's effectiveness in a large population and to evaluate the presence of adverse events. Again, at least one large RCT showing positive results is generally required to obtain regulatory approval [17].

7.2.3.2 Level of evidence to justify a trial during public health crises

In the context of a public health emergency, special consideration must be given to the level of evidence required to justify a clinical trial that includes pregnant women. Indeed, when outbreaks of diseases threaten the lives of pregnant women and their unborn children, the level of evidence required to justify a clinical trial can be lowered. In this context, the potential benefits of each molecule targeting the disease must be carefully weighed against its potential risks. When sound biological rationale and animal studies indicate a potential benefit of a molecule against a lethal disease, consideration may be given to "short-circuiting" the drug development pipeline, and in such cases, it may be unethical to deprive any patient population from a potentially life-saving drug [3].

The best example of this approach is the rapid approval of zidovudine to prevent vertical transmission of HIV. In 1991, a multicenter RCT was launched in the United States and in France to evaluate the efficiency and safety of zidovudine. The study was based only on animal studies and Phase I evidence. The results showed that zidovudine lowered vertical transmission of HIV by two thirds when compared with placebo [18]. Based on the interim results of this study, the CDC recommended the use of zidovudine in pregnant women to prevent vertical transmission of HIV in August 1994, three months before the publication of the trial results [19].

The importance of including pregnant women in pharmaceutical trials of agents targeting lethal diseases is further supported by the example of the Ebola epidemic. During the 2013−2016 Ebola outbreak, pregnant women were excluded from all 16 randomized clinical trials of antiviral treatments or vaccines. Trial investigators justified their decision based on potential embryotoxicity and teratogenicity of the therapeutic agents. The case fatality rate of Ebola in pregnant women is 55%, and only one live birth from a pregnant woman infected with Ebola has ever been reported [20]. Excluding pregnant woman from pharmaceutical trials for a disease whose natural course is maternal and fetal death, based on the fear of causing fetal harm, is both absurd and unacceptable. Investigators have the ethical duty to ensure that pregnant women are given fair access to any trial of a pharmaceutical agent targeting a disease from which they might suffer [6]. In the case of deadly diseases, teratogenic potential alone is not a sufficient reason to preclude the inclusion of pregnant women in research.

Despite serious concerns raised by the scientific community [21,78−81], pregnant and lactating women have been almost systematically excluded from pharmaceutical research in the current covid-19 pandemic [77]. Pregnant women were excluded from phase III RCTs for all the commercially available vaccines [81]. With recent evidence showing increased risks of morbidity and mortality from covid-19 infection in pregnancy [82], this population has become eligible for vaccination in several countries (such as the United States of America, Canada and United Kingdom), but definitive evidence on efficacy and safety in pregnancy is lacking. Most strikingly, pregnant and lactating patients were even excluded from trials of agents known to be innocuous in pregnancy such as hydroxychloroquine and colchicine [22,78]. This situation highlights the need for public policies to mandate the inclusion of pregnant and lactating women in pharmaceutical trials.

7.2.4 Resource allocation in the context of limited research funding

Phase III trials are costly, and as such, the number that can be conducted is limited— far fewer than the number of current and potential treatment approaches that could be tested. When the scientific community gives the green light for a given trial, they are in some ways "saying no" to others, as funds are limited and not every clinical question warrants its own trial. This outlines the importance of evaluating every trial protocol thoroughly before authorizing it, to ensure that both equipoise and sufficient preliminary evidence are available to justify the trial. Trials that move forward should also be methodologically robust to ensure that they are feasible and that their results will be interpretable.

Indeed, negative trials have a variety of costs, including financial costs and the exposure of participants to the potential toxicity of unproven experimental treatments without associated benefits. Nevertheless, negative trials cannot be completely avoided, and they give us important information to abandon the use of ineffective therapies and to help direct future research [11].

7.3 Including pregnant women in pharmaceutical trials for nonobstetrical conditions

7.3.1 The dearth of evidence on the innocuity and efficiency of drugs in the pregnant population

Pregnant women have historically been excluded from pharmaceutical research, and as a result, limited Class I evidence is available on the safety and efficiency of common medications in pregnancy. In 2002, Lo and Friedman reported that more than 90% of the drugs approved by the FDA between 1980 and 2000 had unknown teratogenic potential [23]. This issue is still relevant today, as a 2013 study revealed that 95% of industry-sponsored phase IV pharmaceutical trials for treatment of diseases likely to affect pregnant women excluded this population [4]. This is particularly problematic as it has been estimated that 80% to 90% of women use at least one type of medication during pregnancy [24–27]. Thus, pregnant women are often prescribed medications which have not been adequately studied in this population, with lack of available data on adequate dosage in pregnancy, and on potential teratogenicity in humans. In addition, women now become pregnant at more advanced ages, and with more medical comorbidities than they did in the past [27,28]. The lack of evidence on the use of medications to treat chronic diseases places women at risk of receiving suboptimal treatment for their conditions during pregnancy [29], and of suffering from short- and long-term complications as a result.

7.3.2 Human pharmaceutical trials including pregnant women are required

To fill the knowledge gaps on the innocuity and efficiency of common drugs in the obstetrical population, rigorous human trials are required. While animal studies are an important first step in identifying the potential risks and teratogenic effects of a molecule [30], these data are insufficient to evaluate the full safety profiles of drugs [31]. Indeed, the translation of teratogenic effects between species is not entirely reliable [32]. This is best demonstrated by the example of thalidomide, which causes no specific teratogenic effects in mice, but produces significant limb reduction defects in humans [33]. Results from animal studies are also limited by the drug dosage used, which is not always comparable to the dosage human pregnant patients and their fetuses would be exposed to [32].

Studies are also needed to determine the best dose and the efficiency of medications in the pregnant population. Indeed, pregnancy causes several physiological changes which can significantly alter drug bioavailability and metabolism [34]. Drug dosage and efficiency cannot be extrapolated from studies in men and nonpregnant women and should be established based on pharmacokinetic studies, pharmacodynamic studies, and clinical trials conducted specifically in the pregnant population [35]. The placental passage of drugs also needs to be established in human subjects, and potential benefits or harm to the neonate need to be systematically compiled [34].

7.3.3 Strategies to include pregnant women in pharmaceutical trials for nonobstetrical conditions

7.3.3.1 Public policies to promote pharmaceutical trials in the pregnant population

While we have highlighted that clinical trials are needed to establish the safety profile, adequate dosage, and efficiency of common medications in pregnant women, the pharmaceutical industry is still reluctant to include pregnant women in pharmaceutical trials. Potential solutions can be found by examining the example of the pediatric population [36]. Similar to pregnant women, children and adolescents compose an ethically and scientifically complex population. Children constitute a vulnerable population and their physiology differs from that of adults, which can have impacts on pharmacokinetics and pharmacodynamics [37]. This complexity has led to a long-standing history of exclusion of pediatric patients from pharmaceutical trials [38]. In 1997, the FDA included an exclusivity incentive as part of the *Food and Drug Administration Modernization Act*. This incentive provides a six-month prolongation of patent protection and marketing exclusivity in exchange for conducting pharmaceutical studies in the pediatric population. In 2002, the *Best Pharmaceuticals for Children Act* allowed the NIH to sponsor clinical trials of off-patent drugs in the pediatric population. In 2003, the *Pediatric Research Equity Act* gave the FDA the authority to require pediatric drug studies for molecules likely to be used in the pediatric population [39]. These regulations have been permanently reauthorized as part of the *FDA Safety and Innovation Act* of 2012 and the *FDA Reauthorization Act of 2017* [39,40]. Since their inception, these regulations have substantially increased the amount of pharmaceutical research in the pediatric population and have led to labeling changes for more than 600 pharmaceutical agents [39]. This new body of evidence has led to safer use of medication in children, and has provided economic benefits both for the pharmaceutical industry and government [38]. Similar economical and legal incentives should be adopted to increase the inclusion of pregnant women in pharmaceutical research [41].

7.3.3.2 Innovative designs to determine the safety and efficiency of drugs in the pregnant population

To remedy some of the limitations of registries and case reports, researchers have proposed innovative study designs which allow fair inclusion of pregnant women in pharmaceutical research while optimizing the risk-benefit ratio.

In their 2018 article, Roes et al. proposed that phase I studies can be conducted in the pregnant population at the time of phase II or III study in the general population. This design ensures that specific safety, pharmacokinetic, and pharmacodynamic information can be obtained for pregnant patients, but only for drugs which have proven to be sufficiently safe in the general population. Phase III trials including pregnant participants can then be used to confirm adequate dosage and efficiency of the study drug. The authors propose the inclusion of pregnant women in phase III trials through two scenarios. If sufficient safety and efficacy data are already available, pregnant women can be included as a subpopulation of general phase III trials. If this information is not available at the time of study inception, an adaptive design can be put in place where pregnant women are only enrolled in the phase III trial after preliminary data analysis has confirmed drug efficacy in the general population. For drugs which have already been approved for use in the general population, the authors support the implementation of specific pregnancy phase I trials if observational data are insufficient to determine safety, with subsequent inclusion of pregnant women in postmarketing phase III RCTs to confirm adequate dosage and efficiency [42].

In 2015, Briggs et al. outlined a framework for the fair inclusion of reproductive age and pregnant women in phase IV clinical trials. This framework would apply to drugs likely to be used for acute or chronic conditions in women of child-bearing age, which have not been reported to pose teratogenic risks. They propose conducting of "postapproval" RCTs in a population comprising women of child-bearing age and pregnant women comparing the safety and efficiency of the study drug with that of current standard therapy [41].

These new adaptive designs could help fill the knowledge gaps on the use of medication in pregnancy, and in turn improve the quality and safety of care for pregnant women.

7.4 Improving the success of drug trials for obstetrical conditions

7.4.1 Drug development failures in obstetrics

Failure of a drug to complete the phased process of drug development is not uncommon, and a 2004 review revealed that only 11% of drugs developed between 1991 and 2000 had successfully completed this process. When comparing rates of "success"—from first in-human studies to drug approval, studies conducted in Women's Health had the lowest across sectors, at less than 5% [43]. This is even more concerning, as there are few drug trials conducted in pregnancy, representing only 0.32% of all active registered clinical trials in a 2016 review [44]. Only 7% of these studies were funded by the pharmaceutical industry, and only three new molecules under investigation had been developed specifically for a pregnancy indication [44]. A 2008 review of the Pharmaprojects database also revealed that only three drugs were under preclinical development for obstetrical conditions, five times less than were being studied for the rare disease amyotrophic lateral sclerosis [45].

Even when preclinical studies have been successfully completed and drugs show potential in early clinical studies, they often fail in phase III. In a 2016 review of two large pharmaceutical databases, 54% of agents failed at the phase III level. The most common identified reasons for failure were lack of efficacy and safety concerns, accounting for 57% and 17% of failures, respectively [46].

The scarcity of drug trials in obstetrics, the lack of industry investment, and the high risk of failure in drug development creates an urgent need to "get it right": to invest in the evaluation of treatments for which there is a high probability of success. This begs the question: Can reasons for the failure of seemingly promising pregnancy drug trials be identified? We posit that a better selection of target molecules, appropriate research questions and outcomes, and rigorous study designs can help increase the odds of successful drug trials in obstetrics.

7.4.2 The importance of biological rationale

The high costs of drug development with a perceived low return on investment and high legal risks in the field of obstetrics have resulted in the pharmaceutical industry developing few new drugs for obstetrical diseases [47]. Because of this, the process of "obstetrical drug development" is essentially "a repurposing" [48]. Nevertheless, novel treatments for conditions such as preterm birth and preeclampsia are urgently needed as these diseases are frequent and cause significant morbidities [44]. Whether novel molecules or repurposed ones are being evaluated, drug development in obstetrics should follow the same rigorous steps proposed in other fields, with added considerations unique to pregnancy [48]. Potential molecules should be identified based on a good understanding of disease processes and targeted mechanisms of action. Preclinical studies in animals will then serve to establish drug activity on disease processes in vivo, identify potential toxicity, and establish whether the drug traverses the placenta [47−50]. Only drugs which are shown to be both efficient and safe in animal models should be allowed to move on to early human testing. Phase I studies in pregnancy should serve to establish drug pharmacodynamics and pharmacokinetics, and to confirm potential transplacental passage of the target drug [48]. Only with strict compliance with these steps of development can we expect to lower the odds of failure at the time of human phase II and III clinical trials.

7.4.3 Using adequate design and outcomes in phase II trials

Testing the biological activity, dosage, and safety profile of the drug in question requires thoroughness. An important risk factor for failure in phase III is a phase II clinical trial that has not been done or that has been poorly conducted [50].

While single arm studies with historical controls have often been used in phase II, RCTs have become the norm for rigorous phase II evaluation programs [51]. This design limits selection bias and confounding factors, thus reducing the odds of overestimating treatment effects in phase II [52]. The goal of phase II trials is to determine if drug efficacy can be measured by a number of objective or subjective endpoints and how well this activity compares to that of a placebo or active control. The example of the drug atosiban, an oxytocin antagonist used for tocolysis in preterm labor, outlines the importance of choosing an adequate comparator. A multicenter RCT published in 2000 showed that compared to the beta-agonist ritodrine, atosiban had similar efficacy to prevent birth within 48 hours of admission [53]. However, a large RCT of ritodrine versus placebo published in 1992 had shown no benefit of ritodrine on perinatal mortality, prolongation of pregnancy to term, or birthweight [54]. As a result, atosiban was never approved in North America.

Determination of the most effective drug dose and the collection of information pertinent to the design of a phase III program are other goals of phase II studies. Safety remains a strong component of phase II programs. Serious toxicities may be observed for the first time in a phase II trial.

The choice of the primary outcome for phase II RCTs is critical. A good primary outcome is one that is objective, reproducible, related to the disease process, and relevant to patient health [55]. The biggest challenge in primary outcome selection for phase II is to choose a variable that either is a clinically relevant outcome, or is predictive of one, and for which changes can be detected within a limited population or time frame. Indeed, while phase II studies should help to reliably predict phase III success, they should not be as extensive or resource-consuming as the multicenter RCTs used in phase III. Potential solutions to this challenge are the use of surrogate endpoints.

Surrogate endpoints are variables which are involved in the causal pathway toward development of a disease. Identifying good surrogate outcomes is difficult because significant preliminary data must have demonstrated that "achievement of substantial effects on the surrogate endpoint reliably predicts achievement of clinically important effects on a clinically meaningful endpoint" [56]. For instance, viral load is a good surrogate for HIV studies because reducing viral load reliably leads to a reduced prevalence of AIDS. On the contrary, increased bone mineral density proved to be a poor surrogate outcome for osteoporotic fracture risk in studies of fluoride. Bone mass increases under fluoride treatment, but the bone also becomes brittle and is more prone to fractures [57]. These examples outline that while surrogate endpoints can be extremely useful, they should only be used when sufficient data are available to demonstrate that they reliably predict the outcome of clinical interest [56].

7.4.4 Calculating the sample size for phase III randomized controlled trials

Phase II trials are generally considered to be successful if a statistically significant difference in the primary outcome favoring the experimental treatment is identified. These results are used to justify moving on to phase III trials, and to help calculate their sample size [58]. Phase III trials impose great financial and human burdens, and as such important consideration must be given to trial logistics in order to increase the probability of obtaining informative results.

One key aspect to consider is the calculation of sample size. Estimating sample size requirement based on phase II trial results poses several challenges. First, the phase II primary outcome may not be the clinically relevant primary outcome used for the phase III trial. Secondly, the effect size estimated from a small population is imprecise and may lead to an overestimation of the treatment effect.

Lastly, phase III clinical trials include more diverse populations and treatment settings than phase II trials. All these factors lead to a potentially smaller treatment effects in phase III trials than in phase II [59,60].

Furthermore, phase III trials must be adequately powered to detect minimally important differences in clinically relevant outcomes [61]. For severe outcomes such as death, small differences between treatment groups can lead to changes in practice, and studies must have sufficient power to detect these changes [11]. For instance, in the SWEPIS RCT which compared induction of labor at 41 weeks with expectant management and induction of labor at 42 weeks, a 0.4% increase in perinatal mortality in the expectant management group led to early trial termination and a recommendation to induce labor at 41 weeks [62].

For all these reasons, sample sizes for phase III RCTs must be calculated conservatively. Potential solutions include using an alpha error of 2.5% and 90% power, adjusting the effect size estimate with Bayesian assurance or frequentist-conservatist estimation, or basing the effect size on the minimal clinically important difference rather than phase II estimates [60,63].

Poor recruitment or high-attrition rates may also be problematic, and dropout rates must be realistically estimated and accounted for in sample size calculation [59].

The use of conservative assumptions for the purpose of sample size calculation for phase III RCTs can therefore help lower the risk of failure of a drug at the phase III level because of type II error.

7.4.5 Integrating precision medicine in obstetrics

The explosion of knowledge in genetics, cell, and systems biology has completely changed our understanding of disease pathophysiology and treatment. Diseases which were once thought to be homogenous, such as cancer, can now be subdivided into subgroups based on genetic characteristics [64]. Precision medicine aims to delineate subpopulations of patients with a disease which share common characteristics—either social, clinical, genetic, microbiome profiles, or biomarkers—that make them more susceptible to respond to a given treatment. In breast cancer, for instance, patients whose tumor is human epidermal growth factor receptor 2 (HER-2) positive can receive the monoclonal antibody trastuzumab which directly targets the HER-2 protein and dramatically improves survival [65].

Despite the potential of precision medicine in several areas of medicine, development of targeted therapies by industry has been slow, with only 66 products in late-stage development in a 2013 study. More than 80% of these products had been developed for the treatment of cancer, and none targeted obstetrical diseases [66].

The development of precision medicine in obstetrics seems particularly promising, as many pathologies of pregnancy are clinically and biologically heterogeneous and do not respond well to treatment. This is the case for preterm birth and preeclampsia, which both have various clinical presentations and causes [67–70]. Further research will be required to delineate subpopulations of patients with these diseases, and to understand the precise physiopathology behind each clinical presentation [70–73]. Only with this knowledge, can we hope to make significant progress in the prevention and treatment of preterm birth and preeclampsia. While precision medicine has the potential to impact on the design of trials, there have been few obstetrical trials to date that have used genetic or biological markers or risk factors to select or to stratify participants.

7.4.6 The example of the antioxidant trials

The importance of sound biological rationale and of the choice of primary outcome in phase II trials is further supported by the failure of phase III clinical trials to demonstrate effectiveness of antioxidants in the prevention of preeclampsia.

Oxidative stress is believed to play a role in a number of clinical disorders in obstetrics, including preeclampsia, a major contributor to maternal mortality and maternal and perinatal morbidity. There is a substantial body of evidence linking oxidative stress to preeclampsia, although it remains uncertain whether this is a primary or a secondary phenomenon. In 1999, Chappell et al. reported the results of a phase II trial of the effects of the prophylactic administration of antioxidant vitamins C and E in pregnant women. Women with risk factors for preeclampsia were included in the trial, the most frequent being a positive screen on uterine artery Doppler. The trial was stopped before the full sample size could be achieved, as the proportion of women experiencing preeclampsia, as observed in an interim analysis, was reduced in the active treatment group. In fact, a biochemical indicator of endothelial dysfunction (PAI-1:PAI-2), and not preeclampsia, was the major endpoint of this phase II trial [73]. However, the relationship of this marker to clinical disease was unclear. Furthermore, at the time that the study was initiated, little information was available as to whether the doses of vitamin C and E administered were those most likely to produce an antioxidant effect. Thus, while the findings of this phase II study were encouraging, it suffered from those limitations that placed subsequent phase III studies at high risk of failure: absence of data on dose-finding, uncertain mechanism of action, and high risk of alpha error due to early stopping of the phase II trial. Subsequently, nine large multicenter trials, including patients at high risk of preeclampsia and those where nulliparity was the only identified risk factor, were conducted to assess the role of Vitamins C and E in the prevention of preeclampsia [74]. All yielded negative results. One of the trials was led by the senior author of the current chapter (WDF) and was stopped before recruitment was completed due to concerns raised in the intercurrent reporting of a separate trial about possible effects of the intervention on the risk of low birth weight [75]. Could this have been avoided? In retrospect, given the limitations of the initial phase II study, the most prudent approach might have been to simply attempt to replicate the findings using a rigorous design and predesigned stopping rules, while collecting more data on possible biological mechanisms. Or, at the very least, through international collaboration, could a single trial have been conducted rather than separate trials in Canada, the UK, the US, Australia, and Brazil? The decision to conduct phase III studies in such a context should be based on a cross disciplinary consensus, involving both basic scientists and clinical trialists. From a global perspective, in order to optimize the use of scarce resources, international expertise and collaboration should be brought to bear on prioritizing research questions, so that only studies meeting the most rigorous criteria at the phase II level are given priority for phase III research. The result of this "cumulative" failure has been that even those who have been longstanding leaders and supporters of clinical research in preeclampsia expressed a skepticism regarding the impact of large trials. "Thus for over a decade now, many large and expensive multicentre randomized trials have failed to show significant reductions in the incidence of preeclampsia, or, when positive results occurred, the significance was small and the number to treat large" [76].

7.5 **Summary**

Pregnant women should be considered for inclusion in the study of any pharmaceutical agent expected to provide important benefits in the treatment of a disease that affects reproductive age women. Exposing pregnant women and fetuses to new pharmaceutical agents is considered to be acceptable by the FDA if direct benefit to the woman or fetus is expected, and if enough preliminary evidence in animals or humans is available to anticipate potential risks. Prior to conducting a clinical trial, evidence must be carefully evaluated using systematic reviews that sufficiently take into account the potential for publication bias and type I error in individual studies. In the context of public health emergencies, it is acceptable to conduct a clinical trial with limited preliminary evidence.

Pregnant women are still widely excluded from pharmaceutical trials for diseases that affect reproductive aged women. Potential solutions to increase the inclusion of pregnant women in these trials include legal and financial incentives, and innovative study designs such as phase I pregnancy studies imbricated in phase II or III general population trials, and postmarketing phase III RCTs in the pregnant population.

Few molecules are developed specifically to treat obstetrical conditions, and many drugs fail to successfully complete the drug development process. To improve the success of pharmaceutical research in pregnancy, new or repurposed molecules should be selected based on a good comprehension of disease processes and on a specific mechanism of action. The drug development pipeline should be followed rigorously, and in-human phase I trials should only be realized after both safety and efficacy have been demonstrated in animal models. Phase II studies need to be carefully planned to increase the likelihood of success at the phase III level. These studies should be RCTs with an adequate comparator (placebo or standard treatment), the primary outcome should be objective and relevant—either the disorder itself or on a marker that has been confirmed to be part of disease pathophysiology, and the study should determine the dosage most likely to provide clinical benefit. To lower the risk of type II error in phase III studies, the sample size should be calculated conservatively to detect minimally clinically important differences in the primary outcome. Precision medicine appears as a promising solution to treat heterogeneous diseases such as prematurity and preeclampsia, as it allows to select the participants most likely to benefit from a given intervention.

Further collaboration between both basic science and clinical trial researchers across centers, as well as open dialog between all experts in the field could go a long way in optimizing the use of scarce resources in the area of obstetrical drug trials. For this reason, we urge all researchers active in this discipline to participate in evaluating and critiquing the studies published by their peers. Critical review of small or preliminary studies should make clear their merits and faults; this would undoubtedly aid in identifying promising avenues for further research and minimizing the risk for failure of any subsequent trials.

References

[1] Spilker B. Guide to drug development: a comprehensive review and assessment. Philadelphia: Wolters Kluwer Health/Lippincott Williams & Wilkins; 2009. p. 1277.

[2] White A. Accelerating the paradigm shift toward inclusion of pregnant women in drug research: ethical and regulatory considerations. Semin Perinatol November 2015;39(7): 537−40.

[3] Merkatz RB, Temple R, Sobel S, Feiden K, Kessler DA. Women in clinical trials of new drugs − A change in food and drug administration policy. N Engl J Med July 22, 1993; 329(4):292−6.

[4] Shields KE, Lyerly AD. Exclusion of pregnant women from industry-sponsored clinical trials. Obstet Gynecol November 2013;122(5):1077−81.

[5] Blehar MC, Spong C, Grady C, Goldkind SF, Sahin L, Clayton JA. Enrolling pregnant women: issues in clinical research. Wom Health Issues January 2013;23(1):e39−45.

[6] The American College of, Obstetricians and Gynecologists. Committee Opinion No. 646: ethical considerations for including women as research participants. Obstet Gynecol November 2015;126(5):e100−7.

[7] Pregnant FDA. Women: scientific and ethical considerations for inclusion in clinical trials guidance for industry, vol. 14; 2018.

[8] van der Graaf R, van Delden JJ. Equipoise should be amended, not abandoned. Clin Trials J Soc Clin Trials August 2011;8(4):408−16.

[9] Stark AR, Tyson JE, Hibberd PL. Variation among institutional review boards in evaluating the design of a multicenter randomized trial. J Perinatol March 2010;30(3): 163−9.

[10] Field D, Elbourne D. The randomized controlled trial. Curr Paediatr November 2004; 14(6):519−24.

[11] Strand M, Jobe AH. The multiple negative randomized controlled trials in perinatology—why? Semin Perinatol August 2003;27(4):343−50.

[12] Morley R, Farewell V. Methodological issues in randomized controlled trials. Semin Neonatol May 2000;5(2):141−8.

[13] Villar J, Carroli G, Belizán JM. Predictive ability of meta-analyses of randomised controlled trials. Lancet March 1995;345(8952):772−6.

[14] LeLorier J, Grégoire G, Benhaddad A, Lapierre J, Derderian F. Discrepancies between meta-analyses and subsequent large randomized, controlled trials. N Engl J Med August 21, 1997;337(8):536−42.

[15] Hopewell S, Loudon K, Clarke MJ, Oxman AD, Dickersin K. Publication bias in clinical trials due to statistical significance or direction of trial results. In: Cochrane Methodology Review Group, editor. Cochrane database syst rev; January 21, 2009 [Cited 2020 May 3]; Available from: http://doi.wiley.com/10.1002/14651858. MR000006.pub3.

[16] Hall R, de Antueno C, Webber A. Publication bias in the medical literature: a review by a Canadian research ethics board. Can J Anesth May 2007;54(5):380−8.

[17] Ciociola AA, Cohen LB, Kulkarni P, Kefalas C, Buchman A, Burke C, et al. How drugs are developed and approved by the FDA: current process and future directions. Am J Gastroenterol May 2014;109(5):620−3.

[18] Connor EM, Sperling RS, Gelber R, Kiselev P, Scott G, O'Sullivan MJ, et al. Reduction of maternal-infant transmission of human immunodeficiency virus type 1 with zidovudine treatment. N Engl J Med November 3, 1994;331(18):1173−80.

[19] CDC. Recommendations of the U.S. Public Health Service Task Force on the use of zidovudine to reduce perinatal transmission of human immunodeficiency virus. MMWR Recomm Rep Morb Mortal Wkly Rep Recomm Rep August 5, 1994;43(RR-11):1–20.

[20] Gomes MF, de la Fuente-Núñez V, Saxena A, Kuesel AC. Protected to death: systematic exclusion of pregnant women from Ebola virus disease trials. Reprod Health December 2017;14(S3):172.

[21] Buekens P, Alger J, Bréart G, Cafferata ML, Harville E, Tomasso G. A call for action for COVID-19 surveillance and research during pregnancy. Lancet Glob Health April 2020. https://doi.org/10.1016/S2214-109X(20)30206-0.

[22] Indraratna PL, Virk S, Gurram D, Day RO. Use of colchicine in pregnancy: a systematic review and meta-analysis. Rheumatology February 1, 2018;57(2):382–7.

[23] Lo W. Teratogenicity of recently introduced medications in human pregnancy. Obstet Gynecol September 2002;100(3):465–73.

[24] Lupattelli A, Spigset O, Twigg MJ, Zagorodnikova K, Mårdby AC, Moretti ME, et al. Medication use in pregnancy: a cross-sectional, multinational web-based study. BMJ Open February 2014;4(2):e004365.

[25] Mitchell AA, Gilboa SM, Werler MM, Kelley KE, Louik C, Hernández-Díaz S. Medication use during pregnancy, with particular focus on prescription drugs: 1976–2008. Am J Obstet Gynecol July 2011;205(1):51.e1–8.

[26] Bérard A, Abbas-Chorfa F, Kassai B, Vial T, Nguyen KA, Sheehy O, et al. The French Pregnancy Cohort: medication use during pregnancy in the French population. In: Lupattelli A, editor. PLos One. vol. 14; July 17, 2019. e0219095. 7.

[27] D'Alton ME, Bonanno CA, Berkowitz RL, Brown HL, Copel JA, Cunningham FG, et al. Putting the "M" back in maternal–fetal medicine. Am J Obstet Gynecol June 2013;208(6):442–8.

[28] Hirshberg A, Srinivas SK. Epidemiology of maternal morbidity and mortality. Semin Perinatol October 2017;41(6):332–7.

[29] Morgan MA, Cragan JD, Goldenberg RL, Rasmussen SA, Schulkin J. Management of prescription and nonprescription drug use during pregnancy. J Matern Fetal Neonatal Med August 2010;23(8):813–9.

[30] Scialli AR. Animal studies and human risk. Reprod Toxicol November 1993;7(6):533–4.

[31] Friedman JM. How do we know if an exposure is actually teratogenic in humans? Am J Med Genet C Semin Med Genet August 15, 2011;157(3):170–4.

[32] Brent RL. Utilization of animal studies to determine the effects and human risks of environmental toxicants (drugs, chemicals, and physical agents). Pediatrics April 2004; 113(4 Suppl. l):984–95.

[33] Kim JH, Scialli AR. Thalidomide: the tragedy of birth defects and the effective treatment of disease. Toxicol Sci July 2011;122(1):1–6.

[34] Sheffield JS, Siegel D, Mirochnick M, Heine RP, Nguyen C, Bergman KL, et al. Designing drug trials: considerations for pregnant women. Clin Infect Dis December 15, 2014;59(Suppl. 1_7):S437–44.

[35] Pariente G, Leibson T, Carls A, Adams-Webber T, Ito S, Koren G. Pregnancy-associated changes in pharmacokinetics: a systematic review. In: Chappell LC, editor. PLOS Med. vol. 13; November 1, 2016. e1002160. 11.

[36] Ren Z, Zajicek A. Review of the Best Pharmaceuticals for Children Act and the Pediatric Research Equity Act: what can the obstetric community learn from the pediatric experience? Semin Perinatol November 2015;39(7):530–1.

[37] Rivera DR, Hartzema AG. Pediatric exclusivity: evolving legislation and novel complexities within pediatric therapeutic development. Ann Pharmacother March 2014; 48(3):369−79.

[38] Vernon JA, Shortenhaus SH, Mayer MH, Allen AJ, Golec JH. Measuring the patient health, societal and economic benefits of US pediatric therapeutics legislation. Pediatr Drugs October 2012;14(5):283−94.

[39] Califf RM. Best Pharmaceuticals for Children Act and Pediatric Research Equity Act. July 2016 status report to Congress. Department of Health and Human Services Food and Drug Administration; July 2016.

[40] Walden G. FDA Reauthorization Act of 2017. Law No: 115−52 Aug 18, 2017.

[41] Briggs GG, Polifka JE, Wisner KL, Gervais E, Miller RK, Berard A, et al. Should pregnant women be included in phase IV clinical drug trials? Am J Obstet Gynecol December 2015;213(6):810−5.

[42] Roes KCB, van der Zande ISE, van Smeden M, van der Graaf R. Towards an appropriate framework to facilitate responsible inclusion of pregnant women in drug development programs. Trials December 2018;19(1):123.

[43] Kola I, Landis J. Can the pharmaceutical industry reduce attrition rates? Nat Rev Drug Discov August 2004;3(8):711−6.

[44] Scaffidi J, Mol B, Keelan J. The pregnant women as a drug orphan: a global survey of registered clinical trials of pharmacological interventions in pregnancy. BJOG Int J Obstet Gynaecol January 2017;124(1):132−40.

[45] Fisk NM, Atun R. Market failure and the poverty of new drugs in maternal health. PLoS Med January 22, 2008;5(1):e22.

[46] Hwang TJ, Carpenter D, Lauffenburger JC, Wang B, Franklin JM, Kesselheim AS. Failure of investigational drugs in late-stage clinical development and publication of trial results. JAMA Intern Med December 1, 2016;176(12):1826.

[47] David A, Thornton S, Sutcliffe A, Williams P. Developing new pharmaceutical treatments for obstetric conditions. R Coll Obstet Gynaecol Guidel May 2015;50.

[48] Malek A, Mattison DR. Drug development for use during pregnancy: impact of the placenta. Expet Rev Obstet Gynecol July 2010;5(4):437−54.

[49] Chappell LC, David AL. Improving the pipeline for developing and testing pharmacological treatments in pregnancy. PLoS Med November 1, 2016;13(11):e1002161.

[50] Addeo A, Weiss GJ, Gyawali B. Association of industry and academic sponsorship with negative phase 3 oncology trials and reported outcomes on participant survival: a pooled analysis. JAMA Netw Open May 10, 2019;2(5):e193684.

[51] Seymour L, Ivy SP, Sargent D, Spriggs D, Baker L, Rubinstein L, et al. The design of phase II clinical trials testing cancer therapeutics: consensus recommendations from the clinical trial design task force of the national cancer Institute investigational drug steering committee. Clin Cancer Res March 15, 2010;16(6):1764−9.

[52] Sharma MR, Stadler WM, Ratain MJ. Randomized phase II trials: a long-term investment with promising returns. JNCI J Natl Cancer Inst July 20, 2011;103(14):1093−100.

[53] Moutquin J-M, Sherman D, Cohen H, Mohide PT, Hochner-Celnikier D, Fejgin M, et al. Double-blind, randomized, controlled trial of atosiban and ritodrine in the treatment of preterm labor: a multicenter effectiveness and safety study. Am J Obstet Gynecol May 2000;182(5):1191−9.

[54] The Canadian Preterm Labor Investigators Group. Treatment of preterm labor with the beta-adrenergic agonist ritodrine. N Engl J Med July 30, 1992;327(5):308−12.

[55] Sherman M. Design and endpoints of clinical trials, current and future. Dig Dis Sci April 2019;64(4):1050—7.

[56] Fleming TR, Powers JH. Biomarkers and surrogate endpoints in clinical trials. Stat Med November 10, 2012;31(25):2973—84.

[57] Grimes DA, Schulz KF. Surrogate end points in clinical research: hazardous to your health. Obstet Gynecol May 2005;105(5, Part 1):1114—8.

[58] Götte H, Schüler A, Kirchner M, Kieser M. Sample size planning for phase II trials based on success probabilities for phase III. Pharmaceut Stat November 2015;14(6): 515—24.

[59] Wang S-J, Hung HMJ, O'Neill RT. Adapting the sample size planning of a phase III trial based on phase II data. Pharmaceut Stat April 2006;5(2):85—97.

[60] De Martini D. Empowering phase II clinical trials to reduce phase III failures. Pharmaceut Stat May 2020;19(3):178—86.

[61] Tarnow-Mordi W, Cruz M, Morris J. Design and conduct of a large obstetric or neonatal randomized controlled trial. Semin Fetal Neonatal Med December 2015;20(6): 389—402.

[62] Wennerholm U-B, Saltvedt S, Wessberg A, Alkmark M, Bergh C, Wendel SB, et al. Induction of labour at 41 weeks versus expectant management and induction of labour at 42 weeks (Swedish Post-term Induction Study, SWEPIS): multicentre, open label, randomised, superiority trial. BMJ November 20, 2019:l6131.

[63] King MT. A point of minimal important difference (MID): a critique of terminology and methods. Expert Rev Pharmacoecon Outcomes Res April 2011;11(2):171—84.

[64] Precision medicine. Health Aff May 2018;37(5):688—9.

[65] König IR, Fuchs O, Hansen G, von Mutius E, Kopp MV. What is precision medicine? Eur Respir J October 2017;50(4):1700391.

[66] Milne C-P, Garafalo S, Bryan C, McKiernan M. Personalized medicines in late-stage development. Nat Rev Drug Discov May 2014;13(5):324—5.

[67] Newnham JP, Kemp MW, White SW, Arrese CA, Hart RJ, Keelan JA [Cited 2020 May 27]. Applying precision public health to prevent preterm birth. Front public health [Internet], vol. 5; April 4, 2017. Available from: http://journal.frontiersin.org/article/10.3389/fpubh.2017.00066/full.

[68] Quinney SK, Patil AS, Flockhart DA. Is personalized medicine achievable in obstetrics? Semin Perinatol December 2014;38(8):534—40.

[69] Luizon MR, Palei AC, Cavalli RC, Sandrim VC. Pharmacogenetics in the treatment of pre-eclampsia: current findings, challenges and perspectives. Pharmacogenomics April 2017;18(6):571—83.

[70] Burris HH, Wright CJ, Kirpalani H, Collins Jr JW, Lorch SA, Elovitz MA, et al. The promise and pitfalls of precision medicine to resolve black—white racial disparities in preterm birth. Pediatr Res January 2020;87(2):221—6.

[71] Eidem HR, Ackerman WE, McGary KL, Abbot P, Rokas A. Gestational tissue transcriptomics in term and preterm human pregnancies: a systematic review and meta-analysis. BMC Med Genom December 2015;8(1):27.

[72] Gao Q, Tang J, Li N, Liu B, Zhang M, Sun M, et al. What is precise pathophysiology in development of hypertension in pregnancy? Precision medicine requires precise physiology and pathophysiology. Drug Discov Today February 2018;23(2):286—99.

[73] Chappell LC, Seed PT, Briley AL, Kelly FJ, Lee R, Hunt BJ, et al. Effect of antioxidants on the occurrence of pre-eclampsia in women at increased risk: a randomised trial. Lancet September 1999;354(9181):810—6.

[74] Rumbold A, Duley L, Crowther CA, Haslam RR. Antioxidants for preventing pre-eclampsia. In: Cochrane Pregnancy and Childbirth GROUP, editor. Cochrane database syst rev [Internet]; January 23, 2008 [Cited 2020 May 18]; Available from: http://doi.wiley.com/10.1002/14651858.CD004227.pub3.

[75] Fraser WD, Audibert F, Bujold E, Leduc L, Xu H, Boulvain M, et al. The vitamin E debate: implications for ongoing trials of pre-eclampsia prevention. BJOG Int J Obstet Gynaecol June 2005;112(6):684−8.

[76] Lindheimer MD, Sibai BM. Antioxidant supplementation in pre-eclampsia. Lancet April 2006;367(9517):1119−20.

[77] Whitehead CL, Walker SP. Consider pregnancy in COVID-19 therapeutic drug and vaccine trials. The Lancet 2020 May;395(10237):e92.−22.

[78] Dashraath P, Nielsen-Saines K, Madhi SA, Baud D. COVID-19 vaccines and neglected pregnancy. The Lancet 2020 Sep;396(10252):e22.

[79] Heath PT, Le Doare K, Khalil A. Inclusion of pregnant women in COVID-19 vaccine development. Lancet Infect Dis 2020 Sep;20(9):1007−8.

[80] Klein SL, Creisher PS, Burd I. COVID-19 vaccine testing in pregnant females is necessary. J Clin Invest 2021 Mar;1131(5):e147553.

[81] Rasmussen SA, Kelley CF, Horton JP, Jamieson DJ. Coronavirus Disease 2019 (COVID-19) Vaccines and Pregnancy: What Obstetricians Need to Know. Obstet Gynecol. 2021 Mar;137(3):408−14.

[82] Villar J, Ariff S, Gunier RB, Thiruvengadam R, Rauch S, Kholin A, et al. Maternal and Neonatal Morbidity and Mortality Among Pregnant Women With and Without COVID-19 Infection: The INTERCOVID Multinational Cohort Study. JAMA Pediatr [Internet]. 2021 Apr 22 [cited 2021 Jun 17]; Available from: https://jamanetwork.com/journals/jamapediatrics/fullarticle/2779182.

Pharmacogenomics in pregnancy*

8

David M. Haas, Jennifer L. Grasch, David A. Flockhart

Indiana University School of Medicine, Indianapolis, IN, United States

8.1 Pharmacogenomics

If it were not for the great variability among individuals, medicine might as well be a science and not an art.

Sir William Osler (1892).

While much drug development and many clinical practice guidelines do not directly address variability in drug response, and in many cases assume that the effects of drugs on patients can generally be predicted, the evidence indicates otherwise. Significant numbers of patients do not respond to many medications, and adverse events that accompany drug therapy often compromise the quality of life of patients, limiting compliance with therapy, and can even be fatal in rare circumstances. The reasons for this variability in drug response often lie in easily accessible clinical factors including disease severity, age, weight, gender, ethnicity, or drug–drug interactions. Other factors may also be important, however, and in situations where readily available clinical predictors such as these are inadequate, alternative biomarkers of drug response can be used. In many situations the need for new biomarkers is urgent, perhaps most clearly in the case of diseases such as psychiatric disease or cancer, where considerable morbidity is incurred when therapy is ineffective or impossibly toxic for individual patients.

While improved efficacy is clearly a goal of the new era of "personalized medicine" heralded by the development of increasingly sophisticated new biomarkers of drug response, the occurrence of unanticipated adverse effects is also of great concern. It is clear that considerable damage is done to the public health by such adverse events. In one of the largest studies of in-hospital morbidity published to date, the incidence of serious adverse drug reactions (ADRs) was 6.7%, of fatal ADRs was 0.32%, and it was estimated that of 2 million patients, 216,000 experienced serious ADRs and over 100,000 had fatal ADRs in 1 year, making these reactions between the fourth and sixth leading cause of death [1]. The cost was

---

* We wish to thank and recognize Dr. David A. Flockhart's contribution to the original version of this chapter and for his continued inspiration of advancing pharmacogenomics and individualized pharmacotherapy in pregnancy even after his passing.

Clinical Pharmacology During Pregnancy. https://doi.org/10.1016/B978-0-12-818902-3.00001-4

estimated at more than 100 billion dollars per year in 1994. Even with advances in alerts, electronic records, and other safety checks, it is estimated that ADRs cause an increase of over $5 billion to US health-care payers from injectable drugs alone [2]. It follows that biomarkers that can *predict*, and also *prevent* adverse events, would also be of great potential value.

Biomarkers of drug response in clinical practice are far from new. Tests such as the international normalized ratio (INR) used to monitor warfarin response, the presence of estrogen or progesterone receptors on breast tumors used to guide anti-estrogenic therapy, and the testing of patients with HIV or hepatitis C for viral loads are all a routine part of daily practice that health-care professionals have become comfortable with. We have learned that clinically useful biomarkers of drug response are of most value in situations where there is great variability in response, and a clear clinical decision, such as a change in drug, dose, or therapeutic approach, results from a test. It is equally clear that a test must have iterative value over existing easily available clinical predictors in order to be useful. For example, a test designed to predict the efficacy of an antihypertensive agent that had less predictive ability than routine measurement of blood pressure would be of little value.

The advent of genomics has brought a series of powerful new tools to this predictive science. While proteomics and metabolomics show great promise, it is with germline genomics, the study of the genetic sequence that we inherit from our parents, that we have the most experience. There are a number of reasons why the science of pharmacogenetics (or pharmacogenomics) appears valuable in this context. Not least among these are the simple facts that DNA is very stable and easy to amplify, and that there exists a map of the human genome and of the international hapmap (http://www.genome.gov/10001688). In addition, the cost of DNA testing continues to drop dramatically.

While many definitions of the differences between the science of pharmacogenetics and that of pharmacogenomics have been put forward, a useful distinction appears to be simply that "pharmacogenetics" refers to the study of individual candidate genes, while "pharmacogenomics" refers to the study of whole pathways of genes, and indeed the entire genome.

8.2 Genetics and polymorphisms

Genetic variation in the sequence of about 3 billion nucleotide pairs that make up our DNA comes in many forms, but the most common differences between people are in the form of single-nucleotide polymorphisms (SNPs). These are single letter nucleotide changes and they are referred to as a "polymorphism" if they occur in 1% or more of the population. This is because variants that are that common tend to be stably present in a given population, whereas variants present at less than 1% tend to drift out. There are 12–15 million of such variants, and they have been meticulously cataloged by the Human Genome Project in the publicly available database called dbSNP (http://www.ncbi.nlm.nih.gov/projects/SNP/). Since SNPs are the most common and easily accessible form of variability, they form the basis of the first genome-wide association studies (GWASs) testing that has been used to test for associations between common variants in the genome and nearly every form of human pathology (http://www.genome.gov/gwastudies/).

Other important forms of variation include deletions and insertions of sequence, variable number tandem repeats of short sequences that are clustered together and oriented in the same direction [3], and copy number variation: regions of the sequence that are copied with high fidelity within the genome itself. It has been estimated that such regions constitute up to 12% of the entire sequence in the genome [4].

Since only about 1.5% of the human genome sequence is used for the ~24,000 genes that code for proteins in humans, we presume that not all of it is relevant to therapeutic response, and that not all of this variability has functional or clinically meaningful consequence. That said, large numbers of variants that influence function via "nonsynonymous" changes in coding SNPs (cSNPs) have been found, and a growing number of functionally important variants in intronic and regulatory regions have also been identified [5].

The use of GWASs to identify new genetic associations between SNPs and drug response has begun and already a significant number of important discoveries have resulted. These include the discovery of the SLC transporter with the muscle toxicity incurred by the use of the statin class of drugs [6], and of a gene in the IL-17 pathway with the musculoskeletal toxicity associated with the use of aromatase inhibitors in patients with breast cancer [7]. It is widely appreciated that a large number of new patterns of multiple genetic associations will result from this effort [8], such that tests that involve large numbers of variants organized into a predictive pattern will become commonplace. The use of such predictive patterns is already commonplace in breast cancer, where arrays that test for 20−100 RNA species in a tumor at once are routinely used to predict the value of chemotherapy in individual patients [9]. Additionally, there has been exciting work at implementing CPAC-recommended pharmacogenetic information related to treatments into health record problem lists to help guide clinicians [10].

Within this large field of research, our understanding of genetic factors that affect drug disposition far exceeds our understanding of the factors affecting response. This is in part because pharmacokinetic changes are relatively easy to measure whereas the "phenotype" of overall drug response is more complex. In addition, cloning of most drug-metabolizing enzymes and drug transport proteins within the past 20 years combined with the genetic polymorphism information generated by the sequencing of the human genome and cataloged in dbSNP have allowed a comprehensive characterization of variability in drug metabolism and transport. As the practice of searching for, identifying, and then using determined genetic characteristics as predictors of drug effect becomes more common, it is clear that the entire community of health-care providers—physicians, pharmacists, and nurses—will have to play an increasing role as the value of carefully defined, valuable clinical phenotypes and their individual genetic and genomic associations increases.

8.3 Genes that influence pharmacokinetic variability

It is well recognized that pharmacokinetic variability is most apparent for drugs that are metabolized, and that the majority of this variability is in turn due to inconsistencies in the ability of enzymes in the liver and gastrointestinal tract to carry out drug metabolism. A growing body of literature also makes clear that differences in the activity of drug transporters in the kidney, blood−brain barrier, liver, and at the level of individual tissues between people contribute significantly to pharmacokinetic variability [11].

In terms of metabolic variation, the key enzymes involved include the cytochrome P450 family of drug-metabolizing enzymes that carry out phase I drug metabolism. Phase II enzymes, including the enzymes that carry out acetylation, glucuronidation, sulfation, methylation, and the addition of glutathione, are also important as they increase the solubility of hydrophobic small molecules, and catalyze their removal from the body. Genetic variation in many of these pathway enzymes contribute to drug concentrations and effects [12].

The first genetic associations with drug therapy observed were those involving glucose-6-phosphate dehydrogenase (G6PDH) and sulfa drugs in African American soldiers, and in N-acetyl transferase in patients taking isoniazid for tuberculosis. Since then, 50 years of research on drugs metabolized by the cytochrome P450 enzymes has clearly documented CYP2B6, CYP2C9, CYP2D6, CYP2C19, and CYP3A5 as the most important enzymes that exhibit important genetic alterations (https://cpicpgx.org/guidelines/).

Cytochrome 2B6 is the primary metabolic route for the metabolism of drugs used in the treatment of HIV, including the NNRTIs (nonnucleoside reverse transcriptase inhibitors), nevirapine, and efavirenz [13], but also contributes importantly to the metabolism of methadone [14], cyclophosphamide [15], and ketamine [16]. The enzyme has reduced function in patients who carry the *6 allele [13], and this variant has been associated with reduced rates of metabolism, and higher concentrations of all these drugs.

CYP2C9 is widely recognized as the principal enzyme involved in the clearance of the active S-enantiomer of warfarin. Genetic variants that notably reduce activity result in higher S-warfarin concentrations and in turn lower required warfarin doses, and this effect was obvious even when a GWAS testing thousands of genes was carried out as identified [17].

CYP2D6 is the most studied of the genetically variable cytochrome P450 enzymes. This is one of the most highly polymorphic CYP enzymes, with over 100 allelic variants and subvariants identified [18]. Variants that result in complete "knockout" or loss of enzyme activity are present in 7% of Caucasian populations, and in 2%−5% of African and Asian populations [19]. In addition, the *10 allelic variants that decreases but does not eliminate activity is present in more than 40% of Asians, and similarly the *17 alleles reduces activity in 10%−20% of Africans [19]. These polymorphisms result in clinically important changes in the metabolism of ∼20% of drugs including codeine [20], tamoxifen [21], a large number of the beta-blocker class of drugs that are metabolized, and the majority of clinically available antidepressants, including fluoxetine, paroxetine, and venlafaxine. Changes in the concentrations of these drugs and their metabolites brought about by CYP2D6 genetic variability have been intensely investigated [22], and those with venlafaxine appear to be sufficient to result in clinically significant changes and recommendations for dosing changes [23]. A notable example of genetic variation within the CYP2D6 gene is the presence of copy number variation, such that up to 13 copies of the entire gene have been shown to exist in some families, and to be passed down through the generations in a Mendelian manner [24].

CYP2C19 is also genetically variable, with loss-of-function variants designated as *2 and *3 that are present in 15%−30% of Asian populations, and 2%−5% of Caucasians and Africans. While a large number of drugs are metabolized by this enzyme [25], it is the dominant route for the metabolism of clopidogrel to its active metabolite, and this has resulted in a huge amount of attention because of the widespread use of this drug in cardiology. Pharmacogenetic variability in CYP2C19 has been associated with alterations in platelet function during clopidogrel therapy [26] that has been clearly associated with cardiovascular outcomes in a large number of studies [27].

Important variations in the genetics of CYP3A5 that influence concentrations of vincristine [28], cyclosporine, tacrolimus [29], and notably of nifedipine used in tocolysis [30] have been described. These variants associate with higher concentrations of the parent drugs and can result in clinically significant toxicities.

While these genes represent some of those most studied among pharmacogenetic "VIP" genes, recent results of GWASs and targeted approaches across a wide range of genes involved in the specific diseases have resulted in the development of clinical tests. An easily accessible catalog of such genes has been collected by the Pharmacogenetics and Genomics Knowledge Base (PharmGKB) at www.pharmgkb.org. These tests can be utilized in a CPIC guidance-informed panel to help with clinical care [10].

8.4 The current state of pharmacogenetic testing

Pharmacogenetic testing has the potential to aid in the diagnosis and treatment of multiple conditions. A recent explosion of commercially marketed tests has surfaced, often with direct-to-consumer marketing. In fact, as of June 2020, CPIC had specific guidance information for 127 unique genes related to 240 unique drugs (cpicpgx.org/genes-drugs/). Table 8.1 displays drugs noted to have required or recommended testing. An additional 125 drugs had either "actionable" or "informative" pharmacogenetic data (cpicpgx.org/genes-drugs).

Several pharmacogenetic tests have risen to become standard of care in medical therapy. Patients with colon cancer are often treated with anti−epidermal growth factor receptor (anti-EGFR) monoclonal antibody therapy in the form of cetuximab. A mutation in the KRAS gene codon 12 or 13 leads to resistance to cetuximab

Table 8.1 Fifteen drugs/therapies and their available required or recommended pharmacogenetic tests as of June 2020.

Drug/therapy	Test
Abacavir[a]	HLA-B*5701
Ivacaftor[a]	CTFR
Carbamazepine[a]	HLA-B*1502
Carglumic acid[a]	NAGS
Clopidogrel	CYP2C19
Divalproex sodium[a] and valproic acid[a]	POLG
Eliglustat[a]	CYP2D6
Oxcarbazepine	HLA-B
Pegloticase[a]	G6PD
Pimozide[a]	CYP2D6
Primaquine[a]	G6PD
Azathioprine and mercaptopurine	TPMT, NUDT15
Rasburicase[a]	G6PD
Siponimod[a]	CYP2C9
Tafenoquine[a]	G6PD
Terbenazine[a]	CYP2D6
Thioguanine	TPMT, NUDT15
Velaglucerase alfa[a]	GBA

Other commonly used drugs with actionable pharmacogenetic information: warfarin, clopidogrel, peginterferon, tamoxifen, clozapine, 5-fluorouracil, venlafaxine, escitalopram, citalopram, carvedilol, chloroquine, flibanserin, duloxetine, metoclopramide, esomeprazole, glipizide, norfloxacin, nitrofurantoin, phenytoin, tramadol, and codeine. Full list available from CPIC website: cpicpgx.org/genes-drug.
[a] *Standard of care per the CPIC guidelines requires testing before giving the drug.*

therapy [31]. Thus, the American Society of Clinical Oncology (ASCO) has recommended that all patients with metastatic colorectal carcinoma who are candidates for anti-EGFR therapy should have their tumor tested for KRAS mutations. If codon 12 or 13 mutations are detected, then the patients should not receive anti-EGFR therapy as part of their treatment [31].

The cutaneous adverse drug reaction Stevens–Johnson syndrome (SJS) is a serious concern for people taking drugs such as abacavir and carbamazepine [32,33]. Pharmacogenetic screening for the HLA-B*5701 can help identify those who are most at risk for developing this severe adverse drug reaction with abacavir. Carriers of this HLA-B allele should not be given abacavir. This test is now widely used for screening patients in need of abacavir to avoid SJS in the developed world [34]. In addition, HLA-B*1502 testing is becoming standard of care for Asians prescribed carbamazepine to avoid severe cutaneous drug reactions [32].

For those with chronic myelogenous leukemia, imatinib inhibits the BCR-ABL-activated tyrosine kinase, interrupting signal transduction pathways that would otherwise lead to leukemic transformation. In this way, imatinib has led to impressive survival benefits in these patients [35]. However, a mutation in the BCR-ABL gene negates the benefits of imatinib. As imatinib is an expensive therapy, pharmacogenetic testing is employed in this scenario to avoid prescribing a costly therapy that would not be as beneficial in patients with the mutation.

Commercially available pharmacogenetic testing panels such as Oncotype Dx and MammaPrint have been promoted for women about to undergo chemotherapy for breast cancer [36,37]. ASCO and other organizations have included some of these tests in their guidelines as options to predict benefit, particularly from tamoxifen therapy [38]. These are examples of commercially available tests that are not yet standard of care recommendations. Other tests that similarly have data supporting their potential role for individualizing therapy are the CYP2D6 testing for tamoxifen [39,40] or venlafaxine [23], CYP2C19 testing for clopidogrel antiplatelet therapy [27], and CYP2C9 and VKCoR testing for those starting warfarin therapy [41−43].

Other tests are available for different conditions and/or drug therapies. With the advent of new pharmacogenetic tests, pharmacogenetic modeling strategies, and the need for individualized pharmacotherapy to avoid adverse events, pharmacogenetic testing continues to expand, with multiple vendors and labs advertising direct to consumers.

8.5 Potential therapeutic areas for pharmacogenomics in pregnancy

Most pregnant women take drugs for various conditions. Epidemiologic studies have documented that over 90% of pregnant women take a prescription drug, with most taking more than one [44−46]. Even after eliminating prenatal vitamins and supplemental iron, over 70% of pregnant women take a prescription drug during the course of their pregnancies [45,46]. Polypharmacy, defined as taking at least five drugs, is also common in pregnancy [46]. Many of the drugs commonly consumed by pregnant women are potential candidates for pharmacogenetic testing. Based on the drug metabolism pathway or receptors that serve as targets, pregnancy therapeutics may be a ripe area for pharmacogenetics.

As the cause of the majority of neonatal morbidity and mortality, preterm labor is a major focus of obstetric care and research. Two specific pharmacogenetic studies in preterm birth prevention using progestins have been published. One of the studies demonstrated that response to progestin, specifically 17-OHPC, had some variability based on genotype [47]. In fact, women in certain groups with certain haplotypes actually had higher rates of preterm birth when they received 17-OHPC. If replicated, this could have implications for identifying women who might actually be harmed by this preventive therapy. The use of tocolytic medications to stop uterine contractions is commonplace but of varying success [48]. Many tocolytics are substrates for polymorphic drug-metabolizing enzymes. Nifedipine is a calcium channel blocker commonly used in obstetrics to stop contraction and delay birth [49].

Nifedipine is metabolized by the CYP3A family. Recent studies have documented that CYP3A5 polymorphisms and concomitant use of known CYP3A inhibitors can impact the concentration of nifedipine in maternal blood [30]. Another potential pharmacogenetic target in preterm labor therapy includes indomethacin. Indomethacin, a nonsteroidal antiinflammatory drug used to inhibit contractions, is metabolized by the polymorphic CYP2C9 and CYP2C19 [50]. SNPs in these enzymes can affect the concentrations of these tocolytics. As these two drugs may be the better first-line agents for preterm labor [51], these pharmacogenetic implications should be further interrogated. Additionally related to preterm birth, women at risk for preterm delivery are given antenatal corticosteroids to improve neonatal outcomes. Preliminary investigations have documented that for women receiving betamethasone for this indication, some maternal and fetal SNP variants in CYP3A5 and CYP3A7 were associated with differences in neonatal respiratory outcomes [52,53]. Thus, there may be key genetic variants in betamethasone metabolic and response pathways that may aid in understanding variability in newborn outcomes after preterm birth.

Depression is common in pregnant women. The selective serotonin reuptake inhibitors (SSRIs) are the first-line agents to treat depression and other mood disorders in pregnancy. The SSRI drugs are metabolized by many different polymorphic enzymes (Table 8.2). Depression is commonly noted to be undertreated in pregnancy. It is possible that some of the undertreatment may be due to the combination of pregnancy physiology impacting the drug concentration, as well as pharmacogenetic polymorphism causing reduced drug concentrations. The impact of SNPs in these enzymes on the effectiveness of SSRI therapy is an area of active investigation [54,55].

Nausea and vomiting of pregnancy (NVP) affects up to 80% of pregnant women [56,57]. Both mild and severe cases of NVP have a significant impact on the quality of a woman's life and contribute significantly to health-care costs and time lost from work [57,58]. Many antiemetic drugs are used with various mechanisms of action to

Table 8.2 Drug-metabolizing enzymes for SSRIs.

Drug	Enzymes responsible for metabolism
Fluoxetine (Prozac)	CYP2D6, CYP2C9
Sertraline (Zoloft)	CYP2D6, CYP2C9, CYP2b́, CYP2C19, CYP3A4
Venlafaxine (Effexor)	CYP2D6
Paroxetine (Paxil)	CYP2D6
Fluvoxamine (Luvox)	CYP1A2
Bupropion (Wellbutrin, Zyban)[a]	CYP2B6
Citalopram (Celexa)	CYP3A4, CYP2C19
Escitalopram (Lexapro)	CYP3A4, CYP2C19
Duloxetine (Cymbalta, Irenka)	CYP2D6

[a] Bupropion is not an SSRI but rather a serotonin–norepinephrine reuptake inhibitor.

counter NVP. These include vitamin B6, doxylamine, promethazine, metoclopramide, and ondansetron to name a few. Learning from anesthesia research, emesis and the effectiveness of antiemetic drugs are potential pharmacogenetic targets. Ondansetron is metabolized by CYP2D6. Extensive and ultrarapid CYP2D6 metabolizers have been linked to ondansetron failure [59]. Also, the polymorphic serotonin receptor 5HT3 facilitates the role of serotonin as a mediator of nausea and vomiting [60]. Variants in the 5-HT3B receptor are linked to increased nausea and vomiting due to increased response to serotonin binding [61]. 5HT3 receptor variants are also associated with the severity of NVP (personal communication, data from our center). Thus, it is possible that identifying women with receptor variants with NVP may lead providers to utilize different medication to control a woman's NVP. The individualized treatment of NVP using pharmacogenetics is also an area of investigation.

Hypertension and preeclampsia are common complications of pregnancy. The use of antihypertensive drugs during the antenatal and delivery time frame is crucial given these complications contribution to maternal mortality and morbidity [62]. Multiple drugs are used to control hypertension in pregnancy. However, there are few pharmacogenetic studies regarding the response to antihypertensive drugs during pregnancy. Some genes have been shown to associate with overall drug response but less with individual drug responses [63]. As more pregnant women have genotypes available, further investigation into this area should follow.

These are just a few of the areas of drug therapy in pregnancy where pharmacogenetics may play a role [55,64–66]. As obstetrics moves into the genomics era, active pharmacogenetic research to help individualize therapy is ongoing. Maximizing the benefit for the mother and minimizing the risks to both the mother and fetus are the tenets of individualized pharmacotherapy. With both a mother and fetus to consider, optimizing therapeutics in pregnancy is pivotal. As a tool, pharmacogenetics may provide insights to help achieve maximal benefit with minimal risk.

8.6 Study designs and approaches to pharmacogenetics trials

Gathering quality trial data in pharmacogenetics is often difficult. Genetic testing is expensive and new SNPs are discovered frequently. However, there are key components of pharmacogenetic analyses that can help propel the field forward.

In general, analyses of trials focus on the mean changes in outcome measures of two or more groups. The outliers are often eliminated or statistically compensated for. However, in the field of pharmacogenetics, it is often those same outliers, the subjects in the tails of the bell-shaped curve, who are the most important to analyze. The subjects who have the most robust response to a drug or the poorest response to a drug are often the ones who may have a genetic polymorphism in the metabolic or receptor pathway that is causing this. For instance, for subjects who receive no benefit from a drug may have an SNP in an enzyme like CYP2D6 that makes them an ultrarapid metabolizer, and thus not enough drug is available to achieve the desired effect. In that case, knowing the CYP2D6 status ahead of time could lead to either increased dose or choice of a different drug.

Prospectively obtaining genotype information in a randomized clinical trial setting is difficult logistically. While genotyping costs are decreasing, the approach to genotyping needs to be considered. Assaying for particular candidate pathway genes may be efficient but could miss a key contributor. Using genome-wide association assays or full DNA sequencing may be too expensive and give extraneous data. In addition, these become analytically complex. Using a pathway-informed GWASs approach may be a practical way to limit the data needed and improve the efficiency of using the information.

Because of the expense and time needed to genotype a screening population for entry into a trial, newer adaptive trial designs have been utilized to make mid-study adjustments [67]. These adjustments may be based on genotypes. For instance, halfway through a drug trial, the subjects in the study could be genotyped in a batch to save on cost. Then an interim analysis might indicate that subjects with a certain SNP did not benefit at all at current doses. An adaptive trial design can then allow for dose adjustments for subjects with those SNPs for the remainder of the trial. In this way, adaptive trial designs can improve the efficiency of trials, allowing researchers to demonstrate effectiveness or ineffectiveness sooner, improving subject safety and yielding substantial time and cost savings [67].

As pharmacogenetic studies become more prevalent and the cost of genotyping is reduced, clinical trials of individualized pharmacotherapy will become more common. Upfront genotyping and stratified randomization based on genotyping are beginning to appear in studies. In these ways, pharmacogenomics is emerging as an increasingly important tool that will be available for providers in the future for individualizing drug therapy.

References

[1] Lazarou J, Pomeranz BH, Corey PN. Incidence of adverse drug reactions in hospitalized patients: a meta-analysis of prospective studies. Jama 1998;279(15):1200−5.

[2] Lahue BJ, Pyenson B, Iwasaki K, Blumen HE, Forray S, Rothschild JM. National burden of preventable adverse drug events associated with inpatient injectable medications: healthcare and medical professional liability costs. Am Health Drug Benefits 2012;5(7):1−10.

[3] Naslund K, Saetre P, von Salome J, Bergstrom TF, Jareborg N, Jazin E. Genome-wide prediction of human VNTRs. Genomics 2005;85(1):24−35.

[4] Sebat J, Lakshmi B, Troge J, Alexander J, Young J, Lundin P, et al. Large-scale copy number polymorphism in the human genome. Science 2004;305(5683):525−8.

[5] Wang L, Weinshilboum RM. Pharmacogenomics: candidate gene identification, functional validation and mechanisms. Hum Mol Genet 2008;17(R2):R174−9.

[6] Voora D, Shah SH, Spasojevic I, Ali S, Reed CR, Salisbury BA, et al. The SLCO1B1*5 genetic variant is associated with statin-induced side effects. J Am Coll Cardiol 2009; 54(17):1609—16.

[7] Ingle JN, Schaid DJ, Goss PE, Liu M, Mushiroda T, Chapman JA, et al. Genome-wide associations and functional genomic studies of musculoskeletal adverse events in women receiving aromatase inhibitors. J Clin Oncol 2010;28(31):4674—82.

[8] Motsinger-Reif AA, Jorgenson E, Relling MV, Kroetz DL, Weinshilboum R, Cox NJ, et al. Genome-wide association studies in pharmacogenomics: successes and lessons. Pharmacogenet. Genomics 2013;23(8):383—94.

[9] van't Veer LJ, Bernards R. Enabling personalized cancer medicine through analysis of gene-expression patterns. Nature 2008;452(7187):564—70.

[10] Eadon MT, Desta Z, Levy KD, Decker BS, Pierson RC, Pratt VM, et al. Implementation of a pharmacogenomics consult service to support the INGENIOUS trial. Clin Pharmacol Ther 2016;100(1):63—6.

[11] Cropp CD, Yee SW, Giacomini KM. Genetic variation in drug transporters in ethnic populations. Clin Pharmacol Ther 2008;84(3):412—6.

[12] Crettol S, Petrovic N, Murray M. Pharmacogenetics of phase I and phase II drug metabolism. Curr Pharmaceut Des 2010;16(2):204—19.

[13] Ward BA, Gorski JC, Jones DR, Hall SD, Flockhart DA, Desta Z. The cytochrome P450 2B6 (CYP2B6) is the main catalyst of efavirenz primary and secondary metabolism: implication for HIV/AIDS therapy and utility of efavirenz as a substrate marker of CYP2B6 catalytic activity. J Pharmacol Exp Therapeut 2003;306(1):287—300.

[14] Totah RA, Sheffels P, Roberts T, Whittington D, Thummel K, Kharasch ED. Role of CYP2B6 in stereoselective human methadone metabolism. Anesthesiology 2008; 108(3):363—74.

[15] Takada K, Arefayene M, Desta Z, Yarboro CH, Boumpas DT, Balow JE, et al. Cytochrome P450 pharmacogenetics as a predictor of toxicity and clinical response to pulse cyclophosphamide in lupus nephritis. Arthritis Rheum 2004;50(7):2202—10.

[16] Yanagihara Y, Kariya S, Ohtani M, Uchino K, Aoyama T, Yamamura Y, et al. Involvement of CYP2B6 in n-demethylation of ketamine in human liver microsomes. Drug Metab Dispos 2001;29(6):887—90.

[17] Cooper GM, Johnson JA, Langaee TY, Feng H, Stanaway IB, Schwarz UI, et al. A genome-wide scan for common genetic variants with a large influence on warfarin maintenance dose. Blood 2008;112(4):1022—7.

[18] Del Tredici AL, Malhotra A, Dedek M, Espin F, Roach D, Zhu G-D, et al. Frequency of CYP2D6 alleles including structural variants in the United States. Front Pharmacol 2018;9:305.

[19] Bernard S, Neville KA, Nguyen AT, Flockhart DA. Interethnic differences in genetic polymorphisms of CYP2D6 in the U.S. population: clinical implications. Oncol 2006;11(2):126—35.

[20] Caraco Y, Sheller J, Wood AJ. Pharmacogenetic determination of the effects of codeine and prediction of drug interactions. J Pharmacol Exp Therapeut 1996;278(3):1165—74.

[21] Jin Y, Desta Z, Stearns V, Ward B, Ho H, Lee KH, et al. CYP2D6 genotype, antidepressant use, and tamoxifen metabolism during adjuvant breast cancer treatment. J Natl Cancer Inst 2005;97(1):30—9.

[22] Preskorn SH. Pharmacogenomics, informatics, and individual drug therapy in psychiatry: past, present and future. J Psychopharmacol 2006;20(4 Suppl. l):85—94.

[23] Lobello KW, Preskorn SH, Guico-Pabia CJ, Jiang Q, Paul J, Nichols AI, et al. Cytochrome P450 2D6 phenotype predicts antidepressant efficacy of venlafaxine: a secondary analysis of 4 studies in major depressive disorder. J Clin Psychiatr 2010;71(11): 1482−7.

[24] Ingelman-Sundberg M, Sim SC, Gomez A, Rodriguez-Antona C. Influence of cytochrome P450 polymorphisms on drug therapies: pharmacogenetic, pharmacoepigenetic and clinical aspects. Pharmacol Ther 2007;116(3):496−526.

[25] Desta Z, Zhao X, Shin JG, Flockhart DA. Clinical significance of the cytochrome P450 2C19 genetic polymorphism. Clin Pharmacokinet 2002;41(12):913−58.

[26] Beitelshees AL, Horenstein RB, Vesely MR, Mehra MR, Shuldiner AR. Pharmacogenetics and clopidogrel response in patients undergoing percutaneous coronary interventions. Clin Pharmacol Ther 2011;89(3):455−9.

[27] Scott SA, Sangkuhl K, Gardner EE, Stein CM, Hulot JS, Johnson JA, et al. Clinical pharmacogenetics implementation consortium guidelines for cytochrome P450-2C19 (CYP2C19) genotype and clopidogrel therapy. Clin Pharmacol Ther 2011;90(2): 328−32.

[28] Egbelakin A, Ferguson MJ, MacGill EA, Lehmann AS, Topletz AR, Quinney SK, et al. Increased risk of vincristine neurotoxicity associated with low CYP3A5 expression genotype in children with acute lymphoblastic leukemia. Pediatr Blood Cancer 2011; 56(3):361−7.

[29] Ferraris JR, Argibay PF, Costa L, Jimenez G, Coccia PA, Ghezzi LF, et al. Influence of CYP3A5 polymorphism on tacrolimus maintenance doses and serum levels after renal transplantation: age dependency and pharmacological interaction with steroids. Pediatr Transplant 2011;15(5):525−32.

[30] Haas DM, Quinney SK, McCormick CL, Jones DR, Renbarger JL. A pilot study of the impact of genotype on nifedipine pharmacokinetics when used as a tocolytic. J Matern Fetal Neonatal Med 2012;25(4):419−23.

[31] Allegra CJ, Jessup JM, Somerfield MR, Hamilton SR, Hammond EH, Hayes DF, et al. American Society of Clinical Oncology provisional clinical opinion: testing for KRAS gene mutations in patients with metastatic colorectal carcinoma to predict response to anti-epidermal growth factor receptor monoclonal antibody therapy. J Clin Oncol 2009; 27(12):2091−6.

[32] Aihara M. Pharmacogenetics of cutaneous adverse drug reactions. J Dermatol 2011; 38(3):246−54.

[33] Chung W-H, Hung S-I, Chen Y-T. Human leukocyte antigens and drug hypersensitivity. Curr Opin Allergy Clin Immunol 2007;7(4):317−23.

[34] Phillips EJ, Mallal SA. Pharmacogenetics of drug hypersensitivity. Pharmacogenomics 2010;11(7):973−87.

[35] Peterson C. Drug therapy of cancer. Eur J Clin Pharmacol 2011;67(5):437−47.

[36] Chen E, Tong KB, Malin JL. Cost-effectiveness of 70-gene MammaPrint signature in node-negative breast cancer. Am J Manag Care 2010;16(12):e333−42.

[37] Mook S, Van't Veer LJ, Rutgers EJ, Piccart-Gebhart MJ, Cardoso F. Individualization of therapy using Mammaprint: from development to the MINDACT Trial. Cancer Genomics Proteomics 2007;4(3):147−55.

[38] Harris L, Fritsche H, Mennel R, Norton L, Ravdin P, Taube S, et al. American Society of Clinical Oncology 2007 update of recommendations for the use of tumor markers in breast cancer. J Clin Oncol 2007;25(33):5287−312.

[39] Borges S, Desta Z, Jin Y, Faouzi A, Robarge JD, Philips S, et al. Composite functional genetic and comedication CYP2D6 activity score in predicting tamoxifen drug exposure among breast cancer patients. J Clin Pharmacol 2010;50(4):450−8.

[40] Higgins MJ, Rae JM, Flockhart DA, Hayes DF, Stearns V. Pharmacogenetics of tamoxifen: who should undergo CYP2D6 genetic testing? J Natl Compr Cancer Netw 2009; 7(2):203−13.

[41] Grossniklaus D. Testing of VKORC1 and CYP2C9 alleles to guide warfarin dosing. Test category: pharmacogenomic (treatment). PLoS Curr 2010;2.

[42] Moreau C, Pautas E, Gouin-Thibault I, Golmard JL, Mahe I, Mulot C, et al. Predicting the warfarin maintenance dose in elderly inpatients at treatment initiation: accuracy of dosing algorithms incorporating or not VKORC1/CYP2C9 genotypes. J Thromb Haemostasis 2011;9(4):711−8.

[43] Zambon CF, Pengo V, Padrini R, Basso D, Schiavon S, Fogar P, et al. VKORC1, CYP2C9 and CYP4F2 genetic-based algorithm for warfarin dosing: an Italian retrospective study. Pharmacogenomics 2011;12(1):15−25.

[44] Glover DD, Amonkar M, Rybeck BF, Tracy TS. Prescription, over-the-counter, and herbal medicine use in a rural, obstetric population. Am J Obstet Gynecol 2003; 188(4):1039−45.

[45] Refuerzo JS, Blackwell SC, Sokol RJ, Lajeunesse L, Firchau K, Kruger M, et al. Use of over-the-counter medications and herbal remedies in pregnancy. Am J Perinatol 2005; 22(6):321−4.

[46] Haas DM, Marsh DJ, Dang DT, Parker CB, Wing DA, Simhan HN, et al. Prescription and other medication use in pregnancy. Obstet Gynecol 2018;131(5):789−98.

[47] Manuck TA, Lai Y, Meis PJ, Dombrowski MP, Sibai B, Spong CY, et al. Progesterone receptor polymorphisms and clinical response to 17-alpha-hydroxyprogesterone caproate. Am J Obstet Gynecol 2011;205(2):135.e1−9.

[48] ACOG practice bulletin. Management of preterm labor. Number 43, May 2003. Obstet Gynecol 2003;101:1039−47.

[49] Haas DM, Caldwell DM, Kirkpatrick P, McIntosh JJ, Welton NJ. Tocolytic therapy for preterm delivery: systematic review and network meta-analysis. BMJ 2012;345:e6226.

[50] Nakajima M, Inoue T, Shimada N, Tokudome S, Yamamoto T, Kuroiwa Y. Cytochrome P450 2C9 catalyzes indomethacin O-demethylation in human liver microsomes. Drug Metab Dispos 1998;26(3):261−6.

[51] Haas DM, Imperiale TF, Kirkpatrick PR, Klein RW, Zollinger TW, Golichowski AM. Tocolytic therapy: a meta-analysis and decision analysis. Obstet Gynecol 2009; 113(3):585−94.

[52] Haas DM, Dantzer J, Lehmann AS, Philips S, Skaar TC, McCormick CL, et al. The impact of glucocorticoid polymorphisms on markers of neonatal respiratory disease after antenatal betamethasone administration. Am J Obstet Gynecol 2013;208(3): 215.e1−6.

[53] Haas DM, Lai D, Sharma S, Then J, Kho A, Flockhart DA, et al. Steroid pathway genes and neonatal respiratory distress after betamethasone use in anticipated preterm birth. Reprod Sci 2016;23(5):680−6.

[54] Porcelli S, Drago A, Fabbri C, Gibiino S, Calati R, Serretti A. Pharmacogenetics of antidepressant response. J Psychiatry Neurosci 2011;36(2):87−113.

[55] Haas DM, Hebert MF, Soldin OP, Flockhart DA, Madadi P, Nocon JJ, et al. Pharmacotherapy and pregnancy: highlights from the second international conference for individualized pharmacotherapy in pregnancy. Clin Transl Sci 2009;2(6):439−43.

[56] Emelianova S, Mazzotta P, Einarson A, Koren G. Prevalence and severity of nausea and vomiting of pregnancy and effect of vitamin supplementation. Clin Invest Med 1999; 22(3):106−10.

[57] Mazzotta P, Maltepe C, Navioz Y, Magee LA, Koren G. Attitudes, management and consequences of nausea and vomiting of pregnancy in the United States and Canada. Int J Gynaecol Obstet 2000;70(3):359−65.

[58] Mazzotta P, Stewart D, Atanackovic G, Koren G, Magee LA. Psychosocial morbidity among women with nausea and vomiting of pregnancy: prevalence and association with anti-emetic therapy. J Psychosom Obstet Gynaecol 2000;21(3):129−36.

[59] Candiotti KA, Birnbach DJ, Lubarsky DA, Nhuch F, Kamat A, Koch WH, et al. The impact of pharmacogenomics on postoperative nausea and vomiting: do CYP2D6 allele copy number and polymorphisms affect the success or failure of ondansetron prophylaxis? Anesthesiology 2005;102(3):543−9.

[60] Andrews PL, Bhandari P. The 5-hydroxytryptamine receptor antagonists as antiemetics: preclinical evaluation and mechanism of action. Eur J Cancer 1993;29A(Suppl. 1): S11−6.

[61] Krzywkowski K, Davies PA, Feinberg-Zadek PL, Brauner-Osborne H, Jensen AA. High-frequency HTR3B variant associated with major depression dramatically aug-ments the signaling of the human 5-HT3AB receptor. Proc Natl Acad Sci U S A 2008;105(2):722−7.

[62] Hypertension in pregnancy. Report of the American College of Obstetricians and Gynecologists' Task Force on Hypertension in Pregnancy. Obstet Gynecol 2013; 122(5):1122−31.

[63] Luizon MR, Palei AC, Cavalli RC, Sandrim VC. Pharmacogenetics in the treatment of pre-eclampsia: current findings, challenges and perspectives. Pharmacogenomics 2017; 18(6):571−83.

[64] Haas DM, Gallauresi B, Shields K, Zeitlin D, Clark SM, Hebert MF, et al. Pharmaco-therapy and pregnancy: highlights from the third international conference for individu-alized pharmacotherapy in pregnancy. Clin Transl Sci 2011;4(3):204−9.

[65] Haas DM, Renbarger JL, Denne S, Ahmed MS, Easterling TR, Feibus K, et al. Pharma-cotherapy and pregnancy: highlights from the first international conference for individ-ualized pharmacotherapy in pregnancy. Clin Transl Sci 2009;2(1):11−4.

[66] Manuck TA. Pharmacogenomics of preterm birth prevention and treatment. BJOG 2016;123(3):368−75.

[67] Cirulli J, McMillian WD, Saba M, Stenehjem D. Adaptive trial design: its growing role in clinical research and implications for pharmacists. Am J Health Syst Pharm 2011; 68(9):807−13.

Anesthetic drugs

Harry Soljak, Sarah Armstrong
Frimley Park Hospital, Surrey, United Kingdom

9.1 Introduction

The challenges of general and regional anesthesia in pregnancy are to optimize maternal physiological function, preserve uteroplacental blood flow and oxygen delivery while avoiding unwanted effects of fetal exposure to drugs.

The likelihood of maternal and fetal exposure to anesthetic drugs is not insignificant. Current evidence suggests that between 1% and 2% of pregnant women will undergo a nonobstetric surgical procedure during pregnancy in developed nations [1]. If absolutely necessary, surgery should be delayed to the second trimester of pregnancy to reduce the risk of both teratogenicity and miscarriage, although there is currently no firm evidence to support this approach. Elective surgery and therefore anesthesia should be avoided in pregnancy if at all possible. Postnatally, surgery should ideally take place only after the first six postpartum weeks to allow resolution of the physiological changes of pregnancy. Emergency surgery must proceed regardless of gestational age in order to preserve the life of the mother with the possible adverse effects to the fetus included in the consent process.

At delivery, intervention rates involving the use of general or local anesthetics vary widely across the world. Overall epidural rates (including operative delivery and labor analgesia) are as high as 95% in some regions in the United States. There is also an increasing overall rate of caesarean delivery worldwide, with the Dominican Republic delivering 58.1% of babies via cesarean section [2]. The increasing incidence of these procedures means more women are exposed to anesthetic drugs. For cesarean delivery, regional anesthesia is preferred where possible as it minimizes the risks associated with general anesthesia including pulmonary aspiration of gastric contents, failed intubation, inappropriate maternal awareness, maternal gastric ileus postoperatively, and fetal exposure to drugs. No studies have shown a beneficial effect on the outcome of pregnancy after regional anesthesia compared to general anesthesia. Before the initiation of any anesthetic technique, resuscitation facilities should be available for both mother and fetus.

Clinical Pharmacology During Pregnancy. https://doi.org/10.1016/B978-0-12-818902-3.00020-8

9.2 General anesthesia

General anesthetics may be divided into intravenous (IV) and inhaled volatile anesthetics. Indications for general anesthesia in pregnancy are listed in Table 9.1 and include urgency of delivery due to maternal or fetal indications, or operative delivery where regional anesthesia is not appropriate. As stated in other chapters, pharmacokinetic and pharmacodynamic profiles are altered in pregnancy and drugs for general anesthesia should be titrated as a result.

The uteroplacental circulation is not autoregulated and so fetal perfusion is critically dependent on maternal systolic driving pressure. Hypotension in general anesthesia is common. This is due to the combination of decreased systemic vascular resistance in pregnancy due to progesterone, which is exacerbated by volatile or IV anesthetic agents, and aortocaval compression from the gravid uterus. This is further exacerbated if the patient is in the supine position. Obstetric patients after the first trimester should undergo general anesthesia in the supine position with 15° left lateral tilt to reduce aortocaval compression. Meticulous attention should be paid to the maintenance of maternal systolic blood pressure through the use of IV fluids and vasopressors to ensure adequate placental flow.

9.3 Inhalational anesthetics

The minimum alveolar concentration (MAC) of volatile agents is a term used to describe the potency of anesthetic vapors. It is defined as the concentration that prevents movement in response to skin incision in 50% of unpremedicated subjects studied at sea level (1 atm), in 100% oxygen. Hence, it is inversely related to potency, and the more potent the agent, the lower the MAC value.

Although it is more than 160 years since the first use of modern anesthetics, the mechanism of action of volatile anesthetics still remains elusive [3]. Inhaled anesthetic agents act in different ways at the level of the central nervous system with pre- and postsynaptic effects found. They may disrupt synaptic transmission by interfering with the release of excitatory or inhibitory neurotransmitters from the presynaptic nerve terminal, by altering the reuptake of neurotransmitters or by changing the binding of neurotransmitters to the postsynaptic receptor sites [4]. There is a high correlation between lipid solubility and anesthetic potency

Table 9.1 Indications for general anesthesia in pregnancy.

- Maternal disease/trauma requiring emergency surgery unsuitable for regional technique
- Urgent delivery of fetus (fetal or maternal threat)
- Maternal refusal of regional techniques
- Contraindications to regional technique (e.g., coagulopathy, local, or systemic infection)
- Failed or inadequate regional technique
- Delivery if at risk of obstetric major hemorrhage (e.g., placenta praevia or accreta)

suggesting inhalational anesthetics have a hydrophobic site of action and direct interaction with the neuronal plasma membrane is likely.

In pregnancy, neural tissues show increased sensitivity to effects of volatile anesthetics. The MAC is reduced by 30% under the influence of progesterone and endogenous endorphins [5,6]. The 25% increased alveolar minute volume from the first trimester [caused by both increases in respiratory rate (by 15%) and tidal volume (by 40%)] leads to a more rapid induction of general anesthesia than in the nonpregnant population if an inhalational induction technique were to be used. In most cases of general anesthesia in the parturient, preoxygenation with 100% oxygen precedes rapid sequence IV induction with cricoid pressure to secure the airway and to reduce the likelihood of pulmonary aspiration. This is followed by maintenance with 0.5—1.0 MAC of volatile anesthetic agents in either an air/oxygen or nitrous oxide/oxygen mix. Nitrous oxide has a rapid alveolar uptake and remains an important adjunct to reduce the risk of awareness during emergency cesarean delivery. Nitrous oxide, if administered in high concentrations for long periods (more than 50% concentration for over 24 h), has been shown to be a weak teratogen in rodents. Studies voicing concerns regarding nitrous oxide teratogenicity are not supported in clinical practice to date [7]. Insufficient general anesthesia or analgesia may cause awareness and substantial maternal catecholamine release which is generally considered to be more detrimental to the fetus. Awareness during cesarean section is much more likely than during other procedures. The fifth National Audit Project (NAP5) in the United Kingdom found an incidence of awareness of 1:670 during cesarean section compared to 1:20,000 for all procedures combined [8].

The high lipid solubility and low-molecular weight of all commonly used volatile anesthetics (isoflurane, sevoflurane, and desflurane) facilitate rapid transfer across the uteroplacental unit to the fetus. Prolonged induction to delivery time has been shown to result in lower Apgar scores in the fetus [9]. Low doses of volatile anesthetics in combination with nitrous oxide may improve uterine blood flow but may also induce uterine relaxation. After the fetus is delivered, increasing concentrations of nitrous oxide, systemic opioids and IV oxytocin may be used to reduce the amount of volatile anesthetic required and to encourage uterine contraction. Nitrous oxide is poorly soluble and may be eliminated from the blood into the alveoli very rapidly. This effectively dilutes alveolar air, and available oxygen, so that when room air is inspired hypoxia may result. This "diffusion hypoxia" may occur in the neonate after delivery and so it would seem prudent to administer supplemental oxygen to any neonate exposed to high concentrations of nitrous oxide immediately before delivery [10].

9.4 Intravenous anesthetics

Rapid sequence induction (RSI) is the administration of a potent IV anesthetic agent to induce unconsciousness followed by a rapidly acting neuromuscular blocking agent to achieve motor paralysis for tracheal intubation. The choice and dose of

IV induction agent is crucial to ensure a balance between excellent intubating conditions with minimal maternal recall, and high maternal blood concentrations with subsequent adverse maternal haemodynamic effects and fetal transfer. The lipophilic characteristics of IV anesthetic agents enhance their transfer across the placenta.

9.4.1 Thiopentone

Thiopentone is the most extensively studied IV anesthetic agent and has been shown to be safe in obstetric patients. It is administered in a dose of 3—7 mg/kg with 4 mg/kg being generally agreed to be unlikely to lead to fetal depression, while doses in excess of 7 mg/kg are liable to do so [11]. Thiopentone rapidly crosses the placenta and has been detected in umbilical venous blood within 30 seconds of administration. However, as a result of rapid equilibration in the fetus, thiopentone does not produce fetal neuronal levels high enough to sedate the neonate. Approximately 80% of thiopentone is protein-bound, and both maternal-fetal and fetomaternal transfer is strongly influenced by maternal and fetal protein concentrations. High fetal/maternal ratios suggest that thiopentone is freely diffusible but many factors must be involved in placental transfer as demonstrated by a wide intersubject variability in umbilical cord concentrations at delivery [12]. Thiopentone does however have some significant disadvantages. It has been linked to maternal deaths during cesarean section when dosing has been inappropriately high. This has been most commonly attributed to precalculated doses being used when the anesthetist has underestimated the severity of hypotension or cardiovascular compromise in emergency situations [13]. It requires reconstituting, a process that can take time and is an unwanted delay in an emergency situation. Another disadvantage is that once reconstituted, it looks very similar to antibiotics commonly used in cesarean section. The similarity of the two drugs in syringes has been seen as a contributing factor to administration errors at the time of induction [14].

9.4.2 Propofol

Propofol is the most widely used drug in general anesthesia and produces a rapid, smooth induction. It attenuates the cardiovascular response to laryngoscopy and intubation more effectively than thiopentone resulting in a more cardiovascular stable induction and intubation [15]. Increased maternal blood flow increases placental tissue uptake and facilitates rapid transfer of propofol across the placenta [16]. It is highly protein-bound and so placental transfer may be increased by reduced protein concentrations in the maternal blood. Some studies have shown that propofol use may result in lower Apgar scores when compared to thiopentone even at lower doses where maternal awareness is a distinct possibility. As a result there are currently no major clinical advantages to its use over thiopentone in pregnancy [17]. However, propofol is the agent used most commonly by anesthetists outside of obstetrics. This familiarity with the drug, and now relative inexperience using thiopentone may mean that junior anesthetists are more comfortable using propofol instead of thiopentone for induction of general anesthetic in the obstetric population. These factors along with the disadvantages of thiopentone mentioned above mean that there is now growing momentum toward a shift to propofol for obstetric general anesthetics [18].

9.4.3 Ketamine

This phencyclidine derivative is used at a dose of 1—2 mg/kg for induction in obstetric patients in <2% of general anesthetics [19]. It has a rapid onset providing analgesia, hypnosis, and reliable amnesia and may be useful in patients with asthma or modest hypovolaemia. It rapidly crosses the placenta and a dose of 1 mg/kg appears to not be associated with an increase in uterine tone unlike larger doses. Its use is limited in preeclampsia and hypertension due to its sympathomimetic effects, and due to the risk of increased uterine tone and asphyxia, it should not be used in the first two trimesters. There are practical concerns regarding hallucinations and emergence phenomena although both are dose-related and are thought to occur less frequently in obstetric patients [20]. Apgar scores and umbilical cord gases appear to be similar as with other IV induction agents.

9.4.4 Etomidate

This carboxylated imidazole has been used in patients who are hemodynamically unstable when it is important to maintain baseline systolic blood pressure. However, there are currently no adequate and well-controlled studies in pregnant women. Potential side effects include pain on injection, postoperative nausea, myoclonus, and suppression of the adrenal suppression. Etomidate should be used during pregnancy only if the potential benefit justifies the potential risks to the fetus.

9.4.5 Benzodiazepines

This class of drugs is rarely used as sole anesthetic agents due to their relatively slow maternal onset and offset and neonatal depressive actions. They may be used as coinduction agents. Benzodiazepines have been associated with cleft lip and palate in animal studies, but the association in humans is controversial and a single dose has not been associated with teratogenicity [21,22]. Long term use should be avoided due to the association with neonatal withdrawal.

9.4.6 Systemic opioids in pregnancy

One of the most common forms of analgesia in labor is intramuscular (IM) opioids. Around 33% of laboring women are administered IM pethidine (Meperidine) in the United Kingdom [23]. Pethidine is a synthetic phenylpiperidine opioid which is highly lipid soluble so easily able to cross the placenta. It has a 10% potency when compared to morphine and is metabolized to the toxic metabolite norpethidine, which is less lipid soluble. It has been used safely for decades, but it is not without significant side effects including nausea and vomiting, pruritis, sedation, respiratory depression, urinary retention, and constipation. It has also been suggested that its mechanism of action is more to do with its sedating effects rather than its analgesic effects [24].

Another IM opioid commonly used is diamorphine. It is a synthetic diacetylated derivative of morphine. It acts as a prodrug, being metabolized in the liver and plasma to monoacetylmorphine which is more lipid soluble. It crosses the blood–brain barrier before being converted, by removal of the acetyl group, to morphine after which it can have its therapeutic effect. It is 1.5 times as potent as morphine with a faster onset and shorter duration of action. IM diamorphine has been shown to be mildly superior to IM pethidine as an analgesic in labor, but has also been associated with increased duration of labor [25].

Neuraxial anesthesia or analgesia may be contraindicated or refused in labor or at cesarean delivery necessitating the use of IV patient-controlled analgesia using opioids drugs such as alfentanil, fentanyl, or remifentanil.

Remifentanil is one of the most extensively studied opioids for use in labor analgesia. It is a short-acting mu-opioid receptor agonist [26] with the advantage of a rapid onset and offset of action (context-specific half-life of 3 min in both maternal and neonatal studies). It is hydrolyzed by nonspecific tissue esterases and excreted in the urine. The RESPITE study showed that the use of remifentanil patient-controlled analgesia (PCA) instead of IM pethidine can reduce the number of women who then go on to require epidural analgesia in labor thus reducing the potential for complications from neuraxial analgesia [27]. However, patient satisfaction from epidurals is still higher than using a remifentanil PCA [28]. Both remifentanil and pethidine can cause significant respiratory depression with remifentanil being far more likely to cause apnoea. It is mandatory that all laboring women using either treatment have adequate supervision and that those receiving remifentanil receive constant monitoring with maternal pulse oximetry and fetal heart rate monitoring.

As part of general anesthesia, short and long-acting systemic opioids may be administered for analgesia, facilitation of intubation, and attenuation of the stress response to surgery. Placental transfer to the fetus of systemic opioids is passive; however, opioids such as pethidine have been safely used for pain relief in pregnancy for decades.

Morphine rapidly crosses the placenta and has shown to be associated with a reduction in neonatal apgar scores [29]. Fentanyl is highly lipophilic and rapidly transferred to the placenta. It has been shown in early pregnancy to be detected in both the placenta (which acts as a drug depot) and fetal brain [30]. Maternal alfentanil administration has been associated with a reduction of one-minute Apgar scores despite a relatively low fetal/maternal ratio [31,32]. Alfentanil and remifentanil have shown to reduce the pressor response to laryngoscopy reducing the systolic and mean arterial blood pressures as well as heart rate during induction and intubation [33]. Maternal sufentanil administration results in a very high fetal/maternal ratio of 0.81. Human placental studies have confirmed this rapid transfer across the placenta which is influenced by fetal pH and differences in maternal and fetal plasma protein binding [34].

9.5 **Neuromuscular blocking agents**

In pregnancy, individual drug metabolism is heterogeneous, reflecting the separate pregnancy-related changes in each drug-metabolizing organ system. Neuromuscular blocking agents are required for general anesthesia in cases where endotracheal intubation is required and may be depolarizing or nondepolarizing agents. They are highly polar, fully ionized molecules that do not cross the placenta in significant amounts, and fetal blood concentrations of muscle relaxants are 10%−20% of that of maternal blood [35]. Neonatal hypotonia is rarely seen following induction of general anesthesia with muscle relaxation.

- Depolarizing muscle relaxants include suxamethonium which acts by depolarizing the plasma membrane of the skeletal muscle fiber making it resistant to further stimulation by acetylcholine. It induces rapid paralysis (within 30−90 sec) with a short offset time (2−5 min) in order to safely facilitate tracheal intubation in the presence of increased risk of aspiration, as found in the second and third trimesters. It is metabolized by plasma cholinesterases.
- Nondepolarizing neuromuscular blocking agents act by competitively blocking the binding of acetylcholine to its postsynaptic receptors. This class of drugs includes the aminosteroids (pancuronium, vecuronium, and rocuronium) and the benzylisoquinolines (atracurium, doxacurium, and mivacurium). These drugs have a longer onset time (1.5−3 min) and offset time (20−60 min) compared to suxamethonium. The aminosteroids in general undergo a combination of hepatic and renal metabolism and excretion. Atracurium is broken down to inactive metabolites by ester hydrolysis (the minority) and spontaneous Hoffman degradation (the majority) to laudanosine.

The marked physiological reduction of plasma cholinesterase levels in pregnancy (by 30% from early in the first trimester to several weeks postpartum) theoretically causes suxamethonium to have a prolonged effect. This is however counterbalanced by the increased maternal volume of distribution. Maternal doses of more than 300 mg (recommended dose 1−2 mg/kg) are required before the drug can be detected in umbilical venous blood [36]. Fetal pseudocholinesterase deficiency or repeated high doses of suxamethonium may lead to neonatal neuromuscular blockade [37]. Rocuronium demonstrates an unaltered onset time at a dose of 0.6 mg/kg but shows a longer duration of action in pregnancy [38] whereas vecuronium shows a faster onset at a standard dose of 0.2 mg/kg but also an extended duration of action [39]. The use of rocuronium in place of suxamethonium at a dose of 1 mg/kg has been shown to be safe in the obstetric population with no significant differences in outcomes for mothers and no change in the 5 or 10 min apgar scores for the neonate [40]. Nondepolarizing muscle relaxants are often administered in bolus form which may result in an increase in fetal blood concentration over time even though the transfer rates are relatively low [41].

At cesarean delivery, usually only a single dose of suxamethonium is needed but may be followed by small boluses of a short-acting nondepolarizing neuromuscular blocking agent to maintain neuromuscular blockade and facilitate surgery. For other surgery requiring neuromuscular blockade, longer-acting nondepolarizing neuromuscular blockers may be employed, but time should be allowed for adequate reversal of effects. Monitoring of neuromuscular function is recommended in all cases. Magnesium sulfate is known to decrease requirements of nondepolarizing neuromuscular blockers and prolong their effects, and this should be considered in cases of severe preeclampsia and eclampsia where magnesium infusions may be indicated. The combination of rocuronium at a dose of 1 mg/kg, reversed by sugammadex at the end of the procedure, has also shown to be safe in the obstetric population [42]. Sugammadex is a gamma cyclodextrin developed specifically to reverse the aminosteroid nondepolarizing agents rocuronium and vecuronium. For routine reversal, it is given at a dose of 2—4 mg/kg. It can also be given at a dose of 16 mg/kg for the immediate reversal of neuromuscular blockade including after administration of an RSI dose of rocuronium. It works by encapsulating rocuronium or vecuronium preventing it from binding to the acetylcholine receptor at the neuromuscular junction.

9.6 Regional anesthesia

The advantages of maternal regional anesthesia for both incidental surgeries in pregnancy, analgesia in labor and for operative delivery, are substantial and are listed in Table 9.2. Infiltration of local anesthetic may be employed, for example, in episiotomies and paracervical blocks. It should be noted that there are significant contraindications and complications associated with regional techniques and of which the patient should be made aware when consenting for regional anesthesia.

Local anesthetic drugs are weak bases and exist predominantly in the ionized form at physiological pH as their pKa exceeds 7.4. Each possesses both an aromatic lipophilic group and a hydrophilic group, and they are classified as either esters or

Table 9.2 Advantages of regional anesthesia in obstetrics.

Greater maternal satisfaction
Facilitates instrumental delivery, avoiding cesarean section
Reduces maternal catecholamines and potentially improves placental blood flow
For operative anesthesia:
- Reduces risk of GA (higher risk of maternal aspiration, ileus, awareness, and fetal exposure to anesthetic drugs)
- Improved maternal respiratory function
- Reduced intraoperative blood loss
- Improved maternal bonding, earlier breast-feeding, and reduced incidence postnatal depression
- Good postoperative analgesia

Increased mobility with low-dose epidural (e.g., 0.125% bupivacaine and 2 mcg/mL fentanyl)

amides, the name describing the linkage between the groups. Commonly used local anesthetics in obstetrics have low-molecular weight, high-lipid solubility, and low ionization and include bupivacaine, levobupivacaine, lidocaine and ropivacaine (amides), and chloroprocaine (ester). These agents work by binding to the receptor sites of sodium channels and blocking ion movement across nerve cell membranes. Consequently they prevent the initiation and propagation of the action potential and subsequent sensory nerve transmission. Local anesthetics cross the placenta by simple diffusion. Due to a relative fetal acidosis, there is fetal accumulation of local anesthetic (also known as "ion trapping"). Transfer to the fetus is also affected by total dose, site of administration, and use of adjuvants such as epinephrine.

Choice and concentration of local anesthetic depends on the onset time of block required, the desired indication [operative (incidental surgery or for delivery) or labor analgesia] as well as maternal and fetal conditions. Bupivacaine has a pKa of 8.1 compared lidocaine's pKa of 7.9. This means that at physiological pH, bupivacaine consists of a greater fraction in the ionized form which is unable to penetrate the phospholipid membrane, resulting in a slower onset of action. The duration of action is correlated with the extent of protein binding. Those drugs that are highly protein-bound will have a lower materno-fetal transfer attributed to restricted placental transfer (for example, bupivacaine is 90% protein-bound to lidocaine's 50%). In pregnancy, altered protein binding (physiological hypoalbuminaemia combined with an increase in α_1-glycoprotein concentration) changes the unbound fraction of the drug and reduces the doses required and at which toxicity may occur. The sensitivity of neural tissue to local anesthetics also increases, and this contributes to the risk of toxicity.

The volume of the subarachnoid and epidural spaces is reduced in pregnancy due to compression of the inferior vena cava causing distension of the epidural venous plexus. This results in a greater risk of inadvertent intravascular injection and leads to more extensive spread of local anesthetic in central neuraxial blockade, both of which may increase the subsequent risk of complications.

9.6.1 Bupivacaine

About 0.125%−0.5% bupivacaine is used frequently in both epidural and subarachnoid blocks. The higher the concentration, the greater the motor blockade. It has a slower onset and longer duration than lidocaine (approximately 120−180 min). Bupivacaine toxicity has been associated with refractory ventricular fibrillation leading to the isolation and commercial preparation of the S (−) enantiomer of bupivacaine, levobupivacaine. This has been shown to be less neuro- and cardiotoxic than racemic bupivacaine.

9.6.2 Lidocaine

Lidocaine has an intermediate onset time between 2-chloroprocaine and bupivacaine, and concentrations of 1.5%−2% are often used in neuraxial (predominantly epidural) anesthesia. Epinephrine is often used with lidocaine as an adjunct to decrease systemic absorption, prolong the duration of the block, and increase the intensity of the blockade (both sensory and motor). Without it there may be an increased risk of inadequate anesthesia and a risk of local anesthetic toxicity especially with additional lidocaine doses. Bicarbonate may also be used to buffer lidocaine, increasing the amount of unionized drug and speeding its penetration into the nerve tissue. The addition of bicarbonate and epinephrine to 1.8% lidocaine has been shown to half the onset time of epidural top up for cesarean section compared to 0.5% levobupivacaine [43]. Some studies have found differences in neonatal neuro-behavior following lidocaine compared to bupivacaine in epidural anesthesia, but these differences have been shown to be not clinically significant [44,45].

9.6.3 2-Chloroprocaine

As an ester local anesthetic, 2-chloroprocaine is rapidly metabolized and placental transfer is limited compared to amide local anesthetics. As a result, it is used widely in the United States in the situation of epidural analgesia requiring conversion to anesthesia for instrumental or operative delivery with a decompensating fetus as it has an extremely rapid onset (approximately 5 min), and it is less likely to participate in ion trapping and there is less risk of toxicity. It should not be used in the subarachnoid space due to the risk of adhesive arachnoiditis.

9.6.4 Ropivacaine

This amide anesthetic has an onset intermediate between lidocaine and bupivacaine, and its safety in cesarean delivery has been established [46]. It has a duration similar to bupivacaine (120−180 min) but exhibits less cardiac toxicity as it is supplied in the S(−) enantiomer form. Ropivacaine may provide anesthesia and analgesia with less motor blockade when compared to bupivacaine but the clinical significance of this in practice is uncertain [47].

9.6.5 Adjuvant opioids

The rationale behind using opioids in obstetric regional anesthesia is to minimize maternal systemic and fetal effects of both local anesthetics and opioids. There have been extensive numbers of studies in both human and animal studies confirming the synergism between opioids and local anesthetics in neuraxial anesthesia which may reduce the required local anesthetic dose by up to 30%. This may reduce both the risk of local anesthetic toxicity and the incidence of motor blockade which may be undesirable for the laboring parturient. Neuraxial opioids improve the quality of analgesia and are thought to exert their effects via a direct action on spinal and supraspinal opioids receptors. Dose ranges of commonly used opioids are shown below in Table 9.3.

When considering specific opioids, fentanyl is the most commonly used and most widely studied adjuvant neuraxial opioid in obstetric anesthesia. It is a highly

Table 9.3 Dose ranges of commonly used neuraxial opioids.

Opioid	Epidural Dose	Intrathecal Dose
Fentanyl	50–100 mcg	10–25 mcg
Sufentanil	25–50 mcg	2.5–15 mcg
Morphine	2.0–3.0 mg	100–200 mcg
Diamorphine	4.0–6.0 mg	200–400 mcg

potent lipophilic phenylpiperidine derivative that rapidly binds dorsal horn receptors in the spinal cord after neuraxial administration leading to rapid analgesia within 5 min intrathecally and 10 min epidurally. Cephalad migration and the incidence of central respiratory depression are reduced compared to less lipid-soluble opioids such as morphine. Sufentanil has an analgesic potency that is around five times more potent than fentanyl and has an even more rapid onset. Early respiratory depression however may occur due to rapid systemic absorption of these drugs, and the side effects are equipotent with equivalent doses of either drug. Their fast onset of action makes these opioids desirable for labor analgesia and emergency delivery but limits their use for postoperative analgesia after a single dose.

Morphine is a hydrophilic phenanthrene derivative which is approximately 100 times less potent that fentanyl. It has a slower onset (15 min intrathecally and 30 min epidurally) compared to fentanyl and sufentanil and a significantly longer duration of action (12–24 h). Poor lipid solubility leads to a delay in binding to dorsal horn receptors in the spinal cord and may contribute to the accumulation of free drug within the cerebrospinal fluid (CSF) which may then migrate cranially and cause delayed respiratory depression; however, the clinical significance of this is limited. In both intrathecal and epidural anesthesia, morphine has been shown to have a ceiling effect (at 100 mcg intrathecally and 3.75 mg epidurally) above which there is little analgesic benefit and an increased incidence of adverse effects [48,49]. Neuraxial morphine has been shown to be as effective as fentanyl for labor and cesarean delivery analgesia and more effective than fentanyl in postoperative pain relief. However, the increased incidence and magnitude of side effects such as nausea, vomiting, sedation, urinary retention, respiratory depression, and pruritis when compared to fentanyl limit its effect.

Diamorphine is a suitable alternative to intrathecal morphine and is primarily used in the United Kingdom. It is more lipophilic than morphine and therefore has a faster onset of action. Despite a short half-life in the CSF, it is metabolized into its active components (morphine and 6-acetylmorphine) increasing its duration of action. Intraoperative analgesia is of similar quality to fentanyl with the additional advantage of prolonged postoperative analgesia [50]. Side effects however are dose-dependent with pruritis occurring in up to 90% of women after a 200 mcg dose at cesarean delivery [51]. A dose of 400 mcg has been established as the optimal dose, with higher doses giving no significant analgesic benefit, but greatly increasing the undesirable side effects [52].

9.6.6 Fetal effects of neuraxial opioids

Spinal and epidural opioids will diffuse into the maternal bloodstream and will be rapidly transported to the uterus. All commercially available opioids have low-molecular weights and rapidly cross the placenta by diffusion. The risk of neonatal depression with morphine increases with reduced interdosing interval and with increasing dose due to higher maternal systemic morphine levels. The risk of neonatal depression with fentanyl appears less and has only been reported at very high repeated epidural doses leading to maternal systemic accumulation [53].

9.7 Summary

General anesthesia utilizes pharmacological agents to render the parturient unconscious and unaware. It requires a RSI with neuromuscular blockade to secure the airway after the first trimester due to the risk of aspiration. These drugs cross the placenta in varying amounts and may be implicated in neonatal depression. IV agents should be carefully titrated to minimize fetal exposure while ensuring maternal anesthesia and analgesia. In most cases, regional anesthesia and analgesia may be more appropriate with less potential risk of harm to both mother and fetus.

References

[1] Rasmussen AS, Christiansen CF, Uldbjerg N. Obstetric and non-obstetric surgery during pregnancy: a 20-year Danish population-based prevalence study. BMJ Open 2019;9: e028136. https://doi.org/10.1136/bmjopen-2018-028136.

[2] Boerma T, Ronsmans C, Melesse DY. Global epidemiology of use of and disparities in caesarean sections. Lancet 2018;392(10155):1341–8. https://doi.org/10.1016/S0140-6736(18)31928-7.

[3] Sear JW. What makes a molecule an anaesthetic? Studies on the mechanisms of anaesthesia using a physicochemical approach. Br J Anaesth 2009;103:50–60.

[4] Hemmings Jr HC. Sodium channels and the synaptic mechanisms of inhaled anaesthetics. Br J Anaesth 2009;103:61–9.

[5] Chan MT, Mainland P, Gin T. Minimum alveolar concentration of halothane and enflurane are decreased in early pregnancy. Anesthesiology 1996;85:782–6.

[6] Gin T, Chan MT. Decreased minimum alveolar concentration of isoflurane in pregnant humans. Anesthesiology 1994;81:829–32.

[7] Crawford JS, Lewis M. Nitrous oxide in early human pregnancy. Anaesthesia 1986;41: 900–5.

[8] Pandit J, et al. NAP5 accidental awareness during anaesthesia in the UK and Ireland. 2014.

[9] Lumley J, Walker A, Marum J, Wood C. Time: an important variable at caesarean section. J Obstet Gynaecol Br Commonw 1970;77:10–23.

[10] Mankowitz E, Brock-Utne JG, Downing JW. Nitrous oxide elimination by the newborn. Anaesthesia 1981;36:1014–6.

[11] Crawford JS. Principles and practice of obstetric anaesthesia. 5th ed. Oxford: Blackwell Science; 1984.

[12] SE C. Nonobstetric surgery during pregnancy. In: DH C, editor. Obstetric anesthesia: principles and practice. 2nd ed. St Louis: Mosby; 1999. p. 279.

[13] Knight M, et al., MBRRACE-UK. Saving lives, improving mothers' care—lessons learned to inform future maternity care from the UK and Ireland confidential enquiries into maternal deaths and morbidity. 2019.

[14] Yentis SM, Randall K. Drug errors in obstetric anaesthesia: a national survey. Int J Obstet Anesth 2013;12:246—9.

[15] Gin T, Gregory MA, Oh TE. The haemodynamic effects of propofol and thiopentone for induction of caesarean section. Anaesth Intensive Care 1990;18:175—9.

[16] Zakowski. The placenta: anatomy, physiology and transfer of drugs. In: Chestnut, editor. Obstetric anaesthesia: principles and practice; 2004.

[17] Gin T. Propofol during pregnancy. Acta Anaesthesiol Sin 1994;32:127—32.

[18] Lucas D. Unsettled weather and the end of thiopental? Obstetric general anaesthesia after the NAP5 and MBRRACE-UK reports. Anaesthesia 2015. https://doi.org/10.1111/anae.13034.

[19] Paech MJ, Scott KL, Clavisi O, Chua S, McDonnell N. A prospective study of awareness and recall associated with general anaesthesia for caesarean section. Int J Obstet Anesth 2008;17:298—303.

[20] Schultetus RR, Hill CR, Dharamraj CM, Banner TE, Berman LS. Wakefulness during cesarean section after anesthetic induction with ketamine, thiopental, or ketamine and thiopental combined. Anesth Analg 1986;65:723—8.

[21] Safra MJ, Oakley Jr GP. Association between cleft lip with or without cleft palate and prenatal exposure to diazepam. Lancet 1975;2:478—80.

[22] Rosenberg L, Mitchell AA, Parsells JL, Pashayan H, Louik C, Shapiro S. Lack of relation of oral clefts to diazepam use during pregnancy. N Engl J Med 1983;309:1282—5.

[23] Redshaw M, Rowe R, Hockley C, Brocklehurst P. Recorded delivery: a national survey of women's experience of maternity care 2006. Oxford: National Perinatal Epidemiological Unit, University of Oxford; 2007.

[24] Olofsson C, Ekblom A, Ekman-Ordeberg G, Hjelm A, Irested L. Lack of Analgesic effect of systemically administered morphine or pethidine on labour pain. Br J Obstet Gynaecol 1996;103:968—72.

[25] Wee M, Tuckey J, Thomas P, Burnard S. A comparison of intramuscular diamorphine and intramuscular pethidine for labour analgesia: a two-centre randomised blinded controlled trial. Br J Obstet Gynaecol 2013;121(4):447—56.

[26] Hinova A, Fernando R. Systemic remifentanil for labor analgesia. Anesth Analg 2009; 109:1925—9.

[27] Wilson M, MacArthur C, et al. Intravenous remifentanil patient-controlled analgesia versus intramuscular pethidine for pain relief in labour (RESPITE): an open-label, multi centre, randomised controlled trial. Lancet 2018;392(10148):662—72. https://doi.org/10.1016/S0140-6736(18)31613-1.

[28] Weibel S, Jelting Y, Afshari A. Patient-controlled analgesia with remifentanil versus alternative analgesic methods for pain relief in labour. Cochrane Library 2017. https://doi.org/10.1002/14651858.CD011989.pub2.

[29] Kopecky EA, Ryan ML, Barrett JF, Seaward PG, Ryan G, Koren G, Amankwah K. Fetal response to maternally administered morphine. Am J Obstet Gynecol 2000;183:424—30.

[30] Cooper J, Jauniaux E, Gulbis B, Quick D, Bromley L. Placental transfer of fentanyl in early human pregnancy and its detection in fetal brain. Br J Anaesth 1999;82:929−31.

[31] Gin T, Ngan-Kee WD, Siu YK, Stuart JC, Tan PE, Lam KK. Alfentanil given immediately before the induction of anesthesia for elective cesarean delivery. Anesth Analg 2000;90:1167−72.

[32] Gepts E, Heytens L, Camu F. Pharmacokinetics and placental transfer of intravenous and epidural alfentanil in parturient women. Anesth Analg 1986;65:1155−60.

[33] White L, et al. Induction opioids for caesarean section under general anaesthesia: a systematic review and meta-analysis of randomised controlled trials. Int J Obstet Anaesth 2019;40:4−13. https://doi.org/10.1016/j.ijoa.2019.04.007.

[34] Johnson RF, Herman N, Arney TL, Johnson HV, Paschall RL, Downing JW. The placental transfer of sufentanil: effects of fetal pH, protein binding, and sufentanil concentration. Anesth Analg 1997;84:1262−8.

[35] Ni Mhuireachtaigh R, O'Gorman DA. Anesthesia in pregnant patients for nonobstetric surgery. J Clin Anesth 2006;18:60−6.

[36] Kvisselgaard N, Moya F. Investigation of placental thresholds to succinylcholine. Anesthesiology 1961;22:7−10.

[37] Owens WD, Zeitlin GL. Hypoventilation in a newborn following administration of succinylcholine to the mother: a case report. Anesth Analg 1975;54:38−40.

[38] Puhringer FK, Sparr HJ, Mitterschiffthaler G, Agoston S, Benzer A. Extended duration of action of rocuronium in postpartum patients. Anesth Analg 1997;84:352−4.

[39] Baraka A, Jabbour S, Tabboush Z, Sibai A, Bijjani A, Karam K. Onset of vecuronium neuromuscular block is more rapid in patients undergoing caesarean section. Can J Anaesth 1992;39:135−8.

[40] Kosinova M. Rocuronium versus suxamethonium for rapid sequence induction of general anaesthesia for caesarean section: influence on neonatal outcomes. Int J Obstet Anaesth 2017;32:4−10.

[41] Iwama H, Kaneko T, Tobishima S, Komatsu T, Watanabe K, Akutsu H. Time dependency of the ratio of umbilical vein/maternal artery concentrations of vecuronium in caesarean section. Acta Anaesthesiol Scand 1999;43:9−12.

[42] Wiliamson R. Rocuronium and sugammadex for rapid sequence induction of obstetric general anaesthesia. Acta Anaesthesiol Scand 2011. https://doi.org/10.1111/j.1399-6576.2011.02431.x.

[43] Allam J. Epidural lidocaine-bicarbonate-adrenaline vs levobupivacaine for emergency Caesarean section: randomised controlled trial. Anaesthesia 2008;63(3):243−9.

[44] Kileff ME, James 3rd FM, Dewan DM, Floyd HM. Neonatal neurobehavioral responses after epidural anesthesia for cesarean section using lidocaine and bupivacaine. Anesth Analg 1984;63:413−7.

[45] Abboud TK, D'Onofrio L, Reyes A, Mosaad P, Zhu J, Mantilla M, Gangolly J, Crowell D, Cheung M, Afrasiabi A, et al. Isoflurane or halothane for cesarean section: comparative maternal and neonatal effects. Acta Anaesthesiol Scand 1989;33:578−81.

[46] Stienstra R. Techniques in regional anaesthesia and pain management. Ropivacaine Obstet Use 2001. https://doi.org/10.1053/trap.2001.23682.

[47] Beilin Y, Halpern S. Focused review: ropivacaine versus bupivacaine for epidural labor analgesia. Anesth Analg 2010;111:482−7.

[48] Palmer CM, Emerson S, Volgoropolous D, Alves D. Dose-response relationship of intrathecal morphine for post-cesarean analgesia. Anesthesiology 1999;90:437−44.

[49] Palmer CM, Nogami WM, Van Maren G, Alves DM. Post-cesarean epidural morphine: a dose-response study. Anesth Analg 2000;90:887—91.

[50] Lane S, Evans P, Arfeen Z, Misra U. A comparison of intrathecal fentanyl and diamorphine as adjuncts in spinal anaesthesia for caesarean section. Anaesthesia 2005;60: 453—7.

[51] Wrench IJ, Sanghera S, Pinder A, Power L, Adams MG. Dose response to intrathecal diamorphine for elective caesarean section and compliance with a national audit standard. Int J Obstet Anesth 2007;16:17—21.

[52] Saravanan S. Minimum dose of intrathecal diamorphine required to prevent intraoperative supplementation of spinal anaesthesia for caesarean section. Br J Anaseth 2003; 91(3):368—72.

[53] Hughes SC. Respiratory depression following intraspinal narcotics: expect it! Int J Obstet Anesth 1997;6:145—6.

The management of asthma during pregnancy

Jennifer A. Namazy[1], Michael Schatz[2]

[1]*Scripps Clinic, San Diego, CA, United States;* [2]*Kaiser Permanente, San Diego, CA, United States*

10.1 Introduction

Asthma is one of the most common potentially serious medical problems to complicate pregnancy, and may adversely affect both maternal quality of life and perinatal outcomes. Optimal management of asthma during pregnancy (MAP) is thus important for both mother and baby. While the management of asthma in pregnancy relies on guidelines that were based on studies of nonpregnant populations, special considerations regarding the safety of medications are required.

10.2 Effect of pregnancy on the course of asthma

The prevalence of asthma during pregnancy is estimated to be 5%−8% based on US Health surveys [1]. The prevalence of asthma also appears to be increasing in childbearing−aged women. An analysis of US Health plans between 2001 and 07 shows that the prevalence was 5.5% in 2001 and 7.8% in 2007 [2].

Since the prevalence of asthma is increasing in child-bearing−aged women, it is important to understand how to provide adequate treatment of asthma during pregnancy.

Asthma course may worsen, improve, or remain unchanged during pregnancy, and the overall data suggest that these various courses occur with approximately equal frequency.

In a large prospective study of 1739 pregnant asthmatic women, severity classification (based on symptoms, pulmonary function, and medication use) worsened in 30% and improved in 23% of patients during pregnancy [3]. Asthma also appears to be more likely to be more severe or to worsen during pregnancy in women with more severe asthma before becoming pregnant [4].

In a recent report from US health care claims databases, between 2011 and 2015, about 19% had severe asthma [5]. 28% of pregnant women with asthma who have public insurance have uncontrolled asthma during pregnancy. Supporting this finding are results of a cohort of inner-city pregnant women who experienced severe prenatal asthma exacerbation. The authors found that pregnant asthmatics in this cohort had a higher prevalence of long acting beta-agonist/inhaled corticosteroid

Clinical Pharmacology During Pregnancy. https://doi.org/10.1016/B978-0-12-818902-3.00002-6

and leukotriene modifier prescriptions. They also had a higher prevalence of cigarette smoking and upper respiratory infections [6].

The course of asthma may vary by stage of pregnancy. The first trimester is generally well tolerated in asthmatics with infrequent acute episodes. Increased symptoms and more frequent exacerbations have been reported to occur between weeks 17 and 36 of gestation. In contrast, asthmatic women in general tend to experience fewer symptoms and less frequent asthma exacerbations during weeks 37–40 of pregnancy than during any earlier gestational period [7].

In a prospective study of 50 enrolled women in the MAP program, 13 women had a total of 16 exacerbations in the year followed. Having more pronounced airway hyperresponsiveness and nonatopic state appeared to characterize these women as having a higher risk of exacerbations during pregnancy [8].

The mechanisms responsible for the altered asthma course during pregnancy are unknown. The myriad of pregnancy-associated changes in levels of sex hormones, cortisol, and prostaglandins may contribute to changes in asthma course during pregnancy. In addition, exposure to fetal antigens, leading to alterations in immune function, may predispose some pregnant asthmatics to worsening asthma [4]. Even fetal sex may play a role, with some data showing increased severity of symptoms in pregnancies with a female fetus [5].

There are additional factors that may contribute to the clinical course of asthma during pregnancy. Pregnancy may be a source of stress for many women, and this stress can aggravate asthma. Adherence to therapy can change during pregnancy with a corresponding change in asthma control. Most commonly observed is decreased adherence as a result of a mother's concerns about the safety of medications for the fetus. One study found that women with asthma significantly decreased their asthma medication use from 5 to 13 weeks of pregnancy. During the first trimester, there was a 23% decline in inhaled corticosteroid prescriptions, a 13% decline in short-acting beta-agonist prescriptions, and a 54% decline in rescue corticosteroid prescriptions [6].

Physician reluctance to treat may also affect the severity of asthma during pregnancy. A recent study found that less than 40% of women who classified themselves as "poorly controlled" reported use of a controller medication during pregnancy [7]. Another study identified 51 pregnant women and 500 nonpregnant women presenting to the emergency department with acute asthma. Although asthma severity appeared to be similar in the two groups based on peak flow rates, pregnant women were significantly less likely to be discharged on oral steroids (38% vs. 64%). Presumably related to this undertreatment, pregnant women were three times more likely than nonpregnant women to report an ongoing exacerbation 2 weeks later [8,9].

More recent reassuring data have come from the Pregnancy Risk Assessment Monitoring System which collected data from 34 US states of over 40, 000 women. The prevalence of counseling on medications safe to take during pregnancy was about 89.2% (95%CI 88.7–89.7). Counseling was more common in women who used prescription medications before pregnancy and who reported having asthma before pregnancy [10].

Infections during pregnancy can certainly affect the course of gestational asthma. Some degree of decrease in cell-mediated immunity may make the pregnant patient more susceptible to viral infection, and upper respiratory tract infections have been reported to be the most common precipitants of asthma exacerbations during pregnancy [11]. Sinusitis, a known asthma trigger, has been shown to be six times more common in pregnant compared with nonpregnant women [12]. In addition, pneumonia has been reported to be greater than five times more common in asthmatic than nonasthmatic women during pregnancy [13]. A recent study tried to determine whether a diagnosis of upper respiratory infection or sinusitis was more common during pregnancy and whether pregnant women were more likely to receive a prescription for antibiotics. This study did not confirm the prior finding that sinusitis or antibiotic use for upper respiratory infections is increased in pregnancy. The report did find that respiratory comorbidities, such as asthma, increased the risk of antibiotic use during pregnancy [14].

Obesity has been shown to be an inflammatory state that may play an important role in asthma initiation and control. Obesity during pregnancy has been associated with adverse perinatal outcomes including the following: gestational diabetes, preeclampsia, thromboembolic disorders, postpartum hemorrhage, large for gestational age, fetal death, and congenital anomalies. Higher body mass index (BMI) and gestational weight gain have been associated with an increased risk for asthma exacerbations in both nonpregnant and pregnant women [15].The mechanisms leading to these outcomes are thought to be due to a heightened inflammatory response [16]. In a follow-up study of the same group of pregnant asthmatics, asthma treatment was adjusted according to FeNO and symptoms. Authors report the benefits of a FeNO-based management are attenuated among obese mothers and those with excess gestational weight gain [17].

Population-based studies have shown a relationship between smoking and airway hyperresponsiveness [18,19], implying that smoking is a risk factor for asthma. Asthma exacerbations during pregnancy are more common and more severe in current and former smokers than in never smokers [20]. The potential for maternal smoking to both increase the risk of uncontrolled asthma and to directly adversely affect pregnancy suggests that discontinuation of smoking should be a high priority goal during pregnancy.

10.3 Effect of asthma on pregnancy

One of the largest controlled studies that have evaluated outcomes of pregnancy described 36,985 women identified as having asthma in the Swedish Medical Birth Registry. These outcomes were compared with the total of 1.32 million births that occurred during the years of the study (1984−95). Significantly increased rates of preeclampsia (OR 1.15), perinatal mortality (OR 1.21), preterm births (OR 1.15), and low birth weight infants (OR 1.21), but not congenital malformations (OR 1.05), were found in pregnancies of asthmatic versus control women [21]. The risks appeared to be greater in patients with more severe asthma, which was confirmed in a more recent Swedish Medical Birth Registry report [22]. A metaanalysis, derived from a substantial body of literature spanning several decades and including very large numbers of pregnant women (over 1,000,000 for low birth weight and over 250,000 for preterm labor), indicates that pregnant women with asthma are at a significantly increased risk of a range of adverse perinatal outcomes including low birth weight, small for gestational age, preterm labor and delivery, and pre-eclampsia [23].

A recent study based on nationwide Finnish register—based cohort between 1996 and 2012 of over 25,000 pregnant asthmatics found that maternal asthma was associated with perinatal mortality 1.24(95%CI 1.05—1.46), preterm birth 1.18 (1.11—1.25), low birth weight 1.29 (1.21—1.37), fetal growth restriction (SGA) 1.32 (1.24—1.40), and asphyxia 1.09(1.02—1.17) [24].

Mechanisms postulated to explain the possible increase in perinatal risks in pregnant asthmatic women demonstrated in previous studies have included [1] hypoxia and other physiologic consequences of poorly controlled asthma [2], medications used to treat asthma, and [3] pathogenic or demographic factors associated with asthma but not actually caused by the disease or its treatment, such as abnormal placental function.

Several prospective studies [25—33] have shown that the pregnant asthmatic with mild to moderate severity can have excellent maternal and fetal outcomes. In contrast, suboptimal control of asthma or more severe asthma during pregnancy may be associated with increased maternal or fetal risk [17,20,21]. A recent prospective cohort study highlighted recurrent uncontrolled asthma as a greater contributor to poor perinatal outcomes than asthma exacerbations [34].

10.4 Asthma management

The ultimate goal of asthma therapy in pregnancy is maintaining adequate oxygenation of the fetus preventing hypoxic episodes in the mother. The management of asthma can be summarized in four categories: assessment and monitoring, education of patients, control of factors contributing to severity, and pharmacologic therapy.

The first step is assessment of severity (in patients not already on controller medications) or assessment of control (in patients already on controller medications). Severity is assessed in untreated patients based on the frequency of daytime and nighttime symptoms, rescue therapy use, activity limitation, and pulmonary function (ideally spirometry, minimally peak flow rate) (Table 10.1). Based on this, severity assessment controller therapy is initiated. Patients should be monitored monthly for asthma control (Table 10.2), and if not responding adequately to treatment should have their level of treatment adjusted (Table 10.3).

Table 10.1 Classification of asthma severity in pregnant patients[a].

Asthma severity	Symptom frequency	Night time awakening	Interference with normal activity	FEV$_1$ or peak flow (predicted percentage of personal best)
Intermittent	2 days per week or less	Twice per month or less	None	More than 80%
Mild persistent	More than 2 days per week, but not daily	More than twice per month	Minor limitation	More than 80%
Moderate persistent	Daily symptoms	More than once per week	Some limitation	60%–80%
Severe persistent	Throughout the day	Four times per week or more	Extremely limited	Less than 60%

FEV$_1$, forced expiratory volume in the first second of expiration.
[a] Data from Dumbrowski MP, Schatz M. ACOG Committee on Practice Bulletins - Obstetrics. ACOG practice bulletin: clinical management guidelines for obstetrician -gynecologists number 90, February 2008: asthma in pregnancy. Obstet Gynecol 2008; 111:457–464.

Table 10.2 Assessment of asthma control in pregnant women[a].

Variable	Well-controlled asthma	Asthma not well controlled	Very poorly controlled asthma
Frequency of symptoms	≤2 days/week	>2 days/week	Throughout the day
Frequency of night time awakening	≤2 times/month	1–3 times/week	≥4 times/week
Interference with normal activity	None	Some	Extreme
Use of short-acting β-agonist for symptoms control	≤2 days/week	>2 days/week	Several times/day
FEV$_1$ or peak flow (% of the predicted or personal best value)	>80	60–80	<60
Exacerbation requiring use of systemic corticosteroid (no.)	0–1 in the past 12 months	≥2 in the past 12 months	≥2 in the past 12 months

[a] Data from Schatz M, Dombrowski M. Asthma in pregnancy. N Engl J Med 2009;360:1862–69.

Table 10.3 Steps of asthma therapy during pregnancy[a].

Step	Preferred controller medication	Alternative controller medication
1	None	—
2	Low dose ICS	LTRA, theophylline
3	Medium dose ICS	Low dose ICS + either LABA, LTRA or theophylline
4	Medium dose ICS + LABA	Medium dose ICS + LTRA or theophylline
5	High dose ICS + LABA	—
6	High dose ICS + LABA + oral prednisone	—

ICS, *inhaled corticosteroids;* LABA, *long-acting beta-agonists;* LTRA, *leukotriene receptor antagonists.*
[a] *Data from Schatz M, Dombrowski M. Asthma in pregnancy. N Engl J Med 2009;360:1862–69.*

10.5 Pharmacologic therapy

Assignment of pregnancy risk letter categories, A, B, C, D, or X, was instituted by the U.S. Food and Drug Administration (FDA) over 30 years ago to help clinicians interpret the human and animal data on pregnancy safety for an approved drug. However, in practice, there was concern about the unintended application of these letter categories as an oversimplified grading system.

* To address the need for updated risk categories, in December of 2014, the FDA published a final rule entitled "Content and Format of Labeling for Human Prescription Drug and Biological Products: Requirements for Pregnancy and Lactation Labeling," which is also known simply as the "Pregnancy and Lactation Labeling Rule" or PLLR. The PLLR removes the pregnancy letter categories A, B, C, D, and X for all drugs. The PLLR also requires the label to be updated when information becomes outdated. As revised, the new format includes a narrative summary which includes available human, animal, and any pharmacological data regarding pregnancy risk. Also included is information about risk of the underlying maternal disease and/or risks of undertreatment of that disease during pregnancy. In 2018, the membership of the American Academy of Allergy, Asthma, and Immunology (AAAAI) was surveyed as to the value, awareness, and understanding of the new PLLR. Most respondents were not aware of the removal of the letter category system and did not find the new narrative summary to be clear or useful [35].

Asthma medications generally are divided into long-term control medications and rescue therapy. Long-term control medications are used for maintenance therapy to prevent asthma manifestations and include inhaled corticosteroids, long-acting beta-agonists, leukotriene receptor antagonists, and asthma biologics. Rescue therapy, most commonly inhaled short-acting beta-agonists, provides immediate relief of symptoms. Oral corticosteroids can either be used as a form of rescue therapy or as chronic therapy for severe persistent asthma.

10.5.1 Inhaled corticosteroids

Inhaled corticosteroids are the mainstay of controller therapy during pregnancy. The prevalence of its use in the United States is estimated to be about 34% (among pregnant asthmatics) [36]. Many studies have shown no increased perinatal risks (including preeclampsia, preterm birth, low birth weight, and congenital malformations) associated with inhaled corticosteroids [37–39]. One study of over 4000 women who used inhaled corticosteroids during pregnancy found no increased risk of perinatal mortality associated with inhaled corticosteroid use during pregnancy [40]. Several large studies support the lack of association of inhaled corticosteroid use with total or specific malformations. One study has suggested a relationship between high dose–inhaled corticosteroids and total malformations, but confounding by severity is a possible explanation, based on the relationships between exacerbations and congenital malformations demonstrated by the same group [21].

Because it has the most published human gestational safety data, budesonide is considered the preferred inhaled corticosteroid for asthma during pregnancy. That is not to say that the other inhaled corticosteroid preparations are unsafe. Therefore, inhaled corticosteroids other than budesonide may be continued in patients who were well controlled by these agents prior to pregnancy, especially if it is thought that changing formulations may jeopardize asthma control. Doses of inhaled corticosteroids are categorized as low, medium, and high (Table 10.4).

Table 10.4 Comparative daily doses for inhaled corticosteroids[a,b].

Corticosteroid	Amount	Low dose	Medium dose	High dose
Beclomethasone	40 mcg per puff	2–6 puffs	More than 6–12 puffs	More than 12 puffs
HFA	80 mcg per puff	1–3 puffs	More than 3–6 puffs	More than 6 puffs
Budesonide	90 mcg per inhalation	2–6 puffs	More than 6–12 puffs	More than 12 puffs
	180 mcg per inhalation	1–3 puffs	More than 3–6 puffs	More than 6 puffs
Ciclesonide	80 mcg per actuation	2–4 puffs	More than 4–8 puffs	More than 8 puffs
	160 mcg per actuation	1–2 puffs	More than 2–4 puffs	More than 4 puffs
Flunisolide HFA	80 mcg per puff	4 puffs	More than 4–8 puffs	More than 8 puffs
Fluticasone HFA	44 mcg per puff	2–6 puffs	–	–
	110 mcg per puff	2 puffs	More than 2–4 puffs	More than 4 puffs
	220 mcg per puff	1 puff	More than 1–2 puffs	More than 2 puffs

Continued

Table 10.4 Comparative daily doses for inhaled corticosteroids[a,b].—cont'd

Corticosteroid	Amount	Low dose	Medium dose	High dose
Fluticasone DPI	50 mcg per inhalation	2—6 puffs	—	—
	100 mcg per inhalation	1—3 puffs	More than 3—5 puffs	More than 5 puffs
	250 mcg per inhalation	1 puff	More than 1—2 puffs	More than 2 puffs
Mometasone	110 mcg per actuation	2 puffs	3—4 puffs	More than 4 puffs
	220 mcg per actuation	1 puff	2 puffs	More than 2 puffs

DPI, *dry powder inhaler;* HFA, *hydrofluoroalkane.*
[a] *Total daily puffs are usually divided into a twice-per-day regimen.*
[b] *Data from Ref. Expert Panel Report 3 (EPR-3): Guidelines for the diagnosis and management of asthma-summary report 2007. J Allergy Clin Immunol 2007;120:S94—S138. and Kelly HW Comparison of inhaled corticosteroids: an update. Ann Pharmacother 2009;43:519—27.*

10.5.2 Inhaled beta-agonists

Inhaled short-acting beta-agonists are the rescue therapy of choice for asthma during pregnancy. Inhaled albuterol is the first-choice short-acting beta-agonist for pregnant women because it has been studied the most extensively [23], although other agents may be used if uniquely helpful or well tolerated. Lin et al. using data from the US multicenter case control study of the National Birth Defects Prevention Study, reported the use of bronchodilators to be associated with an increased risk of esophageal atrophy among infants (OR, 2.39%; 95% confidence interval (CI), 1.23—4.66) 41]. The limitation of this study is that the results could be a result of confounding by indication. Also, in another cohort study involving 4558 women, there was an increased risk of cardiac defects exposed to bronchodilators during pregnancy (OR, 1.4; 95% CI, 1.1—1.7) [30]. However, this observation may also be a result of confounding. Asthma exacerbations may be associated with both increased use of bronchodilators and congenital malformations. In addition, factors such as obesity or lower household socioeconomic status may be associated with both more severe asthma requiring more bronchodilators and congenital malformations. A recent study showed that elevated BMI and gestational weight gain was associated with an increased risk of asthma exacerbations during pregnancy [42] In general, patients should use up to two treatments of inhaled albuterol (two to six puffs) or nebulized albuterol at 20-minute intervals for most mild to moderate symptoms; higher doses can be used for severe symptom exacerbations.

The use of long-acting beta-agonists is the preferred add-on controller therapy for asthma during pregnancy. This therapy should be added on when patients' symptoms are not controlled with the use of medium-dose inhaled corticosteroids. Because long-acting and short-acting inhaled beta-agonists have similar pharmacology and toxicology, long-acting beta-agonists are expected to have a safety profile similar to that of albuterol. Two long-acting beta-agonists are available:

salmeterol and formoterol. Limited observational data exist on their use during pregnancy. A possible association between long-acting beta-agonists and an increased risk of severe and even fatal asthma exacerbations has been observed in nonpregnant patients. As a result, long-acting beta-agonists are no longer recommended as monotherapy for the treatment of asthma and are available in fixed combination preparations with inhaled corticosteroids. Data are limited on safety of long-acting beta-agonists during pregnancy. Cossette et al. reported in a large retrospective cohort that the lLABA use was not associated with an increased risk of congenital malformation and that the outcomes of low birth weight, preterm birth, and small for gestational age were similar between commonly used LABA, formoterol, and salmeterol [43]. Expert panels suggest that the benefits of the use of long-acting beta-agonists appear to outweigh the risks as long as they are used concurrently with inhaled corticosteroids [44].

10.5.3 Leukotriene modifiers

Both zafirlukast and montelukast are selective leukotriene receptor antagonists indicated for the maintenance treatment of asthma. Data on the use of leukotriene receptor antagonists during pregnancy are more limited than for inhaled corticosteroids. In a recent retrospective insurance claims, cohort analysis of 1535 exposed infants shows a risk of congenital malformations to be similar to those pregnant women without asthma [45]. Montelukast is available as a once daily medication with doses variable based on age. For adults, the typical dose is 10 mg daily.

10.5.4 Cromolyn and theophylline

Given the superiority of inhaled corticosteroids over cromolyn and theophylline in the prevention of asthma symptoms, the latter are considered alternative treatments for mild persistent asthma. Theophylline is also an alternative, but not preferred, add-on treatment for moderate to severe persistent asthma. Reassuring data on the use of cromolyn and theophylline in pregnant women have been published [44]. Theophylline use is also limited by its many adverse side effects and potential drug interactions resulting in possible toxicity. Serum levels should be monitored during pregnancy and maintained between 5 and 12 mcg/mL. Cromolyn is now only available as a nebulizer solution.

10.5.5 Oral corticosteroids

Some patients with severe asthma may require regular oral corticosteroid use to achieve adequate asthma control. Oral corticosteroids are also typically part of the discharge regimen after an acute asthma episode. Doses are typically 40–60 mg in a single dose or two divided doses for 3–10 days. Oral corticosteroid use has been associated with an increased risk of preterm birth [18,23] and low birth weight infants [23] in 52–185 exposed women. In fact, a metaanalysis of cohort studies between 1975 and 2012 found that pregnant asthmatic who used oral corticosteroids during pregnancy had an increased risk of preterm delivery and low birth weight infants [46]. An increased risk of orofacial clefts was reported in a metaanalysis of case—control studies [47], but this increased risk was not confirmed in a large cohort study [31]. In addition, the National Birth Defects Prevention case control study recently reported no evidence of a link between oral clefts and oral corticosteroids [48]. Since these risks would be less than the potential risks of a severe asthma exacerbation, which include maternal or fetal mortality, oral corticosteroids are recommended when indicated for the management of severe asthma during pregnancy [44].

10.5.5.1 Asthma biologics

In 2003, Omalizumab became one of the treatment options for moderate to severe persistent allergic asthma. It is a recombinant DNA-derived humanized IgG1k monoclonal antibody that specifically binds to free human immunoglobulin E in the blood. It currently is the only asthma biologic with limited available human safety data from the EXPECT pregnancy registry. It was a single arm observational study of 250 pregnant asthmatic women exposed to omalizumab within 8 weeks prior to conception or at any time during pregnancy reported no increased risk of congenital malformations or low birth weight. The rates of prematurity (<37 weeks gestation) and small for gestational age were not unlike those seen in other studies of severe pregnant asthmatics. More recent data compared those patients enrolled in EXPECT to a disease-matched external cohort of moderate to severe asthmatics. There was no significant difference in rate of congenital malformations between the two groups [49].

Other newer medications include the following: tiotropium, mepolizumab, reslizumab, and dupilumab. There are no human data available for any of these medications. Animal studies are reassuring for tiotropium, with no congenital malformations in 800 times the maximum human daily dose. Mepolizumab has reassuring animal data with no fetal harm at 30 times human dose administered intravenously. There are pregnancy registries through the Mother to Baby network currently enrolling exposed pregnant women to mepolizumab, dupilumab, and benralizumab (mothertobaby.org).

10.6 Conclusion

Asthma is a common medical problem that may worsen during pregnancy. In addition to affecting maternal quality of life, uncontrolled asthma may lead to adverse perinatal outcomes. Awareness of proper treatment options for asthma during pregnancy is important for clinicians who care for pregnant patients. However, there are significant gaps in knowledge regarding commonly used asthma medications.

One of the most important needs for the future is the availability of additional safety information for asthma medications used during pregnancy that can also account for asthma control.

10.6.1 The vaccine and medication surveillance study

The Vaccines and Medication in Pregnant Surveillance System (VAMPSS) is coordinated by the AAAAI and has three research arms and an independent advisory committee. Funding has been provided by government agencies and individual pharmaceutical companies to employ a range of observational study designs. This includes the prospective cohort study, the case control study, and the database retrospective cohort study. The final component of VAMPSS is the independent Advisory Committee which is comprised of representatives from government, professional organizations as well as a consumer representative. This surveillance system was developed to provide safety information on the wide range of vaccines and medications taken by pregnant women.

References

[1] Schatz M, Dombrowski M, Wise R. Asthma morbidity during pregnancy can be predicted by severity classification. J Allergy Clin Immunol 2003;112:283−8.

[2] Belanger K, Hellenbrand M, Holford T, Bracken M. Effect of pregnancy on ma- ternal asthma symptoms and medication use. Obstet Gynecol 2010;115:559−67.

[3] Schatz M, Zeiger RS, Harden KM, Hoffman CP, Forsythe AB, Chilingar LM, et al. The course of asthma during pregnancy, post-partum, and with successive pregnancies: a prospective analysis. J Allergy Clin Immunol 1988;81:509−17.

[4] Gluck J, Gluck P. The effect of pregnancy on the course of asthma. Immunol Allergy Clin 2000;20:729−43.

[5] Murphy VE, Gibson PG, Smith R, Clifton VL. Asthma during pregnancy: mechanisms and treatment implications. Eur Respir J 2005;25:731−50.

[6] Enriquez R, Wu P, Griffin MR, Gebretsadik T, Shintani A, Mitchel E, et al. Cessation of asthma medication in early pregnancy. Am J Onstet Gynecol 2006;195:149−53.

[7] Louik C, Schatz M, Hernandez-Diaz S, Werler MM, Mitchell AA. Asthma in pregnancy and its pharmacologic treatment. Ann Allergy Asthma Immunol 2010;105:110−7.

[8] Cydulka R, Emerman C, Schreiber D, Molander K, Woodruff P, Camargo C. Acute asthma among pregnant women presenting to the emergency depart- ment. Am J Respir Crit Care Med 1999;160:887−92.

[9] McCallister J, Benninger C, Frey H, Phillips G, Mastronarde J. Pregnancy related treatment disparities of acute asthma exacerbations in the emergency department. Respir Med 2011;105:1434−40.

[10] Murphy V, Namazy J, Powell H, Schatz M, Chambers C, Attia J, et al. A meta-analysis of adverse perinatal outcomes in women with asthma. BJOG 2011;118:1314−23.

[11] Triche EW, Saftlas AF, Belanger K, Leaderer BP, Bracken MB. Association of asthma diagnosis, severity, symptoms, and treatment with risk of preeclamp- sia. Obstet Gynecol 2004;104:585−93.

[12] Jana N, Vasishta K, Saha SC, Khunnu B. Effect of bronchial asthma on the course of pregnancy, labour and perinatal outcome. J Obstet Gynaecol 1995;21:227−32.

[13] Stenius-Aarniala BS, Hedman J, Teramo KA. Acute asthma during pregnancy. Thorax 1996;51:411−4.

[14] Minerbi-Codish I, Fraser D, Avnun L, Glezerman M, Heimer D. Influence of asthma in pregnancy on labor and the newborn. Respiration 1998;65:130−5.

[15] Mihrshahi S, Belousova E, Marks GB, Peat JK, Childhood Asthma Prevention Team. Pregnancy and birth outcomes in families with asthma. J Asthma 2003;40:181−7.

[16] Stenius-Aarniala B, Piirila P, Teramo K. Asthma and pregnancy: a prospective study of 198 pregnancies. Thorax 1988;43:12−8.

[17] Dombrowski MP, Schatz M, Wise R, Momirova V, Landon M, Mabie W, et al. Asthma during pregnancy. Obstet Gynecol 2004;103:5−12.

[18] Bracken MB, Triche EW, Belanger K, Saftlas A, Beckett WS, Leaderer BP. Asthma symptoms, severity, and drug therapy: a prospective study of effects on 2205 pregnancies. Obstet Gynecol 2003;102:739−52.

[19] Schatz M, Zeiger RS, Hoffman CP, Harden K, Forsythe A, Chilingar L, et al. Perinatal outcomes in the pregnancies of asthmatic women: a prospective controlled analysis. Am J Respir Crit Care Med 1995;151:1170−4.

[20] Firoozi F, Lemiere C, Ducharme FM, Beauchesne MF, Perreault S, Berard A, et al. Effect of maternal moderate to severe asthma on perinatal outcomes. Respir Med 2010; 104:1278−87.

[21] Blais L, Forget A. Asthma exacerbations during the first trimester of pregnancy and the risk of congenital malformations among asthmatic women. J Allergy Clin Immunol 2008;121:1379−84. 1384 e1371.

[22] Expert Panel Report 3 (EPR-3). Guidelines for the diagnosis and management of asthma-summary report 2007. J Allergy Clin Immunol 2007;120:S94−138.

[23] Schatz M, Dombrowski MP, Wise R, Momirova V, Landon M, Mabie W, et al. The relationship of asthma medication use to perinatal outcomes. J Allergy Clin Immunol 2004; 113:1040−5.

[24] Schatz M, Zeiger RS, Harden K, Hoffman CC, Chilingar L, Petitti D. The safety of asthma and allergy medications during pregnancy. J Allergy Clin Immunol 1997;100: 301−6.

[25] Norjavaara E, de Verdier MG. Normal pregnancy outcomes in a population- based study including 2,968 pregnant women exposed to budesonide. J Allergy Clin Immunol 2003; 111:736−42.

[26] Martel MJ, Rey E, Beauchesne MF, Perreault S, Lefebvre G, Forget A, et al. Use of inhaled corticosteroids during pregnancy and risk of pregnancy in- duced hypertension: nested case−control study. BMJ 2005;330:230.

[27] Kallen B, Rydhstroem H, Aberg A. Congenital malformations after the use of inhaled budesonide in early pregnancy. Obstet Gynecol 1999;93:392−5.

[28] Bakhireva LN, Jones KL, Schatz M, Johnson D, Chambers CD, Organization of Teratology Information Services Research Group. Asthma medication use in pregnancy and fetal growth. J Allergy Clin Immunol 2005;116:503−9.

[29] Breton MC, Beauchesne MF, Lemiere C, Rey E, Forget A, Blais L. Risk of peri- natal mortality associated with inhaled corticosteroid use for the treatment of asthma during pregnancy. J Allergy Clin Immunol 2010;126. 772−77.e2.

[30] Kallen B, Otterblad Olausson P. Use of anti-asthmatic drugs during preg- nancy. 3. Congenital malformations in the infants. Eur J Clin Pharmacol 2007;63:383−8.

[31] Hyiid A, Molgaard-Nielesen D. Corticosteroid use during pregnancy and the risk of orofacial clefts. CMAJ (Can Med Assoc J) 2011;183:796−804.

[32] Blais L, Beauchesne MF, Rey E, Malo JL, Forget A. Use of inhaled corticoste- roids during the first trimester of pregnancy and the risk of congenital malfor- mations among women with asthma. Thorax 2007;62:320—8.

[33] Blais L, Beauchesne MF, Lemiere C, Elftouh N. High doses of inhaled cortico- steroids during the first trimester of pregnancy and congenital malformations. J Allergy Clin Immunol 2009;124:1229—34. e1224.

[34] Lin S, Munsie J, Herdt-Losavio M. Maternal asthma medication use and the risk of gastroschisis. Am J Epidemiol 2008;168:73—9.

[35] Lin S, Herdt-Losavio M, Gensburg L, Marshall E, Druschel C. Maternal asth- ma medi- cation use and the risk of congenital heart defects. Birth Defects Res (Part A) 2009;85: 161—8.

[36] Robijn AL, Jensen ME, mclaughlin K, Gibson PG, Murphy VE. Inhaled corticoste- roid use during pregnancy among women with asthma: A systematic review and meta-analysis.Clin Exp Allergy 2019;49(111):1403—17.

[37] Bakhireva LN, Jones KL, Schatz M, Klonoff-Cohen HS, Johnson D, Slymen DJ, et al. Safety of leukotriene receptor antagonists in pregnancy. J Allergy Clin Immunol 2007; 119:618—25.

[38] Sarkar M, Koren G, Kalra S, Ying A, Smorlesi C, DeSantis M, et al. Montelu- kast use during pregnancy; a multicentre, prospective, comparative study of infant outcomes. Eur J Clin Pharmacol 2009;65:1259—64.

[40] Breton MC, Beauchesne MF, Lemiere C, Rey E, Forget A, Blais L. Risk of perinatal mortality associated with inhaled corticosteroid use for the treatment of asthma during pregnancy. J Allergy Clin Immunol 2010;126(4):772—7.

[41] Labor S, Dalbello AM, Plavec D, et al. What is safe enough - asthma in pregnancy - a review of current literature and recommendations. Asthma Res Pract 2018;4:11.

[42] Murphy VE, Jensen ME, Powell H, Gibson PG. Influence of maternal body mass index and macrophage activation on asthma exacerbations in pregnancy. J Allergy Clin Immunol Pract 2017;5(4):981—7.

[43] Cossette B, Forget A, Beauchesne MF, et al. Impact of maternal use of asthma- controller therapy on perinatal outcomes. Thorax 2013;68:724—30.

[44] Busse WW. NAEPP expert panel report. Managing asthma during pregnancy: recom- mendations for pharmacologic treatment — 2004 update. J Allergy Clin Immunol 2005;115:34—46.

[45] Nelsen LM, Shields KE, Cunningham ML, et al. Congenital malformations among infants born to women receiving montelukast, inhaled corticosteroids, and other asthma medications. J Allergy Clin Immunol 2012;129:251.

[46] Murphy VE, Namazy JA, Schatz M, Chambers C, Attia J, Gibson PG. A meta-analysis of adverse perinatal outcomes in women with asthma. BJOG 2011;118(11):1314—23.

[47] Park-Wyllie L, Mazzotta P, Pastuszak A, Moretti ME, Beique L, Hunnisett L, et al. Birth defects after maternal exposure to corticosteroids: prospec- tive cohort study and meta- analysis of epidemiologic studies. Teratology 2000;62:385—92.

[48] Bandoli G, Palmsten K, Forbess Smith CJ, Chambers CD. A review of systemic corti- costeroid use in pregnancy and the risk of select pregnancy and birth outcomes. Rheum Dis Clin North Am 2017;43(3):489—502.

[49] Namazy JA, Blais L, Andrews EB, et al. The Xolair Pregnancy Registry (EXPECT): Peri- natal outcomes among pregnant women with asthma treated with omalizumab (Xolair) compared against those of a cohort of pregnant women with moderate-to-severe asthma. J All Clin Immunol 2019;143(2).

Nausea and vomiting of pregnancy

11

Carolyn Bottone-Post
University of Northern Colorado, Greeley, CO, United States

11.1 Nausea and vomiting of pregnancy

One of the most frequently encountered common discomforts related to pregnancy is nausea and vomiting. Nausea and vomiting of pregnancy (NVP) is often most difficult to deal with, often debilitating to patients, relationships, work performance, and severely impacts quality of life (QOL) if untreated or poorly controlled. While likely multifactorial in nature, there is no "magic bullet" or formula which may be successfully applied to all women; treatments for afflicted women must be considered on an individual basis [51], and prevention is likely the best approach [28]. It is understood that NVP and hyperemesis gravidarum (HG) decrease absorption of many drugs resulting in diminished therapeutic concentrations, while pH changes in the stomach alter drug bioavailability [41]. Drug distribution is further altered due to increased maternal plasma volume; a decrease in plasma protein during pregnancy may result in more unbound, metabolically active drug levels which affect drug excretion [41].

11.2 Prevalence

Statistics vary regarding prevalence, but many authors agree NVP occurs in up to 70—91% of pregnancies [11,16,36]. Authors may differentiate nausea from retching and actual vomiting and agree this debilitating process may occur anytime of the day or night [10]. A challenge to the study of this malady is lack of consistent definitions used among researchers [14] and data collection challenges related to inconsistencies in ICD-10 hospital coding [25].

NVP often begins in the fourth to sixth week of pregnancy, reaching peak prevalence during weeks 8—12, and diminishing by week 20 [7,51], although approximately 10% of women continue to experience NVP throughout pregnancy [11]. Women who experience severe and prolonged NVP are said to have HG, the most severe form of the problem. Although this extreme form of NVP occurs in only approximately 1%—3% of the pregnant population [10,16,36], it is quite challenging to deal with and recurs in about 75% of subsequent pregnancies [63].

HG is generally defined as severe, persistent, and prolonged NVP beginning before 20 weeks of pregnancy and associated with dehydration, ketonuria, and loss of $\geq 5\%$ loss of body mass index (BMI), often requiring hospitalization to achieve symptom relief [14,17,79]. Electrolyte disturbances and abnormalities in liver function occur in approximately 50% of HG sufferers [2]. As the most common reason for hospitalization in the first half of pregnancy [2], the effects of HG severely impact QOL, often result in orthostatic BP and heart rate changes, and may portend postpartum depression [2,17,63]. Rarely, women with HG experience Wernicke encephalopathy, splenic avulsion, esophageal rupture, and pneumothorax [48]; as such, it is suggested when administering IV fluids they be of lactated ringers solution with added thiamine (B-1) to prevent Wernicke encephalopathy [65]. Because NVP is such a common occurrence, providers, family members, and employers may minimize its significance [33], leading women to feel unsupported and labeled lazy or complainers and ultimately experiencing feelings of being dismissed and not heard by providers and family. Those who equate NVP with a protective response to preserve pregnancy may, unfortunately, undertreat patients [3].

NVP and HG have global significance, affecting relationships with significant others, caretaking other children, and employment. Women experience emotional sequelae and economic burdens from these conditions and may ultimately consider termination of the current pregnancy and prevention of any future pregnancies [18]. Women with severe NVP or HG experience diminished QOL as their symptom severity increases; however, even mild symptoms impact women's ability to perform in the workplace, care for their children, and maintain satisfying relationships with friends or partners [11,30,77]. These women may decide to delay or decline future pregnancies and even consider termination if symptoms are severe and unrelenting [77]. Health care professionals may dismiss symptoms as trivial [32]; however, it is critical to intervene early to prevent development of HG [3].

11.3 Etiologies and pathogenesis
11.3.1 Genetic influences

NVP is highly heritable, impacting duration, severity, and recurrence. Women with HG have a greater risk of recurrence with future pregnancies, compounded further in those whose mothers or sisters experienced this problem [11]. Women with prepregnancy mental health disorders may be at higher risk for HG [2]; further, there is an increased risk of postpartum depression in women experiencing NVP or HG [8,16]. Pregnant teens aged 16−19 with NVP or HG were found to have worse Edinburgh Postpartum Depression Scores than those without symptoms and suffered higher rates of prenatal depression related to fatigue, insomnia, and starvation [70]. There appears to be increased incidence of NVP in women with comorbid conditions, such as diabetes (pregestational or gestational), hypertension (HTN) (chronic or gestational), hyperlipidemia, anemia, or thyroid dysfunction [23,76], although linkages are unclear.

11.3.2 Hormonal influences

NVP and HG are frequently thought to result from higher hCG levels, as the peak times of occurrence often correlate to rising hCG; women at risk for NVP and HG often have higher levels due to multiple gestations, molar pregnancies, and those with larger placental volume. However, higher hCG levels have not been found to consistently equate to more pronounced. However, higher hCG levels have not been found to consistently equate to more pronounced nausea symptoms, rather, be associated with receptor sensitivity or differences in hCG isoforms [62]. Studies are not consistent evaluating hCG effects on NVP or HG.

Progesterone is implicated in changes in gastrointestinal (GI) motility, exerting inhibitory effects on GI contractility. Normally, electrical cycles of the GI tract occur at two to four times per minute; however, with delayed cycling (bradygastria), transit time is significantly slowed, resulting in more nausea [10,11,39]. Women with preexisting conditions associated with gastric dysrhythmia, such as reflux disorders, Crohn's disease, celiac disease, and irritable bowel syndrome or women receiving progesterone may experience more NVP [39].

Estrogen also negatively impacts development of NVP; women in hyperestrogenic states, such as multifetal gestations or those with high BMI, often experience more NVP or worse symptoms [11]. Estrogen induces nitric oxide production resulting in relaxation of smooth muscle and delayed gastric transit time [24,31]; further, sex hormone levels dramatically change esophageal, gastric, and small bowel motility impacting NVP [45]. While the role of hCG in NVP is unclear, some suggest NVP is a relative imbalance in acidic isoforms of the hormone, rather than absolute hCG level [11].

Women at risk for HG have demonstrated higher serotonin levels [2,16], a hormone which also modulates GI motility. This suggests serotonin receptor antagonists might be more effective in controlling NVP; however, there is no consistent symptom improvement seen with such medications [11]. Additionally, women experiencing HG may demonstrate heightened sensitivity to estrogen rather than serotonin, worsening symptoms [26].

Pregnancies characterized by NVP or HG may have transient hyperthyroid states because of similarities in the beta-subunits of hCG and thyroid-stimulating hormone [55]. During pregnancy, rising hCG levels can physiologically stimulate the thyroid, resulting in a mild hyperthyroidism which does not require treatment. However, the prevalence of overt thyroid dysfunction during pregnancy is estimated by some at 2%−3% [11,31,51].

Relaxin levels also contribute to slow GI transit times by provoking electrical cycle dysregulation during pregnancy [14]. In addition, relaxin progressively reduces lower esophageal sphincter pressure throughout pregnancy, increasing incidence of GI upset and potential GERD symptoms [10].

11.3.3 *Helicobacter pylori*

90% of HG sufferers are suspected to have *H. pylori* infections as compared with a control group rate of 50% when mucosal samples are compared [10,11]. Severity of symptoms seems to correlate with density of infection; however, blood testing alone fails to identify remote or current infections. Diagnostic testing may be helpful in women without significant NVP or HG symptom improvement [62]. Stool antigen testing may be helpful in identifying current infection; in the presence of a known current infection, dual antibiotic therapy is suggested with 2 weeks treatment with a proton pump inhibitor (PPI) [7].

11.4 Burden of the disease

Many authors agree NVP and HG are leading causes of hospitalization in early pregnancy [32,51,65]. The economic burden of NVP was estimated at $1827 per pregnancy by Ref. [63] and/or approximately $1.8 billion in 2012 in the United States [11,17]. Multiple unscheduled visits to care providers, telephone contacts, and utilization of ambulance or EMT services increase costs for caring for NVP and HG patients [25,53]. Diminished job effectiveness and time lost from work contribute to the economic and psychological burden women suffered [48]. Negative experiences HG may meet criteria for posttraumatic stress disorder [32], suggesting a relationship between degree of symptoms, hospitalization, and risk of prenatal and postpartum anxiety and depression [37].

While the impact on QOL is more difficult to measure, most authors agree there are significant negative effects on partner and parenting relationships, job performance, and fulfillment of household responsibilities [11,30]. However, QOL studies related to NVP and HG are subject to profound recall bias complicating research [64]. Providers must acknowledge grieving processes associated with loss of normal, uncomplicated pregnancy experiences and instead offer support to deal with disruption of QOL by significant symptoms [68]. Heitman et al. [77] reported while even mild NVP negatively impacted women's lives, with severe symptoms, women were less likely to consider future pregnancies. Authors agreed all modes of therapeutic management should be utilized before therapeutic abortion is considered [23]. Evaluating length of stay per hospital admission and improved quantification of symptom severity assist approximations of current cost burden [21,25], as use of incorrect diagnosis codes may result in underreporting admissions for NVP, compounding errors in determining financial burden [23].

11.5 Cultural implications

It is interesting to note some cultures lack words to describe NVP; as a result, diminished self-worth and self-esteem and being thought of negatively by family may result [29]. Difficulty describing the experience of NVP and HG among pregnant women in some cultures is made more difficult by food insecurities, taboos, cultural mores, and norms. Precluding pregnant women from consuming potentially tainted foods, especially meat, milk, and vegetables, may be perceived as problematic, especially younger women with less education, subject to direction from powerful and influential family members. Women may not know or understand the basis of foods recommended or prohibited; however, adherence may be rooted in cultural and evolutionary factors [18]. NVP occurs more commonly in women from India, Pakistan, Asian, and New Zealand compared to other populations [11]. Some authors attribute NVP to an evolutionary mechanism resulting in better precautions around behaviors and intake and promoting additional social support [3,45,53]; however, this may result in undertreatment of symptoms.

11.6 Risk factors

NVP occurs more often in women who are obese, younger, primigravidas, and non-smokers [63]. Other risk factors include multiple gestations, molar pregnancies and pregnancies with female infants, and factors related to an increase in hCG levels [7,53]. Younger women had a higher risk of NVP and had a two times higher likelihood of hospital admission [23]. Smoking seems to exert a protective effect against NVP [11], perhaps due to decreased placental size [23] suggested lower socioeconomic status (SES) as a risk for worse NVP; others, however, found no evidence of association of SES, BMI, or smoking status with NVP [7]. Additionally, women with a history of motion sickness or migraines may experience worse symptoms; avoiding flickering lights and high-humidity environments may be helpful preventive tactics [3,65].

11.7 Quantification

The PUQE, or Pregnancy Unique Quantification of Emesis scoring system, is a frequently employed system used to assess the severity of NVP based on the presence of nausea, vomiting, and retching during a 24-h period. It has been repeatedly validated for use [11,33,50]. This three-question survey differentiates between nausea, vomiting, and retching, with a maximum of 15 points possible, helping categorize severity of NVP into "mild" ($\leq$6 points), "moderate" (7−12 points), and "severe" ($\geq$13 points). It also contains a QOL question with no points attached (see Fig. 11.1). Rhodes Index Score (see Fig. 11.2) is also a valid and reliable tool for self-quantification of postoperative nausea and vomiting and is also used to determine the extent of NVP [20]. Future work includes the MinSafeStart mobile

PUQE form:

Pregnancy-Unique Quantification of Emesis and nausea

Circle the answer that suit the best your situation for the last 24 hours.

1. On average in a day, for how long do you feel nauseated or sick to your stomach?

> 6 hours 5 points	4-6 hours 4 points	2-3 hours 3 points	$\leq$1 hour 2 points	Not at all 1 point

2. On average in a day, how many times do you vomit or throw up?

$\geq$7 times 5 points	5-6 times 4 points	3-4 times 3 points	1-2 times 2 points	Not at all 1 point

3. On average in a day, how many times have you had retching or dry heaves without bringing anything up?

$\geq$7 times 5 points	5-6 times 4 points	3-4 times 3 points	1-2 times 2 points	Not at all 1 point

Total score (sum of replies to 1, 2, and 3): mild NVP $\leq$6; moderate NVP, 7-12; severe NVP $\geq$13.

Quality of life question:
On a scale of 0 to 10, how would you rate your well-being:_____
0 (worst possible) 10 (As good as you felt before pregnancy)

PUQE form modified from: Koren G, Boskovic R, Hard M, Maltepe C, Navioz Y, Einarson A. Motherisk-PUQE (pregnancy-unique quantification of emesis and nausea) scoring system for nausea and vomiting of pregnancy. American journal of obstetrics and gynecology. 2002;186:S228-31, with permission.

FIGURE 11.1

Pregnancy Unique Quantification of Emesis scoring system.

application, currently being developed in Norway, to help quantify symptoms of NVP and optimize treatment [47].

11.8 Effects on fetus

Some authors purport no association between HG and lower APGAR scores or perinatal mortality [2]. [3] implies a possible but unclear connection between the severity of NVP and low birthweight (LBW), small for gestational age (SGA), and preterm births. While there are multifactorial etiologies suspected, children of women with severe NVP and HG may experience developmental disabilities such as seen with Autism Spectrum Disorder including impaired social, verbal, and nonverbal communication abilities [66].

Scores	4	3	2	1	0
1. In the last N hours, I threw up __ times.	7 or more	5–6	3–4	1–2	I did not throw up
2. In the last N hours, from retching and dry heaves, I felt __ distress.	Severe	Great	Moderate	Mild	No
3. In the last N hours, from vomiting or throwing up, I have felt __ distress.	Severe	Great	Moderate	Mild	No
4. In the last N hours, I have felt nauseated or sick to my stomach __.	More than 4 hours	2–3 hours	1–2 hours	1 hour less	Not at all
5. In the last N hours, because of nausea/sickness, I have felt __ distress.	Severe	Great	Moderate	Mild	No
6. In the last N hours, each time I threw up, I produced a __ amount.	Very large (3 cups or more)	Large (2–3 cups)	Moderate (1/2–2 cups)	Small (up to 1/2 cup)	I did not throw up
7. In the last N hours, I have felt nauseated or sick to my stomach __ times.	7 or more	5–6	3–4	1–2	No
8. In the last N hours, I have had periods of retching or dry heaves without bringing anything up __ times.	7 or more	5–6	3–4	1–2	No

FIGURE 11.2

Rhodes index rhodes-index-of-nausea-vomiting-and-retching-3.png.

11.9 Late complications related to NVP

Authors suggested there was an increased risk of preeclampsia, proteinuria, and/or HTN with NVP, which appeared related to elevated hCG levels; however, there appeared to be a lower risk for LBW or SGA infants with NVP [14], while other authors suggested that mild-to-moderate NVP was associated with improved outcomes, such as fewer miscarriages and fetal malformations, less prematurity, and better attainment of developmental milestones [17,34].

11.10 Approaches to treatment

Generally, authors agree treatment must be individualized for every patient and could relate to individual metabolic activity as well as differences in drug bioavailability [11]; 1- [23,30]; further, authors agree that prevention and early treatment of symptoms is better than identifying which treatments are effective after symptoms arise [33,39]. It is appropriate to utilize simpler interventions, such as lifestyle changes, before employing higher level interventions such as pharmaceuticals [63]. However, there is a dearth of evidence-based study related to effective lifestyle changes [39] and few medication studies that included the vulnerable population of pregnant women. This results from regulatory change following the Thalidomide disaster in 1961 [67]. While there are adverse drug events websites for reporting complications around drugs used in pregnancy, most premarketing human clinical trials exclude pregnant women, promoting reliance on less rigorous studies [69].

Authors generally agree that avoidance of medications in the first trimester is advisable [10,11]; however [23], studies suggest nearly half the women who were admitted for symptomatic control of NVP had not previously received a prescription medication. Clinicians following treatment guidelines may prevent initial or recurrent hospital admissions and related resource utilization [56]. Following a logical, stepwise plan using antiemetics and additional strategies will be helpful to combat NVP and HG [36].

11.11 Lifestyle alterations

NVP is described as a self-limiting problem for many for which authors recommend lifestyle alterations. These may include avoiding known triggers, such as certain foods, heated foods, cooking odors, perfumes, or activities which provoke NVP for the individual [2,7,28]. Frequent small, bland, low-fat meals and snacking on carbohydrate-rich items such as crackers and dry toast may be helpful, while others suggest consumption of a small protein meal at bedtime may reduce symptoms [33,65]. Other recommendations include separating food intake from fluid intake so as not to overfill the stomach and avoiding overly sweet or very cold beverages [5,7]. Pregnant women often begin prenatal vitamin supplements in early pregnancy, but may find relief taking two children's chewable vitamins daily instead, supplementing with folic acid, and temporarily stopping oral iron preparations may help prevent GI upset [3,7,10,65]. Avoiding extreme fatigue and excessive stress may be helpful; additionally, consuming high-protein liquids especially to prevent dehydration or consuming electrolyte solutions, eating fresh fruits and vegetables, and consuming cold foods may prevent or correct gastric dysmotility syndromes [10,11,28]. While bland, simple carbohydrates are usually well tolerated, these may provoke rapid blood sugar fluctuations, and protein foods or beverages should be additionally offered [28].

Women who experience signs of circulatory disturbances, such as dizziness, may experience symptom improvement when wearing medium range compression hose (23−32 mm Hg at the ankle), which should be applied before arising each morning for maximum relief [45]. It was suggested women make the most of the times when symptom free and increase rest when symptoms are prominent [53], as rest helps diminish symptoms [68].

11.12 Complementary and alternative medicine

11.12.1 Nonpharmacologic treatments

Acupressure, massage, and hypnotherapy have been suggested for decreasing NVP [7,11,28,73,74]; however, some conclude there is insufficient evidence that hypnotherapy helps NVP [65]. Proponents of hypnosis cite several small studies with encouraging results where hypnosis was helpful to reduce sensitivity of nausea centers in the brain; however, training may be cost prohibitive [28]. Mindfulness therapy is suggested in conjunction with B-6 use [12]. Acupressure especially is considered safe, easy to self-administer, cost-effective, and helpful to some women. Application of Sea Bands is easy for patients, who place their middle three fingers on inside of the wrist with the edge of the third finger on the wrist crease. The appropriate pressure point known as the Nei-Kuan or P-6 point is just under the edge of the index finger between the two central tendons. Sea Bands are applied with the button exerting downward pressure on both wrists at the Nei-Kuan point [23]. Authors suggest additional research is needed to assure the efficacy of acupuncture and acupressure in pregnancy. While there is safety in providing acustimulation or mild electrical stimuli to the P-6 pressure point for the treatment of NVP, there are mixed results on the effectiveness [28,46,65]. Aromatherapy has not been demonstrated effective for treatment of NVP, except for lemon aroma [22].

11.12.2 Vitamins

Authors agree use of vitamin B-6, or pyridoxine, may be helpful primarily in preventing onset of nausea and may be used in doses up to 200 mg daily [2,7,57]. B-6 levels are related to protein and not caloric consumption [31] and may exert a synergistic effect with antihistamines; others suggest dosages up to 1000 mg daily may be used [28]. Similarly, the use of folic acid supplements in place of prenatal vitamin use or changing to two children's chewable vitamins without iron is suggested [23].

11.12.3 Herbal supplements

Herbal treatments employed for NVP generally have an associated and unfounded perception of gentleness and safety, such as using chamomile (*Matricaria chamomilla*) for reducing nausea [2,28], or cranberry and raspberry leaf [35]. Herbal treatments must be treated as seriously as medications since they contain chemically active ingredients that have indications, precautions, and contraindications much like their prescription counterparts, with risks that may include allergy, dehydration, hypotension, arrhythmia, or anticoagulant effects [28,59].

11.12.4 Ginger (*Zingiber officinale*)

Pharmaceutical grade ginger is considered a safe and effective remedy for NVP [7]. Ginger contains gingerols and shogaols which act as dopamine and serotonin antagonists and improve gastric motility and transit time. While the exact mechanism of action is not known, studies suggest anticholinergic and antiserotonergic properties, which improve gastric tone, motility, and transit time [43,51], may be helpful to decrease nausea but not overall vomiting episodes [28]. It is available as a tea, syrup, candied, or in fresh root form, but levels of the active herb vary widely depending on preparations; the highest dosage of gingerols is found in dried ginger powder (7—14 mg/gm), followed by fresh ginger (2—2.8 mg/gm) and powdered tea products (0.8 mg/gm) [43]. Dosages of 200—1000 mg daily in divided doses have been recommended [10,41] however, dosages from 600 to 2500 mg daily may also be used [34]. Studies have found ginger to be very helpful in NVP, but caution it may provoke heartburn [20,57]. Interpretation of study results is hampered by differences in herb preparation and form [43]. Results from a small study suggest the combination of ginger with B-6 is more effective than placebo, but there were no significant differences when participants were treated with one of these supplements alone [58]. Ginger should be avoided by women on anticoagulants as it may inhibit their action leading to more bleeding [11]; however, other studies have not demonstrated any effects on platelet aggregation or interactions with anticoagulants [43]. While there is no evidence of fetal risk associated with use of ginger [65], more research on safety and efficacy is suggested [23].

11.12.5 **Lemon**

Formulations containing lemon, whether in drops, oils, or candies, have been found helpful for nausea in a variety of settings, but conflict regarding timing of doses, formulations, and delivery presents a barrier to use [5,63]. Lemon aroma has been found helpful for combating NVP and nausea in bone marrow transplant patients. In a small study, lemon consumption and inhalation was found helpful for nausea without causing harm; further, oral use may reduce halitosis associated with ketonuria for symptom improvement [9].

11.12.6 **Pomegranate and spearmint**

Pomegranate (*Punica granatum* L.) and spearmint (*Mentha spicata* L.) have been used extensively in traditional Persian medicine for their unique properties. Pomegranate syrup is purported to improve gastric tone and act as a remedy against *H. pylori* and ulcers. It is reported to decrease platelet dysfunction and reduce oxidative stress in the placenta, although there have been no well-constructed studies confirming these properties. Spearmint underwent a small randomized control, double-blind study utilizing oil disbursed in a bowl of water and placed near a bed before sleep. The study suggested while there was improvement of NVP in the spearmint group, it was not significant [1]. While not well studied, mint is reported to reduce smooth muscle spasm and improve dysmotility symptoms [28]. Utilizing mint essential for its aroma was found to significantly decrease NVP, but no impact on maternal anxiety was noted [6].

11.12.7 **Quince (*Cydonia oblonga*)**

This highly astringent fruit is employed successfully in Iranian traditional medicine and is endorsed for antioxidant, antifungal, antibacterial, and antiinflammatory properties, and may be consumed as a raw fruit, concentrated paste, or syrup [35]. In a multicentered randomized controlled trial, quince performed better in preventing and treating NVP than B-6 [35].

11.13 **Pharmacologic therapies**

In general, treatment for NVP soon after presentation of symptoms may halt or delay the appearance of HG. Women who have previously experienced HG should begin treatment early before the onset of symptoms, with consideration of alternate administration routes when treatment is begun. Further, if several medications are used simultaneously, clinicians must be diligent to avoid adverse or compound drug reactions [3].

11.13.1 **Fluid rehydration**

This may be helpful for refractory vomiting or in HG associated with ketonuria, weight loss, and electrolyte disturbances [7,51,53]. Use of lactated ringers or normal saline solutions, not glucose solutions alone, was recommended for fluid replacement [23]. Due to significant risk of serious complications such as infection, thromboembolic events, bacteremia, and sepsis, PICC line placement is not recommended [65].

11.13.2 Enteral versus parenteral nutrition

Authors suggest enteral feedings provide more relief than parenteral feedings [2,65] and promote use of Pedialyte or sports beverages when no evidence of severe dehydration exists [53]. Parenteral hydration should be considered if enteral feedings fail but should be used as a last resort [28].

11.13.3 Diclegis

This is the only medication used for NVP which holds a Food and Drug Administration (FDA) indication and approval since 2013. The formulation includes 10 mg doxylamine and 10 mg Vitamin B-6 in a timed-release formula; it seems more effective if started early in pregnancy to prevent NVP rather than for relieving acute symptoms [7,40]. Diclegis inhibits the action of histamine at H-1 receptor sites and studies suggest no increase in fetal malformations when used in the first trimester [40]. Proponents of the drug suggest Diclegis is one of the most extensively studied medications for pregnancy use, with most evidence suggesting its efficacy due to an abundance of data from the market withdrawal of Bendectin in 1983 [44]. Diclegis does not contain Dicyclomine, a component not found efficacious and was subsequently removed.

Since most women take between two and four tablets daily, Diclegis is costly, ranging from about $220.00 to $570.00 for 100 tablets [27,60] and $136.00 for a generic version [27]. The components of Diclegis may be bought separately as 10 mg Doxylamine and 10 mg B-6 for significantly less but lack the timed-release of Doxylamine and may be less effective. Common side effects include dizziness, dry mouth, and fatigue; less common side effects include urinary retention, vertigo, tinnitus, insomnia, and facial dyskinesia. It should be used cautiously in women with asthma, narrow-angle glaucoma, ulcer, GI obstruction, or bladder neck obstruction (Drug and Therapeutic Bulletin, 2019).

11.13.3.1 Bonjesta

This medication was approved by the FDA in 2016 and has a dual action of a rapid release phase of medication providing appreciable blood levels quickly then employs a delayed release phase providing extended relief [38,51]. It is composed of an enteric coated core of 10 mg each doxylamine and pyridoxine, covered by an immediate release layer of the same, providing a total of 20 mg doxylamine and 20 mg pyridoxine. It appears both bonjesta and diclegis have similar side effect profiles, including somnolence, headache, dizziness, and dry mouth.

11.13.3.2 Antacids

While there are no teratogenic effects from this group, they have limited effect on NVP [7]. Pregnant women should avoid bicarbonate of soda formulation because of the potential for causing systemic pH changes. Calcium, aluminum, and magnesium-based products are considered safe in pregnancy [10]; however, prolonged use of magnesium trisilicate (Gaviscon) has been associated with the formation of renal stones, hypotonia, and fetal respiratory distress [11].

11.13.3.3 Diphenhydramine/dimenhydrinate/meclizine

Benadryl, Dramamine, and Meclizine are H-1 receptor antagonist antihistamines, which are considered safe for use in pregnancy; however, since they may cause excessive drowsiness, they are often used primarily for episodes of breakthrough NVP [7,23]. They additionally provide indirect action on the vestibular system, providing some inhibition of muscarinic receptors to diminish stimulation of brain vomiting centers [11,57]. Other common side effects include drowsiness, restlessness, dry mouth, and constipation [57]. While there appears to be no increased risk of major malformations related to use, there is also no manufacturers support for use of the produce in pregnancy [39].

11.13.3.4 Cimetidine/ranitidine

These H-2 receptor antagonists were generally considered safe for use in pregnancy as there is no known risk for major malformations [7,10,11]. However, in September of 2019, the generic form of Ranitidine was recalled by the manufacturer because testing found low levels of N-nitrosodimethylamine in the drug, a known carcinogen.

11.13.3.5 Omeprazole

Prilosec is a PPI used in pregnancy for treating reflux disease; additionally, it may be helpful in reducing NVP and mitigating the effects of recurrent vomiting episodes [7]; however, there may be an association with dose-related embryonic and fetal development [10]. When *H. pylori* is suspected, PPIs may be employed [23].

11.13.3.6 Metoclopramide

Reglan is a dopamine and serotonin receptor antagonist which may improve gastric dysrhythmia [2,11]. Gastric emptying time is more rapid due to the release of acetylcholine at the neuromuscular junctions [57]. It is considered safe for use in the first trimester but may incite significant drowsiness and dry mouth [7,10]. Patients may experience more dystonia or increased risk of tardive dyskinesia with chronic use, especially if taken after 12 weeks gestation [11,57]. While it appears that no significant risk of malformations occurs with exposure in pregnancy, we must remember there is no manufacture support for use of the product in pregnancy [39,52]. Trimethobenzamide, commonly known as Tigan, is another dopamine antagonist not as commonly used in pregnancy because of increased risk of maternal hepatotoxicity, depression, and extrapyramidal symptoms [57].

11.13.3.7 Promethazine

Phenergan is a dopamine antagonist which may promote improvements in gastric dysrhythmia [2]. An advantage to this medication is its availability in both oral and rectal suppository forms, enabling patients with more severe symptoms to utilize the drug at home. Sedation is a significant but expected side effect. Three clinical trials speak to its safety and effectiveness during pregnancy; side effects include restlessness, tenseness, tardive dyskinesia, muscular rigidity, or dystonia [7] however, it is suggested for cautious use after the first trimester due to its slower excretion from neonatal and fetal tissue [10]. It should be used with caution in patients with seizure disorders, as it may lower the seizure threshold [57]. Dosage recommendations vary but typically include 12.5 mg rectal suppository or 25 mg orally every 4–6 h [28].

11.13.3.8 Droperidol

Droperidol, known commonly as Inapsine is a dopamine antagonist which may positively impact gastric dysrhythmia [2]; however, it is rarely used during pregnancy because of potential maternal safety issues. It is associated with maternal QT prolongation and/or torsades de pointes in higher doses [61].

11.13.3.9 Mirtazapine

Mirtazapine, known as "Remeron" and used as an antidepressant in major depressive disorders, is a Serotonin–Norepinephrine Reuptake Inhibitor (SNRI) which stimulates certain noradrenergic, serotonergic, histaminic, and muscarinic receptors to produce positive effects on mood, reduction of anxiety and nausea, as well as stimulate the appetite without increasing the risk of birth defects [2]. Animal studies have shown adverse fetal effects; however, there are no well-controlled human studies for corroboration. Older case reports recommend Remeron for intractable symptoms of HG. However, it is recommended for use if clear patient benefits override potential risks [54]. Rare side effects may include anxiety, agitation, and suicidal ideation; case reports suggest a higher chance of serotonin syndrome, especially if multiple serotonergic medications are used simultaneously [2]. Symptoms of serotonin syndrome include diarrhea, hyperreflexia, diaphoresis, fever, confusion, ataxia, tremor, and rarely, rhabdomyolysis.

11.13.3.10 Ondansetron/zofran

This is one of the most effective and highly used antiemetics during pregnancy [2] and one more controversial, due to a perception of high teratogenic risk when used in pregnancy [39]. It is a serotonin antagonist at the 5HT3 receptor which blocks serotonin action in the small bowel and is often used for severe nausea related to chemotherapy. It is proposed that cardiac defects in humans may be related to dysrhythmias and disruption of the hERG channel during critical periods of embryonic development [19]. Researchers reevaluated data from the National Birth Defects Prevention study and Birth Defects study evaluating over 12,000 and 20,000 patients in two case control studies looking at 30 major anomalies in live births; results suggest ondansetron use has not been found to increase open neural tube defects or anencephaly and hypospadias; however, there was a small increase in cleft palate (adjusted OR 1.6) and renal agenesis (adjusted OR 1.8) [49].

While found more effective than other antiemetic medications, use during pregnancy is considered off-label and is only approved for nausea and vomiting resulting from chemotherapy, radiation, and surgery [49,57]. Common side effects include headache, constipation and fatigue and rarely serotonin syndrome and prolongation of QT interval in women with undiagnosed cardiac defects [40]. The dysrhythmia-promoting potential of ondansetron, even when used as recommended, is associated with ventricular arrhythmia, such as torsades de pointes [19].

Oral Zofran tablets or orally disintegrating tablets and transdermal patches are suitable for home and outpatient use, while IV and SQ formulations help hospitalized patients achieve rapid symptom relief [7,11]. Weekly applications of the Granisetron transdermal patch suggested better compliance with similar symptom improvements [42]. There is debate regarding the safety of 5HT3 antagonists; limited data suggest a possible risk of cleft palate and cardiac anomalies [7,11,72], while others suggest its safety [30,39]. Conservative use of ondansetron includes avoidance of use earlier than 10 weeks gestation, and using after other treatments fail, following patient discussion regarding the risk versus benefits [3,15,73,72].

Use of ondansetron may pose maternal risk for cardiac rhythm disturbances, particularly when NVP or HG results in metabolic derangement such as low potassium levels [19]. Patients may also have a higher risk of serotonin syndrome with concomitant use of SSRIs, SNRIs, and MAO inhibitors [61]. It remains one of the more expensive treatments for NVP/HG; however, patients may use discount coupons for significant savings. There is no manufactures support for use in pregnancy [39].

11.13.3.11 Glucocorticoids

Authors vary on the utility of glucocorticoids for HG. It has not been shown to reduce hospitalization rates for severe, refractory HG, and may carry with it an increased risk of oral clefts when used in the first trimester [2,7,11,57]. Generally, steroids should be utilized as adjuvant therapy for women with intractable NVP or HG [57]; typical use includes methylprednisolone 16 mg orally every 8 h for 2 weeks (taper); use for more than 6 weeks is discouraged [28].

11.13.3.12 Hospitalization considerations

There are two categories of severity of NVP and HG: the milder grade demonstrates nausea and vomiting without significant weight loss or metabolic changes. Women with the more severe grade experience more than three daily episodes of vomiting combined with profound feelings of sickness, continual feelings of nausea, and weight loss of more than 3 Kg or 5% of body weight, with metabolic derangements including dehydration, ketonuria, alkalosis from chloride loss, and potentially low potassium levels [57,62]. Once patients are normovolemic and able to tolerate oral feedings, they may be discharged to home with a suitable prescription for anti-emetics and instructions to follow-up with their obstetric provider [57,61].

11.13.3.13 Marijuana use

As more states legalize marijuana (MJ), the risk exists that pregnant women suffering from NVP and HG will equate legalized with "safe" in pregnancy. Indeed, MJ lobbying efforts have been successful in many areas to prevent signage in pot shops cautioning pregnant women from using MJ. MJ lobbyists and related organizations generate significant dollars for their efforts; in 2015, $295,000 was spent on lobbying efforts, while in 2019, $5.32 million was generated and spent [13]. A study of 279,000 women by Kaiser Permanente conducted in California and utilizing universal screenings reflected changes in MJ use among pregnant woman suffering from NVP. The baseline self-reported use rate during the year before pregnancy was 8.3%; prevalence rate for mild NVP was 15.3% with this group having an adjusted odds ratio (OR) of 2.37 for MJ use; prevalence rate for severe NVP was 2.3% with this group having adjusted OR for MJ use of 3.8 [71]. It is prudent therefore that women presenting with symptoms of cyclic vomiting and compulsive bathing have cannabinoid hyperemesis syndrome (CHS) added to their differential diagnoses [4,78]. MJ is not recommended for use during pregnancy or lactation.

11.14 Differential diagnoses

Women presenting in the early first trimester of pregnancy should be evaluated via ultrasound for molar pregnancies, multiple fetuses, and GERD [62]. Women presenting with nausea and vomiting after 9 weeks gestation should be evaluated for other diagnoses not related to NVP, particularly in the presence of abdominal pain, fever, headache, or abnormal neurologic exam [57]. If present, other clinical symptoms must be evaluated, such as thyroid goiters, GI viral syndrome and severe constipation or diarrhea, HTN, and preeclampsia, to facilitate proper treatment. Finally, as MJ use in pregnancy escalates, CHS should be considered [36,62].

11.15 Conclusion

Because there is a lack of evidence from clinical trials, we lack consensus on the effectiveness of various modalities for combating NVP and HG. Nonpharmacologic, herbal, vitamins, and pharmacologic remedies for NVP must undergo more rigorous evaluations in parallel clinical trials to determine efficacy [15,63]. Further, FDA consideration of pregnant women in postmarketing clinical trials could be ethically feasible and positively impact care and provide crucial data about this vulnerable population [69]. Additionally, as our ability to quantify NVP and HG improves, our ability to determine the financial impact and burden of disease will improve [25].

Updates to clinical practice guidelines will help in treatment of NVP and HG; however, clinicians need further encouragement to follow them [50]. We must carefully attend to any mental health issue, preexisting or evoked by intensity of NVP symptoms [68]. Further, nontraditional modalities, such as homeopathy and traditional Chinese medicine should be considered, especially for those with fewer symptoms [28,75]. We must remind patients there are no safety data on MJ use in pregnancy [36]. Finally, an individual approach to NVP, guided by efficacy and safety data, corresponding to expert guidelines will benefit patients as they navigate this problem.

References

1. Abdolhosseini S, Hashem-Dabaghian F, Mokaberinejad R, Sadeghpour O, Mehrabani M. Effects of pomegranate and spearmint syrup on nausea and vomiting during pregnancy: a randomized controlled clinical trial. Iran Red Crescent Med J 2017;19(10):e135–142. https://doi.org/10.5812/ircmj.13542.
2. Abramowitz A, Miller ES, Wisner KL. Treatment options for hyperemesis gravidarum. Arch Wom Ment Health 2017;20(3):363–72. https://doi.org/10.1007/s00737-016-0707-4.
3. ACOG practice bulletin no. 189: Nausea and vomiting of pregnancy. Obstet Gynecol 2018;131(1):e15–30. https://doi.org/10.1097/AOG.0000000000002456.
4. Andrews KH, Bracero LA. Cannabinoid hyperemesis syndrome during pregnancy: a case report. J Reprod Med 2019;60(9–10):430–2.
5. Argenbright CA. Complementary approaches to pregnancy induced nausea and vomiting. Int J Childbirth Educ 2017;32(1):6–9.
6. Amzajerdi A, Keshavarz M, Montazeri A, Bekharadi S. Effect of mint aroma on nausea, vomiting and anxiety in pregnant women. J Fam Med Prim Care 2018;19(8):2597–601. https://doi.org/10.4103/jfmpc.jfmpc_480_19:10.4103/jfmpc.jfmpc_480_19.
7. Azzam H, Barrett J, Biringer A, Campbell K, Duperron L, Dy J, et al. The management of nausea and vomiting of pregnancy: clinical practice guideline. J Obstet Gynaecol Can 2016;38(12):1127–37.
8. Bahadirli A, Sonmez MB, Cagdas OM, Bahadirli NB, Memis SD, Dogan B, Sevincok L. The association of temperament with nausea and vomiting during early pregnancy. J Obstet Gynaecol 2019;39(7):969–74.
9. Biyik I, Keskin F. The lollipop with lemon aroma may be promising in nausea and vomiting in pregnancy. Gynecol Obstetr Reproduct Med 2019;1. https://doi.org/10.21613/GORM.2019.973.
10. Body CMD, Christie JAMD. Gastrointestinal diseases in pregnancy. Gastroenterol Clin N Am 2016;45(2):267–83. https://doi.org/10.1016/j.gtc.2016.02.005.
11. Bustos M, Venkataramanan R, Caritis S. Nausea and vomiting of pregnancy - what's new? Auton Neurosci: Basic and Clinical 2016;202:62–72. https://doi.org/10.1016/j.autneu.2016.05.002.
12. Campbell K, Rowe H, Azzam H, Lane CA. The management of nausea and vomiting of pregnancy. J Obstet Gynaecol Can 2016;38(12):1127–37. https://doi.org/10.1016/j.jogc.2016.08.009.

13. Center for Responsive Politics. Open secrets website. 2020. Retrieved from, https://www.opensecrets.org/federal-lobbying/industries/summary?id=N09.

14. Chortatos A, Haugen M, Iversen PO, Vikanes Å, Eberhard-Gran M, Bjelland EK, et al. Pregnancy complications and birth outcomes among women experiencing nausea only or nausea and vomiting during pregnancy in the Norwegian mother and child cohort study. BMC Pregnancy Childbirth 2015;15(1):138. https://doi.org/10.1186/s12884-015-0580-6.

15. Collins KL, Wilson M, Vincent EC, Safranek S. How safe and effective is ondansetron for nausea and vomiting in pregnancy. J Fam Pract 2019;68(7):e12–14.

16. Colodro-Conde L, Cross SM, Lind PA, Painter JN, Gunst A, Jern P, et al. Cohort profile: nausea and vomiting during pregnancy genetics consortium (NVP genetics consortium). Int J Epidemiol 2017;46(2):e17. https://doi.org/10.1093/ije/dyv360.

17. Colodro-Conde L, Jern P, Johansson A, Sánchez-Romera J, Lind PA, Painter JN, et al. Nausea and vomiting during pregnancy is highly heritable. Behav Genet 2016;46(4): 481–91. https://doi.org/10.1007/s10519-016-9781-7.

18. Craig R, Jeyanthi Pelto G, Willford AC, Stoltzfus RJ. Using a cultural-ecological framework to explore dietary beliefs and practices during pregnancy and lactation among women in Adivasi communities in the Nilgiris Biosphere Reserve, India. Ecol Food Nutr 2018;57(3):165–86. https://doi.org/10.1080/03670244.2018.1445088.

19. Danielsson B, Webster WS, Ritchie HE. Ondansetron and teratogenicity in rats: evidence for a mechanism mediated via embryonic hERG blocade. Reprod Toxicol 2018;81: 237–45.

20. Dass A, Satyanarayan N, Rajjapan S. Implementing standardized Rhodes Index to measure the efficacy of ginger extract (*Zingiber officinale*) in pregnancy induced nausea and vomiting. Int J Pharmacol Res 2015;5(10):222–5. https://doi.org/10.7439/ijpr.v5i10.2589.

21. Einarson TR, Piwko C, Koren G. Prevalence of nausea and vomiting of pregnancy in the USA: a meta analysis. J Populat Therap Clin Pharmacol 2013;20(2):e163. Retrieved from: https://www.ncbi.nlm.nih.gov/pubmed/23863545.

22. Fattah A, Hesarinejad Z, Gharaii NJ, Nasibi M. The effect of aromatherapy on nausea and vomiting during pregnancy: a systematic review and meta-analysis. Int J Pediatr 2019;7(3):9061–70.

23. Fiaschi L, Nelson-Piercy C, Deb S, King R, Tata L. Clinical management of nausea and vomiting in pregnancy and hyperemesis gravidarum across primary and secondary care: a population-based study. BJOG An Int J Obstet Gynaecol 2019;126(10):1201–11. https://doi.org/10.1111/1471-0528.15662.

24. Fredette NC, Meyer MM, Prossnitz ER. Role of GPER in estrogen-dependent nitric oxide formation and vasodilation. J Steroid Biochem Mol Biol 2018;176:65–72. doi. org/10.1016/j.jsbmb.2017.05.006.

25. Gadsby R, Rawson V, Dziadulewicz E, Rousseau B, Collongs H. Nausea and vomiting of pregnancy and resource implications: the NVP Impact Study. Br J Gene Pract 2019; 69(680):e217–23. https://doi.org/10.3399/bjgp18X700745. Mar;.

26. Gadsby R, Barnie-Adshead AM. What causes the nausea and vomiting of pregnancy and hyperemesis gravidarum. 2014. Semantic Scholar retrieved from: https://www.semanticscholar.org/paper/What-Causes-the-Nausea-and-Vomiting-of-Pregnancy-E-Gadsby-Barnie-Adshead/57dbfd2de39c8c7d7b7daf4134ec20ebca92bf9a.

27. Good R. Retrieved from: https://www.goodrx.com/diclegis?dosage=10mg-10mg&form=tablet&label_override=doxylamine+%2F+pyridoxine&quantity=100; 2020.

28. Gordon A, Love A. Chapter 54 - nausea and vomiting in pregnancy. Integr Med 2018: 542−9. https://doi.org/10.1016/B978-0-323-35868-2.00054-2. Elsevier Inc.

29. Groleau D, Benady-Chorney J, Panaitoiu A, Jimenez V. Hyperemesis gravidarum in the context of migration: when the absence of cultural meaning gives rise to blaming the victim. BMC Preg Childbirth 2019;19(1):197. https://doi.org/10.1186/s12884-019-2344-1.

30. Haas DM. Helping pregnant women and clinicians understand the risk of ondansetron for nausea and vomiting during pregnancy. J Am Med Assoc 2018;320(23):2425−6. https://doi.org/10.1001/jama.2018.19328.

31. Hassan A, Dubey AK, Bhat MP. Pyridoxine: the 'Ba.Six of use in nausea and vomiting of pregnancy. J Clin Diagn Res 2019;13(5):BE01−6.

32. Havnen GC, Truong MB, Do MH, Heitmann K, Holst L, Nordeng H. Women's perspectives on the management and consequences of hyperemesis gravidarum − a descriptive interview study. Scand J Prim Health Care 2019;37(1):30−40. https://doi.org/10.1080/02813432.2019.1569424.

33. Heitmann K, Solheimsnes A, Havnen GC, Nordeng H, Holst L. Treatment of nausea and vomiting during pregnancy —a cross-sectional study among 712 Norwegian women. Eur J Clin Pharmacol 2016;72(5):593−604. https://doi.org/10.1007/s00228-016-2012-6.

34. Hinkle SN, Mumford SL, Grantz KL, Silver RM, Mitchell EM, Sjaarda LA, et al. Association of nausea and vomiting during pregnancy with pregnancy loss: a secondary analysis of a randomized clinical trial. JAMA Inter Med 2016;176(11):1621−7. https://doi.org/10.1001/jamainternmed.2016.5641.

35. Jafari-Dehkordi E, Hashem-Dabaghian F, Aliasl F, Aliasl J, Taghavi-Shirazi M, Sadeghpour O, et al. Comparison of quince with vitamin B6 for treatment of nausea and vomiting in pregnancy: a randomized clinical trial. J Obstet Gynaecol 2017;37(8): 1048−52. https://doi.org/10.1080/01443615.2017.1322046.

36. King TK, Brucker MC, Jevitt C, Osborne K, editors. Varney's midwifery. 6th ed. Burlington, Massachusetts: Jones & Bartlett Learning; 2019.

37. Kjeldgaard H, Eberhard-Gran M, Benth J, Vikanes Å. Hyperemesis gravidarum and the risk of emotional distress during and after pregnancy. Arch Wom Ment Health 2017; 20(6):747−56. https://doi.org/10.1007/s00737-017-0770-5.

38. Koren G. P56 Breakthrough in the treatment of nausea and vomiting of pregnancy; the first dual release combination of doxylamine-pyridoxine. Arch Dis Child 2019;104(6): e40. https://doi.org/10.1136/archdischild-2019-esdppp.94.

39. Koren G. Safety considerations surrounding use of treatment options for nausea and vomiting in pregnancy. Expet Opin Drug Saf 2017;16(11):1227−34. https://doi.org/10.1080/14740338.2017.1361403.

40. Koren G. Treating morning sickness in the United States—changes in prescribing are needed. Am J Obstet Gynecol 2014;211(6):602−6. https://doi.org/10.1016/j.ajog.2014.08.017.

41. Lassiter NT, Manns-James LE. Pregnancy. In: Brucker MC, King T, editors. Pharmacology for women's health. 2nd ed. 2017. p. 1025−44.

42. Le TN, Adler MT, Ouillette H, Berens P, Smith JA. Observational case series evaluation of the granisetron transdermal patch system (sancuso) for the management of nausea/vomiting of pregnancy. Am J Perinatol 2017;34(9):851−5. https://doi.org/10.1055/s-0037-1598652.

43. Lete I, Allue J. The effectiveness of ginger in the prevention of nausea and vomiting during pregnancy and chemotherapy. Integr Med Insights 2016;11:11−7.

44. Madjunkova S, Maltepe C, Koren G. The delayed-release combination of doxylamine and pyridoxine (diclegis®/diclectin®) for the treatment of nausea and vomiting of pregnancy. Pediatr Drugs 2014;16(3):199−211. https://doi.org/10.1007/s40272-014-0065-5.

45. Mendoza E, Amsler F. A randomized crossover trial on the effect of compression stockings on nausea and vomiting in early pregnancy. Int J Wom Health 2017;9:89−99. https://doi.org/10.2147/IJWH.S120809.

46. Moon HY, Kim MR, Hwang DS, Jang JB, Lee J, Shin JS, Ha I, Lee YJ. Safety of acupuncture during pregnancy: a retrospective cohort study in Korea. Br J Obstet Gynaecol 2020;127:79−86.

47. Ngo E. Use of a mobile application to promote better treatment of nausea and vomiting in pregnancy. Reprod Toxicol 2018;80:143−4. https://doi.org/10.1016/j.reprotox.2018.07.035.

48. Oliveira L, Capp S, You W, Riffenburgh R, Carstairs S. Ondansetron compared with doxylamine and pyridoxine for treatment of nausea in pregnancy: a randomized controlled trial. Obstet Gynecol 2014;124(4):735−42. https://doi.org/10.1097/AOG.0000000000000479.

49. Parker SE, Van Bennekom C, Anderka M, Mitchell AA. Ondansetron for treatment of nausea and vomiting of pregnancy and the risk of specific birth defects. Obstet Gynecol 2018;132(2):385−94.

50. Persaud N, Meaney C, El-Emam K, Moineddin R, Thorpe K. Doxylamine-pyridoxine for nausea and vomiting of pregnancy randomized placebo controlled trial: prespecified analyses and reanalysis. PloS One 2018;13(1):e0189978. https://doi.org/10.1371/journal.pone.0189978.

51. Pontius E, Vieth JT. Complications in early pregnancy. Emerg Med Clin 2019;37(2):219−37. https://doi.org/10.1016/j.emc.2019.01.004.

52. RCOG Green Top Guidelines. The management of nausea and vomiting in pregnancy and hyperemesis gravidarum. 2016. Retrieved from: https://www.rcog.org.uk/globalassets/documents/guidelines/green-top-guidelines/gtg69-hyperemesis.pdf.

53. Revell MA. Self-care of nausea and vomiting in the first trimester of pregnancy. Int J Childbirth Educ 2017;32(1):35.

54. Rohde A, Dembinski J, Dorn C. Mirtazapine (Remergil) for treatment resistant hyperemesis gravidarum: rescue of a twin pregnancy. Arch Gynecol Obstet 2003;268:219−21. https://doi.org/10.1007/s00404-003-0502-0.

55. Ross DL. September 4). Hyperthyroidism during pregnancy: clinical manifestations, diagnosis, and causes. In: Post TW, editor. UpToDate. Waltham, MA: WoltersKluwer Health; 2018. Available from: http://www.uptodate.com.

56. Sabbatini AK, Kocher KE, Basu A, Hsia RY. In-hospital outcomes and costs among patients hospitalized during a return visit to the emergency department. Jama 2016;315(7):663−71. https://doi.org/10.1001/jama.2016.0649.

57. Saborio OEG, Hines BK, Wesselman J. Safe management of nausea and vomiting during pregnancy in the emergency department. Adv Emerg Nurs J 2019;41(4):336−47.

58. Sharifzadeh F, Kashanian M, Koopayehzadeh J, Rezaian F, Sheikhansari N, Eshraghi N. A comparison between the effects of ginger, pyridoxine (vitamin B-6) and placebo for the treatment of the first trimester nausea and vomiting of pregnancy. J Matern Fetal Neonatal Med 2018;31(19):2509−14.

59. Shawahna R, Taha A. Which potential harms and benefits of using ginger in the management of nausea and vomiting of pregnancy should be addressed? a consensual study

among pregnant women and gynecologists. BMC Compl Alternative Med 2017;17(1): 204. https://doi.org/10.1186/s12906-017-1717-0.

60. Shenvi C. Diclegis: drug makes a 30-year comeback. MEDPAGE Today; January 4, 2015. Retrieved from: https://www.medpagetoday.com/emergencymedicine/emergencymedicine/49368.

61. Smith JA, Fox KA, Clark S. Nausea and vomiting of pregnancy: treatment and outcome. In: Post TW, editor. UpToDate. Waltham, MA: WoltersKluwer Health; February 20, 2020. Available from: http://www.uptodate.com.

62. Smith JA, Fox KA, Clark S. Nausea and vomiting of pregnancy: clinical findings and evaluation. In: Post TW, editor. UpToDate. Waltham, MA: WoltersKluwer Health; February 20, 2020. Available from: http://www.uptodate.com.

63. Sridharan K, Sivaramakrishnan G. Interventions for treating nausea and vomiting in pregnancy: a network meta-analysis and trial sequential analysis of randomized clinical trials. Expet Rev Clin Pharmacol 2018;11(11):1143–50. https://doi.org/10.1080/17512433.2018.1530108.

64. Temming L, Franco A, Istwan N, Rhea D, Desch C, Stanziano G, Jpy S. Adverse pregnancy outcomes in women with nausea and vomiting of pregnancy. J Matern Fetal Neonatal Med 2014;27(1):84–8.

65. Tsakridis I, Mamopoulos A, Athanasiadis A, Dagklis T. The management of nausea and vomiting of pregnancy: synthesis of national guidelines. Obstet Gynecol Surv 2019; 74(3):161–9.

66. Whitehouse AJO, Alvares GA, Cleary D, Harun A, Stojanoska A, Taylor LJ, et al. Symptom severity in autism spectrum disorder is related to the frequency and severity of nausea and vomiting during pregnancy: a retrospective case-control study. Mol Autism 2018;9(1):37. https://doi.org/10.1186/s13229-018-0223-7.

67. Willey C, Calip GS. How did research on medication safety in pregnancy define, develop and advance the field of pharmacoepidemiology? Clin Therapeut 2019;41(12):2464–6. https://doi.org/10.1016/j.clinthera.2019.11.004.

68. Wise J. Women with nausea and vomiting in pregnancy should be offered more support, say RCOG guidelines. Br Med J June 23, 2016. https://doi.org/10.1136/bmj.i3509.

69. Wood ME, Andrade SE, Toh S. Safe expectations: current state and future expectations. Clin Therapeut 2019;41(12):2467–76.

70. Yilmaz E, Yilmaz Z, Cakmak B, Karsli MF, Gultekin IB, Guneri Dogan N, et al. Nausea and vomiting in early pregnancy of adolescents: relationship with depressive symptoms. J Pediatr Adolesc Gynecol 2016;29(1):65–8. https://doi.org/10.1016/j.jpag.2015.06.010.

71. Young-Wolff KC, Sarovar V, Tucker L, Avalos LA, Tucker L, Conway A, Armstrong MA, Goler N. Association of nausea and vomiting in pregnancy with prenatal marijuana use. JAMA Internal Med 2018;178(10):1423–4. https://doi.org/10.1001/jamainternmed.2018.3581.

72. Zambelli-Weiner A, Via C, Yuen M, Weiner DJ, Kirby RS. First trimester ondansetron exposure and risk of structural birth defects. Reprod Toxicol 2019;83:14–20. https://doi.org/10.1016/j.reprotox.2018.10.010.

73. Adlan A, Chooi KY, Mat Adenan NA. Acupressure as adjuvant treatment for the inpatient management of nausea and vomiting in early pregnancy: A double-blind randomized controlled trial. J Obstet Gynaecol Res 2017;43(4):662–8. https://doi.org/10.1111/jog.13269.

74. Allais G, Chiarle G, Sinigaglia S, Airola G, Schiapparelli P, Bergandi F, et al. Acupuncture treatment of migraine, nausea, and vomiting in pregnancy. Neurol Sci 2019;40(S1): 213−5. https://doi.org/10.1007/s10072-019-03799-2.

75. Dean E. Morning sickness. Nurs Stand 2016;30(50):15. https://doi.org/10.7748/ns.30.50.15.s16.

76. Fiaschi L, Nelson-Piercy V, Tata LJ. Hospital admission for hyperemesis gravidarum: a nationwide study of occurrence, reoccurrence and risk factors among 8.2 million pregnancies. Hum Reprod 2016;31(8):1675−84. https://doi.org/10.1093/humrep/dew128.

77. Heitmann K, Nordeng H, Havnen GC, Solheimsnes A, Holst L. The burden of nausea and vomiting during pregnancy: severe impacts on quality of life, daily life functioning and willingness to become pregnant again − results from a cross-sectional study. BMC Pregnancy Childb 2017;17(1):75. https://doi.org/10.1186/s12884-017-1249-0.

78. Young-Wolff KC, Sarovar V, Tucker L, Avalos LA, Alexeeff S, Conway A, et al. Trends in marijuana use among pregnant women with and without nausea and vomiting in pregnancy, 2009−2016. Drug Alcohol Depend 2019;196:66−70. https://doi.org/10.1016/j.drugalcdep.2018.12.009.

79. World Health Organization International Statistical Classification of Diseases and Related Health Problems 10th Revision (ICD-10)-WHO Version for 2016. Retrieved from: https://icd.who.int/browse10/2016/en#/O20-O2.

Clinical pharmacology of anti-infectives during pregnancy

12

Jeremiah D. Momper, Brookie M. Best

University of California, Skaggs School of Pharmacy and Pharmaceutical Sciences, San Diego, CA, United States

Serious infections can occur during pregnancy and must be treated to prevent maternal and fetal adverse outcomes. While some anti-infectives have been studied in pregnancy, many agents have inadequate data available to evaluate safety, efficacy, and appropriate dosing, posing a challenge for drug and dose selection. Important safety data have been summarized elsewhere [1,2]. This chapter focuses on pharmacology and pharmacokinetic studies for drugs used to treat or prevent infections in pregnancy. Drug disposition characteristics that may alter drug exposure in pregnancy should be considered in selecting a treatment regimen. For drugs that are primarily renally eliminated, clearance may increase later in pregnancy yielding lower plasma concentrations of the drugs [3]. For drugs primarily metabolized by the liver or by a combination of pathways, changes in exposure during pregnancy may or may not occur depending on the specific enzyme systems involved [3]. Further, drug interactions are a major concern when simultaneously treating multiple infections, such as HIV and tuberculosis. For drugs that are highly protein bound, the dilutional effect on albumin in late pregnancy may increase the free or unbound drug concentration. Finally, the duration of exposure for both the mother and the fetus when a drug is given during pregnancy should be considered when selecting therapy, as about five half-lives must pass for most of the drug to be eliminated from the body. Drugs with short half-lives for which clearance is increased during pregnancy may need to be dosed more frequently. These alterations in disposition can be additive or antagonistic, complicating attempts to predict whether drug exposure will change significantly in pregnancy. Therefore, pharmacokinetic studies in pregnant women are necessary to fully understand changes in exposure and the implications for appropriate dose selection. In the absence of pharmacokinetic studies in pregnant women, close monitoring of drug therapy is warranted, including measurement of plasma concentrations and individual optimization of doses when possible.

Clinical Pharmacology During Pregnancy. https://doi.org/10.1016/B978-0-12-818902-3.00022-1

12.1 Antibacterial therapy

Penicillins are the antibiotics of choice during pregnancy. They cross the placenta and small amounts are excreted in breast milk. *Penicillin G and V* are 45%−68% and 75%−89% bound to plasma proteins, respectively, are partially metabolized (<30%) to inactive metabolites, and parent drug and metabolites are excreted in the urine via filtration and tubular secretion. One pharmacokinetic study of a dose of one million international units (IU) of penicillin G intravenously (IV) every 4 h in pregnant women concluded that this produced adequate maternal penicillin concentrations for prophylaxis against Group B *Streptococcus* [4]. Current guidelines recommend an initial dose of 5 million IU, followed by 2.5−3 million IU every 4 h [5]. Another study of a single 2.4 million IU intramuscular dose of penicillin G for prevention of congenital syphilis showed high variability and some subtherapeutic concentrations; authors suggested that higher doses may need to be studied [6]. Current syphilis treatment guidelines in pregnancy recommend use of penicillins, but state optimal doses are unknown [7]. A study of a single oral dose of penicillin V in both pregnant and nonpregnant (control) women demonstrated significantly decreased area under the concentration time curve (AUC—a measure of overall exposure), shorter half-life, and increased penicillin clearance in pregnant women. The authors concluded shorter dose intervals (1 million IU every 6 h instead of every 8 h) or higher doses of penicillin V may be needed during pregnancy [8]. Studies of higher than standard doses have not been described. In pregnant women with a penicillin allergy history, desensitization protocols have been safely applied [9].

Amoxicillin, ampicillin, dicloxacillin, and *ticarcillin* are all mainly eliminated via renal filtration and tubular secretion, with about 10% metabolized. *Oxacillin* is about half metabolized and half eliminated unchanged in the urine. *Piperacillin* is 10%−20% excreted via bile into the feces, with the rest eliminated unchanged in the urine. *Nafcillin*, unlike all the other penicillins, is 60% metabolized, undergoes enterohepatic recirculation, and both parent and metabolites are excreted in the bile. Plasma protein binding is about 20% for amoxicillin, ampicillin, and piperacillin, is about 50% for ticarcillin, and is 70%−99% for nafcillin, oxacillin, and dicloxacillin. One study of a single oral 500 mg dose of amoxicillin in pregnant women for post-exposure prophylaxis against anthrax showed increased clearance during pregnancy compared to postpartum, and concluded that anthrax preventative concentrations will not be feasible in pregnant women [10]. Studies of IV amoxicillin have recommended a dose during labor or during preterm premature rupture of membranes of 2 g followed by 1 g every 4 h [11−13]. Two older reported studies of ampicillin pharmacokinetics following 500 mg doses during pregnancy found decreased exposure and suggested increased loading doses (because of the large increase in distribution volume) were likely needed [14,15]. Finally, two studies of piperacillin−tazobactam in pregnant women found increased clearance and distribution volume during pregnancy, and suggested that higher than standard doses may be needed during pregnancy [16,17].

Cephalosporins can be safely used to treat various infections during pregnancy, and older agents are preferred due to more data and experience in pregnancy. Specific doses depend on the infection site and offending microbe. They are classified by anti-bacterial activity. Examples of first-generation agents are: *cefadroxil, cephalexin, cephradine,* and *cefazolin*; second-generation agents: *cefoxitin, cefotetan, cefaclor, cefprozil, cefuroxime, cefuroxime axetil*; and third/fourth/fifth-generation agents: *cefotaxime, ceftazidime, ceftriaxone, ceftizoxime, cefixime, cefditoren, cefdinir, cefpodoxime, ceftibuten, cefepime,* and *ceftaroline*. As a class, they all cross the placenta well [18−20], and small amounts are found in breast milk. Many are 60% −90% protein bound in plasma, except for cefaclor, cephalexin, cefadroxil, cefpodoxime, cefotaxime, ceftizoxime, ceftazidime, and cefuroxime, which are less than 50% protein bound.

For first-generation agents, one study of cephalothin in pregnant women concluded that pregnancy alterations in exposure were insignificant and no dose changes were warranted [21]. Cephalothin is 10%−40% metabolized, with the rest excreted unchanged in urine, while the other first-generation agents are not metabolized and are wholly excreted unchanged in urine. In contrast, studies of cephradine and cefazolin in pregnant women showed increased clearance and distribution volumes, decreased AUCs and shorter half-lives, concluding that doses in pregnancy should be increased, possibly by reducing dose intervals rather than by increasing dose amounts [22,23].

Cefuroxime, a second-generation cephalosporin, has lower plasma concentrations and a shorter half-life during pregnancy compared to postpartum [20]. For cefoxitin, at 19−21 weeks gestation, plasma concentrations were similar to those seen in nonpregnant adults [24], while at term, clearance of cefoxitin is significantly increased [25]. The second-generation agents are primarily excreted unchanged in the urine.

Several later generation cephalosporins have been studied in pregnant women. Cefoperazone at term showed a larger distribution volume, lower peak concentration, and decreased protein binding (74% vs. 88%) during pregnancy compared to nonpregnant adults, but also showed that pregnancy did not greatly affect clearance, half-life, or trough concentrations (C_{trough}) [26]. Of note, unlike most other cephalosporins, cefoperazone is metabolized in the liver and excreted in the bile. Ceftazidime clearance increases and concentrations decrease throughout pregnancy compared to postpartum; clearance is primarily renal excretion of unchanged drug [24,27]. Ceftazidime readily crosses the placenta [28]. Cefotaxime is metabolized to an active metabolite, and both parent drug and metabolite are eliminated in urine. All other cephalosporins are not appreciably metabolized, and are primarily excreted unchanged in the urine. While increased dose amounts and more frequent dosing have been proposed to attain adequate drug concentrations for many cephalosporins, pharmacokinetic studies of such increased doses are lacking.

Carbapenems *imipenem-cilastatin* and *meropenem* cross the placenta, have low protein binding, and are excreted mainly unchanged in the urine. Little is known about breast milk penetration. A case report of a breast-feeding mother receiving meropenem for treatment of a postpartum urinary tract infection calculated an infant daily exposure from breast milk of 97 μg/kg/d corresponding to an infant weight-adjusted percentage of maternal dosage of 0.18% [29]. Clearance and distribution volume of imipenem after a single 500 mg IV dose were significantly increased in early and late pregnancy compared to postpartum, and increased doses may be needed in pregnancy [30]. No pharmacokinetic studies of meropenem, doripenem, and ertapenem in pregnancy are reported. Carbacephems *aztreonam* and *loracarbef* pharmacokinetics have not been studied in pregnancy either. Loracarbef is 25% protein bound, is not metabolized, and is excreted unchanged in the urine. Placental and breast milk penetration are unknown. Aztreonam is about 60% protein bound and is mainly eliminated unchanged in the urine, with 6%−16% metabolized. It crosses the placenta well [31], and breast milk penetration is unknown. Beta-lactamase inhibitors, given in combination with penicillins or cephalosporins, include *sulbactam, tazobactam*, and *clavulanic acid*. All are about 30% protein bound. Sulbactam and tazobactam cross the placenta and undergo some metabolism while most drug is excreted unchanged in urine. Both have significantly decreased exposure during pregnancy [16,32]. For clavulanic acid, half is metabolized, half is excreted in urine, and low amounts cross the placenta [33].

Macrolides, such as *erythromycin, azithromycin*, and *clarithromycin*, are used to treat various infections in pregnant women. Placental concentrations are less than 7% of maternal concentrations [34,35]. Erythromycin breast milk concentrations are about 50% of maternal concentrations, and it is compatible with breastfeeding. It is 73%−81% protein bound, is a substrate and inhibitor of both cytochrome P450 (CYP) 3A4 and permeability glycoprotein (Pgp), concentrates in bile and liver, and is excreted in the bile. Clarithromycin is also a substrate and inhibitor of CYP 3A4 and Pgp, while azithromycin is not metabolized and has no effect on CYP enzymes. Limited information is available on penetration of azithromycin and clarithromycin into breast milk, and both have low protein binding. A study on transfer of azithromycin into breast milk estimated an absolute infant dose of 4.5 mg/kg of body weight (95% prediction interval: 0.6−7.0 mg/kg) and a relative cumulative infant dose of 15.7% of the maternal dose (95% prediction interval: 2.0%−27.8%) [36]. One pharmacokinetic study of azithromycin found increased distribution volume but unchanged AUC and elimination half-life in pregnancy versus nonpregnant women, suggesting standard doses should be appropriate in pregnancy [37]. No data are available on the clinical pharmacology of fidaxomicin in pregnant women.

Vancomycin is used for gram-positive bacterial infections. It is administered intravenously to treat systemic infections, widely distributed, 55% protein bound, and excreted renally. It crosses the placenta at concentrations similar to maternal concentrations [38]. It is excreted in breast milk; infants would likely not absorb vancomycin, but their gut flora may be altered. Data in pregnancy are limited, so use should be reserved for serious infections. Other polypeptides, *colistin, polymyxin B*, and *teicoplanin*, have even less data regarding use in pregnancy, and should only be used for compelling indications.

Chloramphenicol is well absorbed and widely distributed, is 60% bound to plasma proteins, with higher placental than maternal concentrations [39]. It is hepatically glucuronidated, and is a potent CYP 3A4 and 2C19 inhibitor. Due to neonatal toxicity, "gray baby syndrome" and agranulocytosis, use during pregnancy, especially near term, should be avoided unless absolutely necessary.

Tetracyclines, including *tetracycline, demeclocycline, doxycycline, minocycline, omadacycline, eravacycline*, and *sarecycline*, are generally not recommended in pregnancy due to strong binding to developing teeth and bones. Tetracycline and doxycycline are enterohepatically recirculated and eliminated mainly in feces (doxycycline) or urine (tetracycline). Minocycline is partially hepatically metabolized. These agents chelate cations, cross the placenta, and penetrate into breast milk, but are considered compatible with breastfeeding. No pharmacokinetic studies in pregnancy have been reported.

Lincomycin and *clindamycin* are hepatically metabolized, cross the placenta with 25%−50% of maternal concentrations found in cord blood, and cross into breast milk but are considered compatible with breastfeeding. Clindamycin, given at 900 mg every 8 h for Group B *Streptococcus*, was evaluated in pregnant women. The authors found that this standard dose may be subtherapeutic [40]. Higher doses have not been studied in this population. These drugs should be avoided during pregnancy unless other first-line agents are ineffective or not tolerated.

Linezolid and *tedizolid* are oxazolidinone antibiotics used to treat gram-positive infections. *Linezolid* is widely distributed, metabolized by both enzymatic (presumably CYP-mediated) and nonenzymatic processes, and about 30% is eliminated unchanged in the urine. Data in pregnancy are very limited. A case report of a pregnant patient with multidrug-resistant TB showed lower linezolid exposure during pregnancy relative to postpartum [41]. Placental and breast milk penetration in humans are unknown. No pharmacokinetic data in pregnancy are available for *tedizolid*. *Dalfopristin-quinupristin* is also used for gram-positive infections. Both agents are metabolized to several active metabolites by non-CYP processes, but these agents potently inhibit CYP 3A4. The parent compounds and metabolites are mainly eliminated in the feces, with 15%−20% of each parent drug eliminated unchanged in the urine. Placental and breast milk transfer are unknown, and no pharmacokinetic studies in pregnancy are available.

Aminoglycosides, including *streptomycin, neomycin, kanamycin, amikacin, gentamicin, tobramycin*, and *plazomicin*, are administered intravenously and eliminated unchanged in the urine. They cross the placenta, and may accumulate in the fetus [42,43]. Gentamicin clearance and dose requirements are increased during pregnancy, which corresponded more with increased distribution volumes than increased renal function [44]. If used, plasma concentration monitoring is necessary to individualize doses. These agents should be avoided in pregnancy unless needed for life-threatening infections because of fetal oto- and nephrotoxicity risks.

Sulfonamides, including *sulfisoxazole, sulfadiazine, sulfamethoxazole, sulfasa-lazine, and sulfadoxine* (see malaria section), are generally used in combination with other antibiotics for various infections, and may be used in pregnancy if penicillins and cephalosporins are not effective. Near term, these drugs should be avoided due to increased risk of hyperbilirubinemia in the neonate; likewise, they are contraindicated in nursing. They readily cross the placenta [45,46] and mostly also penetrate into breast milk. Sulfonamides are hepatically acetylated and are substrates and inhibitors of CYP 2C9.

Trimethoprim is used alone or in combination with sulfamethoxazole for various infections. It is extensively distributed, it inhibits CYP 2C8, and is mostly eliminated unchanged in the urine. It is slowly transported in low concentrations across the placenta [45], but breast milk concentrations are higher than maternal plasma concentrations and caution should be exercised in lactating women. Trimethoprim is a second-line agent that can be used in pregnancy if first-line agents are ineffective. Folic acid supplementation (0.5 mg daily) should be used along with trimethoprim in the first trimester.

Fluoroquinolones include *ciprofloxacin, gatifloxacin, levofloxacin, lomefloxacin, moxifloxacin, norfloxacin, ofloxacin, sparfloxacin, delafloxacin, gemifloxacin, cinoxacin,* and *nalidixic acid.* Absorption of fluoroquinolones is decreased with concomitant cation administration, including calcium, magnesium, iron, and zinc. Lomefloxacin, levofloxacin, norfloxacin, and ofloxacin are mainly excreted unchanged in the urine. Sparfloxacin is metabolized by CYP 1A2. Grepafloxacin is glucuronidated by uridine diphosphate glucuronosyltransferase (UGT) enzymes and metabolized by CYP 1A2. Delafloxacin is glucuronidated by UGT 1A1, UGT 1A3, and UGT 2B15 and renally eliminated. Moxifloxacin is glucuronidated and sulfated, but does not undergo CYP metabolism. Ciprofloxacin is partially excreted unchanged, is partially metabolized by CYP 1A2, and is an inhibitor of CYP 1A2. Low amounts of quinolones cross the placenta [47], while much higher amounts penetrate into breast milk [48]. No other pharmacokinetic studies in pregnancy are available. Because of arthropathy risks, quinolones should be avoided in pregnancy and lactation unless needed for complicated, resistant infections.

Metronidazole is used in pregnancy for treatment of symptomatic bacterial vaginosis or asymptomatic disease in women at high risk for preterm delivery. It is effective for eradication of infection, but does not decrease risk of preterm birth [49,50]. It is well absorbed, widely distributed including fetal [51] and breast milk concentrations as high as maternal concentrations [52−54], and is both oxidized and glucuronidated in the liver by unknown enzymes. Pharmacokinetic studies in early pregnancy and at term showed 15%−30% reductions in AUC compared to historical controls [55,56], but a study in 20 pregnant women taking 500 mg twice daily for 3 days showed weight-corrected exposure was similar in different stages of pregnancy and to reported values in nonpregnant adults [57]. *Nimorazole, tinidazole,* and *ornidazole* do not have enough data in human pregnancy to assess appropriate use.

Nitrofurantoin has been used in pregnancy for decades for urinary tract infections. It undergoes some hepatic metabolism, but is mostly concentrated unchanged in urine. Less than 1% crosses into breast milk [58], and placental exposure is also low. It is contraindicated near term due to risk of hemolytic reactions, particularly in glucose-6-phosphatase dehydrogenase (G6PD) deficiency. *Fosfomycin* is used as a single 3 g dose for uncomplicated urinary tract infections. It is not metabolized, and is excreted unchanged in urine and feces. No pharmacokinetic studies in pregnancy have been reported, though an observational cohort study did not find an increased risk of an adverse pregnancy outcome after first-trimester fosfomycin exposure [59]. *Methenamine mandelate* and *methenamine hippurate* are antiseptics used for urinary tract infections. They cross the placenta, into breast milk, and are excreted unchanged in urine. Experience in pregnancy is very limited, and they should be avoided.

Atovaquone (see malaria section) and *pentamidine* are used for *Pneumocystis jirovecii* infections. Pentamidine crosses the placenta in animals; breast milk penetration is unknown. Elimination is mainly renal, but several metabolites formed by unknown pathways are also present. The half-life is 2−4 weeks. Pharmacokinetic studies of atovaquone in pregnancy have shown more than 50% lower exposure in pregnant women compared to healthy volunteers [60,61]. Higher doses of atovaquone during pregnancy have been suggested [62].

12.2 Antifungal therapy

For treatment of fungal infections, topical therapy with older agents is considered safe in pregnancy. For topical and mucosal use, *nystatin, clotrimazole,* and *miconazole* are drugs of choice, with negligible systemic absorption. Other topical "-azoles" are second line, and other topical antifungals should be avoided due to lack of data in pregnancy. Systemic treatment with *fluconazole, ketoconazole, itraconazole,* and *miconazole* should be avoided unless the indication is compelling. No pregnancy pharmacokinetic studies are available. *Voriconazole, posaconazole,* and *isavuconazonium* are teratogenic in rodents. A case report is available describing a pregnant woman who received voriconazole for life-threatening refractory invasive aspergillosis in the second and third trimesters. No adverse fetal outcome was noted at birth or at 6-month follow-up [63]. However, voriconazole remains contraindicated in pregnancy, and should be considered only in life-threatening cases when no alternatives are available. For treatment of vaginal candidiasis after local treatment has failed, low-dose oral fluconazole (150 mg once daily) may be tried. For serious, disseminated fungal infections, amphotericin B is preferred.

Amphotericin B is poorly absorbed and administered intravenously for systemic fungal infections. Its metabolism is unknown, and it is eliminated slowly with a 1−15 day half-life. It crosses the placenta and may be retained in placental and other tissues. Pharmacokinetics of the original or the liposomal formulations in pregnancy have not been studied. Use should be limited in pregnancy to dangerous systemic mycoses.

Flucytosine is active against *Cryptococcus neoformans* and candida species. It is widely distributed, and mostly eliminated unchanged in the urine. No pregnancy studies are available. Use during pregnancy should be reserved for severe disseminated fungal infection. *Griseofulvin* and *terbinafine* should not be used orally during pregnancy because data for systemic therapy during pregnancy with these agents are limited and skin mycoses do not require urgent oral treatment.

12.3 Malaria

Pregnancy increases susceptibility to and severity of malaria, and maternal malaria increases risks for prematurity, low birth weight, spontaneous abortion, and stillbirth. Prophylaxis and treatment medications must be tailored to the local pattern of antimalarial drug resistance [64,65]. The goal for prophylaxis and treatment regimens is >95% efficacy, but many regimens are associated with much lower cure rates during pregnancy; failure rates >10 or 15% are common [66].

Chloroquine (CQ) is a drug of choice for malaria during pregnancy if the parasite is sensitive. It is well absorbed orally and distributes widely throughout the body. CQ crosses the placenta easily and penetrates into breast milk, delivering low infant doses of ~3%, compatible with breastfeeding [67,68]. It is partially metabolized hepatically by CYP 3A4 and 2D6, and inhibits activity of 2D6. The major metabolite, desethylchloroquine (DECQ) has some activity. The half-life is 1−2 months. CQ should be given with food to minimize gastrointestinal upset. Pharmacokinetic studies in Tanzania and Papua New Guinea demonstrated significantly lower exposure (25%−45%) to CQ and DECQ during pregnancy, suggesting higher doses may be warranted [69,70]. A study in Thailand showed nonsignificant 11%−18% exposure decreases during pregnancy [71]. Above standard CQ doses in pregnancy have not been studied.

Proguanil (PG) alone or combined with CQ is a prophylaxis drug of choice in some regions. It is a prodrug, converted by CYP 2C19 to the active compound, cycloguanil (CG). CYP 2C19 poor metabolizers cannot make enough active metabolite for effective use. About 3% of Caucasians and 20% of Asians and Kenyans are poor metabolizers. The half-life is 12−21 h, but longer in poor metabolizers. Four pharmacokinetic studies in pregnant women from the Western border of Thailand and Zambia all demonstrate increased clearance and reduced plasma concentrations of CG by about twofold in pregnancy [60,61,72,73]; one study recommends increasing PG dose by 50% in late pregnancy, though no data are available for this suggested dose in pregnancy [72]. One postulated mechanism for decreased CG in late pregnancy is inhibition of CYP 2C19 by estrogen. *Atovaquone* is often combined with PG, and exposure is approximately half in pregnancy versus nonpregnant [60,61].

Mefloquine is used for CQ/PG-resistant malaria. It is well absorbed and widely distributed, including penetration into breast milk. It is partially hepatically metabolized by CYP 3A4, and is a substrate and inhibitor of Pgp. Elimination is very slow, mainly via bile and feces, with a half-life of 13−33 days. Two studies have reported decreased plasma mefloquine concentrations during pregnancy, suggesting higher pregnancy doses need to be evaluated [74,75].

Sulfadoxine-Pyrimethamine is used in combination as a second choice antimalarial in the second and third trimesters of pregnancy. Sulfadoxine should be avoided near term due to risk of infant kernicterus. Both are widely distributed and cross the placenta and into breast milk. Both are metabolized; sulfadoxine half-life is 200 h, while pyrimethamine is 80−123 h. Three different pharmacokinetic studies showed

30%−40% decreased sulfadoxine concentrations in pregnancy, and suggested increased doses need to be studied in pregnancy [76−78]. These same three studies conflicted in respect to pyrimethamine, with one showing increased concentrations in pregnancy, one showing no change, and one showing decreased concentrations. *Dapsone* is also used in combination with pyrimethamine. It is well absorbed, widely distributed, and undergoes enterohepatic recirculation. It is metabolized by CYP 3A4 and 2C9, with a 30 h half-life. Large quantities are excreted in breast milk and can cause hemolytic anemia in infants with G6PD deficiency. No pharmacokinetic studies in pregnancy have been conducted.

Quinine may be used for CQ-resistant malaria in pregnancy. It distributes into placenta and breast milk at 10%−50% of maternal concentrations [79]; the American Academy of Pediatrics reports it as compatible with breastfeeding. It is extensively metabolized by CYP 3A4 and others, may inhibit 3A4 and 2D6, and is prone to drug−drug interactions. Half-life is 8−21 h. Large quinine doses are ototoxic. Pregnancy does not significantly affect quinine exposure, and standard doses are recommended [80,81].

Artemether-lumefantrine is a widely used potent antimalarial combination. Artemether is rapidly metabolized by CYP 3A4 to the active metabolite, dihydroartemisinin (DHA), and may induce CYP 3A4/5. Lumefantrine is metabolized by CYP 3A4, inhibits CYP 2D6 in vitro, and has a half-life of 3−6 days. Concentrations of both are decreased in pregnancy, and lumefantrine C_{trough} fall below threshold values associated with treatment failure [82−84]. Artemether and DHA concentrations are decreased by ∼50% in pregnancy [82]. *Artesunate* is another artemisinin derivative rapidly metabolized to DHA. DHA clearance appears increased during pregnancy [85−87]. Increased doses of artemisinin derivatives and lumefantrine are recommended, but the optimum doses have not been determined.

Because of infant toxicity risks and limited data in pregnancy, *primaquine* should be avoided in pregnancy. *Halofantrine* may be necessary for some drug-resistant cases. Its absorption is poor and highly variable. It is metabolized by CYP 3A4 to an active metabolite, and it inhibits CYP 2D6. Breast milk and placental penetration are unknown, and no pharmacokinetic data during pregnancy are available. Additional agents used as drug-resistant strains become more prevalent and include *clindamycin* (described above), *doxycycline* (described above), *amodiaquine*, and *quinacrine*. The latter two are metabolized by CYP 3A4/5. No pregnancy pharmacokinetic data are available.

12.4 Tuberculosis

Treatment recommendations for tuberculosis during pregnancy are the same as in nonpregnant adults. Pregnancy does not seem to alter disease course, but untreated tuberculosis poses hazards to mothers and infants. Because of increasing resistance, multidrug therapy is usually recommended; specific drugs selected depend on the resistance patterns.

Isoniazid is used for prophylaxis and treatment during pregnancy. It is widely distributed, including into placenta and breast milk. It is compatible with breastfeeding, but the infant should be supplemented with pyridoxine. It is acetylated by the liver to inactive metabolites, with a half-life of 1−4 h. It inhibits CYP 1A2, 2A6, 2C9, 2C19, 2D6, and 3A4, yielding many clinically significant drug−drug interactions. Hepatitis from isoniazid is more common in pregnancy, so monitoring is warranted. The effects of pregnancy on the pharmacokinetics of isoniazid were investigated via population pharmacokinetic modeling in pregnant women with tuberculosis and HIV. No significant pregnancy-related changes were seen in isoniazid pharmacokinetic parameters [88].

Rifampicin is another drug of choice for tuberculosis during pregnancy. It does cross the placenta and into breast milk, and prophylactic vitamin K should be administered to the mother and the infant. It is deacetylated in the liver to an active metabolite, and enterohepatically recycled, with 60% eliminated in feces via biliary excretion and 30% eliminated in the urine. It is a potent inducer of CYP 3A4 and other CYP enzymes and causes numerous drug−drug interactions, often requiring dose increases of concomitant medications. A population pharmacokinetic analysis of rifampicin in pregnant women with TB and HIV showed only a 14% reduction in rifampin clearance during pregnancy and a modest increase in exposure. The authors do not suggest adjusting the dose of rifampin during pregnancy [89].

Ethambutol is first-line treatment in combination with isoniazid and rifampicin. It crosses the placenta at about 30% of maternal concentrations and penetrates breast milk in equal concentrations to maternal plasma; no problems with breastfeeding have been reported. It is partially metabolized in the liver, with parent and metabolite excreted in both the urine and the feces, with a half-life of ∼3.5 h. Clinically important drug−drug interactions are not common. Limited clinical data suggest that pregnancy does not cause clinically relevant changes in ethambutol exposure [88].

Pyrazinamide is often reserved for use in women with documented resistance to the three aforementioned first-line agents or in women who are also HIV+. Its ability to transfer into placenta and breast milk is unknown. It is hydrolyzed in the liver to active metabolites, which are excreted in the urine, and has a 9−10 h half-life. Clinically important drug−drug interactions are rare. Limited clinical data suggest that pregnancy does not cause clinically relevant changes in pyrazinamide exposure [88].

Quinolones are occasionally used as second-line agents in multidrug resistance tuberculosis; *ciprofloxacin* is preferred. *Dapsone* may also be considered in specific cases. Other agents, including *aminoglycosides* (causing fetal ototoxicity), *para-aminosalicylic acid* (causing gastrointestinal intolerance), *ethionamide*, *prothionamide, cycloserine, rifabutin, and rifapentine* (all with no pregnancy use data available) are not recommended for use during pregnancy.

12.5 **HIV**

Treatment for HIV is essential during pregnancy for both primary treatment of maternal HIV infection and to prevent mother-to-infant transmission of the virus.

Combination therapy throughout pregnancy is standard of care in areas with sufficient resources; more limited treatment strategies near and during labor/delivery are used in some limited-resource settings. The selection of an antiretroviral regimen for an individual patient depends upon a variety of factors, including whether the woman is initiating therapy for the first time, continuing a regimen after becoming pregnant, or making changes to a regimen while pregnant. This section reviews current pharmacokinetic data on antiretroviral drugs during pregnancy. Situation-specific recommendations for use of antiretroviral drugs in pregnant women are available within the perinatal treatment guidelines at http://www.aidsinfo.nih.gov/guidelines [90].

Nucleoside/nucleotide reverse transcriptase inhibitors include *abacavir, didanosine, emtricitabine, lamivudine, stavudine, tenofovir disoproxil fumarate (TDF), tenofovir alafenamide (TAF)*, and *zidovudine*. The nucleosides are activated intracellularly and the active triphosphate nucleosides have longer half-lives than the parent drug, have low protein binding, and all but abacavir are eliminated renally. Abacavir is metabolized, but is not a substrate for the CYP enzyme family. Lamivudine and zidovudine have been widely used for HIV treatment in pregnancy. They have high placental transfer to the fetus, readily pass into breast milk (breast milk to plasma ratios of 2.56 for lamivudine and 0.4 for zidovudine), and pharmacokinetics are not significantly altered by pregnancy [91,92]. Pregnancy does not significantly alter the pharmacokinetics of abacavir, didanosine, or stavudine [93−95]. Placental transfer of abacavir and stavudine is high, with moderate transfer of didanosine (cord blood to maternal plasma ratio of 0.38). Breast milk concentrations of these three agents are not known. Maternal exposure to emtricitabine and tenofovir (as TDF) is lower during the third trimester compared to postpartum, but third trimester concentrations still appear therapeutic so no dose adjustments are warranted [96,97]. Both readily cross the placenta, but tenofovir transfer into breast milk is low, while emtricitabine breast milk penetration is unknown. In pregnant women taking TAF, plasma TAF exposures during pregnancy and postpartum were within the range of those typically observed in nonpregnant [98].

Pregnancy-specific pharmacokinetic data are currently available for three integrase strand transfer inhibitors (INSTIs): *dolutegravir, raltegravir*, and *elvitegravir*. Pregnancy data are not yet available for *bictegravir*. All INSTIs bind extensively to plasma proteins—primarily albumin and alpha-1 acid glycoprotein—ranging from 83% bound (raltegravir) to ~99% bound (bictegravir, dolutegravir, and elvitegravir). Dolutegravir is primarily metabolized by UGT1A enzymes to a glucuronide metabolite that is excreted in the urine. A minor metabolic pathway is via CYP3A4. Dolutegravir exposures were significantly lower during pregnancy compared to postpartum (29% and 34% reduction in AUC and C_{trough}, respectively, during the third trimester) [99]. Raltegravir is primarily metabolized by UGT1A1 to a glucuronide metabolite with the majority of the raltegravir dose is excreted in the feces (51%) and urine (32%) [100]. Raltegravir exposures were also significantly lower during pregnancy compared to postpartum (46% and 21% reduction in AUC and C_{trough}, respectively, during the third trimester) [101]. Placental transfer is variable but high, often with cord blood concentrations exceeding maternal concentrations [101−103]. Breast milk transfer is unknown. Elvitegravir is metabolized mainly through oxidative metabolism by CYP3A4, with minor contributions from CYP3A5/CYP1A1. Elvitegravir also undergoes glucuronidation by UGT1A1, and to a lesser extent UGT1A3. Elvitegravir is predominately excreted in the feces. Elvitegravir boosted with cobicistat was studied in pregnant women and showed elvitegravir exposures were significantly lower during pregnancy compared to postpartum (44% and 81% reduction in AUC and C_{trough}, respectively, during the third trimester) [104].

First-generation nonnucleoside reverse transcriptase inhibitors include *delavirdine* (no longer available in the United States), *efavirenz*, and *nevirapine*. Efavirenz is highly protein bound (>99%), is metabolized by CYP 3A4 and 2B6, and induces CYP 3A4, with a terminal half-life of 40−55 h. A small study in 13 Rwandan women showed milk to plasma concentration ratios of 54%, and infant plasma concentrations during breastfeeding were 13% of maternal concentrations, with infant concentrations somewhat lower than concentrations targeted for treatment in adults [105]. Likewise, cord blood concentrations are about 50% of maternal concentrations at delivery [106]. Clearance is increased and C_{trough} are decreased during the third trimester compared to postpartum, but third trimester exposure is still high enough to be therapeutic using standard doses [106]. Nevirapine has been used extensively during pregnancy. It is 60% protein bound, has a half-life with chronic dosing of 25−30 h, is metabolized by CYP 3A4 and 2B6, and induces CYP 3A4 and 2B6. It readily crosses the placenta, and breast milk concentrations are 76% of maternal concentrations. Pharmacokinetics are not significantly altered during pregnancy in studies of US women, and standard doses are recommended [107,108]. A study in Ugandan pregnant women showed significantly decreased exposure during pregnancy compared to postpartum, including 67% of women falling below target C_{trough}, suggesting increased doses may be needed in some populations [109].

Second-generation nonnucleosides include *doravirine*, *rilpivirine*, and *etravirine*. Etravirine is 99.9% protein bound with a terminal half-life of 41 h, is metabolized by CYP 3A4, 2C9, and 2C19, induces CYP 3A4, inhibits 2C9, 2C19, and Pgp, and is subject to many drug−drug interactions. The pharmacokinetics of etravirine at a dose of 200 mg twice daily were studied in 15 pregnant women. Although etravirine AUC was 34% higher in the third trimester compared to paired postpartum data, the authors do not suggest a dose adjustment based upon prior dose-ranging and safety data [110].

Rilpivirine is 99.7% protein bound, is metabolized by CYP 3A4, has a half-life of 50 h, and metabolites are excreted primarily in feces. In a study of 32 pregnant women receiving rilpivirine 25 mg once daily, lower overall exposure and C_{trough} were observed during pregnancy compared to postpartum [111]. 90% of women had minimum concentrations above the protein binding adjusted EC90 for rilpivirine [111]. No pregnancy data are available for doravirine.

Protease inhibitors include *atazanavir, darunavir, fosamprenavir, indinavir, lopinavir, nelfinavir, ritonavir, saquinavir,* and *tipranavir*. All are hepatically metabolized by CYP isoenzymes, including CYP 3A4, and are subject to drug−drug interactions. All except nelfinavir are used with a pharmacokinetic enhancer to boost exposure to therapeutic concentrations in pregnancy. Fosamprenavir, indinavir, lopinavir, saquinavir, and tipranavir may be boosted with low-dose ritonavir. Atazanavir and darunavir may be boosted with either low-dose ritonavir or cobicistat. However, the FDA does not recommend cobicistat during pregnancy due to substantially lower exposures of boosted antiretrovirals (elvitegravir, darunavir, and atazanavir). The majority of protease inhibitors studied to date have decreased concentrations during pregnancy, with lowest exposure seen during the third trimester. Interestingly, early postpartum concentrations on standard doses of ritonavir-boosted lopinavir, fosamprenavir, and atazanavir are higher than seen in nonpregnant adults, so close monitoring for toxicity is warranted. Countries with routine access to therapeutic drug monitoring will often draw C_{trough} throughout pregnancy and will adjust individual patient doses as needed to maintain troughs above recommended minimum concentrations.

Atazanavir is 86%–89% protein bound, has a half-life of 7 h, is extensively metabolized by CYP 3A4, inhibits CYP 3A4, 2C8, and UGT 1A1, and is mostly excreted as metabolites in feces. Placental transfer is 10%–20% of maternal concentrations, and breast milk transfer is unknown. Only when coadministered with ritonavir, it is considered a preferred agent for use in pregnant women in the United States [90]. When boosted with cobicistat in pregnant women, atazanavir C_{trough} in the second and third trimesters of pregnancy were 80% and 85% lower, respectively, than previously reported values in nonpregnant, adult patients living with HIV [112]. A study in 17 Italian women found no difference in pharmacokinetic parameters during pregnancy compared to postpartum with the standard dose of 300 mg atazanavir and 100 mg ritonavir once daily [113]. Three other studies found 21%–45% decreased exposure in the third trimester of pregnancy compared to postpartum [114–116]. The study of mainly South African women recommended the standard dose during pregnancy despite AUC and maximum concentration decreases because minimum concentrations were still in the therapeutic range on the standard dose in pregnancy [114]. The P1026s study team investigated standard dose in second trimester and postpartum, and an increased dose of 400 mg atazanavir/100 mg ritonavir in the third trimester. The increased third trimester dose resulted in concentrations similar to those seen in nonpregnant adults [117]; second trimester concentrations on standard doses were lower than typically seen in nonpregnant adults and may be subtherapeutic especially when coadministered with tenofovir, while postpartum concentrations on standard doses were higher than reported in nonpregnant adults. The manufacturer recommends the standard dose in pregnancy, unless the patient is also taking either tenofovir or a histamine-2 receptor antagonist, in which case an increased dose of 400 mg atazanavir/100 mg ritonavir once daily should be used.

Darunavir boosted with ritonavir is a preferred regimen during pregnancy. However, darunavir boosted with cobicistat is not recommended due to substantially lower darunavir exposures. Darunavir is 95% protein bound, is a substrate and inhibitor of CYP 3A4, and has a 15 h half-life when coadministered with ritonavir. In 29 pregnant women receiving darunavir boosted with cobicistat, darunavir AUC was 33% and 48% lower in the second trimester and third trimester, respectively, relative to paired postpartum data [118]. A study in 31 pregnant women showed significantly decreased darunavir exposure during pregnancy with once or twice daily darunavir boosted with ritonavir (800 mg darunavir/100 mg ritonavir once daily or 600 mg darunavir/100 mg ritonavir twice daily), and concluded that only twice daily doses should be used [119]. A recent study reported that the pharmacokinetics of an increased dose of darunavir (800 mg twice daily) with 100 mg ritonavir failed to significantly increase darunavir exposure compared with 600 mg twice daily [120].

Lopinavir (coformulated with ritonavir in 200 mg lopinavir/50 mg ritonavir tablets) is 98%−99% protein bound, metabolized by CYP 3A4 with most metabolites excreted in the feces, and has a 5−6 h half-life. Placental transfer is 20% of maternal concentrations [121], while breast milk passage is unknown. Multiple pharmacokinetic studies have shown 40%−60% increased lopinavir clearance during pregnancy [121,122]. The fraction of unbound drug increases by 18% in late pregnancy, which is not enough to overcome the decrease in total exposure [123]. Some experts recommend standard (400 mg lopinavir/100 mg ritonavir) twice daily doses during pregnancy in treatment-naïve patients and increased doses (600 mg lopinavir/150 mg ritonavir twice daily) in PI-experienced patients [122], while other experts routinely increase the dose to 600 mg lopinavir/150 mg ritonavir twice daily in the third trimester (30 weeks gestation), decreasing to standard dose just after delivery [121]. Once daily dosing of 800 mg lopinavir/200 mg ritonavir (approved in treatment naïve nonpregnant adults) is not recommended during pregnancy.

Fosamprenavir is a phosphate ester prodrug that is rapidly converted to amprenavir in vivo. It is 90% protein bound, is extensively metabolized by CYP 3A4, 2C9, and 2D6, is a Pgp substrate, inhibits CYP 3A4, and has a half-life of 7.7 h. Similar to other protease inhibitors, exposure is significantly decreased during pregnancy when dosed as 700 mg fosamprenavir/100 mg ritonavir twice daily [124]. However, concentrations on this dose during pregnancy are still higher than concentrations in nonpregnant adults taking one of the approved doses of 1400 mg twice daily without ritonavir, and the standard ritonavir-boosted dose should be adequate for treatment naïve patients. Indinavir is 60% protein bound, a substrate of CYP 3A4, UGT, and Pgp, inhibits CYP 3A4 and has a 2 h half-life. Transplacental passage is minimal, while breast milk passage is unknown. The manufacturer does not recommend use in pregnancy because exposure is markedly decreased during pregnancy [125,126]. If needed, only ritonavir-boosted indinavir should be used [127], at a dose of 800 mg indinavir/100−200 mg ritonavir twice daily [90]. Nelfinavir has been extensively used in pregnant women, and placental transfer is minimal, while breast milk transfer is unknown. It is >98% protein bound, is a substrate of CYP 3A4, 2C19, and Pgp, and inhibits CYP 3A4 and Pgp. The half-life is 3.5−5 h. Exposure is significantly decreased during pregnancy [128,129], and dosing with 625 mg tablets (two tablets, 1250 mg twice daily, n = 27) resulted in subtherapeutic C_{trough} in 85% of patients [130], so higher doses have been studied in pregnancy. In 18 pregnant women receiving increased dose nelfinavir during the third trimester of pregnancy (1875 mg twice daily), nelfinavir exposure during pregnancy was similar to that of standard dosing (1250 mg twice daily) in the postpartum period. The authors conclude that increased dose nelfinavir in pregnancy may be beneficial in certain circumstances [131].

Saquinavir combined with ritonavir is 98% protein bound, has a half-life of 12 h, and is a substrate and inhibitor of CYP 3A4 and Pgp. Pharmacokinetics of older formulations showed decreased exposure to either saquinavir [132,133] or ritonavir [134] during pregnancy compared to postpartum. A study of the 500 mg tablet formulation showed saquinavir concentrations were not significantly different between the second and third trimesters of pregnancy and postpartum [135]. The recommended dose is 1000 mg saquinavir/100 mg ritonavir twice daily.

Tipranavir must be coadministered with ritonavir. It is >99.9% protein bound, is a substrate for CYP 3A4 and Pgp, and induces CYP 3A4 and Pgp. A case report showed therapeutic concentrations in late pregnancy on the standard dose (500 mg tipranavir/200 mg ritonavir twice daily), and a cord blood to maternal concentration ratio of 0.41, higher than other protease inhibitors [136]. No other published data are available.

Enfuvirtide is an entry (fusion) inhibitor administered by subcutaneous injection. It is 92% protein bound, has a 3.8 h half-life, and is a peptide that is hydrolyzed to an inactive metabolite, and expected to be catabolized to amino acids. It does not cross the placenta [137,138], and transfer into breast milk is unknown. Pharmacokinetic data during pregnancy are not available. *Maraviroc*, another entry inhibitor classified as pregnancy category B, is 76% protein bound, a substrate of Pgp and CYP 3A4, has a 14—18 h half-life, and is subject to many drug—drug interactions. In pregnant women, overall maraviroc exposure during pregnancy is decreased, with a reduction in AUC_{tau} and maximum concentration of about 30%. However, C_{trough} was reduced by only 15% and exceeded the minimum C_{trough} target concentration, indicating the standard adult dose is sufficient in pregnancy [139].

12.6 Antivirals

Treatment for genital herpes is generally recommended during pregnancy to prevent neonatal herpes. *Acyclovir* distributes widely in the body, crosses into the placenta and the breast milk at concentrations similar to or greater than maternal plasma, and is excreted unchanged in the urine with a short half-life of 2.5—3.3 h. Oral bioavailability is low (10%—20%). A pharmacokinetic study in pregnant women concluded that 400 mg orally three times daily provided appropriate concentrations, similar to those seen in nonpregnant adults [140]. *Valacyclovir* is a prodrug of acyclovir that is converted to acyclovir by first-pass intestinal or hepatic metabolism, with increased bioavailability (~55% acyclovir bioavailability after valacyclovir administration). A pharmacokinetic study comparing valacyclovir 500 mg twice daily and acyclovir 400 mg three times daily found higher acyclovir exposure (approximately double) with administration of valacyclovir in pregnant women. Both were well tolerated, but insufficient safety and efficacy data (compared to acyclovir) are available to recommend use in pregnancy. Likewise, no pharmacokinetic and limited safety/efficacy data are available for *famciclovir, penciclovir, ganciclovir, valganciclovir, foscarnet, cidofovir, fomivirsen, trifluridine, or vidarabine*. Use of several of these agents to treat cytomegalovirus during pregnancy should be limited to serious/severe infections.

Amantadine, rimantadine, oseltamivir, zanamivir, peramivir, and *baloxavir* are used for the treatment of influenza virus. Safety data are inadequate to determine risks of these medications in pregnancy, but morbidity and mortality from influenza are higher during pregnancy, so these agents may be needed in serious infections. Oseltamivir is hepatically metabolized (but not by the CYP P450 system) to the active form, a carboxylate metabolite, which is excreted in urine. The half-life is 1−3 h, and penetration into breast milk yields concentrations significantly lower than considered therapeutic in infants [141]. Two studies have evaluated pharmacokinetics in pregnant women. In 30 women, carboxylate exposure did not change significantly between the three trimesters of pregnancy [142]. Concentrations were above the typical viral 50% inhibitory concentrations, and the authors concluded that standard doses should be adequate in pregnancy. Beigi and colleagues compared 16 pregnant women to 23 nonpregnant controls and found significantly lower carboxylate metabolite exposure during pregnancy [143]. Given the wide therapeutic window of oseltamivir and the increasing prevalence of viral neuraminidase inhibitor resistance, these authors suggest increasing the treatment dose from 75 mg twice daily for 5 days to 75 mg three times daily in pregnant women to better approximate concentrations seen in nonpregnant patients. Pharmacokinetic studies on this increased dose have not been reported.

Amantadine, peramivir, and *zanamivir* are renally excreted unchanged. *Amantadine* has an 11−15 h half-life, crosses the placenta and into breast milk, and is not recommended in breastfeeding. *Peramivir* has a longer half-life of approximately 20 h; it is unknown whether peramivir is excreted in human milk. *Zanamivir* has a 2.5−5 h half-life. Small amounts cross into placenta; breast milk penetration is unknown. *Rimantadine* and *baloxavir* are primarily metabolized. Placenta and breast milk exposure of these drugs are unknown. Amantadine and rimantadine are no longer first-line agents due to high resistance, but are being used in combination with oseltamivir or zanamivir as neuraminidase inhibitor resistance increases. Pharmacokinetic data are not available for amantadine, peramivir, zanamivir, rimantadine, or baloxavir during pregnancy.

Ribavirin is teratogenic in animals. It is used for hepatitis B and C in combination with *interferons* and should be reserved for life-threatening infections. It is also toxic to nursing animals, and should not be used during breastfeeding.

Direct-acting antivirals (DAAs) for the treatment of hepatitis C virus (HCV) infection include *boceprevir, daclatasvir, elbasvir, glecaprevir, grazoprevir, ledipasvir, pibrentasvir, simeprevir, sofosbuvir, telaprevir, velpatasvir*, and *voxilaprevir*—many of which are available in fixed dose combinations. Information on the efficacy, safety, and optimal dosing of DAAs in pregnancy is lacking [144].

For women of reproductive age with known HCV infection, antiviral therapy is recommended before pregnancy to reduce the risk of HCV transmission. Treatment of HCV infection during pregnancy with DAAs is not currently recommended.

12.7 Parasitic infections

Many parasitic infections are asymptomatic, and treatment is only indicated for severe infections during pregnancy. *Mebendazole* can be used during pregnancy if indicated. It is poorly absorbed and metabolized by CYP P450, but very effective within the intestine. *Flubendazole* is structurally related, with limited data available in pregnancy. *Albendazole* is a broad-spectrum anthelmintic. It is poorly bioavailable with extensive first-pass and systemic hepatic metabolism and a 9 h half-life. It may induce CYP 1A activity and be subject to drug—drug interactions. *Thiabendazole* is also extensively metabolized hepatically and is a substrate and inhibitor of CYP 1A2. No data are available for use during pregnancy.

Praziquantel is a first-line agent for schistosomiasis treatment. It is metabolized hepatically, likely by CYP 3A4, and subject to drug—drug interactions with a short half-life of 0.8—1.5 h. Breast milk concentrations are about a quarter of maternal concentrations. No pharmacokinetic data in pregnancy are available. *Pyrantel* is another broad-spectrum anthelmintic, but is not recommended in pregnancy due to very limited pregnancy use data available. *Ivermectin* and *diethylcarbamazine* are used to treat filariasis and onchocerciasis/onchocercosis. Data for use in pregnancy are lacking; they should only be used for compelling indications. *Paromomycin*, is used for intestinal amebiasis, and is not absorbed systemically after oral ingestion. *Niclosamide* is used to treat tapeworm infections, and is not significantly absorbed from the gastrointestinal tract.

References

[1] Drugs during pregnancy and lactation: treatment options and risk assessment. 2nd ed. London: Elsevier; 2007.

[2] Briggs GG, Freeman RK, Yaffe SJ. Drugs in pregnancy and lactation: a reference guide to fetal and neonatal risk. 9th ed. Philadelphia: Lippincott Williams & Wilkins; 2011.

[3] Feghali M, Venkataramanan R, Caritis S. Pharmacokinetics of drugs in pregnancy. Semin Perinatol 2015;39(7):512—9.

[4] Johnson JR, Colombo DF, Gardner D, Cho E, Fan-Havard P, Shellhaas CS. Optimal dosing of penicillin G in the third trimester of pregnancy for prophylaxis against group B Streptococcus. Am J Obstet Gynecol 2001;185(4):850—3.

[5] Control CfD. Prevention of perinatal group B streptococcal disease: revised guidelines from CDC, 2010. Morb Mortal Wkly Rep 2010;59(No. RR-10):1—33.

[6] Nathan L, Bawdon RE, Sidawi JE, Stettler RW, McIntire DM, Wendel Jr GD. Penicillin levels following the administration of benzathine penicillin G in pregnancy. Obstet Gynecol 1993;82(3):338—42.

[7] Control CD. Sexually transmitted diseases treatment guidelines 2010. Morb Mortal Wkly Rep 2010;59(No. RR-12):1—116.

[8] Heikkila AM, Erkkola RU. The need for adjustment of dosage regimen of penicillin V during pregnancy. Obstet Gynecol 1993;81(6):919—21.

[9] Furness A, Kalicinsky C, Rosenfield L, Barber C, Poliquin V. Penicillin skin testing, challenge, and desensitization in pregnancy: a systematic review. J Obstet Gynaecol Can 2020;42(10):1254—1261.e3.

[10] Andrew MA, Easterling TR, Carr DB, Shen D, Buchanan ML, Rutherford T, et al. Amoxicillin pharmacokinetics in pregnant women: modeling and simulations of dosage strategies. Clin Pharmacol Ther 2007;81(4):547—56.

[11] Muller AE, DeJongh J, Oostvogel PM, Voskuyl RA, Dorr PJ, Danhof M, et al. Amoxicillin pharmacokinetics in pregnant women with preterm premature rupture of the membranes. Am J Obstet Gynecol 2008;198(1):108 e101—106.

[12] Muller AE, Dorr PJ, Mouton JW, De Jongh J, Oostvogel PM, Steegers EA, et al. The influence of labour on the pharmacokinetics of intravenously administered amoxicillin in pregnant women. Br J Clin Pharmacol 2008;66(6):866—74.

[13] Muller AE, Oostvogel PM, DeJongh J, Mouton JW, Steegers EA, Dorr PJ, et al. Pharmacokinetics of amoxicillin in maternal, umbilical cord, and neonatal sera. Antimicrob Agents Chemother 2009;53(4):1574—80.

[14] Philipson A. Pharmacokinetics of ampicillin during pregnancy. J Infect Dis 1977; 136(3):370—6.

[15] Kubacka RT, Johnstone HE, Tan HS, Reeme PD, Myre SA. Intravenous ampicillin pharmacokinetics in the third trimester of pregnancy. Ther Drug Monit 1983;5(1): 55—60.

[16] Bourget P, Sertin A, Lesne-Hulin A, Fernandez H, Ville Y, Van Peborgh P. Influence of pregnancy on the pharmacokinetic behaviour and the transplacental transfer of the piperacillin-tazobactam combination. Eur J Obstet Gynecol Reprod Biol 1998;76(1): 21—7.

[17] Heikkila A, Erkkola R. Pharmacokinetics of piperacillin during pregnancy. J Antimicrob Chemother 1991;28(3):419—23.

[18] Fortunato SJ, Bawdon RE, Welt SI, Swan KF. Steady-state cord and amniotic fluid ceftizoxime levels continuously surpass maternal levels. Am J Obstet Gynecol 1988; 159(3):570—3.

[19] Holt DE, Fisk NM, Spencer JA, de Louvois J, Hurley R, Harvey D. Transplacental transfer of cefuroxime in uncomplicated pregnancies and those complicated by hydrops or changes in amniotic fluid volume. Arch Dis Child 1993;68(1 Spec No): 54—7.

[20] Philipson A, Stiernstedt G. Pharmacokinetics of cefuroxime in pregnancy. Am J Obstet Gynecol 1982;142(7):823—8.

[21] Peiker G, Schroder S, Voigt R, Muller B, Noschel H. The pharmacokinetics of cephalothin during the late stage of pregnancy and in the course of labour (author's transl). Pharmazie 1980;35(12):790—3.

[22] Allegaert K, van Mieghem T, Verbesselt R, de Hoon J, Rayyan M, Devlieger R, et al. Cefazolin pharmacokinetics in maternal plasma and amniotic fluid during pregnancy. Am J Obstet Gynecol 2009;200(2). 170 e171-177.

[23] Philipson A, Stiernstedt G, Ehrnebo M. Comparison of the pharmacokinetics of cephradine and cefazolin in pregnant and non-pregnant women. Clin Pharmacokinet 1987; 12(2):136—44.

[24] Giamarellou H, Gazis J, Petrikkos G, Antsaklis A, Aravantinos D, Daikos GK. A study of cefoxitin, moxalactam, and ceftazidime kinetics in pregnancy. Am J Obstet Gynecol 1983;147(8):914—9.

[25] Flaherty JF, Boswell GW, Winkel CA, Elliott JP. Pharmacokinetics of cefoxitin in patients at term gestation: lavage versus intravenous administration. Am J Obstet Gynecol 1983;146(7):760—6.

[26] Gonik B, Feldman S, Pickering LK, Doughtie CG. Pharmacokinetics of cefoperazone in the parturient. Antimicrob Agents Chemother 1986;30(6):874—6.

[27] Nathorst-Boos J, Philipson A, Hedman A, Arvisson A. Renal elimination of ceftazidime during pregnancy. Am J Obstet Gynecol 1995;172(1 Pt 1):163—6.

[28] Dallmann A, van den Anker J, Pfister M, Koch G. Characterization of maternal and neonatal pharmacokinetic behavior of ceftazidime. J Clin Pharmacol 2019;59(1):74—82.

[29] Sauberan JB, Bradley JS, Blumer J, Stellwagen LM. Transmission of meropenem in breast milk. Pediatr Infect Dis J 2012;31(8):832—4.

[30] Heikkila A, Renkonen OV, Erkkola R. Pharmacokinetics and transplacental passage of imipenem during pregnancy. Antimicrob Agents Chemother 1992;36(12):2652—5.

[31] Obata I, Yamato T, Hayashi S, Imakawa N, Hayashi S. Pharmacokinetic study of aztreonam transfer from mother to fetus. Jpn J Antibiot 1990;43(1):70—80.

[32] Chamberlain A, White S, Bawdon R, Thomas S, Larsen B. Pharmacokinetics of ampicillin and sulbactam in pregnancy. Am J Obstet Gynecol 1993;168(2):667—73.

[33] Fortunato SJ, Bawdon RE, Swan KF, Bryant EC, Sobhi S. Transfer of Timentin (ticarcillin and clavulanic acid) across the in vitro perfused human placenta: comparison with other agents. Am J Obstet Gynecol 1992;167(6):1595—9.

[34] Heikkinen T, Laine K, Neuvonen PJ, Ekblad U. The transplacental transfer of the macrolide antibiotics erythromycin, roxithromycin and azithromycin. Bjog 2000;107(6):770—5.

[35] Witt A, Sommer EM, Cichna M, Postlbauer K, Widhalm A, Gregor H, et al. Placental passage of clarithromycin surpasses other macrolide antibiotics. Am J Obstet Gynecol 2003;188(3):816—9.

[36] Salman S, Davis TM, Page-Sharp M, Camara B, Oluwalana C, Bojang A, et al. Pharmacokinetics of transfer of azithromycin into the breast milk of african mothers. Antimicrob Agents Chemother 2015;60(3):1592—9.

[37] Salman S, Rogerson SJ, Kose K, Griffin S, Gomorai S, Baiwog F, et al. Pharmacokinetic properties of azithromycin in pregnancy. Antimicrob Agents Chemother;54(1):360—366.

[38] Laiprasert J, Klein K, Mueller BA, Pearlman MD. Transplacental passage of vancomycin in noninfected term pregnant women. Obstet Gynecol 2007;109(5):1105—10.

[39] Nau H, Welsch F, Ulbrich B, Bass R, Lange J. Thiamphenicol during the first trimester of human pregnancy: placental transfer in vivo, placental uptake in vitro, and inhibition of mitochondrial function. Toxicol Appl Pharmacol 1981;60(1):131—41.

[40] Muller AE, Mouton JW, Oostvogel PM, Dorr PJ, Voskuyl RA, DeJongh J, et al. Pharmacokinetics of clindamycin in pregnant women in the peripartum period. Antimicrob Agents Chemother;54(5):2175—2181.

[41] Van Kampenhout E, Bolhuis MS, Alffenaar JC, Oswald LM, Kerstjens HA, de Lange WC, et al. Pharmacokinetics of moxifloxacin and linezolid during and after pregnancy in a patient with multidrug-resistant tuberculosis. Eur Respir J 2017;49(3).

[42] Bernard B, Abate M, Thielen PF, Attar H, Ballard CA, Wehrle PF. Maternal-fetal pharmacological activity of amikacin. J Infect Dis 1977;135(6):925–32.

[43] Bourget P, Fernandez H, Delouis C, Taburet AM. Pharmacokinetics of tobramycin in pregnant women. Safety and efficacy of a once-daily dose regimen. J Clin Pharm Therapeut 1991;16(3):167–76.

[44] Zaske DE, Cipolle RJ, Strate RG, Malo JW, Koszalka Jr MF. Rapid gentamicin elimination in obstetric patients. Obstet Gynecol 1980;56(5):559–64.

[45] Bawdon RE, Maberry MC, Fortunato SJ, Gilstrap LC, Kim S. Trimethoprim and sulfamethoxazole transfer in the in vitro perfused human cotyledon. Gynecol Obstet Invest 1991;31(4):240–2.

[46] Ambrosius Christensen L, Rasmussen SN, Hansen SH, Bondesen S, Hvidberg EF. Salazosulfapyridine and metabolites in fetal and maternal body fluids with special reference to 5-aminosalicylic acid. Acta Obstet Gynecol Scand 1987;66(5):433–5.

[47] Polachek H, Holcberg G, Sapir G, Tsadkin-Tamir M, Polachek J, Katz M, et al. Transfer of ciprofloxacin, ofloxacin and levofloxacin across the perfused human placenta in vitro. Eur J Obstet Gynecol Reprod Biol 2005;122(1):61–5.

[48] Giamarellou H, Kolokythas E, Petrikkos G, Gazis J, Aravantinos D, Sfikakis P. Pharmacokinetics of three newer quinolones in pregnant and lactating women. Am J Med 1989;87(5A):49S–51S.

[49] McDonald HM, Brocklehurst P, Gordon A. Antibiotics for treating bacterial vaginosis in pregnancy, vol. 1; 2007.

[50] Carey JC, Klebanoff MA, Hauth JC, Hillier SL, Thom EA, Ernest JM, et al. Metronidazole to prevent preterm delivery in pregnant women with asymptomatic bacterial vaginosis. National institute of child health and human development network of maternal-fetal medicine units. N Engl J Med 2000;342(8):534–40.

[51] Karhunen M. Placental transfer of metronidazole and tinidazole in early human pregnancy after a single infusion. Br J Clin Pharmacol 1984;18(2):254–7.

[52] Erickson SH, Oppenheim GL, Smith GH. Metronidazole in breast milk. Obstet Gynecol 1981;57(1):48–50.

[53] Heisterberg L, Branebjerg PE. Blood and milk concentrations of metronidazole in mothers and infants. J Perinat Med 1983;11(2):114–20.

[54] Passmore CM, McElnay JC, Rainey EA, D'Arcy PF. Metronidazole excretion in human milk and its effect on the suckling neonate. Br J Clin Pharmacol 1988;26(1):45–51.

[55] Amon I, Amon K, Franke G, Mohr C. Pharmacokinetics of Metronidazole in pregnant women. Chemotherapy 1981;27(2):73–9.

[56] Visser AA, Hundt HK. The pharmacokinetics of a single intravenous dose of metronidazole in pregnant patients. J Antimicrob Chemother 1984;13(3):279–83.

[57] Wang X, Nanovskaya TN, Zhan Y, Abdel-Rahman SM, Jasek M, Hankins GD, et al. Pharmacokinetics of metronidazole in pregnant patients with bacterial vaginosis. J Matern Fetal Neonatal Med 2011;24(3):444–8.

[58] Pons G, Rey E, Richard MO, Vauzelle F, Francoual C, Moran C, et al. Nitrofurantoin excretion in human milk. Dev Pharmacol Ther 1990;14(3):148–52.

[59] Philipps W, Fietz AK, Meixner K, Bluhmki T, Meister R, Schaefer C, et al. Pregnancy outcome after first-trimester exposure to fosfomycin for the treatment of urinary tract infection: an observational cohort study. Infection 2020;48(1):57–64.

[60] McGready R, Stepniewska K, Edstein MD, Cho T, Gilveray G, Looareesuwan S, et al. The pharmacokinetics of atovaquone and proguanil in pregnant women with acute falciparum malaria. Eur J Clin Pharmacol 2003;59(7):545–52.

[61] Na-Bangchang K, Manyando C, Ruengweerayut R, Kioy D, Mulenga M, Miller GB, et al. The pharmacokinetics and pharmacodynamics of atovaquone and proguanil for the treatment of uncomplicated falciparum malaria in third-trimester pregnant women. Eur J Clin Pharmacol 2005;61(8):573−82.

[62] Burger RJ, Visser BJ, Grobusch MP, van Vugt M. The influence of pregnancy on the pharmacokinetic properties of artemisinin combination therapy (ACT): a systematic review. Malar J 2016;15:99.

[63] Shoai Tehrani M, Sicre de Fontbrune F, Roth P, Allisy C, Bougnoux ME, Hermine O, et al. Case report of exposure to voriconazole in the second and third trimesters of pregnancy. Antimicrob Agents Chemother 2013;57(2):1094−5.

[64] Control CfD. Treatment guidelines for malaria.

[65] WHO. Malaria treatment guidelines.

[66] McGready R, White NJ, Nosten F. Parasitological efficacy of antimalarials in the treatment and prevention of falciparum malaria in pregnancy 1998 to 2009: a systematic review. Bjog;118(2):123−135.

[67] Akintonwa A, Gbajumo SA, Mabadeje AF. Placental and milk transfer of chloroquine in humans. Ther Drug Monit 1988;10(2):147−9.

[68] Law I, Ilett KF, Hackett LP, Page-Sharp M, Baiwog F, Gomorrai S, et al. Transfer of chloroquine and desethylchloroquine across the placenta and into milk in Melanesian mothers. Br J Clin Pharmacol 2008;65(5):674−9.

[69] Karunajeewa HA, Salman S, Mueller I, Baiwog F, Gomorrai S, Law I, et al. Pharmacokinetics of chloroquine and monodesethylchloroquine in pregnancy. Antimicrob Agents Chemother;54(3):1186−1192.

[70] Massele AY, Kilewo C, Aden Abdi Y, Tomson G, Diwan VK, Ericsson O, et al. Chloroquine blood concentrations and malaria prophylaxis in Tanzanian women during the second and third trimesters of pregnancy. Eur J Clin Pharmacol 1997;52(4):299−305.

[71] Lee SJ, McGready R, Fernandez C, Stepniewska K, Paw MK, Viladpai-nguen SJ, et al. Chloroquine pharmacokinetics in pregnant and nonpregnant women with vivax malaria. Eur J Clin Pharmacol 2008;64(10):987−92.

[72] McGready R, Stepniewska K, Seaton E, Cho T, Cho D, Ginsberg A, et al. Pregnancy and use of oral contraceptives reduces the biotransformation of proguanil to cycloguanil. Eur J Clin Pharmacol 2003;59(7):553−7.

[73] Wangboonskul J, White NJ, Nosten F, ter Kuile F, Moody RR, Taylor RB. Single dose pharmacokinetics of proguanil and its metabolites in pregnancy. Eur J Clin Pharmacol 1993;44(3):247−51.

[74] Na Bangchang K, Davis TM, Looareesuwan S, White NJ, Bunnag D, Karbwang J. Mefloquine pharmacokinetics in pregnant women with acute falciparum malaria. Trans R Soc Trop Med Hyg 1994;88(3):321−3.

[75] Nosten F, Karbwang J, White NJ, Honeymoon N, Bangchang K, Bunnag D, et al. Mefloquine antimalarial prophylaxis in pregnancy: dose finding and pharmacokinetic study. Br J Clin Pharmacol 1990;30(1):79−85.

[76] Green MD, van Eijk AM, van Ter Kuile FO, Ayisi JG, Parise ME, Kager PA, et al. Pharmacokinetics of sulfadoxine-pyrimethamine in HIV-infected and uninfected pregnant women in Western Kenya. J Infect Dis 2007;196(9):1403−8.

[77] Karunajeewa HA, Salman S, Mueller I, Baiwog F, Gomorrai S, Law I, et al. Pharmacokinetic properties of sulfadoxine-pyrimethamine in pregnant women. Antimicrob Agents Chemother 2009;53(10):4368−76.

[78] Nyunt MM, Adam I, Kayentao K, van Dijk J, Thuma P, Mauff K, et al. Pharmacokinetics of sulfadoxine and pyrimethamine in intermittent preventive treatment of malaria in pregnancy. Clin Pharmacol Ther;87(2):226−234.

[79] Phillips RE, Looareesuwan S, White NJ, Silamut K, Kietinun S, Warrell DA. Quinine pharmacokinetics and toxicity in pregnant and lactating women with falciparum malaria. Br J Clin Pharmacol 1986;21(6):677−83.

[80] Abdelrahim II, Adam I, Elghazali G, Gustafsson LL, Elbashir MI, Mirghani RA. Pharmacokinetics of quinine and its metabolites in pregnant Sudanese women with uncomplicated Plasmodium falciparum malaria. J Clin Pharm Therapeut 2007;32(1):15−9.

[81] Mirghani RA, Elagib I, Elghazali G, Hellgren U, Gustafsson LL. Effects of Plasmodium falciparum infection on the pharmacokinetics of quinine and its metabolites in pregnant and non-pregnant Sudanese women. Eur J Clin Pharmacol;66(12): 1229−1234.

[82] McGready R, Stepniewska K, Lindegardh N, Ashley EA, La Y, Singhasivanon P, et al. The pharmacokinetics of artemether and lumefantrine in pregnant women with uncomplicated falciparum malaria. Eur J Clin Pharmacol 2006;62(12):1021−31.

[83] McGready R, Tan SO, Ashley EA, Pimanpanarak M, Viladpai-Nguen J, Phaiphun L, et al. A randomised controlled trial of artemether-lumefantrine versus artesunate for uncomplicated plasmodium falciparum treatment in pregnancy. PLoS Med 2008; 5(12):e253.

[84] Tarning J, McGready R, Lindegardh N, Ashley EA, Pimanpanarak M, Kamanikom B, et al. Population pharmacokinetics of lumefantrine in pregnant women treated with artemether-lumefantrine for uncomplicated Plasmodium falciparum malaria. Antimicrob Agents Chemother 2009;53(9):3837−46.

[85] McGready R, Stepniewska K, Ward SA, Cho T, Gilveray G, Looareesuwan S, et al. Pharmacokinetics of dihydroartemisinin following oral artesunate treatment of pregnant women with acute uncomplicated falciparum malaria. Eur J Clin Pharmacol 2006;62(5):367−71.

[86] Morris CA, Onyamboko MA, Capparelli E, Koch MA, Atibu J, Lokomba V, et al. Population pharmacokinetics of artesunate and dihydroartemisinin in pregnant and non-pregnant women with malaria. Malar J;10:114.

[87] Onyamboko MA, Meshnick SR, Fleckenstein L, Koch MA, Atibu J, Lokomba V, et al. Pharmacokinetics and pharmacodynamics of artesunate and dihydroartemisinin following oral treatment in pregnant women with asymptomatic Plasmodium falciparum infections in Kinshasa DRC. Malar J;10:49.

[88] Abdelwahab MT, Leisegang R, Dooley KE, Mathad JS, Wiesner L, McIlleron H, et al. Population pharmacokinetics of isoniazid, pyrazinamide, and ethambutol in pregnant South African women with tuberculosis and HIV. Antimicrob Agents Chemother 2020;64(3).

[89] Denti P, Martinson N, Cohn S, Mashabela F, Hoffmann J, Msandiwa R, et al. Population pharmacokinetics of rifampin in pregnant women with tuberculosis and HIV coinfection in Soweto, South Africa. Antimicrob Agents Chemother 2015;60(3): 1234−41.

[90] Transmission PoToH-IPWaPoP. Recommendations for use of antiretroviral drugs in pregnant HIV-1-Infected women for maternal health and interventions to reduce perinatal HIV transmission in the United States. September 14, 2011. p. 1−207.

[91] Moodley J, Moodley D, Pillay K, Coovadia H, Saba J, van Leeuwen R, et al. Pharmacokinetics and antiretroviral activity of lamivudine alone or when coadministered with zidovudine in human immunodeficiency virus type 1-infected pregnant women and their offspring. J Infect Dis 1998;178(5):1327−33.

[92] O'Sullivan MJ, Boyer PJ, Scott GB, Parks WP, Weller S, Blum MR, et al. The pharmacokinetics and safety of zidovudine in the third trimester of pregnancy for women infected with human immunodeficiency virus and their infants: phase I acquired immunodeficiency syndrome clinical trials group study (protocol 082). Zidovudine Collaborative Working Group. Am J Obstet Gynecol 1993;168(5):1510−6.

[93] Best BM, Mirochnick M, Capparelli EV, Stek A, Burchett SK, Holland DT, et al. Impact of pregnancy on abacavir pharmacokinetics. Aids 2006;20(4):553−60.

[94] Wang Y, Livingston E, Patil S, McKinney RE, Bardeguez AD, Gandia J, et al. Pharmacokinetics of didanosine in antepartum and postpartum human immunodeficiency virus–infected pregnant women and their neonates: an AIDS clinical trials group study. J Infect Dis 1999;180(5):1536−41.

[95] Wade NA, Unadkat JD, Huang S, Shapiro DE, Mathias A, Yasin S, et al. Pharmacokinetics and safety of stavudine in HIV-infected pregnant women and their infants: pediatric AIDS Clinical Trials Group protocol 332. J Infect Dis 2004;190(12):2167−74.

[96] Best B, Stek A, Hu C, Burchett SK, Rossi SS, Smith E, et al. High-dose lopinavir and standard-dose emtricitabine pharmacokinetics during pregnancy and postpartum. In: 15th conference on retroviruses and opportunistic infections. Boston, MA; 2008.

[97] Burchett SK, Best B, Mirochnick M, Hu C, Capparelli E, Fletcher C, et al. Tenofovir pharmacokinetics during pregnancy, at delivery and postpartum. In: 14th conference on retroviruses and opportunistic infections. Los Angeles, CA; 2007.

[98] Momper JD, Best BM, Wang J, Stek A, Cressey TR, Burchett S, Kreitchmann R, Shapiro DE, Smith E, Chakhtoura N, Capparelli EV, Mirochnick M. Tenofovor alafenamide pharmacokinetics with and without cobicistat in pregnancy. In: 22nd international AIDS conference. Amsterdam, Netherlands; July 26, 2018.

[99] Mulligan N, Best BM, Wang J, Capparelli EV, Stek A, Barr E, et al. Dolutegravir pharmacokinetics in pregnant and postpartum women living with HIV. AIDS 2018;32(6): 729−37.

[100] Kassahun K, McIntosh I, Cui D, Hreniuk D, Merschman S, Lasseter K, et al. Metabolism and disposition in humans of raltegravir (MK-0518), an anti-AIDS drug targeting the human immunodeficiency virus 1 integrase enzyme. Drug Metab Dispos 2007;35(9):1657−63.

[101] Watts DH, Stek A, Best BM, Wang J, Capparelli EV, Cressey TR, et al. Raltegravir pharmacokinetics during pregnancy. J Acquir Immune Defic Syndr 2014;67(4): 375−81.

[102] Best BM, Stek AM, Capparelli E, Burchett SK, Huo Y, Aweeka F, et al. Raltegravir pharmacokinetics in pregnancy. In: Interscience conference on antimicrobial agents and chemotherapy. Boston, MA; 2010.

[103] McKeown DA, Rosenvinge M, Donaghy S, Sharland M, Holt DW, Cormack I, et al. High neonatal concentrations of raltegravir following transplacental transfer in HIV-1 positive pregnant women. Aids;24(15):2416−2418.

[104] Momper JD, Best BM, Wang J, Capparelli EV, Stek A, Barr E, et al. Elvitegravir/cobicistat pharmacokinetics in pregnant and postpartum women with HIV. AIDS 2018; 32(17):2507−16.

[105] Schneider S, Peltier A, Gras A, Arendt V, Karasi-Omes C, Mujawamariwa A, et al. Efavirenz in human breast milk, mothers', and newborns' plasma. J Acquir Immune Defic Syndr 2008;48(4):450–4.

[106] Cressey TR, Stek AM, Capparelli E, Bowonwatanuwong C, Prommas S, Huo Y, et al. Efavirenz pharmacokinetics during the 3rd trimester of pregnancy and postpartum. In: Conference on retroviruses and opportunistic infections. Boston, MA; 2011.

[107] Capparelli EV, Aweeka F, Hitti J, Stek A, Hu C, Burchett SK, et al. Chronic administration of nevirapine during pregnancy: impact of pregnancy on pharmacokinetics. HIV Med 2008;9(4):214–20.

[108] Mirochnick M, Siminski S, Fenton T, Lugo M, Sullivan JL. Nevirapine pharmacokinetics in pregnant women and in their infants after in utero exposure. Pediatr Infect Dis J 2001;20(8):803–5.

[109] Lamorde M, Byakika-Kibwika P, Okaba-Kayom V, Flaherty JP, Boffito M, Namakula R, et al. Suboptimal nevirapine steady-state pharmacokinetics during intrapartum compared with postpartum in HIV-1-seropositive Ugandan women. J Acquir Immune Defic Syndr;55(3):345–350.

[110] Mulligan N, Schalkwijk S, Best BM, Colbers A, Wang J, Capparelli EV, et al. Etravirine pharmacokinetics in HIV-infected pregnant women. Front Pharmacol 2016;7:239.

[111] Tran AH, Best BM, Stek A, Wang J, Capparelli EV, Burchett SK, et al. Pharmacokinetics of rilpivirine in HIV-infected pregnant women. J Acquir Immune Defic Syndr 2016;72(3):289–96.

[112] Momper JD, Stek A, Wang J, Shapiro DE, Smith E, Chakhtoura N, Capparelli EV, Mirochnick M, Best BM. Pharmacokinetics of atazanavir boosted with cobicistat during pregnancy and postpartum. In: 20th international workshop on clinical pharmacology of HIV, hepatitis and other antiviral drugs. Netherlands: Noordwijk; May 16, 2019.

[113] Ripamonti D, Cattaneo D, Maggiolo F, Airoldi M, Frigerio L, Bertuletti P, et al. Atazanavir plus low-dose ritonavir in pregnancy: pharmacokinetics and placental transfer. Aids 2007;21(18):2409–15.

[114] Conradie F, Zorrilla C, Josipovic D, Botes M, Osiyemi O, Vandeloise E, et al. Safety and exposure of once-daily ritonavir-boosted atazanavir in HIV-infected pregnant women. HIV Med 2011;12(9):570–9.

[115] Mirochnick M, Best BM, Stek AM, Capparelli EV, Hu C, Burchett SK, et al. Atazanavir pharmacokinetics with and without tenofovir during pregnancy. J Acquir Immune Defic Syndr 2011;56(5):412–9.

[116] Squibb B-M. Reyataz prescribing information. In.

[117] Mirochnick M, Stek A, Capparelli E, Best B, Rossi SS, Burchett SK, et al. Pharmacokinetics of increased dose atazanavir with and without tenofovir during pregnancy. In: 12th international workshop on clinical pharmacology of HIV therapy. FL: Coral Gables; 2011.

[118] Momper JD, Best BM, Wang J, Stek A, Shapiro DE, George K, Barr E, Rungruengthanakit K, Smith E, Chakhtoura N, Capparelli EV, Mirochnick M. Pharmacokinetics of darunavir boosted with cobicistat during pregnancy and postpartum. In: 22nd international AIDS conference. Amsterdam, Netherlands; July 26, 2018.

[119] Capparelli E, Best B, Stek A, Rossi SS, Burchett SK, Kreitchmann R, et al. Pharmacokinetics of darunavir once or twice daily during pregnancy and postpartum. In: 3rd international workshop on HIV Pediatrics. Rome, Italy; 2011.

[120] Eke AC, Stek AM, Wang J, Kreitchmann R, Shapiro DE, Smith E, et al. Darunavir pharmacokinetics with an increased dose during pregnancy. J Acquir Immune Defic Syndr 2020;83(4):373–80.

[121] Best BM, Stek AM, Mirochnick M, Hu C, Li H, Burchett SK, et al. Lopinavir tablet pharmacokinetics with an increased dose during pregnancy. J Acquir Immune Defic Syndr 2010;54(4):381–8.

[122] Bouillon-Pichault M, Jullien V, Azria E, Pannier E, Firtion G, Krivine A, et al. Population analysis of the pregnancy-related modifications in lopinavir pharmacokinetics and their possible consequences for dose adjustment. J Antimicrob Chemother 2009;63(6):1223–32.

[123] Aweeka FT, Stek A, Best BM, Hu C, Holland D, Hermes A, et al. Lopinavir protein binding in HIV-1-infected pregnant women. HIV Med 2010;11(4):232–8.

[124] Capparelli E, Stek A, Best B, Rossi SS, Burchett SK, Li H, et al. Boosted fosamprenavir pharmacokinetics during pregnancy. In: 17th conference on retroviruses and opportunistic infections. San Francisco, CA; 2010.

[125] Unadkat JD, Wara DW, Hughes MD, Mathias AA, Holland DT, Paul ME, et al. Pharmacokinetics and safety of indinavir in human immunodeficiency virus-infected pregnant women. Antimicrob Agents Chemother 2007;51(2):783–6.

[126] Hayashi S, Beckerman K, Homma M, Kosel BW, Aweeka FT. Pharmacokinetics of indinavir in HIV-positive pregnant women. Aids 2000;14(8):1061–2.

[127] Ghosn J, De Montgolfier I, Cornelie C, Dominguez S, Perot C, Peytavin G, et al. Antiretroviral therapy with a twice-daily regimen containing 400 milligrams of indinavir and 100 milligrams of ritonavir in human immunodeficiency virus type 1-infected women during pregnancy. Antimicrob Agents Chemother 2008;52(4):1542–4.

[128] Bryson YJ, Mirochnick M, Stek A, Mofenson LM, Connor J, Capparelli E, et al. Pharmacokinetics and safety of nelfinavir when used in combination with zidovudine and lamivudine in HIV-infected pregnant women: pediatric AIDS Clinical Trials Group (PACTG) Protocol 353. HIV Clin Trials 2008;9(2):115–25.

[129] Villani P, Floridia M, Pirillo MF, Cusato M, Tamburrini E, Cavaliere AF, et al. Pharmacokinetics of nelfinavir in HIV-1-infected pregnant and nonpregnant women. Br J Clin Pharmacol 2006;62(3):309–15.

[130] Read JS, Best BM, Stek AM, Hu C, Capparelli EV, Holland DT, et al. Pharmacokinetics of new 625 mg nelfinavir formulation during pregnancy and postpartum. HIV Med 2008;9(10):875–82.

[131] Eke AC, McCormack SA, Best BM, Stek AM, Wang J, Kreitchmann R, et al. Pharmacokinetics of increased nelfinavir plasma concentrations in women during pregnancy and postpartum. J Clin Pharmacol 2019;59(3):386–93.

[132] von Hentig N, Nisius G, Lennemann T, Khaykin P, Stephan C, Babacan E, et al. Pharmacokinetics, safety and efficacy of saquinavir/ritonavir 1,000/100 mg twice daily as HIV type-1 therapy and transmission prophylaxis in pregnancy. Antivir Ther 2008; 13(8):1039–46.

[133] Acosta EP, Zorrilla C, Van Dyke R, Bardeguez A, Smith E, Hughes M, et al. Pharmacokinetics of saquinavir-SGC in HIV-infected pregnant women. HIV Clin Trials 2001; 2(6):460–5.

[134] Acosta EP, Bardeguez A, Zorrilla CD, Van Dyke R, Hughes MD, Huang S, et al. Pharmacokinetics of saquinavir plus low-dose ritonavir in human immunodeficiency virus-infected pregnant women. Antimicrob Agents Chemother 2004;48(2):430–6.

[135] van der Lugt J, Colbers A, Molto J, Hawkins D, van der Ende M, Vogel M, et al. The pharmacokinetics, safety and efficacy of boosted saquinavir tablets in HIV type-1-infected pregnant women. Antivir Ther 2009;14(3):443–50.

[136] Weizsaecker K, Kurowski M, Hoffmeister B, Schurmann D, Feiterna-Sperling C. Pharmacokinetic profile in late pregnancy and cord blood concentration of tipranavir and enfuvirtide. Int J Std Aids;22(5):294–295.

[137] Brennan-Benson P, Pakianathan M, Rice P, Bonora S, Chakraborty R, Sharland M, et al. Enfurvitide prevents vertical transmission of multidrug-resistant HIV-1 in pregnancy but does not cross the placenta. Aids 2006;20(2):297–9.

[138] Ceccaldi PF, Ferreira C, Gavard L, Gil S, Peytavin G, Mandelbrot L. Placental transfer of enfuvirtide in the ex vivo human placenta perfusion model. Am J Obstet Gynecol 2008;198(4):e431–432. 433.

[139] Colbers A, Best B, Schalkwijk S, Wang J, Stek A, Hidalgo Tenorio C, et al. Maraviroc pharmacokinetics in HIV-1-Infected pregnant women. Clin Infect Dis 2015;61(10): 1582–9.

[140] Frenkel LM, Brown ZA, Bryson YJ, Corey L, Unadkat JD, Hensleigh PA, et al. Pharmacokinetics of acyclovir in the term human pregnancy and neonate. Am J Obstet Gynecol 1991;164(2):569–76.

[141] Greer LG, Leff RD, Rogers VL, Roberts SW, McCracken GH, Jr, Wendel GD, Jr, et al. Pharmacokinetics of oseltamivir in breast milk and maternal plasma. Am J Obstet Gynecol;204(6):524 e521–524.

[142] Greer LG, Leff RD, Rogers VL, Roberts SW, McCracken GH, Jr, Wendel GD, Jr, et al. Pharmacokinetics of oseltamivir according to trimester of pregnancy. Am J Obstet Gynecol;204(6 Suppl. 1):S89–S93.

[143] Beigi RH, Han K, Venkataramanan R, Hankins GD, Clark S, Hebert MF, et al. Pharmacokinetics of oseltamivir among pregnant and nonpregnant women. Am J Obstet Gynecol;204(6 Suppl. 1):S84–S88.

[144] Freriksen JJM, van Seyen M, Judd A, Gibb DM, Collins IJ, Greupink R, et al. Review article: direct-acting antivirals for the treatment of HCV during pregnancy and lactation - implications for maternal dosing, foetal exposure, and safety for mother and child. Aliment Pharmacol Ther 2019;50(7):738–50.

Chemotherapy in pregnancy

13

Sharon E. Robertson, Jeanne M. Schilder

Department of Obstetrics and Gynecology, Indiana University School of Medicine, Indianapolis, IN, United States

13.1 Introduction

Cancer is the second leading cause of death in women of reproductive age and accounts for 16% of deaths among women between ages 20—44 years [1]. The incidence is commonly reported as 1 per 1000 pregnancies, but because of challenges in capturing population-based data, the numbers are likely to be underreported. The largest studies report 17 cases of cancer per 100,000 live births, and 25—27/100,000 pregnancies, with the incidence rising related to delays in childbearing. The most common malignancies diagnosed during pregnancy vary in order of frequency depending on the country studied and inclusion criteria, but the most common pregnancy-associated malignancies consistently include breast cancer, cervical cancer, lymphoma and leukemia, melanoma, thyroid cancer, and colorectal cancer [2] (Table 13.1) The care of the patient with a malignancy during pregnancy requires a multidisciplinary approach. Maternal, fetal, and obstetric outcomes must be considered during treatment planning.

Due to the lack of pharmacokinetic studies of chemotherapeutic agents in pregnancy, our decisions largely rely on case reports and retrospective reviews. Emerging data from large registries have helped guide oncologic treatment during pregnancy, and treatment has evolved significantly over the past 2 decades. Previously, recommendations supported pregnancy termination or intentional preterm delivery in order to proceed with oncologic treatment in the nonpregnant state. Recent data have not demonstrated improvement in outcomes related to either of these approaches, and standard of care chemotherapy, between 14 and 35 weeks' gestation, with some exceptions, provides optimal outcomes for both the mother and fetus. Chemotherapy should be avoided during the first trimester during the period of organogenesis and should be discontinued in a time frame to allow for recovery of chemotherapy-induced maternal and fetal neutropenia and thrombocytopenia to reduce associated delivery complications.

The ethics of the timing of delivery must balance the risk to the mother's health and the risk to the fetus. When treatment with chemotherapy is required, whether with single or multiple agents, the clinician must have knowledge of the optimal

Clinical Pharmacology During Pregnancy. https://doi.org/10.1016/B978-0-12-818902-3.00006-3

Table 13.1 Incidence of cancers per pregnancies or deliveries [2,48,51].

Cancer type	Incidence
Breast cancer	1:3,000–10,000
Cervical cancer	1:2,000–10,000
Hodgkin's lymphoma	1:1,000–6,000
Melanoma	2–5:100,000
Leukemias	1:75,000–100,000
Ovarian cancer	4–8:100,000
Colorectal cancer	1:13,000
Thyroid cancer	3.6–14:100,000

timing of treatment to ensure an efficacious and safe approach to therapy. This chapter will review the general indications for chemotherapy in pregnancy and the data surrounding the best use of the commonly prescribed chemotherapeutic agents in pregnancy.

13.1.1 Maternal outcomes

Maternal outcomes subsequent to a cancer diagnosis during pregnancy are comparable to those of nonpregnant women when adjusted for equal treatment, age, stage at diagnosis, and other cancer-specific risk factors [3]. Treatment, including systemic therapy, should be offered as clinically appropriate. Delays in initiation of treatment may lead to inferior oncologic outcomes.

13.1.2 Obstetric outcomes

In a large cohort of 1170 women treated with chemotherapy during pregnancy, 88% had a successful live birth and 48% of pregnancies resulted in preterm birth. The majority of the preterm births were iatrogenic (88%) [4].

13.1.3 Fetal outcomes

The low molecular weight of most chemotherapeutic agents allows them to cross the placenta, and most are known to have teratogenic potential. Chemotherapy poses the greatest risks for the developing fetus early in pregnancy. Depending on the type of cancer and the stage of diagnosis, chemotherapy may need to be administered without delay and pregnancy termination may either be recommended, or the inevitable outcome of treatment. When the fetus is exposed to the cytotoxic effects of chemotherapy during the first trimester, pregnancy will likely end in spontaneous abortion, major malformations, and fetal loss [5]. Organogenesis, the critical time of organ formation from 2 to 8 weeks following conception, represents the time when the cardiac and central nervous systems are especially susceptible to insult. However, even following organogenesis, injury may still occur to the eyes, gonads, and central nervous and hematopoietic systems as these organ systems continue to mature over the course of a pregnancy [6]. Treatment with chemotherapy in the second and third trimesters is generally thought to be safer but can be associated with intrauterine growth restriction and low birth weight infants. However, longitudinal follow-up is lacking [5]. In one study of 796 singleton pregnancies exposed to chemotherapy, 21% of infants were small for gestational age and 41% required admission to neonatal intensive care after birth, primarily due to prematurity [4]. In this same cohort, 4% of infants were born with a congenital malformation.

13.2 Overview of chemotherapeutic agents

13.2.1 Antimetabolites

Antimetabolites are characterized by their inhibitory activity during DNA or RNA synthesis. Examples include methotrexate, 5-fluorouracil, thioguanine, cytarabine, cladribine, cladribine, fludarabine, mercaptopurine, pemetrexed, and gemcitabine. Perhaps due to its long history as a chemotherapeutic agent, methotrexate has been used for many illnesses, including acute myeloid leukemia, non-Hodgkin's lymphoma (NHL), osteosarcoma, head and neck cancer, and breast cancer [7,8]. It is known to be an abortifacient and a teratogen. In a review of 42 cases of methotrexate exposure, 23 cases in the first trimester found no abnormalities [6]. Previous reports noted associations with cognitive defects, craniosynostosis, hypertelorism, micrognathia, and limb deformities [7]. It is likely that there is a critical dose above which teratogenicity or spontaneous abortion occurs. Methotrexate used in low doses in rheumatologic disease has not been demonstrated to increase rates of fetal malformation or induce spontaneous abortions [9].

5-Fluorouracil was associated with multiple fetal anomalies in a patient who received chemotherapy for colon cancer beginning at 12 weeks' gestation [7]. 5-Fluorouracil is often used in combination with cyclophosphamide and doxorubicin for the treatment of breast cancer. Generally, first trimester exposure should be avoided if possible.

Cytarabine is typically used in combination with other agents such as vincristine, tioguanine, or doxorubicin to treat acute leukemia. There are reports of limb malformations after first trimester exposure, either alone or in combinations for the aforementioned agents [6,10]. In a report of 89 cases, intrauterine fetal distress (IUFD) was noted to have occurred in 6% and neonatal deaths in two [6]. Cause of death was not identified in these cases. Cytarabine and daunorubicin were used in four cases. Cytarabine and tioguanine were used in five of the six intrauterine fetal demises. The effects of underlying maternal leukemia may also have contributed to the complications [6].

A case report of 6-mercaptopurine given for treatment of acute monocytic leukemia in pregnancy during the first trimester and again in the third trimester was associated with the birth of a premature infant but no malformations were noted [6]. As with methotrexate, much of the recent data regarding the thioprine class of chemotherapeutic agents come from the autoimmune literature where this class of medication is commonly used as immunomodulators. Mercaptopurine has been used in combination with azathioprine in patients with inflammatory bowel disease (IBD), which is estimated to affect 1.4 million Americans, with a peak onset at 15–30 years of age [11]. A retrospective cohort study by Francella identified 15 patients who remained on 6-mercaptopurine/azathioprine for their entire pregnancy for the treatment of IBD. The authors reported that previous data showed a 3.9% congenital anomaly rate for the aforementioned agents, while their study found a 2.5% rate for one case of a congenital anomaly, compared to 4% in the control group [12]. There was no difference in spontaneous abortion rates, major or minor malformations, neonatal infection rates, or prematurity.

13.2.2 Alkylating agents

Alkylating agents are commonly used to treat breast cancer, acute leukocytic leukemia, and lymphoma. Cyclophosphamide is contraindicated in the first trimester due to significant malformations including absent toes, eye abnormalities, low-set ears, and cleft palate [6]. Again, much of the data surrounding the use of cyclophosphamide come from the literature regarding rheumatologic diseases. A case report of a mother who was prescribed cyclophosphamide for systemic lupus erythematosus and had exposure to the agent throughout her entire first trimester resulted in an infant with multiple physical anomalies similar to those findings from animal studies, raising the question of a cyclophosphamide phenotype [13]. In utero exposure during the first trimester may be associated with the cyclophosphamide phenotype characterized as growth deficiency, developmental delay, craniosynostosis, blepharophimosis, flat nasal bridge, abnormal ears, and distal limb defects including hypoplastic thumbs and oligodactyly. Cyclophosphamide use has been reported as safe during the second and third trimesters.

Chlorambucil has been reported to cause cleft palate, skeletal dysplasias, and renal aplasia when administered in the first trimester [7]. A case report of a 36-year-old patient who received chlorambucil to treat her chronic lymphocytic leukemia until her pregnancy was diagnosed at 20 weeks' gestation described no associated fetal malformations or major abnormalities [14]. In a series of 15 pregnant patients with Hodgkin's lymphoma (HL), one patient who received chemotherapy with chlorambucil during the latter half of her pregnancy delivered a full-term infant [15].

Dacarbazine is an alkylating agent with little data in humans. In high doses, it is known to be teratogenic in rats [6]. Dacarbazine has emerged as an agent used in combination with tamoxifen, carmustine, and cisplatin for the treatment of metastatic melanoma during pregnancy. It is also used as part of the ABVD regimen for lymphoma [16]. Dipaola et al. published a case report of a patient who received two cycles of this combination therapy for melanoma prior to delivery of her healthy infant at 30 weeks' gestation [17]. No skeletal defects or cleft palate was observed as had been previously described with dacarbazine. The placental tissue was notable for invasion of malignant melanoma into the intervillous spaces; however, the fetus did not have metastatic disease.

Busulfan use in pregnancy was associated with no anomalies during the first trimester [18]. It was associated with malformations in two cases with second trimester use: in one case, unilateral renal agenesis was noted after combination of busulfan and allopurinol, and in the other case, pyloric stenosis occurred after single therapy [6].

13.2.3 Anthracyclines

The anthracycline agents are typically used as combination agents. A mechanism of action is by intercalating between DNA base pairs. 28 pregnancies exposed to doxorubicin and daunorubicin for treatment of acute myeloid leukemia, acute lymphoblastic leukemia (ALL), non-HL, sarcoma, and breast cancer were summarized in a case series. One elective termination and two spontaneous abortions occurred; all fetuses were noted to be normal. 21 pregnancies were delivered without complications. At birth, one infant had transient bone marrow hypoplasia, and one set of twins presented with diarrhea and sepsis at birth. Two patients expired with the fetus in utero prior to delivery [19]. Doxorubicin had been previously cited to be associated with limb abnormalities in the first trimester; however, it was given in combination with cytarabine [6]. A case report of a spontaneous abortion at 17 weeks occurred after exposure at 13 weeks' gestation to doxorubicin and vincristine for treatment of ALL. Postmortem fetal necropsy was not performed [20]. In another case, respiratory distress syndrome, neonatal sepsis, and bronchopneumonia occurred in a 31-week gestation with a birth weight of 2070 g whose mother had received doxorubicin for breast cancer at 28 weeks' gestation. Follow-up of the offspring at 6 years of age revealed normal development [20].

Of 13 women in which epirubicin was used, three fetuses were affected. One neonatal death occurred after exposure to epirubicin, vincristine, and prednisone and another to epirubicin in combination with cyclophosphamide [20,21]. The combination of exposure to cyclophosphamide, epirubicin, and 5-fluorouracil during the first trimester for treatment of infiltrating ductal breast cancer resulted in limb abnormalities and micrognathia [22]. The patient electively terminated the pregnancy and the fetus was examined subsequently to confirm the findings. Epirubicin has been the agent of choice for breast cancer in Europe where doxorubicin was typically used in the United States during pregnancy. There are inherent problems in comparative reviews of retrospective data; however, the conclusion of the authors was that the two agents, doxorubicin and epirubicin, show similar transplacental transfer rates and toxicity profiles [23].

Daunorubicin has most commonly been used in treatment of acute lymphocytic leukemia. Of 43 cases that were reviewed, IUGR occurred in five fetuses, four suffered from transient myelosuppression, and three IUFDs occurred, two of which were notable for complications by severe preeclampsia at 29 weeks or severe maternal anemia and maternal complications from ALL [6]. The third IUFD was following combination therapy with daunorubicin, idarubicin, cytarabine, and mitoxantrone.

Though doxorubicin is typically used in advanced breast cancer in pregnancy as part of the FAC regimen (5-fluorouracil, doxorubicin, and cyclophosphamide), data surrounding its use in pregnancy are limited. Unless the patient has underlying cardiac disease, this anthracycline-containing combination [5,13] is first-line therapy [24]. Anthracyclines are known to be cardiotoxic in children and adults, but the in utero effects on developing fetuses are not known [25]. Meyer-Wittkopf and colleagues performed fetal echocardiograms every 2 weeks on a pregnant patient who was receiving doxorubicin and cyclophosphamide during the second and third trimesters of pregnancy for treatment of infiltrating ductal carcinoma. Measurements of ventricles of unexposed fetuses aged 20–40 weeks were used as controls. No fetal cardiac changes were noted to suggest cardiotoxicity [26]. In a European study, 20 patients were followed throughout their pregnancy, receiving weekly epirubicin at 35 mg/m2 for treatment of breast cancer at a median gestational age of 19 weeks. No major fetal malformations were noted with the exception of one case of inheritable polycystic kidney disease. Children were reported to be developmentally normal by reports of their parents at 2 years of age [27].

13.2.4 Plant alkaloids

The plant alkaloids, vincristine, vinblastine, and vinorelbine, are considered to have a higher safety profile in pregnancy. One malformation was reported in 29 patients treated during the first trimester with combination therapy of vincristine, doxorubicin, cytarabine, and prednisone, an atrial septal defect and absent fifth digit [6]. Two fetal deaths and two neonatal deaths occurred, all after combination therapy in the second and/or third trimester. Of 111 exposures to vincristine or vinblastine, nine cases of IUGR and seven cases of preterm delivery occurred [19]. Vinorelbine was administered to two subjects in combination with 5-fluorouracil and for another patient epidoxorubicin and cyclophosphamide due to disease progression of her breast cancer in pregnancy. The only fetal effect observed was anemia at 21 days of life, but no fetal malformations were noted [28].

13.2.5 Taxanes

Taxanes have been shown to be teratogenic in animal models, but their use in humans during pregnancy has been limited. Paclitaxel works by disruption of microtubule assembly. It has been shown to be toxic to chick, rat, and rabbit embryos when given during the critical organogenesis period [6]. The use of taxanes has emerged as important in patients with node-positive breast cancer [29,30]. A case report published in Clinical Breast Cancer describes a patient with invasive lobular breast cancer who received weekly paclitaxel from 19 to 33 weeks' gestation. Fetal ultrasound was performed at 6-week intervals and labor was induced at 37 weeks due to onset of preeclampsia. The fetus was of normal weight without malformations or infection at birth [31].

13.2.6 **Hormonal agents**

Metastatic breast cancer during pregnancy poses a challenge for the practitioner in terms of treatment options. Though it had been previously held that survival was poorer for pregnant patients, when matched by stage and age with nonpregnant controls, survival is similar [32]. Research on tamoxifen in the animal literature shows epithelial changes in the neonatal period similar to those observed with diethylstilbestrol (DES). DES was used prior to tamoxifen and aromatase inhibitors (AIs) for estrogen-positive breast cancer. It was also used to prevent miscarriages and as estrogen replacement in estrogen-deficient states after its advent in 1938. It had significant adverse effects both on the women who took it and on exposed fetuses. Studies have shown that female fetuses exposed in utero show structural changes in the uterus, cervix, and upper vagina; classically, the T-shaped uteri and uterotubal anomalies that lead to repeat miscarriages [33]. There is also an increased incidence of clear cell vaginal adenocarcinoma in 1/1000 exposures. The proposed mechanism is altered embryological Mullerian duct formation due to estrogenic alterations to stromal junctions [34]. Specific structural changes and clear cell vaginal adenocarcinoma were not reported in the literature surrounding tamoxifen use in fetuses. It is not clear if DES affects fertility; certainly, structural changes may affect fertility. The teratogenicity of tamoxifen has been suggested to be species specific and reports in humans are limited.

Treatment with AIs improves survival for women with metastatic breast cancer by 10% [35]. In initial studies, AIs did not have a statistically significant survival benefit when compared to tamoxifen; however, the third-generation AIs did demonstrate a survival benefit [36]. AIs are typically not given in pregnancy or in premenopausal women as peripheral inhibition of aromatase would not be able to overcome the estrogen produced by the growing pregnancy or the premenopausal ovary. In the postmenopausal female, AI inhibits the conversion of androgen to estrogen in the adipose tissue, as it occurs on a smaller scale.

13.2.7 **Targeted therapies and immunotherapies**

Human epidermal growth factor receptor 2 (HER2/neu) is amplified in 25%−50% of metastatic breast cancer patients [37]. HER2 positivity is associated with an aggressive subtype of breast cancer. However, targeted therapies significantly improve the prognosis. Trastuzumab is a targeted monoclonal antibody that binds the extracellular domain of the overexpressed HER2/neu receptor in metastatic breast cancer patients. Trastuzumab is associated with reversible fetal oligohydramnios or anhydramnios [38]. In one case, a mother treated with trastuzumab delivered a fetus with oligohydramnios, but no IUGR, and with normal lung and kidney development [38]. The proposed mechanism of oligo- or anhydramnios is believed to be related to trastuzumab effects of vascular endothelial growth factor to inhibit amniotic fluid production in the developing fetal kidney [38]. Aside from fetal oligo- or anhydramnios, no other fetal anomalies have been associated with use to date, although human data are limited.

Beyond monoclonal antibody therapy, alternative therapies for breast cancer may include dual inhibition of epidermal growth factor receptor and HER2 with lapatinib, HKI-272, and pertuzumab; anti-mTOR effects of temsirolimus; anti-Hsp-90, such as 17-AAG [37]; and antiangiogenesis agents, such as bevacizumab. To date, reports of bevacizumab in pregnancy are limited to intravitreal use for neovascularization [39]. Data for these agents are limited and use in pregnancy is currently not recommended.

Despite the number of new agents on the horizon, currently, standard treatment for HER2-positive cancer consists of trastuzumab. Caution must be taken with trastuzumab in terms of maternal health. It is associated with 4% cardiotoxicity when given as a single agent and 27% when given in combination with anthracyclines [40]. The cardiotoxicity is associated with a decrease in left ventricular ejection fraction which is suspected to be reversible. Memorial Sloan Kettering has adapted guidelines for monitoring cardiac dysfunction during trastuzumab use; however, these guidelines have not been adapted for pregnancy [40].

The treatment of metastatic melanoma is rapidly evolving. As the mitogen-activated protein (MAP) kinase pathway is further elucidated, many downstream targets have been identified as effective agents in the treatment of metastatic melanoma. Drugs that inhibit BRAF (vemurafenib, dabrafenib, and encorafenib) and MEK (trametinib, cobimetinib, and binimetinib) are frequently used alone or in combination for the treatment of metastatic melanoma. However, the MAP kinase is directly involved in trophoblastic proliferation and these agents are prohibited in pregnancy [41]. Animal studies confirm the teratogenicity of these agents and case reports confirm adverse pregnancy outcomes [41].

Immune inhibition of the PD1/PDL1 and CTLA4 pathways plays an increasing role in the treatment of many malignancies including melanoma and cervical cancer. However, immune tolerance is an important concept that allows for a successful pregnancy. In particular, the PD1/PDL1 pathway plays a key role in preventing an adverse maternal immune response against foreign fetal tissue [42]. Animal studies confirm the increased risk of spontaneous abortion with the use of PD1/PDL1 inhibitors (pembrolizumab and nivolumab). The role of the CTLA4 pathway in pregnancy immune tolerance is less clear and the effect of CTLA4 inhibitors (ipilimumab) on the fetus is not well understood. In general, it is recommended that these agents be avoided in pregnancy.

13.2.8 Other agents

Cisplatin and carboplatin may be given as a single agent or in combination with other chemotherapeutics. They are considered to have a relatively low toxicity profile. An infant was exposed for 2 weeks to cisplatin, etoposide, and cytarabine during the second trimester for the treatment of maternal HL. Fetal jaundice and nonhemolytic anemia were observed in an otherwise normal child born at 36 weeks [20].

In another case, sensorineural hearing loss was reported in a child born with leukopenia, alopecia, and respiratory distress syndrome at 26 weeks after the child was exposed to cisplatin only 6 days prior to delivery [7]. Complicating factors include severe prematurity of the infant and postnatal treatment with gentamicin. A case report of a patient treated for stage IIIC ovarian cancer with paclitaxel and carboplatin beginning at 16 weeks' gestation resulted in no fetal anomalies or complications [43].

Few case reports and little data exist on gemcitabine, bleomycin, mitoxantrone, dactinomycin, idarubicin, allopurinol, rituximab, etoposide, asparaginase, teniposide, mitoguazone, tretinoin, irinotecan, oxaliplatin, melphalan, altretamine, and erlotinib use in pregnancy due to lack of human exposures in pregnancy; thus, discussion has been limited.

13.3 **Treatment of specific cancers**

A summary of perinatal outcomes for 231 women diagnosed with cancer between their last menstrual period and end of pregnancy who voluntarily enrolled in the Cancer and Pregnancy Registry between the years of 1995 and 2008 reported significant detail on the effects of chemotherapy. In this international registry, 13 women elected termination, 67 did not receive chemotherapy with 70 live births, and 157 neonates were delivered following intrauterine chemotherapy exposure. The mean gestational age at the first cycle of treatment was $20.1 \pm 6/2$ weeks, and the mean gestational age of the last treatment was 29.6 ± 5.7 weeks. Overall, the rate of malformations was 3.8% (6/157 neonates exposed), similar to that of the general population [37]. Neonatal demise was observed in one case (0.7%), and an IUFD was observed in one case (0.7%). In 12 cases (7.6%), IUGR was observed. 9 cases delivered prematurely and transient complications of prematurity occurred in 7 infants [44]. Mean gestational age at delivery was not significantly different in neonates exposed to chemotherapy versus those who were not. A statistical difference was noted in birth weight (2647 ± 713 g vs. 2873 ± 788 g), but the authors noted that this was likely to not be clinically significant.

Longer term outcomes from this registry have been reported, with the plan to continue worldwide collaborative efforts to evaluate a multitude of outcomes in this population, ranging from fetal and maternal outcomes to epigenetic alterations and pathophysiologic placental changes associated with cancer treatment, parental psychological coping strategies, and more. The aim of this group is to optimize obstetric and oncologic care for this challenging clinical condition. Reports from large collaborative efforts and large case series comprise the best current data to guide treatment of cancer during pregnancy, which continues to evolve [44].

13.3.1 **Breast cancer**

Most reports in the literature note a poorer prognosis and more advanced disease in women diagnosed with breast cancer during pregnancy compared with their nonpregnant counterparts. Delays in diagnosis as well as nonstandard treatment contribute to this discrepancy. Some studies have shown a similar receptor expression in pregnant versus nonpregnant breast cancers, while others have demonstrated more aggressive biology associated with pregnancy, with an increased frequency of TNBC, higher expression of potentially relevant tumor targets, and a low prevalence of tumor-infiltrating lymphocytes [27]. However, when a timely diagnosis is achieved, and patients are treated per standard of care, outcomes are similar during pregnancy compared with nonpregnant patients, highlighting the importance of prompt diagnosis and treatment for concurrent breast cancer in pregnancy [4,45].

Apparent localized disease can be managed surgically at any time during pregnancy, with adjuvant anthracycline-based therapy for either localized or metastatic breast cancer beginning in the second trimester when chemotherapy is indicated. Other adjuvant therapies, such as radiation, endocrine, or anti-HER2 therapies, are contraindicated during pregnancy and should be delayed to the postpartum state [46]. In addition, patients should not become pregnant during treatment with chemotherapy or endocrine therapy, or within 6 months of completing anti-HER2 therapy.

The Cancer and Pregnancy Registry described outcomes of 128 women diagnosed with breast cancer during pregnancy [44]. Most tumors in this registry were high-grade invasive ductal carcinoma, larger than their age-matched nonpregnant controls, and positive for lymphovascular invasion, with 60%−80% ER negative, and 28%−58% HER2 positive [47]. Most women were treated with doxorubicin/cyclophosphamide with the mean gestational age of first treatment at 20.3 ± 5.4 weeks. The rate of congenital malformations was 3.8%, and 7.8% were small for gestational age at birth. 13 neonates had complications during the neonatal period involving the following: sepsis and anemia at birth in a prematurity infant, gastroesophageal reflux, difficulty in feeding requiring tube feeding in three, transient tachypnea in three, hyperbilirubinemia or jaundice in three, respiratory distress syndrome in two, and apnea of prematurity in two. Death occurred in a neonate who was diagnosed with a severe rheumatologic disorder, which resulted in her demise at 13 months of age. Long-term reports indicated no neurodevelopmental effects or leukemias.

13.3.2 Cervical cancer

Cervical cancer is approximately 3 times more likely to be diagnosed with early stage disease during pregnancy secondary to the increased frequency of gynecologic exams [48]. Preinvasive disease has an 80% chance of regression and does not require intervention during pregnancy. Appropriate management includes surveillance with biopsies if invasion is suspected. Stage IA1 cervical cancer can be managed with cone biopsy and surveillance if margins are negative. Options for patients with locally advanced disease from IA2-IIA or IA1 with positive margins include surgical management of the gravid uterus, radiation, or neoadjuvant chemotherapy and definitive therapy following delivery. Neoadjuvant chemotherapy during pregnancy typically consists of platinum and taxane-based chemotherapy. Successful treatment with topotecan has been reported in patients intolerant of taxanes. Although PD-L1+ tumors are treated with pembrolizumab in the nonpregnant state, immune checkpoint inhibitors induce spontaneous abortion and are not recommended in pregnancy. If radiation or concurrent chemoradiation is administered, spontaneous abortion typically occurs in 35 days when initiated during the first trimester, and 45 days when given in the second trimester. Intentional delays in treatment of 1−32 weeks to allow for fetal maturation have been reported with few cases of disease progression ([49,50] Amant). If the tumor is still present at the time of delivery, cesarean section is recommended in order to avoid tumor implantation of an episiotomy or vaginal tear [3].

A metaanalysis of 88 patients treated with platinum-based neoadjuvant chemotherapy for cervical cancer during pregnancy noted 97.1% stable disease or response and excellent neonatal outcomes. Ultimately, 84 pregnancies delivered 88 newborns, 71 without any complications [49]. Overall, oncologic outcomes appear to be similar to the nonpregnant state.

13.3.3 Lymphoma

Sparse data exist for treatment of lymphoma during pregnancy, with no specific recommendations included in the NCCN guidelines. Treatment with ABVD (doxorubicin, bleomycin, vinblastine, and dacarbazine) is the current preferred regimen for early stage classic HL and has been administered safely following the first trimester with outcomes similar to nonpregnant patients [3,48]. Vincristine as a single agent can be used until after delivery [51]. For indolent NHL, treatment can be delayed. If treatment is indicated, chlorambucil as a single agent or combined with cyclophosphamide, vincristine, and prednisone with or without rituximab can be administered [51]. Transient cytopenias (leukocytopenia, neutropenia, and/or thrombocytopenia) have been observed in newborns. Selective B-cell depletion has been observed in newborns following maternal rituximab treatment ([42,51] Esposito). This highlights the importance of the multidisciplinary care team, including in the postpartum/neonatal period.

In the Cancer and Pregnancy Registry, lymphoma was diagnosed in 35 patients during pregnancy; 23 were diagnosed with primary HL, 2 with recurrent HL, and 10 with NHL. 30 of those 35 received chemotherapy during pregnancy, none during the first trimester. One child was born with syndactyly, and no other congenital malformations were observed. Two children (6.6%) were small for gestational age (<10%). An IUFD occurred at 28 weeks after CHOP chemotherapy (cyclophosphamide, doxorubicin, vincristine, and prednisone.) Although an autopsy was performed, the cause of death was not identified. One case of speech delay was reported at 4.3 years of age [44].

13.3.4 Leukemia

Treatment of acute leukemia should not be delayed, even if diagnosed in the first trimester of pregnancy, as delays can affect maternal prognosis. A multitude of multiagent chemotherapy regimens may be recommended for induction chemotherapy depending on risk stratification based on immunophenotype, molecular, and cytogenetic markers [46]. Additional management includes consolidation, CNS prophylaxis or treatment, and maintenance regimens, as well as the possibility of hematopoietic stem cell transplantation. Treatment can result in spontaneous abortion related to the teratogenic nature of chemotherapy. Fetal complications may include spontaneous abortion, prematurity, IUGR, and IUFD which may be attributed to maternal anemia and disseminated intravascular coagulation [7]. In cases where first trimester treatment does not result in spontaneous abortion, therapeutic termination can be considered once induction chemotherapy has been administered, and maternal blood counts are appropriate for maternal safety related to the procedure. Profound leukocytosis can be managed safely with leukapheresis during pregnancy. Leukemia is also associated with hypercoagulation, and thromboprophylaxis should be considered when associated with the hypercoagulable state of pregnancy [3]. Chronic myeloid leukemia is commonly managed with imatinib, which has been shown to increase the frequency of spontaneous abortion, as well as profound anomalies including exencephaly, encephalopathies, and abnormalities of the skull bones [42].

Three women in the Cancer and Pregnancy Registry were diagnosed with acute leukemia in pregnancy and two received chemotherapy. Mean gestational age at diagnosis was 24.7 ± 5.1 weeks, and mean gestational age of first chemotherapy treatment was 28.7 ± 1.4 weeks. Neither of the infants had low birth weight, congenital malformations, or long-term complications. One patient was advised to terminate her twin pregnancy at 19 weeks' gestation, but continued the pregnancy without chemotherapy, and delivered at 27 weeks' gestation [44]. Three patients in the registry were diagnosed with chronic myeloid leukemia during pregnancy, although only one received chemotherapy with cytarabine. She delivered a normal infant at 42 weeks without anomalies, pregnancy complications, or long-term complications.

Aviles and colleagues followed 84 children whose mothers were treated for hematologic malignancies during pregnancy (acute leukemia 29, HL 29, and NHL 26), including 38 treated in the first trimester, with a median follow-up of 18.7 years (range 6–29 years.) In all children studied (including 12 second-generation children), birth weight, growth and development, learning, and educational performance were normal, and there were no cases of cancer or acute leukemia, congenital, neurologic, or psychological abnormalities [52]. The authors concluded that if a patient is diagnosed with an aggressive hematologic malignancy during pregnancy, curative-intent full-dose chemotherapy can be administered safely, even during the first trimester. Contrary to these data, one of the largest series evaluating cancer in pregnancy noted 9/11 fetal malformations to be associated with first trimester exposure to chemotherapy. In addition, fetal demise, including IUFD and neonatal death, was noted in 23 cases, 20 of which were associated with hematologic malignancies [7]. The multidisciplinary team approach evaluating maternal and fetal considerations and counseling are important factors in weighing the risk and benefit in these cases.

13.3.5 Ovarian cancer

Malignant germ cell tumors are the most common ovarian malignancies identified during pregnancy. Sex-cord stromal tumors account for only 2%–3% of all ovarian neoplasms and are rarely associated with pregnancy. Epithelial tumors when encountered during pregnancy are more likely to be borderline tumors, and less commonly, invasive epithelial ovarian cancer. Treatment is similar to the nonpregnant state, with diagnostic and/or therapeutic surgical resection, preferably between 14 and 22 weeks' gestation, with debulking, if indicated, reserved for the postpartum state. If surgical resection is deemed inappropriate for gestational age, neoadjuvant chemotherapy can be considered. Concurrent resection at the time of cesarean delivery can be appropriate in some cases. Germ cell tumors are treated with bleomycin, etoposide, and cisplatin, and invasive epithelial tumors are managed with platinum and taxane-based chemotherapy [7]. Carboplatin has been administered safely during pregnancy, but cisplatin may be chosen over carboplatin since carboplatin is less protein bound with higher rates of placental transfer and resulting fetal thrombocytopenia [2]. Antiangiogenesis agents, such as bevacizumab, and poly-ADP ribosome polymerase inhibitors have recently become important agents in the treatment of platinum-sensitive ovarian cancer but are not recommended during pregnancy [49,50].

The Cancer and Pregnancy Registry reported 11 women with ovarian cancer during pregnancy, 7 of whom received chemotherapy including carboplatin, cisplatin, etoposide, prednisone, and bleomycin. IUGR was noted in two neonates, one child was affected with attention deficit disorder and one child was diagnosed with genetic hearing loss (both parents were carriers of a predisposing gene) [44]. 13 patients were treated with platinum and taxane analogues including carboplatin, cisplatin, paclitaxel, and docetaxel in the second and third trimesters, and delivered 13 of 14 healthy neonates with a mean birth weight of 2442 g [49].

13.3.6 Melanoma

Melanoma represents approximately 8% of cancers diagnosed in pregnancy. Despite this frequency, little data exist regarding treatment-associated pregnancy outcomes. Previously, treatment included high-dose interferon and chemotherapy, but these regimens have largely have been replaced by immune checkpoint inhibitors and immunotherapy. Unfortunately, most of these agents are not recommended during pregnancy. Dacarbazine-based chemotherapy was studied in 28 pregnancies with administration in the second and third trimesters, with one minor congenital abnormality (syndactyly) and one IUFD reported [2]. Local excision and sentinel lymph node biopsy can be performed during pregnancy, and if adjuvant therapy is recommended, counseling regarding fetal risks versus elective termination can be considered. Alternatively, treatment can be delayed until postpartum. Outcomes are poor with metastatic disease. Overall, prognosis appears to be similar to the nonpregnant state.

13.3.7 Other malignancies

Other relatively common malignancies associated with pregnancy are thyroid cancer and colorectal cancer, but little data exist for those either. Fortunately, the prognosis of thyroid cancer is often excellent, and chemotherapy can be avoided. Surgical resection and hormonal therapies are the preferred treatments during pregnancy, while radiotherapy is contraindicated [2,48]. Colorectal cancer was reported in seven patients in the International Registry. One patient underwent elective termination, one had a spontaneous abortion, and five were treated with chemotherapy with one case of neonatal lower extremity hemihypertrophy, and no other significant adverse fetal outcomes reported. Four patients received fluorouracil and leucovorin, and one received capecitabine and oxaliplatin. Long-term follow-up is lacking [44].

13.4 Pharmacokinetics in pregnancy

To date, there have not been any pharmacokinetic studies of chemotherapeutic agents in pregnant women. Current data regarding pregnancy-related pharmacokinetics of chemotherapeutic agents in pregnancy come from studies in mice and baboons and human retrospective reviews and case reports [53,54]. The physiologic changes in pregnancy also provide insights regarding maternal and fetal drug exposure. For example, pregnancy results in increased plasma volume and increased extracellular fluid volume, which both contribute to an increase in the volume of distribution and decrease peak plasma concentrations. Drug exposure is also affected by pregnancy-related increases in renal blood flow and glomerular filtration rate. Pregnancy also upregulated the P450 system in the liver, particularly CYP3A4, which is associated with metabolism of many chemotherapy agents [53].

In addition, to maternal physiology, the placenta affects fetal exposure to drugs. Transplacental transfer of chemotherapy agents is greater with medications of lower molecular weight, and those that are less protein bound. Active transport can play a role as well, with lower fetal compartment concentrations of drugs that are substrates of ABC transporters. As a result of these factors, anthracyclines and taxanes remain relatively confined to the maternal circulation with <10% and <2%, respectively, noted in the fetal compartment, whereas 55% of the maternal concentration of carboplatin is found in the fetal compartment [53].

Theoretically, these changes may result in underdosing of patients during pregnancy. In order to achieve doses similar to the nonpregnant state, compensating for these physiologic changes could require an increase of docetaxel by 17% and paclitaxel by 40% [53]. Altering dosing in pregnancy is not currently recommended based on the lack of evidence. In addition, the current literature consistently notes similar outcomes in pregnant patients when compared to nonpregnant patients with similar treatment regimens. Nonetheless, research continues in order to determine the optimal approach [3,54].

References

[1] Leading causes of death-all races and origins-females - United States, 2017. Centers for Disease Control and Prevention, Centers for Disease Control and Prevention; 20 November, 2019. www.cdc.gov/women/lcod/2017/all-races-origins/index.htm.

[2] Voulgaris E, Pentheroudakis G, Pavlidis N. Cancer and pregnancy: a comprehensive review. Surg Oncol 2011;20:e175—85.

[3] Maggen C, Wolters V, Cardonick E, et al. Pregnacy and cancer: the INCIP project. Curr Oncol Rep 2020;22(17):1—10.

[4] Amant F, von Minckwitz G, Han SN, et al. Prognosis of women with primary breast cancer diagnosed during pregnancy: results from an international collaborative study. J Clin Oncol 2013;31(20):2532—9.

[5] de Haan J, Verheecke M, Van Calsteren K, et al. Oncological management and obstetrics and neonatal outcomes for women diagnosed with cancer during pregnancy: a 20-year international cohort study of 1170 patients. Lancet Oncol 2019;19:337—46.

[6] Zemlickis D, Lishner M, Degendorfer P, et al. Fetal outcome after in utero exposure to cancer chemotherapy. Arch Intern Med 1992;152:573—6.

[7] Cardonick E, Iacoboccu A. Use of chemotherapy during human pregnancy. Lancet Oncol 2004;5(5):283—91.

[8] Jolivet J, Cowan KH, Curt GA, Clendeninn NJ, Chabner BA. The pharmacology and clinical use of methotrexate. N Engl J Med 1983;309(18):1094—104.

[9] Abeloff A, Armitage JO, Nieferhaber JE, Kastan MB, KcKenna WG. Abeloff's clinical oncology. Philadelphia: Churchill Livingstone; 2008.

[10] Kozlowski RD, Steinbrunner JV, MacKenzie AH, Clough JD, Wilke WS, Segal AM. Outcome of first-trimester exposure to low-dose methotrexate in eight patients with rheumatic disease. Am J Med 1990;88(6):589—92.

[11] Wagner VM, Hill JS, Weaver D, Baehner RL. Congenital abnormalities in baby born to cytarabine treated mother. Lancet 1980;2:98—9.

[12] Abraham C, Cho JH. Inflammatory bowel disease. N Engl J Med 2009;361(21):2066—78.

[13] Francella A, Dyan A, Bodian C, Rubin P, Chapman M, Present DH. The safety of 6-mercaptopurine for childbearing patients with inflammatory bowel disease: a retrospective cohort study. Gastroenterology 2003;124(1):9—17.

[14] Enns GM, Roeder E, Chan RT, Ali-Khan Catts Z, Cox VA, Golabi M. Apparent cyclophosphamide (cytoxan) embryopathy: a distinct phenotype? Am J Med 1999;86(3):237—41.

[15] Ali R, Ozkalemkas F, Kimya Y, Koksal N, Ozocaman V, Yorulmaz H, et al. Pregnancy in chronic lymphocytic leukemia: experience with fetal exposure to chlorambucil. Leuk Res 2009;33(4):567—9.

[16] Jacobs C, Donaldson SS, Rosenberg SA, Kaplan HS. Management of the pregnant patient with Hodgkin's disease. Ann Intern Med 1981;95(6):669—75.

[17] Dipaola RS, Goodin S, Ratzel M, Florcyzk M, Karp G, Ravikumar TS. Chemotherapy for metastatic melanoma during pregnancy. Gynecol Oncol 1997;66(3):526—30.

[18] Nolan GH, Marks R, Perez C. Busulfan treatment of leukemia during pregnancy. A case report. Obstet Gynecol 1971;38(1):136—8.

[19] Turchi JJ, Villasis C. Anthracyclines in the treatment of malignancy in pregnancy. Cancer 1988;61(3):435—40.

[20] Peres RM, Sanseverino MT, Guimaraes JL, Coser V, Giuliani L, Moreira RK, et al. Assessment of fetal risk associated with exposure to cancer chemotherapy during pregnancy: a multicenter study. Braz J Med Biol Res 2001;34:1551—9.

[21] Giacalone PL, Laffargue F, Benos P. Chemotherapy for breast carcinoma during pregnancy: a French national survey. Cancer 1999;86:2266—72.

[22] Leyder M, Laubach M, Breugelmans M, Keymolen K, De Greve J, Foulon W. Specific congenital malformations after exposure to cyclophosphamide, epirubicin, and 5-fluorouracil during the first trimester of pregnancy. Gynecol Obstet Invest 2011; 71(2):141—4.

[23] Mir O, Berveiller P, Rouzier P, Goffinet F, Goldwasser F, Treluyer JM. Chemotherapy for breast cancer during pregnancy: is epirubicin safe? Ann Oncol 2008;19(10): 1814—5.

[24] Shenkier T, Weir L, Levine M, Olivotto I, Whelan T, Reyno L, et al. Clinical practice guidelines for the care and treatment of breast cancer: treatment for women with stage III or locally advanced breast cancer. Can Med Assoc J 2004;170(6):983—94.

[25] Lipshultz SE, Colan SD, Gelber RD, Perez-Atayde AR, Sallan SE, Sanders SP. Late cardiac effects of doxorubicin therapy for acute lymphoblastic leukemia in childhood. N Engl J Med 1991;324(12):808—15.

[26] Meyer-Wittkopf M, Barth H, Emons G, Schimidt S. Fetal cardiac effects of doxorubicin therapy for carcinoma of the breast during pregnancy: case report and review of the literature. Ultrasound Obstet Gynecol 2001;18(1):62—6.

[27] Peccatori FA, Azim Jr HA, Scarfone G, Gadducci A, Bonazzi C, Gentilini O, et al. Weekly epirubicin in the treatment of gestational breast cancer (GBC). Breast Canc Res Treat 2009;115(3):591—4.

[28] Cuvier C, Espie M, Etra JM, Marty M. Vinorelbine in pregnancy. Eur J Canc 1997; 33(1):168—9.

[29] Buzdar AU, Singletary SE, Valero V, Booser DJ, Ibrahim NK, Rahman Z, et al. Evaluation of paclitaxel in adjuvant chemotherapy for patients with operable breast cancer: preliminary data of a prospective randomized trial. Clin Canc Res 2002;8:1073—9.

[30] Mamounas EP, Bryant J, Lembersky BC, Fehrenbacher L, Sedlacek SM, Fisher B, et al. Paclitaxel (T) following doxorubicin/cyclophosphamide (AC) as adjuvant chemotherapy for node-positive breast cancer: results from NSABP B-28. Proc Am Soc Clin Oncol 2003;22(4a) (Abstract #12).

[31] Gonzalez Angula AM, Walters RS, Carpenter RJ, Ross MI, Perkins GH, Gwyn K, et al. Paclitaxel chemotherapy in a pregnant patient with bilateral breast cancer. Clin Breast Canc 2004;5:317—9.

[32] Isaacs RJ, Hunter W, Clark K. Tamoxifen as systemic treatment of advanced breast cancer during pregnancy — case report and literature review. Gynecol Oncol 2001; 80(3):405—8.

[33] Goodman A, Schorge J, Greene MF. The long-term effects of in-utero exposures — the DES story. N Engl J Med 2011;364(22):2083—4.

[34] Diethylstilbestrol, ACOG Committee Opinion. Committee on gynecologic practice. Int J Gynaecol Obstet 1994;44(2):184. Number 131 — December 1993.

[35] Gibson L, Lawrence D, Dawson C, Bliss J. Aromatase inhibitors for treatment of advanced breast cancer in postmenopausal women. Cochrane Database Syst Rev 2009;4:CD003370.

[36] McArthur HL, Morris PG. Aromatase inhibitor strategies in metastatic breast cancer. Int J Wom Health 2010;1:67—72.

[37] Wiadakowich C, Phuong D, EvandrodeAzambuja A, Martine P-G. HER-2 positive breast cancer: what else beyond trastuzamab-based therapy? Anticanc Agents Med Chem 2008;8:488—96.

[38] Pant S, Landon MB, Blumenfeld M, Farrar W, Shapiro CL. Treatment of breast cancer with trastuzamab during pregnancy. J Clin Oncol 2008;26(9):1567—9.

[39] Tarantola RM, Folk JC, Boldt HC, Mahaian VB. Intravitreal bevacizumab during pregnancy. Retina 2010;30(9):1405—11.

[40] Keefe D. Trastuzumab-associated cardiotoxicity. Cancer 2002;95(7):1592—600.

[41] Ziogas DC, Diamantiopoulos P, Benopoulou O, et al. Prognosis and management of BRAF V600E-mutated pregnancy-associated melanoma. Oncol 2020;25:1—12.

[42] Hepner A, Negrini D, Azeka Hase E, et al. Cancer during pregnancy: the oncologist overview. World J Oncol 2019;10(1):28—35.

[43] Mendez LE, Mueller A, Salom E, Gonzalez-Quintero VH. Paclitaxel and carboplatin chemotherapy administered during pregnancy for advanced epithelial ovarian cancer. Obstet Gynecol 2003;102(5 Pt 2):1200—2.

[44] Cardonick E, Usmani A, Ghaffar S. Perinatal outcomes of a pregnancy complicated by cancer, including neonatal follow-up after in utero exposure to chemotherapy: results of an international registry. Am J Clin Oncol 2010;33(3):221—8.

[45] Litton JK, Warneke CL, Hahn KM, et al. Case control study of women treated with chemotherapy for breast cancer during pregnancy as compared with nonpregnant patients with breast cancer. Oncol 2013;18(4):369—76.

[46] National Comprehensive Cancer Network (NCCN). Clinical practice guidelines in oncology: breast cancer version 5.2020 july 15, 2020; acute lymphoblastic leukemia version 1.2020 january 15, 2020, acute myeloid leukemia version 3.2020, december 23, 2019, chronic lymphocytic leukemia version 4.2020 december 20, 2019, and chronic myeloid leukemia version 2.2021. August 28, 2020.

[47] Berry DL, Theriault RL, Holmes FA, Parisi VM, Booser DJ, Singletary SE, et al. Management of breast cancer during pregnancy using a standardized protocol. J Clin Oncol 1999;17:855—61.

[48] Mitrou S, Zarkavelis G, Fotopoulos G, et al. A mini review on pregnant mothers with cancer: a paradoxical coexistence. J Adv Res 2016;7:559—63.

[49] Korenaga T, Tewari K. Gynecologic cancers in pregnancy. Gynecol Oncol 2020;157: 799—809.

[50] Amant F, Berveiller P, Boere A, et al. Gynecologic cancers in pregnancy: guidelines based on a third international consensus meeting. Ann Oncol 2019;30:1601—12.

[51] Esposito S, Tenconi R, Preti V, et al. Chemotherapy against cancer during pregnancy. A syst Rev Neonat Outcome Med 2016;95:1—6. 38 (e4899).

[52] Aviles A, Neri N. Hematological malignancies and pregnancy: a final report of 84 children who received chemotherapy in utero. Clin Lymphoma 2001;2(3):173—7.

[53] Bell DJ, Kerr DJ. Pharmacokinetic considerations in the use of anticancer drugs during pregnancy: challenges and new developments. Expet Opin Drug Metabol Toxicol 2015; 11(9):1341—4.

[54] Van Calsteren K, Heyns L, De Smet F, et al. Cancer during pregnancy: an analysis of 215 patients emphasizing the obstetrical and neonatal outcomes. J Clin Oncol 2009; 28:683—9.

Substance abuse in pregnancy

14

Kala R. Crobarger

Tanner Health System School of Nursing, University of West Georgia, Carrollton, GA, United States

14.1 Introduction

Reports of substance abuse during pregnancy are recorded in nursing literature as early as the 1980s with an increase in substance use continuing through to the present [1,2]. Data from the National Survey on Drug Use and Health (NSDUH) [3] (SAMHSA) revealed a continued increase from an overall estimate of 1 in 10 Americans in 2016 to an estimated 1 in 5 Americans in 2018 (p. 1). Marijuana use is growing and is now the most commonly used illegal substance in the United States [4,5]. According to a study by Ref. [6], substance use when associated with the use of tobacco is an additional significant public health issue because of the potential additive risk during pregnancy. Substance use in pregnancy of alcohol, tobacco, and other drugs (ATOD) is the single most preventable public health and social problem affecting women. Substance use in pregnancy is significantly underreported as disclosing the use of an illegal substance may lead to possible legal ramifications, child custody concerns, and the stigma associated with a substance use [7]. Due to these concerns, many women delay in seeking prenatal care, which places both mother and fetus at greater risk for pregnancy complications Screening for alcohol use in pregnancy is more socially accepted. Currently, one of the major problems in screening for illicit drug use involves the "validity, reliability, and clinical utility of standardized questionnaires" (p. 3) along with a lack of education and training to administer in a nondiscriminatory and routine manner. This chapter will review the unique issues facing women and especially pregnant women involved with substance use. Treatment plans that involve an interdisciplinary team approach will be discussed, focusing on medicine and nursing.

14.2 Substance use disorders defined

A more enlightened definition perspective of substance abuse has emerged during the last 2 decades and since the implementation of the fifth edition of the *Diagnostic and Statistical Manual of Mental Disorders DSM-V* [8], substance abuse as a disorder has officially been replaced with the term *substance use disorder* [9,10].

The DSM-V notes some distinguishing factors between substance dependence and substance abuse.

Substance Dependence is a pattern of substance use, leading to clinically significant impairment or distress and includes three or more of the following, occurring at any time in the same 12-month period: tolerance, withdrawal, or the substance is taken in larger amounts over a longer period than was intended. A persistent desire exists or unsuccessful efforts to cut down or control use of the substance. An inordinate time is spent in acquiring the substance, use of the substance, or recovery from its effects. Important social, occupational, or recreational activities are given up or reduced. Finally, dependence is continued despite knowledge of having a persistent or recurrent physical or psychological problem that is likely caused or exacerbated by consumption of the substance [8].

Substance abuse is a separate diagnosis from substance dependence. It is a maladaptive pattern of substance use with one or more of the following criteria over a 1-year period: repeated substance use that results in an inability to fulfill obligations at home, school, or work; repeated substance use when it could be dangerous (e.g., driving a car); repeated substance-related legal problems, such as arrests; and continued substance use despite interpersonal or social problems that are caused or made worse by use [8].

14.3 Addiction defined as a disease of the brain

The disease model of addiction is now firmly established based on overwhelming evidence that addiction is a disease of the brain, where a substance or behavior can produce a need to use drugs or behave in a compulsive manner with known adverse consequences [11,12]. It manifests as a chronic relapsing process and successful treatment is comparable to, or better than, compliance with treatment plans for hypertension or diabetes [13]. The National Institute on Drug Abuse (NIDA) defines addiction as "a chronic, relapsing brain disease that is characterized by compulsive drug seeking and continued use despite harmful consequences" (para. 1). Similar to diabetes and hypertension, addiction is an interaction between three vectors:

(a) the substance (ATOD);
(b) the host (genetics, vulnerabilities, comorbid disorders, and
(c) the environment (family, friends, and culture).

Continuous use of drugs changes the anatomy and physiology of brain cells, particularly in the lateral tegmental area and the nucleus accumbens [14–16]. PET/MRI scans have mapped the location in the brain where drugs and behaviors have their effects. Addiction depletes dopamine and the altered brain cannot manufacture sufficient dopamine to function in a normal manner [17]. This process occurs in all addictive drugs and behaviors.

The pharmacological relevance of this disease model is used in the treatment of nicotine dependence. Nicotine activates the nucleus accumbens, releases dopamine, and dopamine is then depleted. Antidepressants that are dopamine reuptake inhibitors are effective in stabilizing dopamine levels by blocking or blunting the effect of nicotine, decreasing cravings, and thus enhancing smoking cessation. Similar antidepressants have also been used in methamphetamine treatment with good results [18].

The American Society of Addiction Medicine (ASAM) redefined addiction that is more consistent with current medical and neurobiological evidence. The society definition states "addiction is a treatable, chronic medical disease involving complex interactions among brain circuits, genetics, the environment, and an individual's life experiences. People with addiction use substances or engage in behaviors that become compulsive and often continue despite harmful consequences" ([19]; pp. 2, para. 1). ASAM describes five characteristics or "ABCs" within its definition:

(a) Inability to consistently Abstain;
(b) Impairment in Behavioral control;
(c) Craving or increased "hunger" for drugs or rewarding experiences;
(d) Diminished recognition of significant problems with one's behaviors and interpersonal relationships; and
(e) A dysfunctional Emotional response.

Moreover, the ASAM definition holds that addiction affects emotional and cognitive behaviors and interpersonal relationships, especially those regarding family, community, and other important aspects of life that may transcend their daily experience. This dovetails well with the perspective of addiction from 12-Step fellowships programs. This is termed as the *relationship view* and simply stated, if the substance use and associated behavior keep the person from the physical and emotional attachments of those who love them, then they are addicted. In these circumstances, this behavior should trigger an intervention. This modern interpretation of substance use disorder [19] may be difficult for some physicians and nurses to assimilate into their healthcare practice. Older established beliefs regarding substance abuse consider treatment and referrals to services as ineffective and time consuming. In fact, treatment works, brief interventions are effective, and spiritual models assist in motivating the patient in recovery [2,20−22].

14.4 The good news: the brain can recover

Current research indicates that recovery in the brain is mediated by adult stem cells, a large source of which is located by the nucleus accumbens [23,24]. The stem cells can migrate relatively large distances and appear to rebuild damaged circuitry. Factors found to stimulate stem cell production include physical exercise and folic acid. It is well established that folic acid supplements are able to prevent neural tube defects and thereby be able to repair other structural damage [7,25]. Thus, folic acid supplementation may become a new pharmacologic strategy to enhance recovery from addiction. An interesting question is whether high dose folic acid supplements can protect against and prevent fetal alcohol syndrome (FAS) and its associated brain damage. A theory for stem cell repair would assert that alcohol damages neurons and abstinence removes the stresses to the central nervous system (CNS). Stem cells would slowly migrate from the lateral tegmental area to rebuild the damaged circuitry. In alcohol recovery, it takes 8–12 months to see distinct mental changes indicating that the stem cell process is slow and that some permanent damage may persist. Another indicator of this process is the relapse rate in alcohol recovery, which is high in the first 3 months but after 9 months of abstinence, relapse rates drop significantly [26]. Pharmacologic therapy in alcohol recovery is well accepted. Double blind placebo-controlled studies indicate naltrexone and acamprosate have significantly reduced relapse rates [27]. Naltrexone is an opioid antagonist and congener of oxymorphone and has a blocking effect on cravings. Acamprosate may act by interacting with glutamate and GABA neurotransmitter systems, with similar effects [23]. These drugs and folic acid appear to have no harmful effects on the fetus and may be used in pregnancy.

14.5 Addiction in women and pregnancy

Opioid and other drug use during pregnancy continues to rise along with perinatal and neonatal complications ([28–30]; March 27). In general, gender does play a critical role in tendencies toward opioid dependence and related mental health issues. Studies reveal that women initiate substance use at an earlier age and will see a more rapid progression in opioid use disorder than men [31,32].

One challenge for the interdisciplinary team is identifying pregnant women who fall into the category of substance dependence or abuse disorders. Many times, they are prone to come late to care due to fear of stigmatization, shame, or concerns over pressure to enroll in addiction treatment programs [21]. Women also have different psychological dynamics operating in their substance use. Defense mechanisms include self-blaming and denial styles include internalizing and rationalizing, while the identity components include the caretaker and selflessness [33,34]. Social differences reflect the double standard where men are expected to be able to hold their liquor and women who drink are easy. And there is a special shame reserved for women who drink in pregnancy, i.e., "how can you do that to your baby?" This is sometimes called the shame-based approach [35]. Other psychosocial issues include "poverty, domestic violence, and comorbid mental health issues, [which] are more prevalent among pregnant women who use drugs and have been associated with delays in receipt of care" ([36]; p. 91).

The inner voice of women echoes a different psychological voice that reflects shame as an internalized oppression in addiction. Self-talk might revolve around such statements as, "I'm not worthy of recovery." "I'm a bad person, not sick." "I can't tolerate my emotional pain without drugs" [37]. Women often use drugs and alcohol in isolation, and the role of shame delays diagnosis and treatment. This isolation response promotes enabling where the family enables by hiding the secret. Most important is the unrecognized role of trauma and PTSD. There is a strong correlation between past sexual trauma and addiction [38]. According to Ref. [21], intravenous drug use (heroin and synthetic opioids) increases the risk for other complications such as cellulitis, endocarditis, chorioamnionitis, HIV, and sexually transmitted infections. Hormonal differences in women may be another factor predisposing women to addiction. Women studied during the follicular phase of their menstrual cycle had peak plasma cocaine levels of 73.2 ± 9.9 ng/mL, which was significantly higher than when they were studied during their luteal phase (54.7 ± 8.7 ng/mL), but there were no differences in their subjective reports of cocaine effects [39].

There are differences in how women respond to addiction with regard to specific drugs. Heroin use is rapidly increasing due to low cost and women develop dependence quicker than men. During pregnancy it readily crosses to the placenta, entering fetal tissues within an hour of maternal substance use. Women using cocaine are more likely to use the IV route, and so the risk for HIV infection is greater [40,41]. Other drugs such as tobacco, marijuana, alcohol, methamphetamines, and both prescriptive or illicit opiates all have a negative impact on maternal pregnancy and fetal outcomes [2,6,20,40,42,43]. Numerous sources within healthcare literature indicate an increase in prescriptive and illicit opioid use over the last 2 decades, with women and pregnancy mimicking the drug abuse rise found within the general population [2,7,28,36,42−45].

14.6 Psychiatric comorbidity

Historically, many pregnant women with a substance use disorder also have a concomitant psychiatric illness. Unger Metz and Fischer note the "majority of opioid-dependent women suffer cooccurring psychiatric disorders with prevalence numbers ranging between 56% and 73%, mainly affective disorders, PTSD, or personality disorders" (2012, p. 1). One critical aspect of effective treatment of substance use disorders is to identify and treat psychiatric comorbid disorders. Some types are more common in women [46] and include bipolar disorders, panic disorder, PTSD, cluster B personality disorders, bulimia, and depression. In pregnancy, physical and sexual abuse are known factors with approximately 25% of women diagnosed with PTSD ([9]; p. 926).

Treatment modalities include pharmacologic and psychosocial interventions. Pharmacologic treatments that enhance recovery from substance use also pose additional problems for the fetus, including need for treatment of the neonate in a neonatal intensive care unit (NICU) for symptom withdrawal [47]. According to a systematic review and metaanalysis by Ref. [48], from inception through 2014, fetal exposure to marijuana use was also indicative of a higher NICU admission rate. Other psychosocial concerns such as poverty, mental health disorders, and domestic violence may also impact entry into care [36]. Early identification through the use of screening tools that includes ATOD is recommended by the [49] government agencies and professional associations such as the US Department of Health and Human Services, the American Academy of Pediatrics [28], and the World Health Organization [50].

14.7 Substances used in pregnancy

The most frequently used substances in pregnancy are alcohol, tobacco, marijuana, cocaine, opioids, and amphetamines [28,49]. Alcohol damages neurons, which results in FAS and fetal alcohol spectrum disorders (FASDs) which are the most common preventable causes of mental retardation. Alcohol is associated with higher rates of still birth, spontaneous abortion, and low birth weight [51,52]. When looking at how drugs can negatively affect placental blood flow through vasoconstriction, cocaine, heroin, nicotine, and marijuana come to mind as majorly impacting fetal and maternal well-being. Nicotine may be seen as having a minor impact on pregnancy outcomes; however, it is associated with a high incidence of miscarriage, low birth weight, and preterm delivery. Other addictive drugs that are known to affect development of the fetal and newborn CNS are opioids, marijuana, cocaine, and methamphetamines [51]. Substance misuse and abuse has skyrocketed over the last 2 decades. Common forms include tobacco, alcohol, cannabinoids (marijuana and hashish), club drugs (methylenedioxymethamphetamine [MDMA] and gamma-hydroxybutyrate [GHB]), dissociative drugs (ketamine and phencyclidine [PCP]), hallucinogenics (lysergic acid diethylamide [LSD] and mescaline), opioids (heroin and opium), and stimulants (cocaine, amphetamine, and methamphetamine) [51,53].

The following sections will describe the maternal, fetal, and newborn effects of the frequently used substances. Pharmacological treatment during pregnancy involves a number of strategies including detoxification, abstinence, maintenance, and treatment of comorbid psychiatric disorders. Diet, nutrition, social service support, and 12-Step groups are essential adjuncts to pharmacologic therapy. Nursing and medicine are both integral to the development and implementation of healthcare to this population.

14.7.1 Alcohol

Alcohol is a known teratogen and there is no known safe level for use in pregnancy [49,51]. Blood alcohol levels in women are higher than men after drinking similar amounts and women are more sensitive to its toxic effects; that is, they get drunk faster. This appears to be due to a lower percentage of body water and lower gastric alcohol dehydrogenase resulting in a reduced first-pass metabolism [54]. Alcohol readily crosses the placenta and is present in amniotic fluid after the mother's level is metabolized to zero. Alcohol damage can occur early in pregnancy before a woman realizes she is pregnant. Fetal toxicity is dose related with the greatest risk occurring early in the first trimester [55].

There are many mechanisms that result in cell death by necrosis or apoptosis including oxidative stress, damage to mitochondria, effects on glial cells, impaired development and function of chemical messenger systems, transport and uptake of glucose, and cell adhesion [56].

In addition to cranio-facial abnormalities and mental retardation associated with FAS (average IQ is 67), for children with FASD, attention deficit hyperactivity disorder is more likely to be earlier onset of the inattention subtype. Other syndrome characteristics include speech and language delays and poor social skills. These children appear to have a disturbance in brain structure, in the corpus callosum, and the response to standard psychostimulant medication can be unpredictable [57,58].

14.7.1.1 Pharmacologic treatment of alcohol use in pregnancy

Treatment is predicated on detoxification and abstinence. During detoxification, benzodiazepines are the drug of choice to reduce the excitatory state of the brain during withdrawal. Carbamazepine, an antiseizure medication, has been used extensively in Europe. As this is a category D drug, it should only be best used in the second and third trimester [59]. Folic acid supplementation is recommended with the use of carbamazepine due to an increased incidence of neural tube defects with this medication [60].

Disulfiram is used to maintain abstinence. It inhibits aldehyde dehydrogenase production. Subsequent use of alcohol leads to accumulation of acetaldehyde. As a result, the patient experiences harsh symptoms including facial flushing, tachycardia, hypotension, nausea, and vomiting. This is a form of negative reinforcement and may not be well tolerated by the pregnant alcoholic in recovery. Reports of fetal anomalies are sporadic and disulfiram appears to be relatively safe [61].

Naltrexone and acamprosate have also been used to support abstinence. Naltrexone is an opiate agonist. It appears to act by blocking opiate receptor activation mediated by alcohol and one effect is to reduce craving. Acamprosate has a similar outcome and the mechanism is thought to modulate NMDA receptors in the brain [61]. There are few data regarding the use of acamprosate in pregnancy. In most cases, the risks of continued alcohol use far outweigh the risks of pharmacologic therapy in pregnancy.

14.7.2 Tobacco; nicotine

Nicotine in the form of tobacco smoke is a double-edged sword for fetal harm. There are more than 4000 chemicals produced during smoking with over 40 of these as known carcinogens [40]. Cigarette smoke contains cyanide, carbon monoxide, and a plethora of toxic hydrocarbons, which affect oxygen transport to the placenta. This results in spontaneous abortion, low birth weight and preterm delivery [50,62,63]. Tobacco use during pregnancy is a commonly used substance with 12% or higher use during pregnancy reported by Ref. [64]. Ref. [65] also note placenta previa, neonatal mortality, and risk for sudden infant death syndrome as risk factors for smoking. Nicotine affects umbilical blood flow, fetal cerebral artery blood flow and potentiates the effects of the smoke [66]. Smoking cessation programs are effective in reducing these effects, especially if started before or early in the pregnancy [67].

Pharmacologic therapy for nicotine use is similar to alcohol focusing on detoxification and abstinence support. Nicotine patches, lozenges, and gums are most often used in conjunction with a smoking cessation program. Nicotine replacement treatment (NRT) helps prevent relapse and removes the effects of the smoke on the fetus. It appears that minimal amounts of nicotine are excreted into breastmilk and that NRT can be used while breastfeeding [68]. It is imperative that patients understand not to smoke while using any NRT program because the combined dose of nicotine substantially increases fetal exposure.

Selective serotonin and dopamine reuptake inhibitors have had some success. Of these, bupropion is the most frequently prescribed antidepressant, with varenicline a more recent choice. Bupropion is a dopamine reuptake inhibitor and blocks cravings. Varenicline is a partial agonist selective for $\alpha4\beta2$ nicotinic acetylcholine receptor subtypes. It also reduces cravings and has a blocking effect. Both may lead to neuropsychiatric symptoms in the mother, and healthcare team providers and nurses should be aware of the black-box warning of these agents [69,70].

14.7.3 Opiates and opioids

Research findings support the association of substance misuse and an increase in psychological distresses that cross all socioeconomic and racial differences. In particular, opioid misuse is linked with poor mental health outcomes [71–73]. Women who are opioid dependent have a prevalence of affective or personality mental health disorders along with PTSD [32,74].

Opiates are alkaloids derived from the opium poppy and include morphine, codeine, and thebaine. Opioids include all opiates plus the semisynthetics, which are derived from the alkaloid family. From thebaine come the semisynthetics: hydrocodone, oxycodone, and heroin. The synthetics include methadone, fentanyl, Nubain, and buprenorphine. At times, these terms may be used interchangeably by healthcare providers.

There has been a major shift in the approach to opiate treatment from detoxification and abstinence to a maintenance program or medication-assisted treatment (MAT). Older practices of withdrawal during pregnancy carry an increased risk for abruption and preterm labor. Best practices for opioid treatment during pregnancy currently involve some form of MAT. The use of an agonist/antagonist treatment, such as methadone or buprenorphine, has been effective in reducing opioid misuse and abuse during pregnancy [31,74]. Buprenorphine has a high binding affinity for the Mi receptor. Thus, if the patient uses another opiate while on buprenorphine, there will be a minimal euphoric response. This effect significantly reduces the abuse potential [75]. It is metabolized by placental aromatase to norbuprenorphine resulting in low placental transfer. This may account for limited fetal exposure and its lower incidence of NAS [76]. Small amounts of buprenorphine are found in breastmilk. However, it has little if any effect on the newborn with no evidence of neonatal withdrawal when breastfeeding is discontinued [77,78]. While both buprenorphine and methadone are categorized as Pregnancy Category C, this treatment plan has been found to be safe and effective [2,20,42,79]. To date, there is no relationship between use of methadone dosing and the severity of NAS. The major maternal risks of opioid misuse during pregnancy are malnutrition, malnutrition, and respiratory depression which can lead to death [80].

14.7.4 Neonatal abstinence syndrome

Neonatal abstinence syndrome is one of the most common complications of opioid use disorder during pregnancy. Newborns born to opioid-dependent mothers are at risk for withdrawal and neonatal abstinence syndrome, which occurs during the first few days after delivery. The main organs affected are the newborn CNS, cardiac and respiratory system, and digestive tract [31].

The Neonatal Abstinence Scoring System was initially devised by Finnegan in 1975 [81] and contains 21 items. It is the most commonly used scoring system over the last 40 years. This scoring system was simplified by a team of researchers, including the original author, focusing on combining some items and value points. The new simplified Finnegan Neonatal Abstinence Scoring System (sFNAS) contains 10 items for scoring purposes. Research results provide a Pearson's correlation of 0.914 with the original scale. These symptoms include the following: cry (high pitched, excessive); tremors (undisturbed or disturbed and mild, moderate, or severe); increased muscle tone; sleep (<1 h, $< 2-3$ h); nasal stuffiness; respiratory rate (>60/min); excessive sucking; poor feeding; feed tolerance (regurgitation, projectile vomiting); and stools (loose or watery) (p. 4). The sFNAS is a valuable tool used by nurses and physicians to manage withdrawal symptoms.

Other neonatal complications associated with opioid misuse during pregnancy are low birth weight, intrauterine growth restriction, microcephaly, and NICU admission along with prolonged hospitalization due to these congenital anomalies and NAS [30,31,51]. Other newborn congenital anomalies including spina bifida, gastroschisis, congenital heart disease (ventricular and atrial septal defects, hypoplastic left heart syndrome), and visual complications have been suggested as associated complications from fetal exposure to opioids [82,83].

14.7.5 Marijuana and THC

Although marijuana is usually grouped with the hallucinogens, it deserves special attention because it is one of the most commonly used psychoactive substances [84]. There is a wide variance in self-reported marijuana use. Metz and Stickrath report a range of 3%−34% (p. 761). States such as Colorado with legalized medical (2000) and recreational (2012) marijuana use continue to see an increase in sales and consumption. Attitudes and beliefs influence use and many perceive it as not so harmful in nature. Data taken from the NSDUH indicate marijuana use in the past month among pregnant women increased by as much as 62% between the years 2002 and 2014 [85]. As these are self-reported values, there is a high probability of under reporting due to perceived stigmatization, fear of legal consequences, or feelings of guilt due to the risk of negative effects on the neonate [86,87].

The active substance in marijuana is delta-9-tetrahydrocannabinol or THC. It is derived from the plant *Cannabis sativa*. Its lipophilic structure allows it to accumulate in fatty tissue and remain for days before it is metabolized in the liver. Marijuana is smoked, usually as a cigarette or in water pipes (bongs) or used in small pipes called a one hitter. Inhalation of smoke is held in the lungs for long periods and results in higher levels of carboxyhemoglobin [88]. Marijuana produces a mild euphoric or hallucinogenic response and affects most major organ systems. In high doses, it may precipitate psychosis. Marijuana increases blood pressure and cardiac output, compromises respiratory function, decreases the immune response, and is perceived by many as a harmless drug [89].

How marijuana affects fetal development is not well understood. Receptors for cannabinoid are present in the placenta and appear in fetal brain tissue around 14 weeks gestation. Because of its lipophilic nature, it crosses from maternal plasma to the placenta. It is also excreted into breastmilk [87]. Cannabinoid receptors are densely packed in the frontal lobe and cerebellum. Some studies have reported an effect on the mesocorticolimbic system, which assists with regulation of emotions. Adverse pregnancy outcomes are associated with marijuana use and include preterm birth, small for gestational age, and may affect glucose and insulin regulation [4,84,86]. Long-term effects include deficits in cognitive functioning, attention span, analytical skills, and problems with visual integration There is an increased likelihood of marijuana use during adolescents as well [90,91].

14.7.6 Cocaine

Cocaine is a highly addictive lipophilic alkaloid extracted from the plant *Erythroxylum coca*. It is generally snorted, smoked, and less frequently injected. As a powerful dopamine, serotonin, and norepinephrine reuptake inhibitor, it produces a profound high experience. The euphoric effect is short lasting, and users try to recapture the same high feeling over and over by using cocaine more frequently [92].

Cocaine is now the fourth most abused substance during pregnancy and is associated with multiple negative effects on maternal and fetal well-being [51]. Cocaine is known to affect CNS development, which begins during the first weeks of pregnancy and continues on after birth. Studies have shown cocaine inhibits dopamine, noradrenalin, and serotonin reuptake at the presynaptic terminals, resulting in an exaggerated effect on the specific terminal organs [93]. Congenital malformations have shown a correlation with cocaine use, particularly of the brain and heart. Other risks in the neonate period include risk for intestinal infarction, bowel atresia or perforation, and limb malformations. Associated complications in the newborn age involve poor response to environmental factors, leading to fever, sweating, irritability, seizures, and vomiting [51,93,94].

Cocaine has sympathomimetic properties which may cause maternal vasoconstriction along with hypertension, tachycardia, and cardiac arrhythmias. This has a detrimental effect on placental blood flow, which leads to an increased risk for abruption, abortion, and preterm birth. Those children exposed to cocaine use in utero may exhibit long-term cognitive deficits, aggressiveness and/or depression, and difficulty in verbalization [93,95].

Pharmacological treatment of cocaine use includes topiramate, and anticonvulsant, and baclofen, a GABA-B receptor agonist. Topiramate raises cerebral GABA levels, facilitates GABA adrenergic neurotransmission, and inhibits glutamatergic activity [96]. It would appear that the risk of cocaine use would outweigh the risks of topiramate use in pregnancy. Baclofen appears to act in a similar manner as topiramate in reducing cravings and substance use. However, baclofen is transferred thorough the placenta and long-term use is associated with a neonatal abstinence syndrome and seizures [97]. Topiramate would appear to be the safer choice for treatment in pregnancy.

14.7.7 Stimulants: amphetamine, methamphetamines; methylphenidate; ephedra; khat

The family of stimulants act similarly to cocaine with dopamine, serotonin, and norepinephrine release and inhibition of uptake. The effects vary from mild euphoria to profound psychosis and violent behavior. They also increase blood pressure, tachycardia, and arrhythmias, which may induce an obstetrical emergency resulting in an unplanned and urgent cesarean delivery [98]. When coming off of a high, there is a profound withdrawal associated with amphetamines and methamphetamines producing depression, anxiety, fatigue, paranoia, and aggression [98,99].

14.7.7.1 Amphetamines and methamphetamines

Amphetamine and methamphetamine have similar adverse effects on the fetus and neonate. These include a higher risk for fetal growth restriction, placental abruption, and preterm labor. Withdrawal symptoms are similar to cocaine and include anxiety, fatigue, depression, and mood disturbances. Stronger psychotic effects involve feelings of paranoia, visual and auditory hallucinations, or delusions [98]. The fetus has a longer elimination half-life than the mother with higher doses remaining in the fetal brain [100]. High doses of methamphetamine in the breastmilk have been associated with fatal levels transferred to the infant [101,102]. Similar to cocaine, long-term effects of methamphetamine suggest a delay in cognitive skills and growth [98,103].

Pharmacologic treatment of amphetamine and methamphetamine is limited in pregnancy with only a few case reports. Randomized, placebo-controlled, double-blind trial of baclofen and gabapentin for the treatment of methamphetamine dependence revealed limited effects [104]. According to the NIDA [98], "the most effective treatments for methamphetamine addiction at this point are behavioral therapies, such as cognitive behavioral and contingency management interventions" (p. 15).

14.7.7.2 Methylphenidate

Methylphenidate is pharmacologically similar to amphetamines. It is used in attention deficit disorders in children and has a high potential for addiction. Acute effects include tachycardia, irritability, and hypertension. Methylphenidate is most often obtained by diversion of a child's prescription, thus causing harm to both parent and child. Effects on the fetus are not well known. Treatment is by gradual weaning and the use of cognitive behavioral therapy and motivational enhancement [105].

14.7.7.3 Ephedra

Ephedra is a naturally occurring stimulant used primarily as a weight loss aid. It may cause stroke, heart attacks, and death [106]. Effects on the fetus and pregnancy are not well known.

14.7.7.4 Khat

Khat is related to amphetamine and is a natural stimulant. It is used primarily in East Africa and the Arabian peninsula [107]. The leaves are chewed releasing the active substance, cathinone, with a resultant psychoactive effect. Vasoconstriction affects the utero-placental blood flow during pregnancy. Fetal outcomes reveal a restriction in weight and growth [108].

14.7.7.5 Hallucinogens: lysergic acid diethylamide and phencyclidine

LSD binds to 5-hydroxytryptamine receptors and causes vivid hallucinations. It is not associated with the onset of dependence and does not cause chromosomal damage [109]. The effects on pregnancy are unknown due to limited research. It does pass into breastmilk and should not be used while breastfeeding [110].

PCP is used as a hallucinogen. It is a dissociative anesthetic and acts as an N-methyl-D-aspartate antagonist at low doses causing methamphetamine-like effects resulting in frequent violent behavior [107,111]. Newborns of users may present with irritability, poor feeding, and hypertonicity. It is readily passed into breastmilk.

14.7.8 Club drugs: MDMA; gamma-hydroxybutyrate; flunitrazepam; ketamine

14.7.8.1 MDMA

MDMA was patented in Germany in 1912 by E. Merck of Darmstadt. Little is known about the history behind this drug and it is said to have been used as an appetite suppressant. Decades later, it resurfaced as ecstasy, which often contains more volatile and toxic amphetamine-like substances [112]. Ecstasy produces highly subjective effects of stimulation, feelings of closeness, and hallucinations. It is similar to cocaine as a nonselective monoamine uptake inhibitor. It does not appear to cause dependence. Adverse effects of this drug can be life threatening and includes lethal hyperthermia and fatal hyponatremia secondary to inappropriate secretion of antidiuretic hormone [113]. The typical side effects are similar to those found with amphetamines. Neurotoxicity has been reported with associated cognitive impairment. In utero exposure may lead to an increased risk of cardiovascular and skeletal abnormalities [114]. Most people stop using ecstasy on their own. Since women who use ecstasy in pregnancy also smoke heavily, as well as use alcohol and other drugs, it is difficult to determine a causal role for MDMA in newborns.

14.7.8.2 Gamma-hydroxybutyrate

GHB is a dissociative anesthetic and is used to treat narcolepsy. It is used for its intoxicating effects, similar to alcohol. It is used by clubbers and has a short half-life and is often used multiple times in an evening. It has a strong addictive potential, and adverse effects include acute intoxication, vomiting, and respiratory depression [115]. It carries a withdrawal syndrome similar to that of benzodiazepines. Fetal and neonatal effects are not well documented but would be expected to be similar to those of the benzodiazepines. Treatment for GHB addiction is similar to alcohol treatment and good success is seen with 12-Step Recovery support.

14.7.8.3 Flunitrazepam

Flunitrazepam or roofies is a long acting benzodiazepine and used outside the United States for the treatment of sleep disorders. It is implicated as a date-rape drug and most often used with alcohol, leading to psychomotor impairment and respiratory depression [116]. Maternal and neonatal effects are typical of the benzodiazepines. It does cross over into breastmilk.

14.7.8.4 Ketamine

Ketamine is a dissociative anesthetic. It produces changes in perception, depersonalization, and hallucination and finds its way to clubbers by diversion from legal sources [117]. The effects include tachycardia, vomiting, amnesia, delirium, and rhabdomyolysis [118]. Although it poses a low risk of overdose, aspiration from vomitus and sedation can be profound. Some evidence suggests it can damage the developing fetal brain [119]. Treatment of ketamine dependence would include detoxification, cognitive behavioral therapy, and 12-Step Recovery support.

14.8 Screening and detection

It is not difficult to improve outcomes in pregnancy. Adequate screening and detection are essential and brief physician interventions are highly effective. Nurses remain an integral part of the interdisciplinary healthcare team as they maintain close interactions with the patient and family during all aspects of care (prenatal, natal, and postnatal). It is important for all interdisciplinary team members to communicate well in caring for this high-risk population.

Historically, a punitive approach to care has been the response with little proven benefit for maternal or infant health. Interventions should remain nonjudgmental in nature, focusing on the care and treatment of a clinical condition rather than a judgmental or biased attitude [2]. A multidisciplinary approach that includes psychosocial services when available may improve successful treatment and positive outcomes [30]. In a study by Ref. [120], after a year of treatment, 65.7% of women who entered treatment while pregnant used no drugs, while only 27.7% of nonpregnant women remained drug free ($P < .0005$). Screening during prenatal care is recommended and should include a validated screening tool such as the 4P's Screening Tool [2] that includes questions focusing on parents, partners, past, and present use of any ATOD. Another screening tool focuses on women 26 years of age or younger and encompasses six questions. The CRAFFT tool looks at substance use while riding in a Car; drug use to Relax or fit in with others; use of drugs when Alone; poor memory or Forgetting things while using alcohol or drugs; Family (or friends) tell you to cut down on use; and getting into Trouble while using drugs or alcohol [30,121]. This assessment should take place in a private location and include a therapeutic communication approach. The desired outcome of a healthy mother and baby should be the focus of all team members. Prenatal substance use intervention reduces neonatal low birth weight and preterm delivery [122]. Guidelines published from the American College of Obstetricians and Gynecologists (ACOG) counsel against using marijuana while trying to get pregnant, during pregnancy, and while they are breastfeeding [15]. There remains a gap in the literature on marijuana use during pregnancy due to insufficient data to evaluate the effect on both fetus and infant. In a systematic review and metaanalyses of the literature by Ref. [48], it was found that women who used marijuana during pregnancy were at greater risk for anemia. Infants who experienced in utero exposure to marijuana had a decrease in birthweight when compared with infants without exposure. A third finding indicated the marijuana exposed infants were more likely to receive care in the NICU.

Wherever care is provided for newborns going through withdrawal, be that during couplet care at the bedside, a newborn nursery, or NICU, protocols and defined procedures are key in planning for care. Each nursery needs a standardized plan that includes evaluation, assessments, and comprehensive treatment whether at risk or showing signs of withdrawal [94]. The approach should include interdisciplinary team members with an open communication approach to provide the best care for the newborn and mother.

14.9 The role of urine and meconium testing

Both urine and meconium testing can be used to determine the prevalence of drug use during pregnancy. Since the 1970s, states have enacted legislature either supporting mandatory priority access to substance use disorder treatment for pregnant women or the opposite, as a punitive action for child abuse [123]. The potential risk of being reported to Child Protective Services (CPS) for reporting substance use during a screening or brief intervention will most likely cause women to underreport use to healthcare providers [124]. In this respect, the results of urine drug screens may also carry legal jeopardy and may deter pregnant substance users from receiving prenatal care [123,125].

Informed decisions are integral to providing quality healthcare. It is important to inform patients that a number of routine screening tests are completed during pregnancy care and these include blood tests, diabetes and genetic screenings, tests for sexually transmitted infections, fetal ultrasound, and urine tests for protein, sugar, infection, and drugs. Given the high incidence of substance use in pregnancy, urine drug screens are appropriate at the first prenatal visit and are especially effective in revealing substance use when coupled with verbal screening [123,124]. Transparency requires informing the patient that she may opt out of any test. Also, important is to let her know that opting out of urine drug screen may then lead to the pediatrician ordering drug screens after the baby is born. State laws tend to be profuse about what constitutes child abuse. A patient who opts out of a urine drug screen creates a reasonable basis to suspect drug use. Thus, pediatricians may legally order urine and meconium tests on the newborn without parental consent. Obstetrical indications for a urine drug screen include any history of drug use, missing prenatal appointments, entering prenatal care late in the pregnancy (only in the third trimester), preterm labor (<37 weeks' gestation), third trimester bleeding due to placental abruption, and fetal growth restriction [126,127]. The major limiting factor of urine drug screens is that, with few exceptions, they only reveal recent drug use. The table below indicates how long a particular drug may be detectable in urine after typical use [128] (Table 14.1).

Table 14.1 Length of time substance is detectable in urine.

Substance		Time
Alcohol		24 h
Amphetamines		48 h
Barbiturates	Short acting	48 h
	Long acting	7 days
Benzodiazepines		72 h
Cocaine		72 h
Marijuana	Single use	72 h
	Chronic use	30–40 days
Opiates	Morphine/Heroin	72 h
	Methadone	96 h
	Codeine	Up to 10 days
Nicotine		3–5 days from last use

14.10 Brief office screening strategies

Universal screening means that every obstetrical patient is asked about substance use at the first prenatal or intake visit, and at least once per trimester thereafter. Thus, there is a clear distinction between urine drug testing and verbal screening. When identified and treated, the rate of abstinence increases and maternal and fetal complications decrease. There is less preterm labor, less placental abruption, and less growth restriction. Treatment is highly cost effective due in part to the reduction in preterm labor and birth, low birth weight, and decrease in extended neonatal intensive care hospitalization services [129].

A simple screening method uses a two-item screen for substance use, takes less than a minute to complete, and has good sensitivity and specificity. It consists of two questions [130]:

1. "In the last year have you ever smoked cigarettes, drunk alcohol, or used any drugs more than you meant to?"
2. "Have you felt you wanted or needed to cut down on your smoking or drinking or drug use in the last year?"

Another practical and validated screening approach is the 4P's Plus method. This screening tool focuses on parent, partner, past, and pregnancy as key words and has been validated for use with pregnant women by the ACOG. Is there a history or present substance use by her parents or partner? This screening tool also looks at prepregnancy and current use during pregnancy [130,131]. This is a verbal screening conducted by a healthcare professional and includes these five questions:

1. "Did either of your PARENTS have a problem with alcohol or drugs?"
2. "Do any of your PEERS have a problem with alcohol or drugs?"
3. "Does your PARTNER have a problem with alcohol or drugs?"
4. "Have you ever drunk beer, wine, or liquor to excess in the PAST?"
5. (Plus, question) "Have you smoked any cigarettes, used any alcohol, or any drug at any time in this PREGNANCY?"

Numerous screening approaches have been developed for alcohol use in women. The T-ACE screening tool is adapted from the classic CAGE questions for alcohol use. It can be used alone or in combination with the 4P's Plus questions. If there was a positive answer to questions about past and current pregnancy in the 4P's Plus, then follow up with the T-ACE screening tool. A score of 2 or more points indicates at-risk drinking in pregnancy [132,133]. The four-item questions are a verbal screening tool:

1. T: Tolerance: "How many drinks does it take you to feel high?" (More than two drinks is a positive response—score 2 points)
2. A: Annoyed: "Have people annoyed you by criticizing your drinking?" (Yes— score 1 point)
3. C: Cut down: "Have you ever felt you ought to cut down on your drinking?" (Yes—score 1 point)

4. E: Eye opener: "Have you ever had a drink first think in the morning to steady your nerves or get rid of a hangover?" (Yes—score 1 point)

TWEAK is used for alcohol screening in the current pregnancy [132,134] and includes these questions:

1. T: Tolerance: "How many drinks does it take you to feel high?" (More than two drinks is a positive response—score 2 points)
2. W: Worried: "Have close friends or relatives worried or complained about your drinking?" (Yes—score 1 point)
3. E: Eye opener: "Have you ever had a drink first thing in the morning to steady your nerves or get rid of a hangover?" (Yes—score 1 point)
4. A: Amnesia: "Has a friend or family member ever told you about things you said or did while drinking that you could not remember?" (Yes—score 1 point)
5. K: Cut down: "Have you ever felt you ought to cut down on your drinking?" (Yes—score 1 point)

With positive answers to the alcohol screens, it is imperative to ask questions about consumption. These questions look at consuming more than one drink a day or more than three drinks per social occasion. At-risk consumption is considered when responses indicate >7/drinks/week or >4 drinks per occasion for women. A positive answer to any question when screening for substance use in pregnancy should trigger a urine drug test. Using a combined verbal screening and urine screening approach to care will yield the best results.

14.11 Brief office interventions

When the patient admits to drug use or a screen is positive, a urine drug screen is indicated. Sharing the laboratory report of a positive urine drug test with the patient is the most effective way to break through the denial that often accompanies substance use. A brief office intervention is immediately indicated. Brief office interventions have proven to be powerful therapeutic approaches with results comparable to more prolonged therapies [135,136]. Overall, consideration should be taken to identify the best screening tool in order to determine women who drink at a level that may prove harmful to the fetus with long-lasting sequelae such as FAS. The goal of a brief intervention is to motivate on an individual, one on one level, aiming toward behavior modification [132,137].

FRAMES was used in a World Health Organization study to assess brief interventions. While the focus of this study evaluated heavy male drinkers, FRAMES also works well with other drug use [138,139]. The interview topics include the following:

■ F − Feedback about the adverse effects of drugs or alcohol. This allows for patient education.

- R — Responsibility for a change in behavior: "Only you can decide that you want to stop using. If you do, how will your life be better?"
- A — Advise to reduce or stop use: "For the next 2 weeks, stop using, and let's see how you feel."
- M — Menu of options: treatment; medications: "If you find that not using for the next 2 weeks is impossible, then we should consider other options."
- E — Empathy is central to the intervention. "I know this may be hard to do."
- S — Self-empowerment: You can change. "I am impressed that you are considering making this change. Your strong determination is going to help you succeed."

In the FRAMES intervention, feedback follows a specific formula that has universal applications. The interviewer uses four issues to clarify the situation: data, feelings, judgments, and what the interviewer wants to happen. Here is an example of how this might progress:

- The data in your urine screen were positive for cocaine.
- I am afraid (feeling) that if you are positive at delivery, CPS will investigate and may put the baby in foster care.
- My opinion (judgment) is that you can stop using.
- I want you to stop using now.

This four-point approach is designed to clarify the issue and share feelings to enhance empathy in the interviewer—patient relationship. This approach also empowers the listener to act and focuses on making the listener less likely to resist this motivationally enhanced intervention [139].

14.12 Long-term care and maintenance

Screening and detection are critical for the treatment of substance use in pregnancy. By identifying the patient, the physician can determine the appropriate path to recovery, which may include detoxification, pharmacologic treatment, and maintenance. Short-term interventions are designed to educate the patient and empower her to change behavior. A number of strategies have evolved to enhance long-term abstinence or maintenance.

Motivational Enhancement Therapy (MET) is the foundation for supporting the substance user as she moves through the stages of recovery. Developed by Ref. [138], its premise is that the responsibility for change rests squarely on the shoulders of the patient. The approach is easy to learn and apply in prenatal care. Basic interviewing skills include the ability to express empathy, to continue forward even when met with resistance, and to empower the patient to move through the changes occurring in her life. This approach has improved maternal and neonatal outcomes in pregnancy [140].

Integrating MET with the Stages of Change approach, developed by Prochaska, creates a powerful therapeutic alliance leading to maintenance of recovery [141,142]. Prochaska describes six stages of change and this model measures progress over time. The goal is to motivate the patient to move from one stage to the next, only when the patient is ready to move forward. Psychosocial support for the recovering addict is critical in maintaining abstinence and preventing relapse. This approach to motivational therapy has also shown improved retention in prenatal care and substance treatment programs.

14.13 Conclusion

The identification and treatment of substance use in pregnancy remains a most challenging prospect for all members of the healthcare team. It requires a thorough evidence-based knowledge of the pharmacologic effects of a plethora of drugs on the mother, fetus, and neonate.

The use of brief interventions during office visits in the prenatal care includes the 4P's Plus method, the FRAMES, or CRAFFT tools. Common themes involve asking about any past history of substance use (e.g., alcohol, cocaine, and methamphetamines), concerns of overindulgence, or lapse in memory after substance use. The FRAMES intervention provides the interviewer an opportunity for demonstrating empathy and encouraging the patient to self-empowerment.

State laws have historically enacted a punitive approach to substance use during pregnancy in an effort to protect the fetus during critical growth and development periods. More recent literature speaks to improved outcomes when provision of substance treatment is made available to women at risk or in use of harmful substances. However, there continues to be limited healthcare coverage and resources for this type of therapy.

Most important is the ability of the physician, and when required, other team members, to form a close and supportive therapeutic relationship with the patient. This relationship has a tremendous potential to transform a patient's lifestyle into a positive and healthy approach to life. Moreover, it can influence the well-being of her children and future generations.

References

[1] Maguire D. Drug addiction in pregnancy: disease not moral failure [Nursing] Neonatal Netw 2014;33(1):11–8. https://doi.org/10.1891/0730-0832.33.1.11Accepted.

[2] Mahoney K, Reich W, Urbanek S. Substance use disorder: prenatal, intrapartum, and postpartum care. Mater Child Nurs 2019;44(5). https://doi.org/10.1097/NMC.0000000000000551.

[3] Substance Abuse and Mental Health Services Administration, SAMSHA. Key substance use and mental health indicators in the United States: results from the 2018 national survey on drug use and health. 2019. Type of work], https://www.samhsa.gov/data/.

[4] Metz TD, Stickrath EH. Marijuana use in pregnancy and lactation: a review of the evidence [Medical] Am J Obstet Gynecol 2015;223(1):761—78.

[5] Substance Abuse and Mental Health Services Administration, SAMSHA. Learn about marijuana risks: marijuana and pregnancy [report]. July 6, 2020. https://www.samhsa.gov/marijuana/marijuana-pregnancy.

[6] Oga ES, Mark K, Coleman-Cowger VH. Cigarette smoking status and substance use in pregnancy [Public health] Matern Child Health J 2018;22(10):1477—83. https://doi.org/10.1007/s10995-018-2543-9.

[7] Reddy UM, Davis JM, Ren Z, Greene MF. Opioid use in pregnancy, neonatal abstinence syndrome, and childhood outcomes: executive summary of a joint workshop by the Eunice Kennedy Shriver National Institute of Child Health and Human Development, American Congress of Obstetricians and Gynecologists, American Academy of pediatrics, Society for Maternal-fetal Medicine, Centers for Disease Control and Prevention, and the March of Dimes Foundation [Medical] Obstet Gynecol 2017; 130(1):10—28. https://doi.org/10.1097/AOG.0000000000002054.

[8] American Psychiatric Association. Diagnostic and statistical manual of mental disorders. 5th ed. 2013.

[9] Ordean AI, Wong SI, Graves L. No. 349-substance use in pregnancy. J Obstet Gynaecol Can 2017;39(10):922—37. https://doi.org/10.1016/j.jogc.2017.04.028.

[10] Reitan T. Substance abuse during pregnancy: a 5-year follow-up of mothers and children. Drugs Educ Prev Pol 2019;26(3):219—28. https://search.ebscohost.com/login.aspx?direct=true&AuthType=ip,shib&db=sph&AN=135909162&site=eds-live&scope=site&custid=wgc1.

[11] Krans EE, Patrick SW. Opioid use disorder in pregnancy: health policy and practice in the midst of an epidemic. Obstet Gynecol 2016;128(1):4—10. https://doi.org/10.1097/AOG.0000000000001446.

[12] Leshner AI. Addiction is a brain disease, and it matters. Science 1997;45(7):278.

[13] McLellen AT, Lewis DC, O'Brien CP, Kleber HD. Drug dependence, a chronic medical illness: implications for treatment, insurance, and outcomes evaluation. J Am Med Assoc 2000;1689(95):284.

[14] NIDA. Cocaine research report: what is cocaine?. 2016. https://www.drugabuse.gov/publications/research-reports/cocaine/what-cocaine.

[15] Thompson R, DeJong K, Lo J. Marijuana use in pregnancy: a review. Obstet Gynecol 2020;74(7):415—28. https://doi.org/10.1097/OGX.0000000000000685.

[16] Willuhn I, Wanat MJ, Clark JJ, Phillips PE. Dopamine signaling in the nucleus accumbens of animals self-administering drugs of abuse. In: Self DW, Staley Gottschalk JK, editors. Behavioral neuroscience of drug addiction. Springer; 2009. p. 29—71.

[17] Wise RA. Addictive drugs and brain stimulation reward. Annu Rev Neurosci 1996; 19(3):19—40.

[18] Anderson AL, Li S-H, Markova D, Holmes TH, Chiang N, Kahn R, Campbell J, Dickerson DL, Galloway GP, Haning W, Roache JD, Stock C, Elkashef AM. Bupropion for the treatment of methamphetamine dependence in non-daily users: a randomized, double-blind, placebo-controlled trial. Drug Alcohol Depend 2015;150:170—4. https://doi.org/10.1016/j.drugalcdep.2015.01.036.

[19] American Society of Addiction Medicine. The definition of addiction (short version). Public Pol Statement 2015. https://www.asam.org/Quality-Science/publications/magazine/public-policy-statements/2019/10/21/short-definition-of-addiction.

[20] Latuskie KA, Andrews NCZ, Motz M, Leibson T, Austin Z. Reasons for substance use continuation and discontinuation during pregnancy: a qualitative study [Pharmacology] Women Birth 2019;32:e57−64. https://doi.org/10.1016/j.wombi.2018.04.001.

[21] McKeever AE, Spaeth-Brayton S, Sheerin S. The role of nurses in comprehensive care management of pregnant women with drug addiction [Nursing] Nurs Women's Health 2020;18(4):284−93. https://doi.org/10.1111/1751-486X.12134.

[22] Patrick SW, Schiff DM. A public health response to opioid use in pregnancy. Pediatrics 2017:e20164070. https://doi.org/10.1542/peds.2016-4070.

[23] Geil CR, Hayes DM, McClain JA, Liput DJ, Marshall SA, Chen KY, Nixon K. Alcohol and adult hippocampal neurogenesis: promisuous drug, wanton effects. Progr Neuropsychopharmacol & Biol Psychiatry 2014;54:103−13. https://doi.org/10.1016/j.pnpbp.2014.05.003.

[24] Nixon K, Morris SA, Liput DJ, Kelso ML. Roles of neural stem cells and adult neurogenesis in adolescent alcohol use disorders. Alcohol 2010;44(1):39−56. https://doi.org/10.1016/j.alcohol.2009.11.001.

[25] Yazdy MM, Mitchell AA, Tinker SC, Parker SE, Werler MM. Periconceptional use of opioids and the risk of neural tube defects. Obstet Gynecol 2013;122(4):838−44. https://doi.org/10.1097/AOG.0b013e3182a6643c.

[26] Milunsky A, Jick H, Jick SS, Bruell CL, MacLaughlin DS, Rothman KJ, Willett W. Multivitamin/folic acid supplementation in early pregnancy reduces the prevalence of neural tube defects. J Am Med Assoc 1989;262(20):2847−52.

[27] Kiefer F, Jahn H, Tarnaske T, Helwig H, Briken P, Holzbach R, Kämpf P, Stracke R, Baehr M, Naber D, Wiedemann K. Comparing and combining naltrexone and acamprosate in relapse prevention of alcoholism: a double-blind, placebo-controlled study. Arch Gen Psychiatr 2003;60(1):92−9.

[28] Azuine RE, Ji Y, Chang H-Y, Kim Y, Ji H, DiBari J, Hong X, Wang G, Singh GK, Pearson C, Zuckerman B, Surkan PJ, Wang X. Prenatal risk factors and perinatal and postnatal outcomes associated with maternal opioid exposure in an urban, low-income, multiethnic us population. JAMA Netw Open 2019;2(6):1−15. https://doi.org/10.1001/jamanetworkopen.2019.6405.

[29] Busch DW. Clinical management of the breast-feeding mother-infant dyad in recovery from opioid dependence. J Addict Nurs 2016;27(2):68−77.

[30] Ecker J, Abuhamad A, Hill W, Bailit J, Bateman BT, Berghella V, Blake-Lamb T, Guille C, Landau R, Minkoff H, Prabhu M, Rosenthal E, Terplan M, Wright TE, Yonkers KA. Substance use disorders in pregnancy: clinical, ethical, and research imperatives of the opioid epidemic: a report of a joint workshop of the Society for Maternal-fetal Medicine, American College of Obstetricians and Gynecologists, and American Society of Addiction Medicine. Soc Mater Fetal Med March 27, 2019. https://doi.org/10.1016/j.ajog.2019.03.022.

[31] Unger A, Metz V, Fischer G. Opioid dependent and pregnant: what are the best options for mothers and neonates? Obstetrics & Gynecol Int 2012;2012:195954. https://doi.org/10.1155/2012/195954.

[32] Unger AMD, Jung EMD, Winklbaur BPD, Fischer GMD. Gender issues in the pharmacotherapy of opioid-addicted women: buprenorphine. J Addict Dis 2010;29: 217−30. https://search.ebscohost.com/login.aspx?direct=true&AuthType=ip,shib&db=ncj&AN=SM252907&site=eds-live&scope=site&custid=wgc1.

[33] Marcenko MO, Spence M, Rohweder C. Psychosocial characteristics of pregnant women with and without a history of substance abuse. Health Soc Work 1994;19(1): 17−22.

[34] Sutter MB, Gopman S, Leeman L. Patient-centered care to address barriers for pregnant women with opioid dependence. Obstet Gynecol Clin N Am 2017;44(1):95−107. https://doi.org/10.1016/j.ogc.2016.11.004.

[35] Dearing RL, Stuewig J, Tangney JP. On the importance of distinguishing shame from guilt: relations to problematic alcohol and drug use. Addict Behav 2005;30(7): 1392−404.

[36] Polak K, Kelpin S, Terplan M. Screening for substance use in pregnancy and the newborn. Fetal & Neonatal Med 2019;24:90−4. https://doi.org/10.1016/j.siny.2019.01.007.

[37] Chavkin W, Breitbart V. Substance abuse and maternity: the United States as a case study. Addiction 1997;92(9):1201−5.

[38] Shenai N, Gopalan P, Glance J. Integrated brief intervention for PTSD and substance use in an antepartum unit [Article] Matern Child Health J 2019;23(5):592−6. https://doi.org/10.1007/s10995-018-2686-8.

[39] Lukas SE, Sholar M, Lundahl LH, Lamas X, Kouri E, Wines JD, Kragie L, Mendelson JH. Sex differences in plasma cocaine levels and subjective effects after acute cocaine administration in human volunteers. Psychopharmacology 1996; 125(4):346−54. https://doi.org/10.1007/BF02246017.

[40] Keegan J, Parva M, Finnegan M, Gerson A, Belden M. Addiction in pregnancy. J Addict Dis 2010;29(2):175−91. https://doi.org/10.1080/10550881003684723.

[41] McCance-Katz EF, Carroll KM, Rounsaville BJ. Gender differences in treatment-seeking cocaine abusers–implications for treatment and prognosis. Am J Addict 1999;8(4):300−11. https://search.ebscohost.com/login.aspx?direct=true&AuthType=ip,shib&db=mnh&AN=10598213&site=eds-live&scope=site&custid=wgc1.

[42] American College of Obstetricians and Gynecologists. Opioid use and opioid use disorder in pregnancy (committee opinion no. 711). Obstet Gynecol 2017;130(2):488−9. https://doi.org/10.1097/AOG.0000000000002229.

[43] American College of Obstetricians and Gynecologists. Opioid use in pregnancy, neonatal abstinence syndrome, and childhood outcomes: executive summary of a joint workshop by the Eunice Kennedy Shriver National Institute of Child Health and Human Development, American Congress of Obstetricians and Gynecologists, American Academy of Pediatrics, Society for Maternal-fetal Medicine, Centers for Disease Control and Prevention, and the March of Dimes Foundation. Obstet Gynecol 2017;130(1): 10−28. https://doi.org/10.1097/AOG.0000000000002054.

[44] Oral R, Koc F, Jogerst K, Bayman L, Austin A, Sullivan S, Ozgur-Bayman E. Staff training makes a difference: improvements in neonatal illicit drug testing and intervention at a tertiary hospital. J Matern Fetal Neonatal Med 2014;27(10):1049−54. https://doi.org/10.3109/14767058.2013.847418.

[45] Substance Abuse and Mental Health Services Administration, SAMSHA. Substance use during pregnancy varies by race and ethnicity. May 10, 2012. http://www.samhsa.gov/data/.

[46] Miles DR, Kulstad JL, Haller DL. Severity of substance abuse and psychiatric problems among perinatal drug-dependent women. J Psychoact Drugs 2002;34(4):339−46.

[47] Malm H, Klaukka T, Neuvonen PJ. Risks associated with selective serotonin reuptake inhibitors in pregnancy. Obstet Gynecol 2005;106(6):1289−96.

[48] Gunn JKL, Rosales CB, Center KE, Nunez A, Gibson SJ, Christ C, Ehiri JE. Prenatal exposure to cannabis and maternal and child health outcomes: a systematic review and meta-analysis. BMJ Open 2016;6(4):1—8. https://doi.org/10.1136/bmjopen-2015-009986.

[49] American College of Obstetricians and Gynecologists. Alcohol abuse and other substance use disorders: ethical issues in obstetric and gynecologic practice (committee opinion no. 633). Obstet Gynecol 2015;125:1529—37.

[50] Wilson CA, Finch CK, Shakespeare J. Alcohol, smoking, and other substance use in the perinatal period. BMJ 2020. https://doi.org/10.1136/bmj.m1627.

[51] Bailey NA, Diaz-Barbosa M. Effect of maternal substance abuse on the fetus, neonate, and child. Pediatr Rev 2018;39(11):550—9. https://doi.org/10.1542/pir.2017-0201.

[52] Riley EP, McGee CL. Fetal alcohol spectrum disorders: an overview with emphasis on changes in brain and behavior. Exp Biol Med 2005;230(6):357—65.

[53] NIDA. Commonly abused drugs: prescription and OTCs. 2015. http://www.drugabuse.gov/drugs-abuse/commonly-abused-drugs.

[54] Baraona E, Abittan CS, Dohmen K, Moretti M, Pozzato G, Chayes ZW, Schaefer C, Lieber CS. Gender differences in pharmacokinetics of alcohol. Alcohol Clin Exp Res 2001;25(4):502—7. https://search.ebscohost.com/login.aspx?direct=true&AuthType=ip,shib&db=mnh&AN=11329488&site=eds-live&scope=site&custid=wgc1.

[55] Ernhart CB, Sokol RJ, Martier S, Moron P, Nadler D, Ager JW, Wolf A. Alcohol teratogenicity in the human: a detailed assessment of specificity, critical period, and threshold. Am J Obstet Gynecol 1987;156(1):33—9. https://search.ebscohost.com/login.aspx?direct=true&AuthType=ip,shib&db=mnh&AN=3799767&site=eds-live&scope=site&custid=wgc1.

[56] Goodlett CR, Horn KH, Zhou FC. Alcohol teratogenesis: mechanisms of damage and strategies for intervention. Exp Biol Med 2005;230(6):394—406. https://search.ebscohost.com/login.aspx?direct=true&AuthType=ip,shib&db=mnh&AN=15956769&site=eds-live&scope=site&custid=wgc1.

[57] Howlett H, Mackenzie S, Strehle EM, Rankin J, Gray WK. A survey of health care professionals' knowledge and experience of foetal alcohol spectrum disorder and alcohol use in pregnancy. Clin Med Insights Reprod Health 2019;13:1—10. https://doi.org/10.1177/1179558119838.

[58] O'Malley PM, Johnston LD. Epidemiology of alcohol and other drug use among American college students. J Stud Alcohol 2002;l14:23—39. https://doi.org/10.15288/jsas.2002.s14.23 [College drinking, what it is, and what do to about it: review of the state of the science].

[59] Mueller TI, Stout RL, Rudden S, Brown RA, Gordon A, Solomon DA, Recupero PR. A double-blind, placebo-controlled pilot study of carbamazepine for the treatment of alcohol dependence. Alcohol Clin Exp Res 1997;21(1):86—92. https://doi.org/10.1111/j.1530-0277.1997.tb03733.x.

[60] Harden CL, Pennell PB, Koppel BS, Hovinga CA, Gidal B, Meador KJ, Hopp J, Ting TY, Hauser WA, Thurman D, Kaplan PW, Robinson JN, French JA, Wiebe S, Wilner AN, Vazquez B, Holmes L, Krumholz A, Finnell R, Shafer PO. Practice parameter update: management issues for women with epilepsy—focus on pregnancy (an evidence-based review): vitamin k, folic acid, blood levels, and breastfeeding: report of the Quality Standards Subcommittee and Therapeutics and Technology Assessment Subcommittee of the American Academy of Neurology and American Epilepsy Society. Neurology 2009;73(2):142—9. https://doi.org/10.1212/WNL.0b013e3181a6b325.

[61] Johnson BA. Update on neuropharmacological treatments for alcoholism: scientific basis and clinical findings [Review Article] Biochem Pharmacol 2008;75(1):34–56. https://doi.org/10.1016/j.bcp.2007.08.005.

[62] Bernstein IM, Mongeon JA, Badger GJ, Solomon L, Heil SH, Higgins ST. Maternal smoking and its association with birth weight. Obstet Gynecol 2005;106(5 part 1): 986–91. https://doi.org/10.1097/01.aog.0000182580.78402.d2.

[63] Khawam I. A cross-sectional study: maternal smoking during pregnancy and its harmful association with neonatal birth weight decrease. Multi-Knowl Electr Compr J Educ & Sci Publ (MECSJ) 2019;24:1. https://search.ebscohost.com/login.aspx?direct=true&AuthType=ip,shib&db=edb&AN=141950715&site=eds-live&scope=site&custid=wgc1.

[64] Tong VT, Dietz PM, Morrow B, D'Angelo DV, Rarr SL, Rockhill KM, England LJ. Trends in smoking before, during, and after pregnancy: pregnancy risk assessment monitoring system, United States, 40 sites, 2000–2010. Morb Mortal Wkly Rep - Surveillance Summ 2013;62(6):1–19.

[65] Hand DJ, Ellis JD, Carr MM, Abatemarco DJ, Ledgerwood DM. Contingency management interventions for tobacco and other substance use disorders in pregnancy. Psychol Addict Behav 2017;31(8):907–21. https://doi.org/10.1037/adb0000291.

[66] Albuquerque CA, Smith KR, Johnson C, Chao R, Harding R. Influence of maternal tobacco smoking during pregnancy on uterine, umbilical, and fetal cerebral artery blood flows. Early Hum Dev 2004;80:31–42.

[67] Higgins ST, Heil SH, Solomon LJ, Bernstein IM, Lussier JP, Abel RL, Lynch ME, Badger GJ. A pilot study on voucher-based incentives to promote abstinence from cigarette smoking during pregnancy and postpartum. Nicotine Tob Res 2004;6(6): 1015–20. https://doi.org/10.1080/14622200412331324910.

[68] Dempsey DA, Benowitz NL. Risks and benefits of nicotine to aid smoking cessation in pregnancy. Drug Safety 2001;24(4):277–322. https://search.ebscohost.com/login.aspx?direct=true&AuthType=ip,shib&db=mnh&AN=11330657&site=eds-live&scope=site&custid=wgc1.

[69] Federal Drug Administration. Fda's postmarketing review of varenicline and bupropion. React Wkly 2009;1236:3. Retrieved 01/24/, from, https://search.ebscohost.com/login.aspx?direct=true&AuthType=ip,shib&db=edb&AN=36289659&site=eds-live&scope=site&custid=wgc1.

[70] Pollock M, Lee J. The smoking cessation aids varenicline (marketed as chantix) and bupropion (marketed as zyban and generics). 2010. http://www.fda.gov/downloads/Drugs/DrugSafety/DrugSafetyNewsletter/UCM107318.pdf.

[71] Chan KT, Trant J. The relationship of psychological distress and living with children and adolescents for adult non-medical prescription opioid users [Article] Child Adolesc Soc Work J 2018;35(4):391–405. https://doi.org/10.1007/s10560-018-0534-8.

[72] Green KM, Zebrak KA, Robertson JA, Fothergill KE, Ensminger ME. Interrelationship of substance use and psychological distress over the life course among a cohort of urban African Americans. Drug Alcohol Depend 2012;123(1):239–48. https://doi.org/10.1016/j.drugalcdep.2011.11.017.

[73] Gyawali B, Choulagai BP, Paneru DP, Ahmad M, Leppin A, Kallestrup P. Prevalence and correlates of psychological distress symptoms among patients with substance use disorders in drub rehabilitation centers in urban Nepal: a cross-sectional study. BMC Psychiatr 2016;16:314–23. https://doi.org/10.1186/s12888-016-1003-6.

[74] Martin PR, Arria AM, Fischer G, Kaltenbach K, Heil SH, Stine SM, Coyle MG, Selby P, Jones HE. Psychopharmacologic management of opioid-dependent women during pregnancy [Article] Am J Addict 2009;18(2):148−56. https://doi.org/10.1080/10550490902772975.

[75] Bridge TP, Fudala PJ, Herbert S, Leiderman DB. Safety and health policy considerations related to the use of buprenorphine/naloxone as an office-based treatment for opiate dependence [Review Article] Drug Alcohol Depend 2003;70(2):S79−85. https://doi.org/10.1016/S0376-8716(03)00061-9.

[76] Deshmukh SV, Nanovskaya TN, Ahmed MS. Aromatase is the major enzyme metabolizing buprenorphine in human placenta. J Pharmacol Exp Therapeut 2003;306(3):1099−105. https://search.ebscohost.com/login.aspx?direct=true&AuthType=ip,shib&db=mnh&AN=12808001&site=eds-live&scope=site&custid=wgc1.

[77] American Academy of Pediatrics. AAP reports breast-feeding by mothers on methadone preferred over infant withdrawal syndrome [Article] Brown Univ Child & Adolesc Psychopharmacol Update 2013;15(10):4. https://search.ebscohost.com/login.aspx?direct=true&AuthType=ip,shib&db=aqh&AN=90402997&site=eds-live&scope=site&custid=wgc1.

[78] Marquet P, Chevrel J, Lavignasse P, Merle L, Lachâtre G. Buprenorphine withdrawal syndrome in a newborn. Clin Pharmacol Ther 1997;62(5):569−71. https://search.ebscohost.com/login.aspx?direct=true&AuthType=ip,shib&db=mnh&AN=9390114&site=eds-live&scope=site&custid=wgc1.

[79] Lavely E, Love H, Shelton M, Nichols TR. Methadone use and pregnancy: lessons learned from developing a reproductive health program for women in drug treatment [Article] Int J Childbirth Educ 2018;33(2):9−12. https://search.ebscohost.com/login.aspx?direct=true&AuthType=ip,shib&db=awh&AN=130741708&site=eds-live&scope=site&custid=wgc1.

[80] Wang MJ, Kuper SG, Sims B, Paddock CS, Dantzler J, Muir S, Harper LM. Opioid detoxification in pregnancy: systematic review and meta-analysis of perinatal outcomes. Am J Perinatol 2019;36(6):581−7. https://doi.org/10.1055/s-0038-1670680.

[81] Gomez Pomar E, Finnegan LP, Devlin L, Bada H, Concina VA, Ibonia KT, Westgate PM. Simplification of the finnegan neonatal abstinence scoring system: retrospective study of two institutions in the USA. BMJ Open 2017;7(9):e016176. https://doi.org/10.1136/bmjopen-2017-016176.

[82] Broussard CS, Rasmussen SA, Reefhuis J, Friedman JM, Jann MW, Riehle-Colarusso T, Honein MA. Maternal treatment with opioid analgesics and risk for birth defects [Article] Am J Obstet Gynecol 2011;204(4). https://doi.org/10.1016/j.ajog.2010.12.039. 314-314.

[83] Hamilton R. Ophthalmic, clinical and visual electrophysiological findings in children born to mothers prescribed substitute methadone in pregnancy [Article] Br J Ophthalmol 2010;94(6):696−700. https://doi.org/10.1136/bjo.2009.169284.

[84] Crume TL, Juhl AL, Brooks-Russell A, Hall KE, Wymore E, Borgelt LM. Cannabis use during the perinatal period in a state with legalized recreational and medical marijuana: the association between maternal characteristics, breastfeeding patterns, and neonatal outcomes [Article] J Pediatr 2018;197:90−6. https://doi.org/10.1016/j.jpeds.2018.02.005.

[85] Brown QL, Sarvet AL, Shmulewitz D, Martins SS, Wall MM, Hasin DS. Trends in marijuana use among pregnant and nonpregnant reproductive-aged women, 2002–2014. J Am Med Assoc 2017;317(2):207–9. https://doi.org/10.1001/jama.2016.17383.

[86] Corsi DJ, Hsu H, Weiss D, Fell DB, Walker M. Trends and correlates of cannabis use in pregnancy: a population-based study in Ontario, Canada from 2012 to 2017. Can J Public Health 2019;110(1):76–84. https://doi.org/10.17269/s41997-018-0148-0.

[87] Roncero C, Valriberas-Herrero I, Mezzatest-Gava M, Villegas JL, Aguilar L, Grau-Lopez L. Cannabis use during pregnancy and its relationship with fetal developmental outcomes and psychiatric disorders. A systematic review. Reprod Health 2020;17:1. https://doi.org/10.1186/s12978-020-0880-9.

[88] Henry JA, Oldfield WLG, Kon OM. Comparing cannabis with tobacco: smoking cannabis, like smoking tobacco, can be a major public health hazard [Research-article] BMJ Br Med J (Clin Res Ed) 2003;326(7396):942. https://search.ebscohost.com/login.aspx?direct=true&AuthType=ip,shib&db=edsjsr&AN=edsjsr.25454338&site=eds-live&scope=site&custid=wgc1.

[89] Ashton CH. Pharmacology and effects of cannabis: a brief review. Br J Psychiatr 2001; 178:101–6. https://doi.org/10.1192/bjp.178.2.101.

[90] Day NL, Goldschmidt L, Thomas CA. Prenatal marijuana exposure contributes to the prediction of marijuana use at age 14. Addiction 2006;101(9):1313–22. https://doi.org/10.1111/j.1360-0443.2006.01523.x.

[91] Gray TR, Eiden RD, Leonard KE, Connors GJ, Shisler S, Huestis MA. Identifying pre-natal cannabis exposure and effects of concurrent tobacco exposure on neonatal growth. Clin Chem 2010;56(9):1442–50. https://doi.org/10.1373/clinchem.2010.147876.

[92] Lester BM, ElSohly M, Wright LL, Smeriglio VL, Verter J, Bauer CR, Shankaran S, Bada HS, Walls HC, Huestis MA, Finnegan LP, Maza PL. The maternal lifestyle study: drug use by meconium toxicology and maternal self-report. Pediatrics 2001;107(2):309–17. https://doi.org/10.1542/peds.107.2.309.

[93] dos Santos JF, de Melo Bastos Cavalcante C, Barbosa FT, Gitaí DLG, Duzzioni M, Tilelli CQ, Shetty AK, de Castro OW. Maternal, fetal and neonatal consequences asso-ciated with the use of crack cocaine during the gestational period: a systematic review and meta-analysis. Arch Gynecol Obstet 2018;298(3):487–503. https://doi.org/10.1007/s00404-018-4833-2.

[94] Hudak ML, Tan RC, The Committee on Drugs and the Committee on Fetus and Newborn. Neonatal drug withdrawal. Pediatrics 2012;129(2):e540. https://doi.org/10.1542/peds.2011-3212.

[95] Burkett G, Bandstra ES, Cohen J, Steele B, Palow D. Cocaine-related maternal death. Am J Obstet Gynecol 1990;163(1 Pt 1):40–1. https://search.ebscohost.com/login.aspx?direct=true&AuthType=ip,shib&db=mnh&AN=2375369&site=eds-live&scope=site&custid=wgc1.

[96] Johnson BA. Recent advances in the development of treatments for alcohol and cocaine dependence: focus on topiramate and other modulators of gaba or glutamate function. CNS Drugs 2005;19(10):873–96. https://search.ebscohost.com/login.aspx?direct=true&AuthType=ip,shib&db=sph&AN=18855551&site=eds-live&scope=site&custid=wgc1.

[97] Czeizel AE, Tomcsik M, Tímár L. Teratologic evaluation of 178 infants born to mothers who attempted suicide by drugs during pregnancy. Obstet Gynecol 1997; 90(2):195−201. https://search.ebscohost.com/login.aspx?direct=true&AuthType=ip, shib&db=mnh&AN=9241292&site=eds-live&scope=site&custid=wgc1.

[98] NIDA. Methamphetamine research report: overview. July 20, 2020. https://www.drugabuse.gov/publications/research-reports/methamphetamine/overview.

[99] Kratofil PH, Baberg HT, Dimsdale JE. Self-mutilation and severe self-injurious behavior associated with amphetamine psychosis. Gen Hosp Psychiatr 1996;18(2): 117−20. https://doi.org/10.1016/0163-8343(95)00126-3.

[100] Won L, Bubula N, McCoy H, Heller A. Methamphetamine concentrations in fetal and maternal brain following prenatal exposure [Article] Neurotoxicol Teratol 2001;23(4): 349−54. https://doi.org/10.1016/S0892-0362(01)00151-9.

[101] Chomchai C, Chomchai S, Kitsommart R. Transfer of methamphetamine (ma) into breast milk and urine of postpartum women who smoked ma tablets during pregnancy: implications for initiation of breastfeeding. J Hum Lactation: Off J Int Lactation Consul Assoc 2016;32(2):333−9. https://doi.org/10.1177/0890334415610080.

[102] Jansson LM. Abm clinical protocol #21: guidelines for breastfeeding and the drug-dependent woman. Breastfeed Med 2009;4(4):225−8. https://doi.org/10.1089/bfm.2009.9987.

[103] Diaz SD, Smith LM, LaGasse LL, Derauf C, Newman E, Shah R, Arria A, Huestis MA, Della Grotta S, Dansereau LM, Neal C, Lester BM. Effects of prenatal methamphetamine exposure on behavioral and cognitive findings at 7.5 years of age [Article] J Pediatr 2014;164(6):1333−8. https://doi.org/10.1016/j.jpeds.2014.01.053.

[104] Heinzerling KG, Shoptaw S, Peck JA, Yang X, Liu J, Roll J, Ling W. Randomized, placebo-controlled trial of baclofen and gabapentin for the treatment of methamphetamine dependence [Article] Drug Alcohol Depend 2006;85(3):177−84. https://doi.org/10.1016/j.drugalcdep.2006.03.019.

[105] Andrade C. Adverse gestational outcomes associated with attention-deficit/hyperactivity disorder medication exposure during pregnancy. J Clin Psychiatr 2018;79(1). https://doi.org/10.4088/JCP.18f12136.

[106] Samenuk D, Link MS, Homoud MK, Contreras R, Theohardes TC, Wang PJ, Estes IIINAM. Adverse cardiovascular events temporally associated with ma huang, an herbal source of ephedrine [Article] Mayo Clin Proc 2002;77(1):12−6. https://doi.org/10.4065/77.1.12.

[107] Ling-Yi F, Battulga A, Eunyoung H, Heesun C, Jih-Heng L. New psychoactive substances of natural origin: a brief review [Article] J Food Drug Anal 2017;25(3): 461−71. https://doi.org/10.1016/j.jfda.2017.04.001.

[108] Hassen K. Khat (*Catha edulis*) chewing as a risk factor of low birth weight among full term newborns: a systematic review [Article] Middle East J Fam Med 2015;13(7): 10−4. https://search.ebscohost.com/login.aspx?direct=true&AuthType=ip,shib&db=a9h&AN=110461398&site=eds-live&scope=site&custid=wgc1.

[109] Long SY. Does LSD induce chromosomal damage and malformations? A review of the literature. Teratology 1972;6(1):75−90. https://search.ebscohost.com/login.aspx?direct=true&AuthType=ip,shib&db=mnh&AN=4626857&site=eds-live&scope=site&custid=wgc1.

[110] Preece PM, Riley EP. Alcohol, drugs and medication in pregnancy: The long-term outcome for the child [Book]. Mac Keith Press; 2011. https://search.ebscohost.com/login.aspx?direct=true&AuthType=ip,shib&db=nlebk&AN=511508&site=eds-live&scope=site&custid=wgc1.

[111] Fishbein DH. Female PCP-using jail detainees: proneness to violence and gender differences [Article] Addict Behav 1996;21(2):155−72. https://doi.org/10.1016/0306-4603(96)00049-4.

[112] Ling LH, Marchant C, Buckley NA, Prior M, Irvine RJ. Poisoning with the recreational drug paramethoxyamphetamine ("death"). Med J Aust 2001;174(9):453−5. https://search.ebscohost.com/login.aspx?direct=true&AuthType=ip,shib&db=mnh&AN=11386590&site=eds-live&scope=site&custid=wgc1.

[113] Hartung TK, Schofield E, Short AI, Parr MJA, Henry JA. Hyponatraemic states following 3,4-methylenedioxymethamphetamine (MDMA, 'ecstasy') ingestion. QJM: Int J Med 2002;95(7):431−7. https://search.ebscohost.com/login.aspx?direct=true&AuthType=ip,shib&db=edo&AN=ejs4627818&site=eds-live&scope=site&custid=wgc1.

[114] McElhatton PR, Bateman DN, Evans C, Pughe KR, Thomas SH. Congenital anomalies after prenatal ecstasy exposure [Article] Lancet 1999;354(9188):1441−2. https://doi.org/10.1016/S0140-6736(99)02423-X.

[115] Miotto K, Davoodi P, Maya S. Gamma-hydroxybutyrate (GHB) and ketamine: effects and treatment of toxicity [Article] Adolesc Psychiatr 2005;29:149. https://search.ebscohost.com/login.aspx?direct=true&AuthType=ip,shib&db=aqh&AN=18809685&site=eds-live&scope=site&custid=wgc1.

[116] Rickert VI, Wiemann CM, Berenson AB. Prevalence, patterns, and correlates of voluntary flunitrazepam use. Pediatrics 1999;103(1):E6. https://search.ebscohost.com/login.aspx?direct=true&AuthType=ip,shib&db=mnh&AN=9917486&site=eds-live&scope=site&custid=wgc1.

[117] Klafta JM, Zacny JP, Young CJ. Neurological and psychiatric adverse effects of anaesthetics: epidemiology and treatment. Drug Safety 1995;13(5):281−95. https://search.ebscohost.com/login.aspx?direct=true&AuthType=ip,shib&db=mnh&AN=8785016&site=eds-live&scope=site&custid=wgc1.

[118] Weiner AL, Vieira L, McKay CA, Bayer MJ. Ketamine abusers presenting to the emergency department: a case series [Article] J Emerg Med 2000;18(4):447−51. https://doi.org/10.1016/S0736-4679(00)00162-1.

[119] Chrysanthy I, Friederike B, Michael M, Petra B, Jessica V, Krikor D, Tanya IT, Vanya S, Lechoslaw T, John WO. Blockade of NMDA receptors and apoptotic neurodegeneration in the developing brain [Research-article] Science 1999;283(5398):70. https://search.ebscohost.com/login.aspx?direct=true&AuthType=ip,shib&db=edsjsr&AN=edsjsr.2897193&site=eds-live&scope=site&custid=wgc1.

[120] Peles E, Adelson M. Gender differences and pregnant women in a methadone maintenance treatment (MMT) clinic. J Addict Dis 2006;25(2):39−45. https://search.ebscohost.com/login.aspx?direct=true&AuthType=ip,shib&db=cin20&AN=106272935&site=eds-live&scope=site&custid=wgc1.

[121] American College of Obstetricians and Gynecologists. Toolkit on state legislation: pregnant women and prescription drug abuse, dependence and addiction. Obstet Gynecol 2017. https://www.acog.org/-/media/Departments/Government-Relations-and-Outreach/NASToolkit.pdf.

[122] Armstrong MA, Gonzales Osejo V, Lieberman L, Carpenter DM, Pantoja PM, Escobar GJ. Perinatal substance abuse intervention in obstetric clinics decreases adverse neonatal outcomes [Article] J Perinatol 2003;23(1):3. https://doi.org/10.1038/sj.jp.7210847.

[123] Subbaraman MS, Thomas S, Treffers R, Delucchi K, Kerr WC, Martinez P, Roberts SCM. Associations between state-level policies regarding alcohol use among pregnant women, adverse birth outcomes, and prenatal care utilization: results from 1972 to 2013 vital statistics. Alcohol Clin Exp Res 2018. https://doi.org/10.1111/acer.13804.

[124] Grekin ER, Svikis DS, Lam P, Connors V, LeBreton JM, Streiner DL, Smith C, Ondersma SJ. Drug use during pregnancy: validating the drug abuse screening test against physiological measures. Psychol Addict Behav 2010;24(4):719–23. https://doi.org/10.1037/a0021741.

[125] Chasnoff IJ, Landress HJ, Barrett ME. Prevalence of illicit-drug or alcohol use during pregnancy and discrepancies in mandatory reporting in pinellas county, Florida, vol. 322; 1990. p. 1202–6. https://search.ebscohost.com/login.aspx?direct=true&AuthType=ip,shib&db=ncj&AN=SM155863&site=eds-live&scope=site&custid=wgc1.

[126] Goler NC, Armstrong MA, Taillac CJ, Osejo VM. Substance abuse treatment linked with prenatal visits improves perinatal outcomes: a new standard [Article] J Perinatol 2008;28(9):597–603. https://doi.org/10.1038/jp.2008.70.

[127] Klawans MR, Northrup TF, Villarreal YR, Berens PD, Blackwell S, Bunag T, Stotts AL. A comparison of common practices for identifying substance use during pregnancy in obstetric clinics. Birth Issues Perinat Care 2019;46(4):663. https://search.ebscohost.com/login.aspx?direct=true&AuthType=ip,shib&db=edb&AN=139725114&site=eds-live&scope=site&custid=wgc1.

[128] Moeller KE, Lee KC, Kissack JC. Urine drug screening: practical guide for clinicians [Review article] Mayo Clin Proc 2008;83(1):66–76. https://doi.org/10.1016/S0025-6196(11)61120-8.

[129] Hubbard RL, French MT. New perspectives on the benefit-cost and cost-effectiveness of drug abuse treatment. NIDA Res Monogr 1991;113:94–113. https://search.ebscohost.com/login.aspx?direct=true&AuthType=ip,shib&db=mnh&AN=1762645&site=eds-live&scope=site&custid=wgc1.

[130] Chasnoff IJ, Wells AM, McGourty RF, Bailey LK. Validation of the 4p's plus© screen for substance use in pregnancy validation of the 4p's plus [Article] J Perinatol 2007;27(12):744–8. https://doi.org/10.1038/sj.jp.7211823.

[131] Oga ES, Peters EN, Mark K, Trocin K, Coleman-Cowger VH. Prenatal substance use and perceptions of parent and partner use using the 4p's plus screener. Matern Child Health J 2019;23:250–7. https://doi.org/10.1007/s10995-018-2647-2.

[132] Burns E, Gray R, Smith LA. Brief screening questionnaires to identify problem drinking during pregnancy: a systematic review [Article] Addiction 2010;105(4):601–14. https://doi.org/10.1111/j.1360-0443.2009.02842.x.

[133] Chan AWK, Pristach EA, Welte JW, Russell M. Use of the tweak test in screening for alcoholism/heavy drinking in three populations. Alcohol Clin Exp Res 1993;17(6): 1188−92. https://doi.org/10.1111/j.1530-0277.1993.tb05226.x.

[134] Bernstein J, Bernstein E, Tassiopoulos K, Heeren T, Levenson S, Hingson R. Brief motivational intervention at a clinic visit reduces cocaine and heroin use [Article] Drug Alcohol Depend 2005;77(1):49−59. https://doi.org/10.1016/j.drugalcdep.2004.07.006.

[135] Babor TF. A cross-national trial of brief interventions with heavy drinkers [Article] Am J Publ Health 1996;86(7). https://doi.org/10.2105/AJPH.86.7.948. 948-948.

[136] Blow FC, Walton MA, Bohnert ASB, Ignacio RV, Chermack S, Cunningham RM, Booth BM, Ilgen M, Barry KL. A randomized controlled trial of brief interventions to reduce drug use among adults in a low-income urban emergency department: the healthier you study [Article] Addiction 2017;112(8):1395−405. https://doi.org/10.1111/add.13773.

[137] Sharma M. Alcohol use in women of childbearing age: implications for practice [Editorial] J Alcohol Drug Educ 2014;58(1):3−6. https://search.ebscohost.com/login.aspx?direct=true&AuthType=ip,shib&db=eft&AN=97519700&site=eds-live&scope=site&custid=wgc1.

[138] Miller WR. Motivational enhancement therapy manual: a clinical research guide for therapists treating individuals with alcohol abuse and dependence. U.S. Dept. of Health and Human Services, Public Health Service, National Institutes of Health, National Institute on Alcohol Abuse and Alcoholism; 1995. https://search.ebscohost.com/login.aspx?direct=true&AuthType=ip,shib&db=cat06551a&AN=wga.993506544602961&site=eds-live&scope=site&custid=wgc1.

[139] Singh K, Srivastava P, Chahal S. Application of motivational enhancement therapy in group settings among patients with substance abuse. Indian J Psychiatr Soc Work 2019;10(1):22−7. https://doi.org/10.29120/IJPSW.2019.v10.i1.105.

[140] Xu X, Yonkers KA, Ruger JP, Xu X. Economic evaluation of a behavioral intervention versus brief advice for substance use treatment in pregnant women: results from a randomized controlled trial. BMC Pregnancy Childbirth 2017;17:1. https://search.ebscohost.com/login.aspx?direct=true&AuthType=ip,shib&db=edb&AN=121676175&site=eds-live&scope=site&custid=wgc1.

[141] Fergie L, Campbell KA, Coleman-Haynes T, Ussher M, Cooper S, Coleman T. Identifying effective behavior change techniques for alcohol and illicit substance use during pregnancy: a systematic review. Ann Behav Med 2019;53(8):769. https://search.ebscohost.com/login.aspx?direct=true&AuthType=ip,shib&db=edb&AN=137542269&site=eds-live&scope=site&custid=wgc1.

[142] Prochaska JO, DiClemente CC, Norcross JC. In search of how people change. Applications to addictive behaviors. Am Psychol 1992;47(9):1102−14. https://search.ebscohost.com/login.aspx?direct=true&AuthType=ip,shib&db=mnh&AN=1329589&site=eds-live&scope=site&custid=wgc1.

Diabetes in pregnancy

15

Kimberly K. Trout[1], Cara D. Dolin[2]

[1]*Department of Family and Community Health, University of Pennsylvania, School of Nursing, Philadelphia, PA, United States;* [2]*Department of Obstetrics and Gynecology, University of Pennsylvania, Perelman School of Medicine, Philadelphia, PA, United States*

15.1 Introduction

Pregnancy imposes unique metabolic demands to provide sustained and sufficient transfer of nutrients to the growing fetus during fasting periods by ensuring adequate nutrient storage during feeding. Hormones produced by the feto-placental unit play a pivotal role in adjusting metabolic features to benefit both mother and fetus. However, in pregnancies complicated by diabetes mellitus (DM), its metabolic consequences for both mother and fetus can be exacerbated by the otherwise adaptive effects of pregnancy per se [1]. The effect of DM on the fetus is determined by two factors: the intrauterine environment provided by the mother and the fetal response to it. Tight glycemic control with exogenous insulin and, to a lesser extent, with oral hypoglycemic drugs, can markedly improve maternal and perinatal outcomes. Evidence from the international, multicentered HAPO study revealed that even mild maternal hyperglycemia can result in poor perinatal outcomes, thus highlighting the importance of maternal treatment [2]. This chapter reviews the clinical diagnosis and effects of a pregnancy affected by diabetes with a focus on therapeutics.

15.2 Epidemiology

Pregestational DM is increasingly prevalent worldwide, principally due to an increase in type 2 diabetes associated with obesity and increasing maternal age. Globally, gestational diabetes mellitus (GDM) is one of the most common complications of pregnancy, with prevalence ranging up to 30% in some countries. Risk factors for GDM include advanced maternal age, geography and ethnicity, modifiable lifestyle factors, and genetics [3]. GDM has the lowest prevalence in Europe (6%), the highest prevalence in the Middle East, some North African countries, and some countries in Southeast Asia (median of 15% of pregnancies). In the United States, the overall prevalence of GDM is approximately 6% [4]. The United States, and other countries with multiracial and multiethnic populations, see a large difference in prevalence between racial and ethnic groups, with higher prevalence in

Clinical Pharmacology During Pregnancy. https://doi.org/10.1016/B978-0-12-818902-3.00005-1

Asian, Latina, and African-Africans when compared with non-Hispanic whites [3]. Findings from genetic studies are inconsistent, although a systematic review and metaanalysis found that the minor alleles of nine single-nucleotide polymorphisms in seven genes involved in regulating insulin secretion were involved in the pathogenesis of GDM. In a genome-wide association study performed in an Asian population, two genetic variants, rs10830962 (near MTRNR1B) and rs7754840 (in CDKA1) were linked with GDM diagnosis [3,5]. However, noting that there has not been a substantial change in the gene pool, modifiable risk factors, such as a Westernized diet, physical activity, and other lifestyle factors, are thought to be largely responsible for the increase in DM that is being seen today [6].

15.3 Classification

Outside of pregnancy, diabetes is classified according to its pathophysiology [7]. Broadly, type 1 DM is due to absolute insulin lack, most commonly due to immune destruction of β-cells, while type 2 DM is characterized by progressive insulin resistance, which leads initially to compensatory hyperinsulinemia, and then to defective insulin secretion as well. While treatment of type 1 DM requires insulin replacement, many type 2 DM patients will also be treated with insulin as adjunctive or primary therapy; thus, the terms insulin-dependent [8] and noninsulin-dependent DM [8] should no longer be used. During pregnancy, women can be categorized as those who were known to have DM prior to pregnancy—pregestational or overt— and those diagnosed during the latter half of pregnancy with GDM [9].

Screening and diagnosis of GDM can be performed by either the one-step approach, a 75 g 2-h oral glucose tolerance test (OGTT) or the two-step approach, a 50 g 1-h screening OGTT followed by the 100 g 3 h diagnostic OGTT, if needed. The American Diabetes Association (ADA) and the American College of Obstetricians and Gynecologists (ACOG) are in agreement that both one-step and two-step OGTT for GDM are acceptable [9,10]. HgbA1C testing for GDM diagnosis is not recommended at this time as there is limited evidence on interpretation and clinical use in pregnancy, as HgbA1C values in pregnancy will be lower than for nonpregnant individuals, primarily due to more rapid red blood cell turnover in pregnancy [9]. The prevalence of GDM differs based on test choice. While the two-step method is typically used in the United States, if the one-step test were applied consistently across the United States, the prevalence of GDM would increase to approximately 18% of pregnancies [10]. Notably, first trimester testing in pregnancy is *not* to test for GDM. The purpose of first trimester testing is to detect previously undiagnosed *overt* diabetes (either type 1 or type 2). For this reason, HgbA1C is an acceptable test for diabetes diagnosis in the first trimester, as well as other endorsed methods for diagnosing diabetes in the nonpregnant population (fasting plasma glucose, random plasma glucose, or 75 g, 2 h glucose tolerance test) [9]. Women who are overweight (BMI ≥ 25 kg/m^2 [9] or obese BMI ≥ 30 kg/m^2) [10] should receive this testing in the first trimester, as well as women with other risk factors for diabetes, such as a family history of diabetes in a first-degree relative, or a personal history of GDM in a previous pregnancy.

Some women who have been classified as having GDM actually have had pregestational DM that had not come to clinical recognition before the more attentive medical evaluation that accompanies antenatal care; ACOG [11] has recently shifted toward the importance of differentiating between gestational and pregestational DM, as advocated by the Expert Committee on the Diagnosis and Classification of Diabetes [7] and away from the White classification [12], which focused on classifying women by the type and severity of diabetic target organ damage.

Pregnancy is associated with resistance to the glucose-lowering effects of insulin resulting in relative postprandial hyperglycemia. It is thought that the endocrine effects of the feto-placental unit play an important role in the development of insulin resistance during pregnancy [13,14]. In fact, pregnant women experience less hypoglycemia in response to exogenous insulin but more fasting hypoglycemia than nonpregnant women [15], and normal pregnant women have exaggerated insulin responses to glucose ingestion compared to nonpregnant women [16]. It is estimated that in healthy pregnant women insulin sensitivity decreases by 40%−56% during the third trimester [17].

To compensate, pregnancy is characterized by an adaptive increase in pancreatic β-cell function [18] that also leads to maternal pancreatic hypertrophy and hyperplasia [19]. GDM results when insulin resistance exceeds the capacity to increase insulin secretion. The absolute or relative insulin deficiency which characterizes type 1 and type 2 DM, respectively, precludes normal pancreatic β-cell compensation during pregnancy, resulting in maternal hyperglycemia sufficient to impact fetal development unless adequate exogenous insulin is provided. Although patients with type 1 DM usually have normal insulin sensitivity when nonpregnant, the insulin resistance of pregnancy leads to a substantial (1.5- to 3-fold) increase in their insulin requirements [20]. Patients with type 2 DM have striking pregestational insulin resistance, leading to insulin requirements higher than women with type 1 DM [21]. Insulin requirements increase throughout gestation until near the end of the third trimester, paralleling the rise in insulin resistance; following birth, they are decreased markedly [20].

15.4 Gestational diabetes

GDM may be mild or may present with more severe hyperglycemia. Women with GDM but without fasting hyperglycemia usually revert to euglycemia following delivery. However, they carry an ∼50% risk of developing DM [22] during the first 5−10 years following an affected pregnancy [23,24]. Women with GDM appear to have underlying (and often, previously unrecognized) insulin resistance that is exacerbated by the additive insulin resistance due to pregnancy [25].

Obesity further increases insulin resistance in many women whose pregnancies are complicated by GDM [26]. Since both insulin resistance and impaired compensatory β-cell function are usually required to manifest either type 2 DM or GDM, it is not surprising that maternal hyperglycemia is associated with insufficient insulin secretion in GDM [27].

15.5 Diabetes management in pregnancy

15.5.1 Nutritional goals and exercise

Lifestyle modifications, including both healthful eating and increased physical activity, remain the first-line therapy for newly diagnosed GDM. Approximately 75%−80% of women diagnosed with GDM can by managed with lifestyle modifications alone [9]. Encouraging well-balanced meals with fresh vegetables and fruits (such as is found in the Mediterranean diet) and a caloric intake that supports Academy of Medicine (formerly Institute of Medicine) weight gain guidelines help to ensure adequate nutrition for fetal growth and maternal health [28].

The dietary reference intake (DRI) for carbohydrates in pregnancy is 175 g/day, the minimal requirement to assure adequate glucose to meet fetal and maternal needs. The DRI for protein is 71 g/day and for fiber, 28 g/day [9]. However, there is not definitive evidence regarding the optimal diet for women with GDM; individualized instructions regarding calorie/carbohydrate recommendations are ideally made in consultation with a Registered Dietician. Since carbohydrates are the macronutrients that have the greatest effect on postprandial blood glucose levels, women are usually advised to monitor carbohydrates more closely than other macronutrients, following an eating plan of approximately 30%−40% complex carbohydrates, eliminating simple sugars, 20% protein, and 40% fats [10]. ACOG notes that a diet consisting of 50%−60% carbohydrate levels often results in excessive weight gain and poor glucose control [10]. To prevent large blood glucose "excursions" (wide fluctuations in BG), three meals a day with two to three snacks are advised, with carbohydrates spaced out between the meals and snacks. If women are not achieving target glucose levels consistently (meeting less than 70% of blood glucose goals) after 1 week of dietary treatment, pharmacologic therapy may be indicated. One important component of nutrition therapy is the provision of an evening snack consisting of approximately 15−30 g carbohydrate. An overnight fast should not exceed 10 h, as prolonged fasting could result in a surge in counterregulatory hormones with a subsequent elevation of fasting glucose.

15.5.1.1 Physical activity

Unless otherwise contraindicated, healthful nutrition should be combined with regular exercise. Thirty minutes of moderate-intensity aerobic exercise at least 5 days per week (for a minimum of 150 min per week) is recommended [10]. Daily simple exercise such as walking, yoga, tai chi, or riding a stationary bike can help to normalize and stabilize BG levels; in some cases, the addition of daily routine physical activity has eliminated the need for medication. For women with sedentary occupations, taking hourly short breaks to stand up and stretch has also reduced backaches and fatigue and contributed to overall improved sense of well-being [29−31].

15.5.2 Glucose monitoring and glycemic control

Monitoring of capillary blood glucose 4−6 times/day, including fasting, preprandial, and postprandial values, is central to tight management for all types of DM during pregnancy. Treatment goals for blood glucose control are as follows: fasting <95 mg/dL, 1 h postprandial <140 mg/dL, and 2 h postprandial <120 mg/dL [32]. Women treated only with lifestyle modifications or with stable and optimal glycemic control may be able to monitor less frequently. For women with type 1 or type 2 diabetes, who are often advised to test even more frequently, the use of continuous glucose monitoring systems (CGMSs) has been especially beneficial in facilitating blood glucose control. The CONCEPTT randomized trial found that CGM use in women with type 1 diabetes in pregnancy resulted in improvements in HgbA1C without an increase in either maternal or neonatal hypoglycemia and with a reduction in large-for-gestational age (LGA) infants [33]. However, studies have also found that CGMS is not as reliable at low blood glucose levels due to shifts in interstitial fluid that occur during pregnancy. Additionally, when blood glucose is rapidly rising or falling (for all individuals, pregnant or nonpregnant), there is a lag time in interstitial fluid values when compared with capillary blood glucose [34]. Therefore, patients are urged to check glucose with capillary blood testing when experiencing symptoms of hypoglycemia or when it is suspected that blood glucose values are rapidly rising or falling.

The use of Smartphone technology has increased the ease of recording blood glucose results. There are several phone Apps available that interface with CGMS and Flash technology (such as the Dexcom and the Abbott systems). These may be especially helpful to clinicians as well, making it much easier to track patients' BG results, preventing the "I forgot my blood glucose log" statement heard sometimes at prenatal care visits.

Tight glycemic control is essential to improve outcomes in all women, whether with severe DM, mild DM, or GDM [35,36]. Despite the variety of effective therapies for DM during pregnancy, treatment barriers persist. There are particular challenges to instituting insulin therapy in pregnant women with DM, in that it is important to control hyperglycemia quickly, yet opportunities for patient education and insulin titration are limited.

15.5.3 Insulin therapy

Exogenous insulin therapy attempts to use glucose monitoring−guided dose adjustment of long and short acting (SA) insulin analogs to mimic the normal profile of insulin in response to diet and metabolic demands in order to maintain euglycemia. Insulin therapy is currently recommended for nearly all women with pregestational diabetes during pregnancy and for women with GDM who fail to achieve glycemic control with diet. Insulin therapy will usually require separate insulin analogs and dosing strategies to mimic the normal basal secretion of insulin as well as the rapid and transient β-cell response to meals. In most women without gastroparesis, essentially all nutrients are absorbed within 90 min after a meal and both plasma glucose and insulin return to premeal values within 2 h [12]. Endogenous insulin is secreted largely from the pancreas into the portal circulation with hepatic extraction of ∼50% [37]. Insulin concentrations in the portal vein exceed those in arterial plasma by approximately threefold. In healthy adults, the rate of basal insulin secretion into the portal system is ∼1 unit/h. With the intake of food, the rate increases by 5—10-fold [37]. Insulin acts in the liver by prompt and efficient inhibition of glycogenolysis [37], beginning within minutes and reaching full effect within hours [38]. Secondarily and subsequently, insulin inhibits hepatic gluconeogenesis, principally by decreasing release and transport of free fatty acids and precursors from fat and skeletal muscle to the liver. The effect on gluconeogenesis is usually delayed and requires more insulin than the effect on glycogenolysis, due to its peripheral sites of action [37,39].

Insulin metabolism is, itself, altered during pregnancy, with 24% and 30% reductions in hepatic insulin extraction noted in women with type 1 DM and GDM, respectively, perhaps due to changes in hepatic blood flow [40,41]. Placental perfusion studies show that only minimal amounts (1%—5%) of maternal insulin is transferred into fetal circulation, likely due to its molecular weight of ∼5800 Da [42]. The fetal pancreas begins to develop at around 5 weeks gestational age, with all pancreatic cell types seen in the fetus by 9—10 weeks and the β-cells functional by 14 weeks. Chronic maternal hyperglycemia results in fetal islet cell hyperplasia and increased insulin secretion [43]. The risk of fetal macrosomia has been linked to high levels of insulin in cord blood and amniotic fluid [44].

Regular human insulin needs to be administered 30—45 min prior to meals to control postprandial hyperglycemia, though its peak effect occurs 2—4 h after injection, likely due to delayed absorption and leading, in some cases, to inadequate control followed by late postprandial hypoglycemia. The delayed absorption may be due to formation of insulin molecular clusters (hexamers) that dissociate slowly, limiting the rate of absorption of active insulin from the subcutaneous space into the systemic circulation [45]. The inconvenience associated with injecting human insulin half an hour prior to a meal often leads to poor compliance and suboptimal glycemic control [46]. These limitations of regular insulin led to the development of analogs with improved characteristics, including SA insulins with faster onset and clearance of long acting (LA) insulins with delayed and prolonged distribution resulting in low sustained levels. The different types of insulin used currently are listed in Table 15.1.

SA analogs attempt to mimic the rapid onset and disappearance of endogenous insulin around a meal.

Lispro and Aspart form hexamers that dissociate more rapidly so they can be administered immediately before or up to 15 min after starting meals. Their effect

Table 15.1 Insulin analogs and pharmacokinetics.

Type	Onset of action	Peak of action (hours)	Duration of action (hours)
[a]Afrezza (insulin inhaled powder)	1—12 min	0.5—1	1.5 (at dose of 4U) 4.5 (at dose of 48U)
Humalog (lispro)	1—15 min	1	2—4
NovoLog (aspart)	1—15 min	1	2—4
Regular insulin	30—60 min	2	4
Humulin N (NPH)	1—3 h	8	8
Lantus (glargine)	1 h	No peak	<24
Levemir (detemir)	3—4 h	No peak	12—24 h (dose dependent)

[a] *Limited data available for use in pregnancy.*

peaks after 1—2 h with peak concentrations twice that of regular insulin [47]. Severe hypoglycemic episodes are less common with SA insulins. Circulating levels of SA insulins mirror the rise and fall in serum glucose following an oral load, leading both to better control of postprandial glucose excursion and to fewer episodes of late postprandial hypoglycemia. Inhaled human insulin powder (Afrezza) has not been studied well in pregnancy, but the average pharmacodynamic profile with its quick onset of action and fast peak of action may make it a desirable choice for elevated postprandial BG levels. The shorter duration of action is potentially beneficial in preventing late postprandial hypoglycemia, although pharmacodynamics profiles can vary significantly by individuals when tested in a euglycemic clamp study [48].

Longer acting agents are needed to complement SA agents in order to mimic basal pancreatic insulin secretion, and maintain euglycemia without hypoglycemic episodes between meals and overnight. NPH (Neutral Protamine Hagedorn), an intermediate acting insulin, is usually administered at bedtime for women with GDM and high fasting blood glucose, but otherwise, normal postprandial BG values. For women with type 1 or type 2 DM, twice daily NPH injections provide 24 h glycemic control in concert with prandial SA insulin. Two LA insulin analogs are also used; glargine and detemir are insulin analogs containing stabilized hexamers that dissociate slowly, resulting in a stable monotonous basal profile decreasing the risk of fasting hypoglycemia [38,49]. LA agents are associated with decreased fasting glucose, HbA1c, and nocturnal hypoglycemia [50]. When compared to NPH insulin, LA agents had similar or lower rates of maternal microvascular morbidity, macrosomia, and neonatal hypoglycemia [51—53]. Placental perfusion studies using glargine and detemir demonstrated negligible placental transfer, and animal studies showed rates of teratogenicity and embryotoxicity similar to human insulin [54,55]. Besides influencing glucose metabolism, insulin acts to alter cellular proliferation, differentiation, and cell apoptosis. At higher concentrations, it promotes growth and proliferation via activation of receptors for insulin-like growth factor type I (IGF-I) [56]. Structural changes in the design of insulin analogs appear

Table 15.2 Daily insulin dose across trimesters for pregestational diabetes.

Gestational period (weeks)	Total daily dose (units/kg[a])
1–18	0.7
18–26	0.8
26–36	0.9
36–40	1
0–6 (postpartum)	0.4

[a] Based on actual weight.

to alter its affinity for IGF-1 receptors [57]. Indeed, glargine has a 6–8-fold increased affinity for IGF-1 receptors when compared to insulin in an osteosarcoma cell line [57]. Lispro has also been shown to have some increase in IGF-1 binding [58]. This interaction could potentially lead to increased fetal growth and other mitogenic effects, though there are no in vivo or clinical data to support these concerns. IGF-1 binding appears not to be increased for other insulin analogs.

Continuous subcutaneous insulin infusions (CSII-aka insulin pumps) deliver insulin in a pattern that closely resembles physiologic insulin secretion and may be used safely in pregnancy. Studies have described similar safety and efficiency as multiple injection therapy with use during pregnancy [59]. An SA insulin (either regular or lispro) is used, with 50%–60% of the total daily dose (which may be calculated as described in Table 15.2) given as the basal rate and the remaining 40%–50% given as premeal/snack boluses. Many women are reluctant to administer multiple insulin injections daily, resulting in limited adherence to treatment. The use of insulin pumps can be beneficial for women who have injection phobia, as infusion sets usually only need to be replaced once every 2–3 days, as opposed to needing multiple injections several times daily [60] Some closed-loop systems are able to temporarily reduce or cease basal insulin based on feedback from CGMS compatible with the pump [61]. However, with these closed-loop systems (FDA approved *outside* of pregnancy), the preset glucose targets of 120 mg/dL are too high for optimal nighttime control in pregnant women [9]. A Cochrane metaanalysis that included five randomized trials involving 153 pregnant women found no clear differences in the use of insulin pumps versus multiple daily injections for any of the reported outcomes (including cesarean section, LGA, perinatal mortality, weight gain during pregnancy, and blood glucose levels) [60].

Insulin requirements vary across trimesters and are illustrated in Table 15.2. Early in pregnancy (9–13 weeks), a decrease in insulin may be needed to adjust for decreased oral intake and vomiting, as well as evidence of enhanced insulin sensitivity in the first trimester [9]. After 14 weeks of gestation, insulin requirements begin to increase steadily (Table 15.2). Maternal obesity increases the insulin requirement by 0.1–0.2 units/kg. Fig. 15.1 illustrates a suggested protocol for insulin dosing during pregnancy and Fig. 15.2 illustrates a protocol for insulin adjustment. It is important to note that treatment-associated hypoglycemia is often

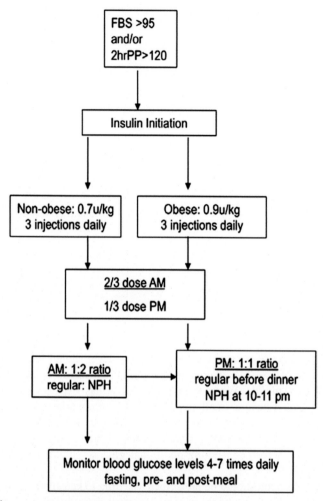

FIGURE 15.1

Insulin protocol during pregnancy. *2hrPP*, 2 h postprandial fingerstick glucose; *FBS*, fasting fingerstick glucose.

the rate-limiting factor in the ability to achieve tight glucose control, especially with type 1 DM where there is greater glucose variability [62]. Patients need to know the symptoms of and how to treat hypoglycemia (blood glucose < 70 mg/dL or blood glucose < 80 mg/dL with symptoms) [9]. These symptoms are shakiness, trembling, cool, clammy skin, anxiety, and/or tachycardia. As soon as hypoglycemic symptoms are noted, instruct the individual to ingest 15–20 g of a quickly absorbed source of glucose. Prompt ingestion of dextrose tablets or gel (available over the counter in most pharmacies), fruit juices, or hard candies should be available for immediate consumption and should always be kept nearby the individual with DM. 15 min after

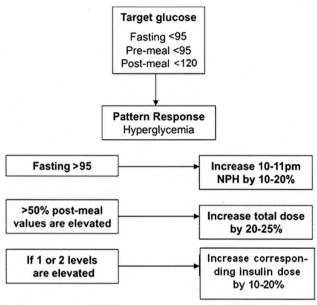

FIGURE 15.2

Insulin adjustment protocol.

ingestion of the glucose source, the blood glucose level should be rechecked. An additional intake of 15−20 g of glucose should be consumed if blood glucose is not higher than 90 mg/dL. When the blood glucose has risen to a normal value, the individual should have a small snack or meal that contains some protein and/ or fat which will help maintain the blood glucose at normal levels. It is also important to be aware of the risk of overtreatment, which is why a wait of 15 min is usually advised before consuming additional glucose subsequent to the initial dose of glucose [9,63].

Emergency glucagon should be prescribed as a drug to keep on hand for any person who takes a medication with the potential to cause hypoglycemia (insulin or oral sulfonylureas, such as glyburide). If a pregnant individual should become unconscious due to hypoglycemia (and this should not occur if oral treatment is initiated soon enough), there should be no attempt to give anything by mouth due to the risk of aspiration; in this instance, an emergency dose of glucagon could be lifesaving. Glucagon kits include emergency glucagon injection instructions and should be provided to partners/family members/close friends of persons with diabetes. Supportive family members should be taught how to administer glucagon in the event that they should find the individual with DM unconscious. In addition to injection kits, glucagon has recently become available in an inhaled form, with excellent results shown in a noninferiority study involving nonpregnant individuals [64]. Severe hypoglycemia (defined as requiring the assistance of another person for treatment) should be followed by an emergency 911 call for transport to the nearest hospital setting for appropriate follow-up. It is always important to try to identify why a hypoglycemic episode may have occurred. Although not always possible to identify the reason why, common etiologies might include a late meal or engaging in vigorous exercise with a "borderline" low blood glucose and not supplementing with a snack beforehand. Although it may not be entirely possible to prevent hypoglycemic episodes completely, determining why the "low blood glucose" occurred will help the individual prevent future occurrences [63].

15.5.4 Oral hypoglycemics

Oral agents are first-line therapy for type 2 DM outside of pregnancy [65]. In pregnancy, however, oral hypoglycemics should *not* be first-line treatment for hyperglycemia when diet and exercise fail to achieve treatment goals, primarily due to unknown long-term fetal effects. Sulfonylureas cross the placenta with concentrations of glyburide found in maternal cord plasma at 50%−70% of maternal levels [66].

Glyburide, a third-generation sulfonylurea oral hypoglycemic agent, acts primarily through specific receptors on the β-cell surface. Drug−receptor binding acts to close adenosine triphosphate-dependent potassium channels, resulting in cellular depolarization, calcium influx, and translocation of insulin secretory granules to the β-cell surface. The resulting release of insulin into the portal vein rapidly suppresses hepatic glucose production and later facilitates peripheral glucose use [67,68]. Insulin resistance commonly diminishes as a secondary result of the reversal of hyperglycemia [68,69]. Because sulfonylureas rely on a preserved β-cell response, they are ineffective in patients with absent or severely diminished β-cell function, as in type 1 DM or advanced type 2 DM. Sulfonylureas increase insulin secretion in direct proportion to plasma glucose levels from 60 to 180 mg/dL, with no effect if glucose is less that 60 mg/dL [70,71]. Despite these data, sulfonylureas, including glyburide, can still lead to symptomatic and severe hypoglycemia, most commonly in the setting of unrecognized renal insufficiency. There is then a minimal lag time between the changes in plasma glucose and the change in insulin secretion rate [72,73]. When given as a single agent, peak plasma glyburide concentrations are achieved within 4 h and absorption is not affected by food. Its elimination $t_{1/2}$ is approximately 10 h in nonpregnant adults and shorter in pregnancy due to increased clearance.

A pharmacokinetic−pharmacodynamic (PK−PD) [74] study of glyburide in 40 women with GDM receiving glyburide monotherapy, and controlled for fasting glucose concentration <95 mg/dL, described 50% lower dose-adjusted plasma drug concentrations in pregnancy, likely due to an increase in hepatic metabolism [75]. One might expect, therefore, that dose increases, perhaps beyond those in nonpregnant labeling might overcome increased glyburide clearance, resulting in better glycemic control. However, the glyburide dose−response relationship is uncertain and a ceiling effect may limit benefits due to higher doses. Indeed, studies in nonpregnant patients with type 2 DM suggest little incremental benefit following increased doses [76,77]. While glyburide normalized insulin secretion in women with GDM following a mixed meal in the glyburide PK—PD study, this was inadequate to compensate fully for their insulin resistance, manifest as imperfect control of postprandial hyperglycemia in those women [75]. A prior study had similarly demonstrated the challenges due to insulin resistance in women with GDM during insulin infusion [78]. Taken together, these results suggest that although some women with GDM may benefit from more aggressive glyburide dose titration, treatment in others may be improved by the use of additional or alternative agents to improve insulin resistance.

Studies of glyburide in pregnancy describe glycemic control and pregnancy outcomes similar to those of insulin in eligible women when dosing was adjusted frequently [55,79], starting at 2.5 mg in the morning titrating to a maximum dose, based on nonpregnant package labeling, of 10 mg twice a day [79]. However, almost 20% of women with GDM treated with glyburide will eventually require insulin therapy; granted, this may have been due to poor dose titration and switching to insulin prior to reaching maximal doses [80].

Neonatal hypoglycemia and macrosomia were seen more often with use of glyburide when compared with insulin or metformin, and long-term safety data for glyburide are not available [9].

Metformin is primarily an insulin sensitizer that reduces hepatic glucose production by suppressing gluconeogenesis [81,82]. It may also augment peripheral glucose uptake, though this may be secondary to reversal of hyperglycemia. Since it does not increase insulin secretion, the risk for hypoglycemia is minimal. Peak metformin plasma concentrations are achieved within 4 h of oral administration and administration with meals decreases drug-induced gastrointestinal discomfort, though it decreases absorption. Metformin's elimination $t_{1/2}$ in nonpregnant adults is approximately 6 h. Its renal clearance increases significantly in mid- and late gestation, in parallel with gestational increases in creatinine clearance [83]. Metformin crosses the placenta readily and has been found to sometimes be at higher levels in umbilical cord blood than maternal serum concentrations [84,85]. There is evidence of decreased neonatal hypoglycemia and less maternal weight gain with use of metformin. However, results of some long-term studies are concerning. One study found that 9-year-olds who had been exposed in utero to metformin were heavier and had a higher waist-to-height ratio and waist circumference than those exposed to insulin [86]. A metaanalysis found that metformin exposure in utero resulted in lower birthweight neonates who subsequently had accelerated postnatal growth and higher childhood BMIs [87].

Studies comparing metformin to insulin or glyburide describe lower rates of achieving euglycemia with metformin [88,89]. The higher rates of failure in women receiving metformin may have been due to inadequate dose adjustment to account for increased renal and total body drug clearance during pregnancy [83]. Metformin and insulin treatment each resulted in similar rates of perinatal morbidity, including metabolic abnormalities, premature birth, and birth trauma, in a randomized trial for the treatment of GDM unresponsive to lifestyle interventions between 28 and 32 weeks' gestation [89]. The starting dose was 500 mg once or twice daily with dose titration every 1–2 weeks to meet glycemic targets [89]. Women receiving both metformin and insulin had lower insulin requirements and gained less weight during pregnancy and during postpartum follow-up than those receiving insulin only [89]. In study subjects, metformin was highly accepted and preferred over insulin [89]. These findings highlight the potential benefits of combination therapy with metformin, either with glyburide or insulin, and suggest that outcomes could be improved with more aggressive dose titration. Despite these concerns, there are some advantages for the oral agents, primarily related to cost and ease of use. Quicker patient learning, lower risk for hypoglycemia, and higher patient adherence make oral agents a more desirable choice for many women.

Further research is underway regarding long-term effects of oral agents. Until those results are available, insulin remains the drug of choice for pharmacologic management of diabetes in pregnancy. It remains unclear whether the benefits of tighter glycemic control in women with GDM exceed those due to potential hypoglycemia. Still, primary or combined therapy with agents that target insulin resistance may be especially useful in improved glycemic control in GDM.

15.5.5 Risk for hypertensive disorders of pregnancy

Women with any type of diabetes are at increased risk of developing a hypertensive disorder in pregnancy (HDP). The pharmacologic management of HDP is detailed in Chapter 16 - Cardiovascular Medications in Pregnancy. Studies have demonstrated that low-dose aspirin may decrease the risk of developing HDP; thus, it is important for women with pregestational diabetes to take low-dose (81–150 mg) aspirin daily, beginning at 12 weeks of gestation [9].

15.5.6 Postpartum metabolic management and preconception care

Insulin requirements decrease immediately after delivery, when women with overt diabetes can either have their insulin dose empirically decreased by 50% or be returned to their prepregnancy regimen. Women with GDM should be reminded about their increased risk for diabetes and the need for screening by OGTT starting at 4–12 weeks after delivery (new ADA recommendation). Breastfeeding should be strongly encouraged, as evidence demonstrates metabolic benefits for both mother and infant that appear to persist well beyond the period of weaning [90]. Despite observations that support the use of combination hormonal contraceptives in women with diabetes, ACOG recommends that their use be limited to nonsmoking, healthy women with diabetes who are younger than 35 years with no evidence of hypertension, nephropathy, retinopathy, or other vascular disease [11]. Long-acting reversible contraceptives are effective and safe in women with diabetes, and current recommendations are to keep them in place until "a woman is prepared and ready to become pregnant" [9].

There is a renewed emphasis on the critical importance of preconception care for the woman with pregestional diabetes.

Maintaining euglycemia around the time of conception and through the critical period of organogenesis (through 8 weeks of gestation) is the most important factor to minimize an increased risk for congenital anomalies. The ADA recommends HgbA1c should optimally be <6.5% just prior to conception. ACOG recommends an even stricter target when trying to conceive: a HgbA1c <6.0%. The risk of congenital anomalies increases with HgbA1C > 7%, particularly neural tube and cardiac defects [91].

Folic acid supplementation to prevent neural tube defects is recommended as a part of preconception care for all women, although, once again, professional societies differ in recommended dosage amounts for women with diabetes. The ADA and ACOG recommend at least 400 µg taken daily preconception, while the Endocrine Society recommends 5 mg be taken daily to begin 3 months before stopping contraception, reduced to 0.4−1.0 mg daily at 12 weeks gestation. Medication adjustment for other chronic conditions may also be warranted. Women who have been taking statin medications, angiotensin-converting enzyme inhibitors, or angiotensin receptor blockers should discontinue these medications under medical supervision and transition to other medications as needed for blood pressure control prior to conceiving as these medications are also associated with teratogenic effects on the fetus [92].

15.6 Conclusion

The number of pregnancies complicated by DM is increasing.

Research evidence suggests that tighter glycemic criteria may improve neonatal outcomes. However, the current treatment strategies for DM during pregnancy are limited. Further research is needed to investigate alternative therapies and to develop pregnancy-specific treatment strategies that would also impact favorably on long-term maternal and offspring health.

References

[1] Friedman JE, Ishizuka T, Shao J, Huston L, Highman T, Catalano P. Impaired glucose transport and insulin receptor tyrosine phosphorylation in skeletal muscle from obese women with gestational diabetes. Diabetes 1999;48:1807−14.

[2] HAPO Study Cooperative Research Group, Metzger BE, Lowe LP, Dyer AR, Trimble ER, Chaovarindr U, et al. Hyperglycemia and adverse pregnancy outcomes. N Engl J Med 2008;358:1991−2002.

[3] McIntyre HD, Catalano P, Zhang C, Desoye G, Mathiesen ER, Damm P. Gestational diabetes mellitus. Nat Rev 2019;5:47.

[4] Deputy NP, Kim SY, Conrey EJ, Bullard KM. Prevalence and changes in preexisting diabetes and gestational diabetes among women who had a live birth - United States, 2012-2016. MMWR Morb Mortal Wkly Rep 2018;67(43):1201.

[5] Kwak SH, Kim SH, Cho YM, et al. A genome-wide association study of gestational diabetes mellitus in Korean women. Diabetes 2012;61:531—41.

[6] Evert AB, Dennison M, Gardner CD, et al. Nutrition therapy for adults with diabetes or prediabetes: a consensus report. Diabetes Care 2019;42:731—54.

[7] Diagnosis and classification of diabetes mellitus. Diabetes Care 2014;33(Suppl. 1): S62—9.

[8] Chiasson JL, Josse RG, Gomis R, Hanefeld M, Karasik A, Laakso M, et al. Acarbose for prevention of type 2 diabetes mellitus: the STOP-NIDDM randomised trial. Lancet 2002;359:2072—7.

[9] American Diabetes Association. 14. Management of diabetes in pregnancy: standards of medical care in diabetes-2020. Diabetes Care 2020;43(Suppl. 1):S183—92.

[10] Committee on Practice Bulletins-Obstetrics. ACOG practice bulletin no. 190: gestational diabetes mellitus. Obstet Gynecol 2018;131(2):e49—64.

[11] ACOG Committee on Practice Bulletins-Gynecology. ACOG practice bulletin. No. 73: use of hormonal contraception in women with coexisting medical conditions. Obstet Gynecol 2006;107:1453—72.

[12] White P. Classification of obstetric diabetes. Am J Obstet Gynecol 1978;130:228—30.

[13] Kuhl C. Etiology and pathogenesis of gestational diabetes. Diabetes Care 1998; 21(Suppl. 2):B19—26.

[14] Butte NF. Carbohydrate and lipid metabolism in pregnancy: normal compared with gestational diabetes mellitus. Am J Clin Nutr 2000;71:1256S—61S.

[15] Burt RL. Peripheral utilization of glucose in pregnancy. III. Insulin tolerance. Obstet Gynecol 1956;7:658—64.

[16] Spellacy WN, Goetz FC. Plasma insulin in normal late pregnancy. N Engl J Med 1963; 268:988—91.

[17] Catalano PM, Tyzbir ED, Roman NM, Amini SB, Sims EA. Longitudinal changes in insulin release and insulin resistance in nonobese pregnant women. Am J Obstet Gynecol 1991;165:1667—72.

[18] Sorenson RL, Brelje TC. Adaptation of islets of Langerhans to pregnancy: beta- cell growth, enhanced insulin secretion and the role of lactogenic hormones. Horm Metab Res 1997;29:301—7.

[19] Kalhan SC, D'Angelo LJ, Savin SM, Adam PA. Glucose production in pregnant women at term gestation. Sources of glucose for human fetus. J Clin Invest 1979;63:388—94.

[20] Jovanovic L, Peterson CM. Optimal insulin delivery for the pregnant diabetic patient. Diabetes Care 1982;5(Suppl. 1):24—37.

[21] Burt RL, Leake NH, Rhyne AL. Glucose tolerance during pregnancy and the puerperium. A modification with observations on serum immunoreactive insulin. Obstet Gynecol 1969;33:634—41.

[22] Kjos SL, Peters RK, Xiang A, Henry OA, Montoro M, Buchanan TA. Predict- ing future diabetes in Latino women with gestational diabetes. Utility of early postpartum glucose tolerance testing. Diabetes 1995;44:586—91.

[23] O'Sullivan JB. Diabetes mellitus after GDM. Diabetes 1991;40(Suppl. 2):131—5.

[24] Metzger BE, Cho NH, Roston SM, Radvany R. Prepregnancy weight and ante- partum insulin secretion predict glucose tolerance five years after gestational diabetes mellitus. Diabetes Care 1993;16:1598—605.

[25] Catalano PM, Tyzbir ED, Wolfe RR, Calles J, Roman NM, Amini SB, et al. Carbohydrate metabolism during pregnancy in control subjects and women with gestational diabetes. Am J Physiol 1993;264:E60—7.

[26] Catalano PM, Bernstein IM, Wolfe RR, Srikanta S, Tyzbir E, Sims EA. Subclinical abnormalities of glucose metabolism in subjects with previous gestational diabetes. Am J Obstet Gynecol 1986;155:1255−62.

[27] Devlieger R, Casteels K, Van Assche FA. Reduced adaptation of the pancreatic B cells during pregnancy is the major causal factor for gestational diabetes: current knowledge and metabolic effects on the offspring. Acta Obstet Gynecol Scand 2008;87:1266−70.

[28] Trout KK. Managing the sugar blues: putting the latest gestational diabetes mellitus guidelines into practice. Wom Health 2019;1(7):37−43.

[29] Brankston GN, Mitchell BF, Ryan EA, Okun NB. Resistance exercise decreases the need for insulin in overweight women with gestational diabetes mellitus. Am J Obstet Gynecol 2004;190(1):188−93.

[30] Halse RE, Wallman KE, Newnham JP, Guelfi KJ. Home-based exercise training improves capillary glucose profile in women with gestational diabetes. Med Sci Sports Exerc 2014;46(9):1702−9.

[31] Anjana RM, Sudha V, Lakshmipriya N, et al. Physical activity patterns and gestational diabetes outcomes-The wings project. Diabetes Res Clin Pract 2016;116:253−62.

[32] Metzger BE, Buchanan TA, Coustan DR, de Leiva A, Dunger DB, Hadden DR, et al. Summary and recommendations of the fifth international workshop- conference on gestational diabetes mellitus. Diabetes Care 2007;30(Suppl. 2):S251−60.

[33] Fieg DS, Donavan LE, Corcoy R, et al. Continuous glucose monitoring in pregnant women with type 1 diabetes (CONCEPTT): a multicenter international randomized controlled trial. Lancet 2017;10110(390):2317−59.

[34] DEXCOM package insert.

[35] Landon MB, Spong CY, Thom E, Carpenter MW, Ramin SM, Casey B, et al. A multicenter, randomized trial of treatment for mild gestational diabetes. N Engl J Med 2009;361:1339−48.

[36] Crowther CA, Hiller JE, Moss JR, McPhee AJ, Jeffries WS, Robinson JS, et al. Effect of treatment of gestational diabetes mellitus on pregnancy outcomes. N Engl J Med 2005;352:2477−86.

[37] Sindelar DK, Balcom JH, Chu CA, Neal DW, Cherrington AD. A comparison of the effects of selective increases in peripheral or portal insulin on hepatic glucose production in the conscious dog. Diabetes 1996;45:1594−604.

[38] Woolderink JM, van Loon AJ, Storms F, de Heide L, Hoogenberg K. Use of insulin glargine during pregnancy in seven type 1 diabetic women. Diabetes Care 2005;28:2594−5.

[39] Poulin RA, Steil GM, Moore DM, Ader M, Bergman RN. Dynamics of glucose production and uptake are more closely related to insulin in hindlimb lymph than in thoracic duct lymph. Diabetes 1994;43:180−90.

[40] Bjorklund AO, Adamson UK, Lins PE, Westgren LM. Diminished insulin clearance during late pregnancy in patients with type I diabetes mellitus. Clin Sci 1998;95:317−23.

[41] Kautzky-Willer A, Prager R, Waldhausl W, Pacini G, Thomaseth K, Wagner OF, et al. Pronounced insulin resistance and inadequate beta-cell secretion characterize lean gestational diabetes during and after pregnancy. Diabetes Care 1997;20:1717−23.

[42] Challier JC, Hauguel S, Desmaizieres V. Effect of insulin on glucose uptake and metabolism in the human placenta. J Clin Endocrinol Metab 1986;62:803−7.

[43] Blackburn ST. Maternal, fetal & neonatal physiology. 4th ed. Maryland Heights, MO: Elsevier, Inc; 2013.

[44] Carpenter MW, Canick JA, Hogan JW, Shellum C, Somers M, Star JA. Amniotic fluid insulin at 14—20 weeks' gestation: association with later maternal glucose intolerance and birth macrosomia. Diabetes Care 2001;24:1259—63.

[45] Mosekilde E, Jensen KS, Binder C, Pramming S, Thorsteinsson B. Modeling absorption kinetics of subcutaneous injected soluble insulin. J Pharmacokinet Biopharm 1989;17: 67—87.

[46] Zinman B. The physiologic replacement of insulin. An elusive goal. N Engl J Med 1989;321:363—70.

[47] Torlone E, Fanelli C, Rambotti AM, Kassi G, Modarelli F, Di Vincenzo A, et al. Pharmacokinetics, pharmacodynamics and glucose counterregulation follow- ing subcutaneous injection of the monomeric insulin analogue [Lys(B28), Pro(B29)] in IDDM. Diabetologia 1994;37:713—20.

[48] AFREZZA package insert.

[49] Price N, Bartlett C, Gillmer M. Use of insulin glargine during pregnancy: a case—control pilot study. BJOG 2007;114:453—7.

[50] Jovanovic L, Ilic S, Pettitt DJ, Hugo K, Gutierrez M, Bowsher RR, et al. Metabolic and immunologic effects of insulin lispro in gestational diabetes. Diabetes Care 1999;22: 1422—7.

[51] Negrato CA, Rafacho A, Negrato G, Teixeira MF, Araujo CA, Vieira L, et al. Glargine vs. NPH insulin therapy in pregnancies complicated by diabetes: an observational cohort study. Diabetes Res Clin Pract 2010;89:46—51.

[52] Fang YM, MacKeen D, Egan JF, Zelop CM. Insulin glargine compared with Neutral Protamine Hagedorn insulin in the treatment of pregnant diabetics. J Matern Fetal Neonatal Med 2009;22:249—53.

[53] Di Cianni G, Torlone E, Lencioni C, Bonomo M, Di Benedetto A, Napoli A, et al. Perinatal outcomes associated with the use of glargine during pregnancy. Diabet Med 2008; 25:993—6.

[54] Kovo M, Wainstein J, Matas Z, Haroutiunian S, Hoffman A, Golan A. Pla- cental transfer of the insulin analog glargine in the ex vivo perfused placental cotyledon model. Endocr Res 2011;36:19—24.

[55] Torlone E, Di Cianni G, Mannino D, Lapolla A. Insulin analogs and pregnancy: an update. Acta Diabetol 2009;46:163—72.

[56] Zelobowska K, Gumprecht J, Grzeszczak W. Mitogenic potency of insulin glargine. Endokrynol Pol 2009;60:34—9.

[57] Kurtzhals P, Schaffer L, Sorensen A, Kristensen C, Jonassen I, Schmid C, et al. Correlations of receptor binding and metabolic and mitogenic potencies of insulin analogs designed for clinical use. Diabetes 2000;49:999—1005.

[58] Jorgensen LN. Carcinogen effect of the human insulin analogue B10 Asp in female rats. In: Didriksen LH, Jorgensen LN, Drejer K, editors. Diabetologia, vol. 35; 1992. A3 (Abstract).

[59] Gabbe SG. New concepts and applications in the use of the insulin pump during pregnancy. J Matern Fetal Med 2000;9:42—5.

[60] Farrar D, Tuffnell DJ, West J, West HM. Continuous subcutaneous insulin infusion versus multiple daily injections of insulin for pregnant women with diabetes. Cochrane Database Syst Rev 2016;(6). Art.No:CD005542.

[61] T-SLIM package insert.

[62] Rama CS, Tay WL, Lye WK, et al. Beyond HbA1c: comparing glycemic variability and glycemic indices in predicting hypoglycemia in type 1 and type 2 diabetes. Diabet Technol Therapeut 2018;20:353—62.

[63] Trout KK, McCool WF, Homko CJ. Person-centered primary care and type 2 diabetes: beyond glucose control. J Midwifery Wom Health 2019;64:312—23.

[64] Rickels MR, Ruedy KJ, Foster NC, T1D Exchange Intranasal Glucagon Investigators. Intranasal glucagon for treatment of insulin-induced hypoglycemia in adults with type 1 diabetes: a randomized crossover noninferiority study. Diabetes Care 2016;39:264—70.

[65] Luna B, Hughes AT, Feinglos MN. The use of insulin secretagogues in the treatment of type 2 diabetes. Prim Care 1999;26:895—915.

[66] Malek R, Davis SN. Pharmacokinetics, efficacy and safety of glyburide for gestational diabetes mellitus. Expet Opin Drug Metabol Toxicol 2016;(6):691—9.

[67] DeFronzo RA, Simonson DC. Oral sulfonylurea agents suppress hepatic glucose production in non-insulin-dependent diabetic individuals. Diabetes Care 1984;7(Suppl. 1):72—80.

[68] Simonson DC, Ferrannini E, Bevilacqua S, Smith D, Barrett E, Carlson R, et al. Mechanism of improvement in glucose metabolism after chronic glyburide therapy. Diabetes 1984;33:838—45.

[69] Rossetti L, Giaccari A, DeFronzo RA. Glucose toxicity. Diabetes Care 1990;13:610—30.

[70] Kahn SE, McCulloch D, Porte Jr D. Insulin secretion in normal and diabetic humans. In: Alberti KGMM, Zimmet P, DeFronzo RA, Keen H, editors. International textbook of diabetes mellitus. 2nd ed. Chichester, UK: Wiley; 1997. p. 337—54.

[71] Mitrakou A, Kelley D, Mokan M, Veneman T, Pangburn T, Reilly J, et al. Role of reduced suppression of glucose production and diminished early insulin release in impaired glucose tolerance. N Engl J Med 1992;326:22—9.

[72] Leahy JL. Natural history of beta-cell dysfunction in NIDDM. Diabetes Care 1990;13:992—1010.

[73] Polonsky KS, Given BD, Hirsch LJ, Tillil H, Shapiro ET, Beebe C, et al. Abnormal patterns of insulin secretion in non-insulin-dependent diabetes mellitus. N Engl J Med 1988;318:1231—9.

[74] Schwartz RB, Feske SK, Polak JF, DeGirolami U, Iaia A, Beckner KM, et al. Preeclampsia-eclampsia: clinical and neuroradiographic correlates and in- sights into the pathogenesis of hypertensive encephalopathy. Radiology 2000;217:371—6.

[75] Hebert MF, Ma X, Naraharisetti SB, Krudys KM, Umans JG, Hankins GD, et al. Are we optimizing gestational diabetes treatment with glyburide? The pharmacologic basis for better clinical practice. Clin Pharmacol Ther 2009;85:607—14.

[76] Groop L, Groop PH, Stenman S, Saloranta C, Totterman KJ, Fyhrquist F, et al. Comparison of pharmacokinetics, metabolic effects and mechanisms of action of glyburide and glipizide during long-term treatment. Diabetes Care 1987;10:671—8.

[77] Coppack SW, Lant AF, McIntosh CS, Rodgers AV. Pharmacokinetic and pharmacodynamic studies of glibenclamide in non-insulin dependent diabetes mellitus. Br J Clin Pharmacol 1990;29:673—84.

[78] Catalano PM, Huston L, Amini SB, Kalhan SC. Longitudinal changes in glucose metabolism during pregnancy in obese women with normal glucose tolerance and gestational diabetes mellitus. Am J Obstet Gynecol 1999;180:903—16.

[79]   Langer O, Conway DL, Berkus MD, Xenakis EM, Gonzales O. A comparison of glyburide and insulin in women with gestational diabetes mellitus. N Engl J Med 2000; 343:1134−8.

[80]   Kahn BF, Davies JK, Lynch AM, Reynolds RM, Barbour LA. Predictors of glyburide failure in the treatment of gestational diabetes. Obstet Gynecol 2006;107:1303−9.

[81]   DeFronzo RA, Goodman AM. Efficacy of metformin in patients with non- insulin-dependent diabetes mellitus. The Multicenter Metformin Study Group. N Engl J Med 1995;333:541−9.

[82]   Stumvoll M, Nurjhan N, Perriello G, Dailey G, Gerich JE. Metabolic effects of metformin in non-insulin-dependent diabetes mellitus. N Engl J Med 1995;333:550−4.

[83]   Eyal S, Easterling TR, Carr D, Umans JG, Miodovnik M, Hankins GD, et al. Pharmacokinetics of metformin during pregnancy. Drug Metab Dispos 2010;38:833−40.

[84]   Vanky E, Zahlsen K, Spigset O, Carlsen SM. Placental passage of metformin in women with polycystic ovary syndrome. Fertil Steril 2005;83(5):1575−8.

[85]   Charles B, Norris R, Xiao V, Hague W. Population pharmacokinetics of metformin in late pregnancy. Ther Drug Monit 2006;1:67−72.

[86]   Rowan JA, Rush EC, Plank LD, et al. Metformin in gestational diabetes: the offspring follow-up (MiG TOFU): body composition and metabolic outcomes at 7-9 Years of Age *BMJ Open*. Diabet Res Care 2018;6(1):e00456.

[87]   Hanem LGE, Stridskev S, Juliusson PB, Vanky E. Metformin use in PCOS pregnancy increases the risk of offspring overweight at 4 years of age: followup of two RCTs. J Clin Endocrinol Metab 2018;103(4):1612−21.

[88]   Moore LE, Clokey D, Rappaport VJ, Curet LB. Metformin compared with glyburide in gestational diabetes: a randomized controlled trial. Obstet Gynecol 2010;115:55−9.

[89]   Rowan JA, Hague WM, Gao W, Battin MR, Moore MP, Mi GTI. Metformin versus insulin for the treatment of gestational diabetes. N Engl J Med 2008;358:2003−15.

[90]   Gunderson EP, Lewis CE, Lin Y, et al. Lactation duration and progression to diabetes in women across the childbearing years: the 30-year CARDIA study. JAMA Intern Med 2018;178(3):328−37.

[91]   Yang P, Reece EA, Wang F, Gabbay-Benziv R. Decoding the oxidative stress hypothesis in diabetic embryopathy through preapoptotic kinase signaling. Am J Obstet Gynecol 2018;132(6):e228−48.

[92]   Yehuda I. Implementation of preconception care for women with diabetes. Diab Spectr 2016;29(2):105−14.

Cardiovascular medications in pregnancy

16

Andrew Youmans*

University of Michigan School of Nursing, MI, United States

16.1 Introduction

Cardiovascular disease is the leading cause of death for women in the United States, and similarly in other countries with developed health systems. Heart disease is the leading cause of death worldwide for men and women. While it is common to think of noncongenital heart disease as one of older populations, women of childbearing age can be affected by any noncongenital cardiovascular condition. The leading cause of maternal death in the United States is cardiovascular disease [17]. When combined with other cardiovascular causes of death, such as hypertensive disorders, thromboembolism, and cerebrovascular accidents (CVAs), nearly half of all maternal deaths in this country can be attributed to these causes [17]. It is also important to understand that metaphorically maternal deaths are just the tip of the iceberg, for every death more women suffer severe morbidity or near misses.

Pregnancy care presents a unique challenge with any pharmacotherapy. Maternal needs have to be balanced with fetal safety and vice versa. This intricate balance is often challenging for those who do not routinely provide maternal healthcare. A similar challenge also applies to maternal healthcare providers in areas such as cardiology where they do not routinely provide care. Some medications used in the treatment of cardiovascular conditions have known adverse fetal effects. For many women with diagnosed cardiovascular disease, such as hypertension or conditions requiring anticoagulation, it may require a strategy of either changing medications starting with preconception care or as soon as pregnancy is known or prescribing alternative medications that are safer for women desiring pregnancy.

Another challenge in maternity care may be the first significant access to the health system as an adult, which means that obstetrical providers cannot rely solely on patient histories to provide care. Patients may have underlying cardiovascular disease that is not readily apparent, even with a physical exam.

For women with known cardiovascular disease (either congenital or noncongenital), the European Society of Cardiology (ESC) recommends that these patients receive an evaluation to include an electrocardiogram (ECG), echocardiogram,

* Funded by Predoctoral Fellowship Training Grant (T32 NR016914. Program Director: Titler) Complexity: Innovations in Promoting Health and Safety.

Clinical Pharmacology During Pregnancy. https://doi.org/10.1016/B978-0-12-818902-3.00009-9

and exercise stress testing. If a patient has a known aortic issue, such as an aneurysm, the ESC Guidelines recommend Computerized Tomography (CT) or Magnetic Resonance (MR) Imaging [70].

There are many known risk factors for various types of CVD. Current recommendations from both American College of Obstetricians and Gynecologists (ACOG) and ESC each have a directed screening algorithm that focuses on patient symptoms, abnormal vital signs, risk factors, and physical exam findings. The California Maternal Quality Care Collaborative (CMQCC) also has an algorithm and toolkit identifying which patients should see a cardiologist versus obstetrical provider management [15]. An area to focus future research is determining if the directed screening is as effective as universal screening. Given the impact of cardiovascular disease on maternal health and lifespan health, it may be time to consider universal screening with a more focused approach to those at higher risk similar to current screening for gestational diabetes in the United States. The current body of literature does not support the practice of universal screening for cardiovascular conditions, instead, focusing on those with certain risk factors.

Electrocardiography and specifically 12-Lead ECG is a powerful diagnostic tool. Beyond the simple assessment of ischemia or infarction, a 12-Lead can provide a wealth of information [35]. It is normal for an ECG to have changes as pregnancy progresses, notably a more leftward axis deviation due to the physical shifting of the heart due to the upward shifting of the uterus. It is important to note that having a baseline 12-Lead ECG increases the diagnostic value of subsequent ECGs.

Cardiovascular disease is a prime example of the medical reasons to focus on preventing unplanned pregnancy. In cases of severe congenital disease or cardiomyopathy with a low ejection fraction carrying a pregnancy not only to term gestation but even to the age of viability for a fetus could prove to be fatal to the woman [91]. Even in patients with unknown cardiovascular disease, prepregnancy screening offers more diagnostic testing and treatment options than screening patients who are already pregnant. CT imaging and invasive cardiovascular testing utilize ionizing radiation, and MR imaging uses high-powered magnetic fields that are not recommended for routine use in pregnant patients. Most transcatheter interventions for heart problems, whether electrophysiology procedures, percutaneous coronary interventions, valvuloplasty, aortic aneurysm repairs, or others, require the use of ionizing radiation that is shown to be harmful to the fetus.

It should be noted that these interventions require the use of fluoroscopy, which emits higher doses of ionizing radiation than a single chest X-ray and, in some cases, CT imaging. Shielding of the abdomen is possible for some areas, and certain procedures like percutaneous coronary intervention can be completed through a radial approach minimizing radiation exposure to the fetus by shifting the brunt of the radiation exposure to the upper extremities and chest. Surgical interventions for cardiovascular problems often require cardiopulmonary bypass, which has evidence of increased risk of fetal mortality, but this could be attributed to the severity of maternal health [46]. The bottom line is that these procedures are often challenging and complex enough without involving pregnancy. It would be ideal to identify these issues prior to pregnancy, where all of the focus can be on the mother's health and after treatment, and while these issues are being managed, women can be counseled on risks to be able to make an informed decision on whether to attempt pregnancy.

Another key point from both ACOG and the ESC guidelines is that a single provider should not be managing pregnancy in patients with cardiovascular disease in isolation. Patients with these conditions require a team approach, including cardiology providers, obstetrical providers, maternal–fetal medicine specialists, and other specialties as needed. In the United States, there are cardiologists and cardiology providers who have a particular interest in sex-specific cardiovascular issues focused on women. Cardio-obstetrics is an area of growing interest in the cardiology and women's health communities [22].

Vaginal delivery is preferred over cesarean when maternal hemodynamics are stable. In cases of hemodynamic instability, a cesarean is preferred [70].

16.2 Resources for guidance

Clinical Guidelines provide the most up-to-date and comprehensive focus on this subject. As this topic is seeing increased research activity by both women's health providers and cardiology providers, these guidelines are likely to be updated again shortly. The ESC and ACOG both have clinical guidelines and practice bulletins published or updated very recently [2,70]. CQMCC has also developed a toolkit for Maternal Cardiovascular Disease that contains valuable clinical information [15]. The CMQCC resource provides algorithms and guidance to help with screening and referral to cardiovascular providers. Pharmacology reference databases also provide updated information on each medication. It is the responsibility of the clinician to evaluate any resource for accuracy and applicability critically.

16.3 Cardiovascular changes in pregnancy

The maternal cardiovascular system is one of the most changed body systems in pregnancy. Blood and plasma volumes increase, creating more strain on the maternal cardiovascular system. Hemodynamics, cardiac outputs, peripheral vascular resistance, and heart rate all change during pregnancy [10,64]. During pregnancy a woman's heart is likely working harder than it will at any other point in her life [92]. Fig. 16.1 shows graphs showing how each of these measures changes throughout pregnancy.

16.3.1 Sedation for invasive procedures and timing of procedures

While not directly cardiovascular related, Cardiac Catheterization, Pacemaker/Implanted Cardiac Defibrillator placement, and transesophageal echocardiogram are just a few examples of often invasive procedures performed with some degree

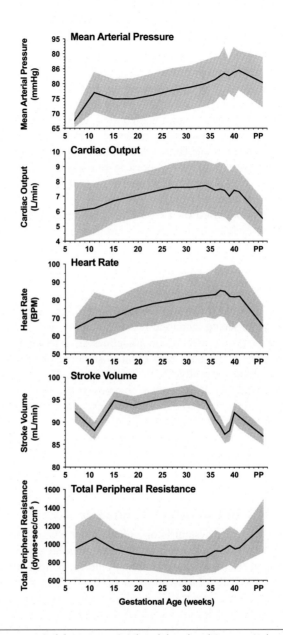

FIGURE 16.1

Cardiac output, mean arterial pressure, total peripheral resistance, stroke volume and heart rate derived from serial measurements in normotensive nulliparous pregnancies: mean ± sd.

of sedation [49]. Commonly, this involves fentanyl and versed. Versed and all benzodiazepines are contraindicated in pregnancy, until birth [13]. It may be possible to complete the procedure with fentanyl only or adding diphenhydramine. It may be helpful to consult or involve anesthesia, as this would allow for a greater number of sedation options [13]. It is currently recommended to wait until the second trimester, if possible, for any procedures requiring the use of radiation to reduce risks to the fetus [70].

16.4 Cardiovascular disease in pregnancy

16.4.1 Hypertension

Hypertension is the most common cardiovascular condition during pregnancy. While many think immediately of preeclampsia when thinking of elevated blood pressure in pregnancy, patients can have chronic hypertension existing before the pregnancy or develop gestational hypertension [1]. Preeclampsia presents with hypertension, proteinuria, and other physical symptom manifestations [3]. Gestational hypertension should not have any physical symptoms or abnormal lab work associated with it [85]. It was once a common belief that preeclampsia was "cured" by delivering the placenta. Postpartum preeclampsia, by definition, completely discredits that belief. Current research is not only highlighting the immediate postpartum impacts of preeclampsia but lifelong cardiovascular impacts [14,39,40,84].

		Features	**Pharmacologic goals**
Chronic hypertension	Existing or hypertension diagnosed prior to 20 wks EGA First diagnosed in pregnancy in first 20 wks EGA and does not resolve postpartum	Likely to require antihypertensive long-term following pregnancy. ACOG recommendation to evaluate liver enzymes, creatinine, potassium, blood urea nitrogen, and blood count. Either a spot protein/creatinine ratio or a 24 h urine can be considered Consider 12-Lead ECG and/or echocardiogram	Maintain blood pressure in normal range, assess and adjust dosage throughout and after pregnancy

		Features	Pharmacologic goals
Gestational hypertension	Occurs after 20 wks EGA	No abnormal labwork or other features associated with preeclampsia other than elevated blood pressure. Should be monitored for hypertension following pregnancy, hypertension likely to resolve after pregnancy. Increased risk of hypertension later in life requires annual evaluation in primary care	Maintain normal blood pressure. Reassess and evaluate for the efficacy of therapy and signs of preeclampsia
Preeclampsia	Occurs after 20 wks EGA	Labwork is abnormal and/or accompanied with features of preeclampsia	Pharmacological goals are to maintain blood pressures in a normal range until birth and the postpartum period. If pharmacological therapies are not effective in maintaining blood pressure in a safe range, consider emergent birth. Magnesium sulfate is used for preeclampsia and not other forms of hypertensive disorders in pregnancy

Hypertension management is a crucial preventative measure in reducing the risk of several disease processes, including cardiovascular disease [93]. Keeping blood pressure in a normal range has been shown to reduce the risk of renal disease, heart disease, stroke, and even dementia. Hypertension is one of the most common chronic conditions worldwide and most often requires lifelong management. Hypertension in nonpregnancy is divided into primary and secondary hypertension. The overwhelming majority of cases in the United States and worldwide are primary hypertension; that is, the hypertension is not caused by another medical condition. In secondary hypertension, the focus is on correcting the cause of the hypertension versus long-term management.

There is not an antihypertensive medication that is free from potential fetal effects. With that said, there are also significant issues relating to hypertension in pregnancy [84]. Maternal risks from hypertension include the risk of CVAs and renal disease in cases of severe hypertension [27]. Preeclampsia has a very different pathology from hypertension and can have even more severe and sudden physiological impacts [84]. Hypertensive disorders of pregnancy can be fatal. From 2011 to 2016, 6.9% of maternal deaths in the United States were due to hypertensive disorders [17]. The fetus is not isolated from maternal hypertension, and preterm birth and fetal growth restriction are only two common fetal impacts from maternal hypertension. In the general population and in the peripartum, severe hypertension or hypertensive emergency has immediate health implications, including hemorrhagic stroke or hypertensive bleeding [72]. Observation of blood pressure in pregnancy has become more common as we are watchful for preeclampsia. In the general population, mild—moderate hypertension chronically shows little short-term impacts, but the chronic impacts are immense. Hypertension has long been called, "the silent killer" because patients are often asymptomatic until they start to show effects of long-term hypertension or blood pressure reaches severe ranges [44]. Pregnancy treatment for mild to moderate hypertension is essential, but care should be made to avoid dropping blood pressures so low that they interfere with placental perfusion [1,85].

Currently, ACOG recommends labetalol or nifedipine as the first-line medications for chronic and gestational hypertension, with hydralazine being recommended only for acute hypertension [2,85].

Both ACOG and ESC recommend keeping maternal blood pressure below 140/90 and to consider blood pressure severe at 160/110. This applies to both the systolic and diastolic. ACOG recommends using the trend of two blood pressures at least 4 hours apart. In sudden onset of hypertension over 160/110, prompt administration of antihypertensives is indicated [27,85]. Hypertensive emergency/crisis, or malignant hypertension, is an abrupt increase in blood pressure. For nonpregnant patients, it is recommended to decrease pressure, but should aim for a target of 160—100. IV antihypertensives are recommended for this purpose [44,94].

In patients with chronic hypertension in pregnancy, antihypertensive treatment is proven to help reduce the occurrence of severe hypertension during pregnancy [80].

For nonpregnant patients, there has been some debate regarding guidelines for hypertension. Some have suggested a more relaxed guideline, and others, specifically the American Heart Association and American College of Cardiology guidelines recommended tighter blood pressure control. While these guidelines have some disagreement, provided a patient is not symptomatic, evidence shows tighter blood pressure control has positive benefits in terms of cardiovascular disease risk reduction.

Guideline and year updated	JNC-8 (2014)	AHA/ACC (2017)	EHA/ESC
BP where medication is initiated	Ages 60+: 150/90 Under 60: 140/90 Also considers lower thresholds for diabetes and CKD	130/80 Lower thresholds based of CVD risk	Based on disease staging and 4-step grading of hypertension 130/85 for those with severe disease 160/100 in those with no risk factors
Has race-specific guidelines	Yes	Yes	Yes (extrapolates on US data)

16.5 Mechanism of action for hypertensive medications

Hypertension is an abnormally elevated blood pressure caused by alterations in the body's standard physiological systems for maintaining homeostasis. The body has several ways to regulate and adjust blood pressure, and pharmacological methods have been developed to alter these processes to achieve modification of the blood pressure to acceptable ranges [90]. The heart's contractile force, rate, and the compliance of arteries and blood vessels all factor in the maintenance of normal blood pressure. The amount of circulating volume can be increased or reduced through hormonal actions to further balance blood pressure.

16.5.1 Medications affecting the renin angiotensin aldosterone system (the kidney−lung pathway)

The kidneys and the lungs are two areas of the body that are sensitive to blood pressure changes. The kidneys especially need adequate perfusion to function. The kidneys produce a substance called renin, which has no significant effect on blood pressure. Renin is converted into Angiotensin I by angiotensinogen, which is produced by the liver. Angiotensin I also has no significant systemic effects. The lungs create Angiotensin-Converting Enzyme (ACE) that converts the relatively inert Angiotensin I into Angiotensin II, a potent vasoconstrictor. Angiotensin II binds with receptors in the arteries causing this vasoconstriction [60]. This pathway is the target of many hypertension medications (ACE Inhibitors, Angiotensin II Receptor Blockers (ARBs), and Direct Renin Inhibitors); however, all of the medications altering this pathway are contraindicated in pregnancy due to risk for fetal renal and other congenital issues [20]. Direct renin inhibitors bind to the renin and prevent angiotensinogen from converting it to Angiotensin I [48]. ACE Inhibitors prevent the ACE from converting the inert Angiotensin I to the potent Angiotensin II. Finally, ARBs block the binding sites where Angiotensin II would bind to induce vasoconstriction. While these medications are not used in pregnancy, they are some of the first-line medications used in hypertension in the general population [43,90]. Drugs in these classes can be used in postpartum/breastfeeding, but it is suggested to observe the infant for signs of hypotension. As ACE Inhibitors are a common first-line medication for the treatment of hypertension, it is possible for someone with an unplanned pregnancy to be on one before pregnancy is diagnosed [43,90]. While a patient should be transitioned to another class of medication promptly, data suggest no significant risk of harm in these cases [6].

16.5.2 Beta-Blockers

Beta-Blockers or Beta-Adrenergic Blocking agents are a family of medications that block the receptor site of naturally occurring beta-adrenergic agonists, such as epinephrine [74].

Beta-blockers, as a class, provide multiple therapeutic effects. The heart beats more slowly and with less force, and there is also a vasodilatory property [34,48]. Beta-blockers also are divided into two categories: selective and nonselective. Our bodies have three different types of beta-adrenergic receptors: B1, B2, and B3 [36]. B1 receptors are located primarily in the heart and kidneys. B2 Receptors are located in most other parts of the body, but most notably in the lungs. B3 receptors are found in adipose tissue, and while they are found in the cardiovascular system, their role is not fully understood. Most selective Beta-blockers target B1 only, while nonselective beta-blockers affect all beta-receptors or at least B1 and B2 [95].

One of the most commonly used antihypertensives in pregnancy is labetalol (Trandate) [85]. Labetalol is a nonselective beta-blocker that also has an alpha-receptor blocking effect. ACOG Guidelines recommend labetalol as a first-line drug to manage both chronic and gestational hypertension [85]. ESC guidelines suggest a Beta-1 Selective Beta-Blocker due to the lack of effects on uterine beta receptors [70].

Carvedilol is currently one of the preferred beta-blockers for the treatment of heart failure and is considered safe in pregnancy.

Breastfeeding: Labetalol and Propranolol are the preferred beta-blockers for use in breastfeeding as both of these medications are significantly bound to plasma proteins and are not found in high levels in breast milk compared to some other beta-blockers such as metoprolol.

16.5.3 Calcium Channel Blockers

Calcium Channel Blockers are commonly used in pregnancy. They provide smooth muscle relaxation in the arteries and decrease vascular resistance [53]. Some calcium channel blockers can be used outside of hypertension management to relax the uterine muscle for tocolysis as well [54]. The uterine relaxation could be to delay labor or to allow for relaxation for an external cephalic version [79].

Calcium channel blockers are also a fantastic option for long-term management instead of ACE Inhibitors or ARBs in women with chronic hypertension desiring future pregnancy. Many formulations also have extended release options that can increase compliance by reducing the number of times per day a patient needs to take medication to be effective [48]. In situations where immediate blood pressure control is needed, IV administration is preferred (hydralazine or labetalol). Oral nifedipine can be used, but only immediate release versions should be used for emergent hypertension management [85]. Following pregnancy, maternal heart rate returns to a normal baseline from the sight tachycardia that is common in late pregnancy. Most calcium channel blockers do not affect heart rate as significantly as beta-blockers, making them an excellent choice for long-term postpregnancy use in women who have a normal baseline heart rate. In both the JNC-8 and AHA/ACC Guidelines, calcium channel blockers are an option for initial therapy in patients of African descent. ACE Inhibitors are not as effective as thiazide diuretics or calcium channel blockers in studies examining black populations in the United States [43,90]. The EHA/ESC guidelines are cautious about this recommendation, as they based their race-specific recommendation on extrapolation from United States' data. They specifically cite several differences in the black populations in Europe compared to the United States, including a socioeconomic difference [82]. The concerns in the EHA/ESC Guideline are a valid consideration in non-United States populations, and clinicians should use their best judgment when selecting medications.

16.5.4 Diuretics

The human body has several hormones that are used to maintain adequate fluid balance; aldosterone, antidiuretic hormone, and others work to maintain this fluid balance. Diuretic medications work to alter that balance by increasing the excretion of fluids. This is primarily done by altering the excretion or retention of certain ion such as sodium or potassium.

Diuretics are the oldest antihypertensive class for long-term use, with Diuril (chlorothiazide), becoming commercially available in the United States in 1958

[8]. Diuretics are not commonly used in pregnancy as there is a concern with inter-rupting uteroplacental blood flow due to volume depletion. Diuretics cause the body to expel intravascular fluid through urination. Hydrochlorothiazide works through inhibition of sodium reabsorption in the distal tubules of the kidney [48]. This causes increased expulsion of water. Furosemide (Lasix) is primarily used for the treatment of heart failure and related edema. Its primary action is on the Loop of Henle in the kidney and causing increased water excretion along with potassium. All diuretics impact the electrolyte balance (primarily sodium and potassium), and it is important to monitor this in patients' levels shortly after initiation and regularly during use. This is particularly true in higher doses and in medications such as furosemide (Lasix) that are notorious for depleting electrolytes. Electrolyte supplementation may be needed for long-term use of some diuretics.

Patients who require hydrochlorothiazide to manage their hypertension before pregnancy can continue to take this medication, but it is not recommended to initiate it as a new medication during pregnancy [85].

16.5.5 Direct vasodilators

Direct vasodilators' primary action is to cause arterial vasodilation through a mech-anism that directly affects the muscle. While calcium channel blockers also cause vasodilation, their mechanism of action is specifically on the inhibition of calcium ions which leads to vasodilation, and it is not a direct effect. Direct vasodilators are excellent for treating severe hypertension quickly; drugs in this category work very quickly. Postural hypotension with these medications is more likely than with other classes.

Hydralazine is an example of a direct vasodilator. While its mechanism of action is not fully understood, it is safe for limited use in pregnancy. The preferred use for hydralazine is for severe hypertension in the inpatient setting [85]. This can be in the setting of preeclampsia or hypertensive emergency. It is recommended to use other agents, if possible, for chronic blood pressure management.

Nitroglycerin is another example of a direct vasodilator. Once absorbed, it is con-verted into nitric oxide, which provides the vasodilatory effect. Nitroglycerin is in no means a first-line antihypertensive but can be used in cases of severe hypertension in pregnancy that does not respond to hydralazine. Patients on intravenous nitroglyc-erin need to be on telemetry. A common side effect with nitroglycerine is a headache that usually resolves upon decreasing the dose or discontinuation.

Quick reference of common antihypertensives in pregnancy

Generic name	Brand Name(s)	Subclass	Recommendation	Pregnancy-related issues	Breastfeeding
Beta-blockers					
Labetalol	Trandate	Nonselective beta-blocker with alpha blocking activity	First line	**Recommended for treatment of chronic hypertension in pregnancy** [2] Fetal risks Bradycardia, hypotension, hypoglycemia, and reduced birth weight Not recommended for use in women with asthma due to risk of bronchoconstriction	**May be safely used in breastfeeding** Medication has significant plasma protein binding and is not expressed in breastmilk in high quantities compared with some other beta-blockers
Propranolol	Inderal	Nonselective beta blocker Class II antiarrhythmic agent	Second or third line	May be used in pregnancy for hypertension. More commonly used for antiarrhythmic properties and migraine prophylaxis. Not recommended for use in patients with asthma If used for migraine prophylaxis, discontinuation 2−3 days before birth is recommended **Fetal risks** Bradycardia, hypotension, hypoglycemia, and reduced birth weight	May be used in breastfeeding. Binds to plasma proteins similarly to labetalol

Drug	Brand	Mechanism of action	Line	Notes	Breastfeeding
Metoprolol	Lopressor	Selective beta-blocker: Beta-1	Second or third line	Not the first-line consideration for pregnancy, but may be considered. ESC guidelines recommend nonselective beta-blockers	Does not bind to plasma proteins like labetalol and is comparatively more available in breastmilk. Estimates of a maximum of 0.1/mg/kg/day of exposure in neonate which is well below therapeutic levels
Calcium channel blockers					
Nifedipine	Procardia Adalat		First line	Considered safe for management of chronic hypertension in pregnancy [2]. May also be used for acute hypertension (immediate release versions) May also be used as a tocolytic	Is excreted in breastmilk, but does not contraindicate breastfeeding
Nicardipine	Cardene		Second line	May be used for treatment of acute and severe maternal hypertension when first-line medications fail. Patient should be continuously monitored while on this medication	Minimally excreted in breastmilk
Direct vasodilators					
Hydralazine	Apresoline	Direct vasodilator unknown mechanism of action	First line (acute)	Hydralazine is a first-line medication for acute hypertension in pregnancy. It is not a recommended agent for chronic hypertension	Excreted in breastmilk. Caution recommended

Continued

—cont'd

Quick reference of common antihypertensives in pregnancy

Generic name	Brand Name(s)	Subclass	Recommendation	Pregnancy-related issues	Breastfeeding
Nitroglycerine	Nitro-big	Vasodilator nitric oxide	Third line	Nitroglycerine is not recommended for treatment of hypertension in pregnancy. Its only indications are for the treatment of preeclampsia w/pulmonary edema and angina	Unknown excretion. Use cautioned in breastfeeding mothers
Alpha-adrenergic agonist					
Methyldopa	Aldomet Dopamet Medopa	Alpha2-adrenergic agonist	Second line (ACOG)	ACOG guidelines do not recommend methyldopa be used during pregnancy. The rationale is not based on fetal effects, but "lack of effectiveness" and "adverse effects" ESC places a higher emphasis on this medication due to it being the only antihypertensive medication with a long-term infant follow-up ESC and ACOG also specifically expresses concerns about the use of this medication in the postpartum due to an increased risk of depression	Methyldopa is considered safe in breastfeeding, but should be avoided in postpartum due to risk of maternal depressive symptoms

ACE Inhibitors, ARB, Direct Renin Inhibitors.
ACE Inhibitors, Angiotensin Receptor Blockers, Direct Renin Inhibitors are not recommended for use in pregnancy.

16.5.6 Considerations for long-term therapy

Antihypertensive use in pregnancy is not the same as used in the general population. Many women using antihypertensives in pregnancy will not need to continue them postpartum. For most nonpregnant patients, antihypertensive medication becomes a lifelong therapy. It is vital to make sure that a patient has the best possible fit with medication to ensure compliance. In women of reproductive age, particularly those desiring future pregnancy, it does not make sense to start them on a therapy that they will need to discontinue if they become pregnant, such as an ACE inhibitor. Antihypertensive medications are not free from side effects. Even mild side effects, such as the dry hacking cough that is common with ACE inhibitors and ARBs, can discourage the patient from taking the medication. Multiple doses increase the risk of a patient missing a dose. Utilization of formulations that have extended, controlled, or slow release medications can help reduce the number of doses.

Sexual dysfunction is an area where research on female populations lags far behind that for males [96]. Hypertension is considered a contributing factor to erectile dysfunction, and some patients report antihypertensive medications causing erectile dysfunction [25]. There is limited information on the impact of hypertension and use of antihypertensives on female sexual function and if it parallels the research information on male patients. Despite this lack of information, it is possible that women with sexual dysfunction could be suffering from side effects of the medication and a change in therapy may be beneficial. This is an area for future research.

16.5.7 Magnesium sulfate

Magnesium sulfate is a unique medication in the obstetrical community. It is a vital medication for the treatment and management of preeclampsia, particularly the neurological effects [3]. Its primary mechanism of action is through cerebral vasodilation. If preeclampsia is suspected, magnesium sulfate should be started promptly [3]. Magnesium sulfate alone may not reduce blood pressure to safe levels. Medications like hydralazine may be used to quickly bring blood pressure to safe levels concurrently with the infusion of magnesium sulfate. For nonobstetric providers, it may seem counterintuitive to administer magnesium sulfate for seizure, where benzodiazepines are a first-line medication in nonpregnant patients and medications like levetiracetam (Keppra) are also used; magnesium sulfate is the primary medication for seizure in pregnant women as it is likely to be related to preeclampsia or eclampsia. Magnesium has several side effects and requires monitoring to ensure serum levels are not exceeding safe thresholds. High magnesium levels can lead to lethargy, decreased reflexes, hypotension, pulmonary edema, and respiratory issues. Most common is a general feeling of malaise.

16.6 Coronary artery disease and Spontaneous Coronary Artery Dissection

Women of even younger and childbearing age can have coronary artery disease. Coronary artery disease can include a variety of problems. Most commonly, we view cholesterol plaque formation as the culprit. This is due to a variety of issues. Certain lifestyle habits, such as tobacco use, promote coronary disease. There is also a strong genetic predisposition for coronary artery disease [29]. Poorly controlled blood sugar, hypertension, and hypercholesterolemia are all key factors promoting traditional coronary disease [29]. Inflammation can also contribute to development of coronary artery disease [19]. It is widely publicized that women present with atypical myocardial infarction presentations than men [62]. The atypical symptoms that women experience may be masked by perimenopause or pregnancy symptoms. This is a reason to keep cardiovascular issues in the differential diagnosis list.

Smoking cessation, blood glucose management, and hypertension management are established standards of practice for maternity care. Hyperlipidemia is not an area that is currently routinely evaluated [81]. This is because many of the medications used to treat this condition are not considered safe for pregnancy and/or breastfeeding. Currently, dietary management is the recommendation during pregnancy for hyperlipidemia. Severe hyperlipidemia has evidence of fetal impacts, but lack of therapies considered safe in pregnancy poses a challenge [81].

The diagnosis of coronary artery disease follows an algorithmic pathway. Chest pain of suspected cardiac origin or cardiovascular-related symptoms are evaluated first with a 12-Lead ECG. If the 12-Lead ECG indicates an acute myocardial infarction, indicated by hallmark ST segment elevations, the patient is transported to the cardiac catheterization lab for emergent angiography and reperfusion by percutaneous coronary intervention or coronary artery bypass grafting [45]. In areas where there will be a significant delay, thrombolytic therapy may be given. Rapid reperfusion is the key to better outcomes. When an ECG does not indicate acute myocardial infarction, the next step is to assess for cardiovascular enzymes; the standard test is troponin at this time, and point-of-care testing for troponin is available. These cardiac enzymes should be assessed serially. Upward trending troponin levels indicate a non-ST elevation myocardial infarction (NSTEMI). Patients with an NSTEMI should have a heparin infusion started immediately and have nonemergent coronary angiography prior to discharge [4]. In patients with an NSTEMI where chest pain remains, nitroglycerin may be administered sublingually, topically, or as an infusion. In patients with normal troponins, a cardiac stress test is the usual next step. Exercise stress testing is the most basic, with nuclear stress testing and other options. Coronary disease is only treated when it is deemed to be clinically significant, and research is indicating that the use of Fractional Flow Reserve testing or instantaneous wave-free ratio is useful in deciding if coronary artery disease is clinically significant and is becoming a more common method to assess the severity of coronary artery disease [97].

There are two main options for percutaneous treatment of coronary artery disease: bare-metal stents and drug-eluting stents. Drug-eluting stents are used, and two commonly used drugs in commercially available stents are Zotarolimus and Everolimus which are immunosuppressant drugs used to help eliminate the occurrence of restenosis inside the newly placed stent [98,99]. With either a bare metal stent or a drug-eluting stent, immediately following placement the stent, exposed stent struts are in the lumen of the coronary artery. These struts are a target for platelet aggregation until the vessel regrows a layer of endothelium, the neo-endothelium. This process occurs more quickly in bare metal stents and more slowly in drug-eluting stents. For this reason, antiplatelet therapy durations are longer in drug-eluting stents.

It is currently recommended to take dual antiplatelet therapy for 30–60 days for bare metal stents and 12 months for drug-eluting stents, though research is suggesting a shorter duration of DAPT in patients with high bleeding risk may be safe [73]. In pregnancy and breastfeeding, clopidogrel has the best safety profile of the currently available medications as it is the oldest [24]. There are limited data on ticagrelor and prasugrel. The second component of antiplatelet therapy is aspirin. Currently, low-dose (81 mg) aspirin is being used for a variety of reasons in pregnancy. The same 81 mg dose is recommended as part of the DAPT. It is important to note the Aspirin functions to permanently affect platelet function for the life of the platelet. Clopidogrel is a P2y12 inhibitor. A key consideration with clopidogrel is that it takes upward of 5 days for platelet function to return to a normal baseline following discontinuation [48]. In the setting of pregnancy, it will be necessary to either bridge to a reversible medication, like heparin, several days before birth is expected or plan for and anticipate additional blood loss in pregnancy. Maternal bleeding risks are much lower in vaginal delivery than cesarean [70].

Additional medications that are commonly used in and around the setting of coronary artery disease are IIb/IIIa inhibitors. One of the most commonly used of these is tirofiban (Aggrastat). There is limited information regarding its use in pregnancy, but it is considered safe for use.

Spontaneous Coronary Artery Dissection (SCAD) is the tearing of the inner lining, the intima, of the coronary arteries [55]. It presents with symptoms similar or identical to myocardial infarction, but can also present as syncope, shortness of breath, and/or angina. SCAD follows the same diagnostic pathway as coronary artery disease, and is not usually diagnosed until a patient has coronary angiography or another form of cardiac imaging. SCAD is the leading cause of myocardial infarction in peripartum women [77]. Pregnant/postpartum women are also the leading demographic for SCAD. It is crucial to differentiate pregnancy-related SCAD from nonpregnancy-related SCAD when discussing this topic as P-SCAD has substantially higher morbidity and mortality than NP-SCAD [78].

SCAD can be obstructive, partially obstructive, or nonobstructive. This guides the management of SCAD. In nonobstructive or partially obstructive SCAD, the preferred management method is to use medical management [57]. Medical management includes heparin, antiplatelet therapy like clopidogrel, medications to control hypertension if present, and possibly a beta-blocker [57,77]. The heparin and antiplatelet therapy try to prevent the formation or growth of clot in the false lumen created by the tear. Percutaneous coronary interventions/assessments require placing a wire down the affected artery. This presents a significant difficulty as this could extend the dissection and it makes it difficult for the interventionalist to determine if the wire is in the true or the false lumen. Percutaneous coronary intervention or coronary artery bypass grafting may be used as the treatment to be determined on an individual basis [57,77].

The effect of certain pregnancy hormones relaxin and progesterone on the connective tissue contributes to SCAD [78]. Those with a connective tissue disorder are at higher risk of dissections of not only the coronary arteries but also the aorta. Connective tissue disorders are also more common in women than in men.

16.7 Coronary Microvascular Disease and angina

Traditional focus on coronary artery disease has been on the major coronary arteries and the larger branches off of these. Due mostly in part to the small size and inability to intervene, the smaller branches and the microvasculature of the coronary arteries have often been ignored. The larger vessels can have endothelial dysfunction as well as the microvasculature, causing spasm that reduces blood flow [66]. Myocardial Infarction with NonObstructive Coronary Arteries (MINOCA) is a recent terminology for when the myocardium is damaged, releasing cardiac biomarkers indicating infarction or having ECG changes characteristic of an ischemia/infarction, but coronary angiography reveals no obstructive disease [65]. Not all cases of microvascular disease and endothelial dysfunction lead to infarction. Most people diagnosed with this have chest pain or shortness of breath and follow the standard pathway for assessing coronary artery disease. Selective coronary angiography of a typical heart catheterization may not reveal evidence of microvascular disease [18]. Not all health systems have the ability to perform the invasive physiological testing that can be used to diagnose microvascular disease, so referral may be needed. Patients may report very classical angina or cardiac symptoms, but they may not be reproducible. A key point for women's healthcare providers is that patients can pass stress testing and even have normal coronary angiography during a heart catheterization and still have endothelial dysfunction or microvascular disease. If women are still having anginal and cardiovascular symptoms, referring them to a cardiologist who focuses on microvascular disease may be beneficial. Both MINOCA and Coronary Microvascular Disease are significantly more common in women than men [52]. Treatment includes a combination of medications to reduce the spasm and increase blood flow. This includes a combination of calcium channel blockers, long acting nitrates, and some other medications such as ranolazine [18,52,100].

16.7.1 Cardiomyopathy/heart failure

While peripartum cardiomyopathy is the most commonly thought of type of heart failure, many different types of heart failure can exist before or develop during pregnancy [51]. Preexisting heart failure or decreased ejection fraction before pregnancy is very serious and is associated with a high degree of maternal morbidity and mortality; this is why the U.S. Centers for Disease Control, separates cardiomyopathy from cardiovascular disease in the reporting of its maternal mortality data. It is vital to screen patients for signs of cardiomyopathy as early as possible in pregnancy and during pregnancy, particularly those with a strong family history. Common pregnancy symptoms are very similar to heart failure symptoms such as the following: edema, shortness of breath with exertion, and difficulty lying flat. It is vital to not dismiss these symptoms without at least a focused cardiovascular exam. Peripartum cardiomyopathy disproportionately affects women of black race, and women of black race also have delayed diagnosis and poorer clinical trajectories [37,42]. While areas like Haiti and SubSaharan Africa have very high incidences of peripartum cardiomyopathy, when examining black populations alone in certain areas of the United States, rates are comparable to these hotspots [37]. Heart failure also disproportionately impacts patients of black race [9].

Another key recommendation from the ESC guidelines is the recommendation to transfer women who are requiring inotropes or vasopressors to a facility that can provide mechanical circulatory support, while transcatheter ventricular assist devices are becoming more common, fewer facilities offer extracorporeal membraneous oxygenation [31].

One challenge with peripartum cardiomyopathy is the timing. Currently, cases are predominately diagnosed in the postpartum, with black women predominantly being diagnosed late postpartum [42]. Most women in the United States are released from maternity care following the sixth postpartum week, and peripartum cardiomyopathy can be diagnosed up to 5 months postpartum. The definition of peripartum cardiomyopathy also provides a bit of ambiguity to the cause of the condition. That is, by definition, peripartum cardiomyopathy has an unknown cause [89]. There are many suggested causes of peripartum cardiomyopathy, and strong links to hypertension and preeclampsia have also been established [7]. The reality is that there are several possible causes for peripartum cardiomyopathy that all have some validity, and until we know the etiology, a focus on earlier recognition is crucial. Also, as the vast majority of women are diagnosed postpartum, there is not a clear recommendation on the preferred route of birth. Coordination with multiple specialties to provide care for a mother suffering from cardiomyopathy is critical [33].

Electrocardiography has some potential in detecting cardiomyopathy [39,40].

16.8 Medications for cardiomyopathy

Diuretics are often the first pharmacological therapy that comes to mind in heart failure. ESC guidelines recommend the use of diuretics only when pulmonary congestion is present. It is essential to monitor for electrolyte imbalances common with the use of diuretics.

Breastfeeding should not be discontinued solely due to the diagonosis of peripartum cardiomyopathy or another form of heart failure. This decision should be made based on the maternal condition. Despite a possible link between prolactin and peripartum cardiomyopathy, breastfeeding can be safely continued [23]. The 2018 ESC guidelines do suggest stopping breastfeeding in severe cases of heart failure citing a reduction in maternal cardiometabolic demands [70]. The use of certain medications can make breastfeeding more difficult. Furosemide (Lasix) was used in the past to assist in the suppression of lactation, a practice that has been discontinued. In each patient, the desire and benefits of breastfeeding should be weighed against the physical needs of the mother. Breastfeeding has numerous documented benefits for the fetus and should be supported if the mother is able to tolerate and is desiring. In some areas, it may be possible to obtain donor breast milk.

In most cases of heart failure, beta-blockers are recommended. This helps to create a slower heart rate, but this slower rate allows for filling in diastole increasing the efficiency of the heart. Diuretics are often necessary to reduce fluid volumes, and depending on the level of heart failure, anticoagulation may be needed in the event or to prevent left ventricular thrombus. Positive inotropes, like milrinone, may be needed in the case of more severe heart failure.

16.9 Electrophysiological

It is normal to have an increase in maternal heart rate as pregnancy progresses [10]. Premature contractions of both the atria and ventricle are common. Any electrophysiological issue can develop in pregnancy that develops in the general population. Electrophysiological problems can be grouped into the following categories: blocks, bradycardia, tachycardia, or arrest rhythms. Immediate stabilization is the key. Heart blocks that are affecting hemodynamics will likely not resolve with pharmacological therapy. Electrical cardioversion or pacing is often the quickest way to restore a normal rhythm and should not be delayed if the patient is hemodynamically unstable. Advanced Cardiac Life Support (ACLS) algorithms should be followed in cases of hemodynamic instability [75]. Placement of implanted cardiac defibrillators, pacemakers, and other electrophysiological devices are best delayed until at least the second trimester, if possible, to minimize fetal risks due to radiation exposure.

16.9.1 Antiarrhythmic medications

There are currently five classes of antiarrhythmic medications, Class I–V. They are classified based on their mechanism of action. Class I affect sodium ion channels and are divided into three subclasses based on the speed of the blocking Ia–Ic, Class II affect the sympathetic nervous system, Class III affect potassium ions, Class IV affects the calcium channels, and Class V are other actions or unknown actions [48].

Many antiarrhythmic medications have other uses. As an example, we have mentioned both beta-blockers (Class II antiarrhythmics) and calcium channel blockers (Class IV antiarrhythmics) for their antihypertensive properties. Nifedipine is the most commonly used calcium channel blocker used in pregnancy, but it does not have much use as an antiarrhythmic medication. Labetalol has some antiarrhythmic effect, though selection depends largely on the specific need. Amiodarone is a medication that should be used with careful consideration. Amiodarone can lead to thyroid and arrhythmia in the fetus. Use of this drug in the ACLS algorithm for pregnant women is debated, and AHA recommends the use of all drugs in the ACLS algorithm be used without concern for fetal effects in the event of a maternal emergency. In a nonemergent setting, amiodarone should be saved for postpartum. As a consideration for use, amiodarone does have an extremely long half-life, up to and exceeding 100 days [41].

Classes of antiarrhythmics		
Class I	Alter Na+	Procainamide (Ia) Lidocaine (Ib) Flecainide (Ic)
Class II	Parasympathetic action	Beta blockers • Esmolol • metoprolol
Class III	Alter K+ channel	Amiodarone
Class IV	Ca + alteration	Verapamil Diltiazem
Class V	Direct nodal or unknown	Adenosine Digoxin Magnesium sulfate

Atrial fibrillation is one of the most common arrhythmias in the word. It is characterized by a quivering (fibrillating) atrial rhythm an irregular ventricular rhythm [34]. The rhythm can present with a normal ventricular response (a rate similar to that of a normal pulse rate), a slow ventricular response, and a rapid ventricular response. In addition to the rate, atrial fibrillation increases the risk of thrombus formation in the atria, notably in the left atrial appendage [34]. Echocardiography may be needed to assess for the presence of clot before cardioversion. Atrial fibrillation is often asymptomatic and may be undetected.

16.9.1.1 Rate control

In atrial fibrillation with rapid ventricular response, it is often necessary to slow the heart rate to a more normal level. Digoxin or a selective beta-blocker like metoprolol or atenolol is recommended starting points. Digoxin is considered safe and the only common fetal issues have been associated with digoxin toxicity, not digoxin use [83]. The use of diltiazem or verapamil is not the recommended first-line therapy due to risk of fetal effects. In nonpregnant individuals, an IV bolus of diltiazem 10−20 mg followed by infusion may be used to reduce the heart rate and aid in converting to a sinus rhythm [12].

16.9.1.2 Anticoagulation with atrial fibrillation

Unique among the arrhythmias is the need for anticoagulation in atrial fibrillation. Atrial fibrillation increases the risk for cerebrovascular events. Traditionally, this has been accomplished with Coumadin in nonpregnant individuals, but newer medications NonVitamin K Oral Anticoagulants (NOACs) or Direct Oral Anticoagulants (DOACs) are now the preferred therapy for stroke prevention in patients with atrial fibrillation over Coumadin per the 2019 AHA/ACC/HRS Guideline for the Management of Patients with Atrial Fibrillation. Two glaring nonobstetric reasons to avoid NOACs are moderate−severe mitral stenosis and the presence of a mechanical heart valve. NOACs have very little data on their safety during pregnancy and Coumadin is a known teratogen causing facial/palate defects and limb malformations when used in the first trimester [30]. There is not consensus on when to use oral anticoagulants (Coumadin) and when to use heparin or low-molecular weight heparin (LMWH). There is no clear guidance on deciding whether to use heparin or Coumadin for atrial fibrillation in a pregnant woman. Ideally, chemical or electrical cardioversion to a sinus rhythm and an appropriate antiarrhythmic therapy would be the stop point, but this is not always the case, as atrial fibrillation can be refractory to both pharmacologic and electrical cardioversion. Electrical cardioversion provides less risk to the fetus than pharmacological therapies [88]. The multidisciplinary pregnancy heart team should make the best recommendation to patients and allow for shared decision-making. Heparin whether unfractionated or LMWH is not an oral medication and will likely require injections multiple times a day during pregnancy. Guidance from Elkayam et al. recommends first trimester heparin therapy for mechanical heart valves and transition to Coumadin in the second trimester (2016). However, others recommend discussions with the patient and find the optimal balance of maternal and fetal risk, with coumadin being more protective for the mother, and heparin having a safer profile for the fetus [26]. Discontinuation of Coumadin is recommended closer to anticipated delivery and transition to standard heparin due to the ability to reverse completely and more efficiently with protamine sulfate [30]. If the Coumadin is not discontinued, the recommendation is for cesarean delivery to avoid fetal bleeding related to trauma from passage through the pelvis.

Coumadin reversal:
Vitamin K infusion is an effective reversal, the usual dose for reversal is 2.5–5 mg.
In emergent reversal for bleeding, a plasma infusion may be needed.
Kcentra is a prothrombin complex concentrate that is effective and quickly reversing when used with vitamin K. Kcentra is extremely expensive, but provides a rapid alternative to plasma (especially noting that it can be stored longer than plasma). Reversal in patients with mechanical valves or atrial fibrillation should not be done routinely as the ramifications from a thrombosed valve or stroke can be very significant.
Heparin reversal
Protamine sulfate is used to reverse both standard heparin and low-molecular weight heparin, though LMWH is not fully reversible with protamine.
Protamine dosage depends on the total number of units of heparin administered and the time since administration.

16.9.1.3 Anticoagulation and antiplatelet therapy

Anticoagulation and antiplatelet therapies are becoming increasingly more common in the obstetrical patients. Outside of traditional obstetrical reasons (risk to fetus/infant), there are many considerations when choosing an anticoagulant or antiplatelet. Included in these considerations are duration of effect and reversibility, as well as the reason for anticoagulation or antiplatelet need. In a pregnant patient, a bleeding event should be anticipated. A birth may have minimal blood loss, but with each birth, there is the potential for hemorrhage, trauma, and the need for emergent surgical intervention. Anticoagulants and antiplatelets increase this bleeding risk. To add to the challenge, traditionally, very few medications in these classes had reversal agents. Coumadin and heparin both have reversal agents that are effective quickly, with heparin being the most easily reversible. Currently, none of the commercial antiplatelet medications are reversible, though ticagrelor's effect is reversible and an agent, PB2452, is in development. Most of these antiplatelet medications affect the IIb/IIIa pathway either directly (tirofiban/eptifibatide) or indirectly through the P2Y12 pathway (clopidogrel, ticagrelor, and prasugrel) and there are no commercially available therapies to reverse drugs affecting this pathway. The current practice for patients on an antiplatelet agent with an emergent bleeding event is to transfuse platelets. This is why patients may be asked to bridge to heparin injections 5–7 days before birth is anticipated and discontinue their oral antiplatelet. The three major DOACs (Eliquis, Xarelto, and Pradaxa) entered the market without reversibility. Providers were required to balance the benefits of consistent dosing and more consisted anticoagulation with an inability to reverse their effects in the event of a major bleeding incident or trauma. Particularly, considering many patients on anticoagulants are of advanced age, minor falls could become major life threatening events. Today, these three DOACs all have a reverse agent increasing the safety of their use [21]. Unfortunately, data are limited on the use of these DOACs in pregnancy or breastfeeding, and none of these medications are considered first-line therapies. It is important to note that most of the reversal agents for these medications are considerably expensive. Vitamin K and protamine sulfate are relatively inexpensive, but medications like Kcentra, Andexxa, or Praxbind can cost upwards of a few thousand dollars a dose [21]. Coumadin and heparin are some of the oldest and most used anticoagulants, but they are far from benign. Coumadin requires frequent lab work to monitor levels; without monitoring, levels could be subtherapeutic or reach toxic levels. Heparin has a rare but unique consideration, heparin-induced thrombocytopenia, an antibody response that attacks platelets [28]. For patients requiring anticoagulation at birth, it may be possible to have technologies for autotransfusion available to avoid or reduce the use of donor blood.

Name	Mechanism of action	Reversal agent	Pregnancy/ Breastfeeding	Considerations
Anticoagulants				
Warfarin (coumadin)	Alters vitamin K utilization	Vitamin K Plasma Prothrombin complex concentrate	Evidence shows risk for teratogenicity when used in first trimester (limb malformations and cleft lip/ palate) Coumadin is being used in pregnancy for those with mechanical heart valves. Heparin may be used for the first trimester Recommendation to discontinue and bridge to heparin close to delivery. Minimal levels of coumadin are present in breast milk and breastfeeding is considered safe	Requires dietary modification Requires frequent monitoring Only oral anticoagulant currently indicated for use with mechanical heart valves
Eliquis (apixaban)	Direct inhibition of factor Xa	Andexxa (coagulation factor Xa recombinant)	No quality data exist on the safety of Eliquis in pregnancy, but animal studies have not revealed any issues There is not any data on the use of Eliquis in	Eliquis is not approved for use with mechanical heart valves

Name	Mechanism of action	Reversal agent	Pregnancy/ Breastfeeding	Considerations
			breastfeeding; it is suggested to "pump and dump" if on Eliquis	
Pradaxa (dabigatran etexilate)	Direct thrombin inhibitor	Praxbind (idarucizumab)	No current data are available on Pradaxa in breastmilk; it is currently recommended to consider another medication if breastfeeding	
Xarelto (rivaroxaban)	Direct factor Xa inhibition	Andexxa (coagulation factor Xa recombinant)	Due to limited data, breastfeeding is not recommended while on this medication	
Heparin (Lovenox - low molecular weight)	Binds and activates antithrombin III	Protamine sulfate (low-molecular weight heparin is not fully reversible)	Heparin is considered safe in pregnancy and breastfeeding	Patients utilizing heparin (either unfractionated or low molecular weight) should be monitored for signs of heparin-induced thrombocytopenia Levels can be monitored using activated clotting time (ACT) in the procedural setting. PTT can also be used to monitor, but increasingly a shift has been made to assess anti-Xa or heparin level

Name	Mechanism of action	Reversal agent	Pregnancy/ Breastfeeding	Considerations
Angiomax (bivalirudin)	Direct thrombin inhibitor	Limited reversal agents due to short half-life of bivalirudin (~1 h). Factor 7a has shown efficacy, but is expensive	There is limited safety data on bivalirudin and pregnancy or breastfeeding. Bivalirudin's short half-life and short-term use makes it reasonable to "pump and dump" and resume breastfeeding when off medication	Bivalirudin is primarily only used in procedural settings. It is IV infusion only

Antiplatelet

Name	Mechanism of action	Reversal agent	Pregnancy/ Breastfeeding	Considerations
Aspirin	Blocks the formation of thromboxane A2 permanently inhibiting platelet aggregation	Platelet transfusion	Use of low-dose aspirin is considered safe in pregnancy and is frequently recommended for use in certain populations. 75–325 mg daily are also considered safe for breastfeeding, doses over 325 mg daily may require discontinuation of breastfeeding	Enteric coated aspirin is preferred for long-term use to reduce initiation to reduce gastric irritation
Plavix (clopidogrel)	Inhibits adenosine diphosphate (ADP) from binding with the P2Y12 (irreversible) receptor. This subsequently inhibits IIb/IIIa	Platelet transfusion	Of the P2Y12 inhibitors commercially available, clopidogrel has the most data to support its safety in pregnancy and it is the preferred medication when antiplatelet therapy is needed in pregnant/ breastfeeding women	Following a loading dose of 300–600 mg, Plavix is shown to be effective in 2 h. It can take upwards of 5 days or more for platelet function to return to normal following discontinuation of Plavix Plavix does

Name	Mechanism of action	Reversal agent	Pregnancy/ Breastfeeding	Considerations
				have a subset of 5%—11% of patients that do not respond to the medication. In patients developing in-stent thrombosis following PCI, lab testing is available or another pharmacological agent may be considered
Brilinta (ticagrelor)	P2Y12 inhibitor (reversible)	Platelet transfusion No commercially available reversal. PB2452 is a recombinant monoclonal antibody medication that is being developed	Adverse pregnancy events have been reported in animal studies	
Effient (prasugrel)	P2Y12 inhibitor (irreversible)		There is limited evidence on pregnancy safety; there have been no adverse events in animal studies	
Aggrastat (tirofiban)	IIb/IIIa inhibitor	No known reversal, platelet transfusion may be helpful	Adverse events have not been reported in animal studies. Aggrastat is most often used in a very short-term manner, usually to bridge to an oral P2Y12 and has a short half-life of 4 h	Intravenous use only; used only short term until bridged to oral P2Y12 medication

Name	Mechanism of action	Reversal agent	Pregnancy/ Breastfeeding	Considerations
Integrilin (eptifibatide)	IIb/IIIa inhibitor	No known reversal, platelet transfusion may be helpful	Adverse events have not been reported in animal studies. Integrilin is most often used in a very short-term manner, usually to bridge to an oral P2Y12 and has a short half-life of 4 h	Intravenous use only; used only short term until bridged to oral P2Y12 medication

16.9.1.4 Long QT syndrome

Beta-blockers are indicated for patients with long QT syndrome.

It is important to note that many medications that are commonly used in pregnancy can cause QT-Prolongation; you should avoid use of these medications in patients with Long QT Syndrome. Ondansetron (Zofran) is a documented example of a common medication that prolongs the QT interval [101]. Other medications commonly used in pregnancy that prolong QT interval are diphenhydramine, erythromycin, and fluoxetine. Providers should assess the potential of any new medications to prolong the QT interval in patients with long QT syndrome prior to prescribing or recommending over-the-counter therapies [76].

16.9.1.5 Antiarrhythmic medications

There are currently five classes of antiarrhythmic medications Class I−V. They are classified based on their mechanism of action. Class 1 affects sodium ion channels, Class II affects the sympathetic nervous system, Class III affects potassium ions, Class IV affects the calcium channels, and Class V are other actions or unknown actions.

Many antiarrhythmic medications have other uses. As an example, we have mentioned both beta-blockers (Class II antiarrhythmics) and calcium channel blockers (Class IV antiarrhythmics). Nifedipine is the most commonly used calcium channel blocker used in pregnancy, but it does not have much use as an antiarrhythmic. It is important to consider the side effects of any medication and implications to patients' health prior to prescribing.

16.9.1.6 Thromboembolic disorders

Thromboembolic disorders are common in pregnancy and the risk is significantly increased cesarean births compared to vaginal birth [61]. Pulmonary embolism and CVA are the most serious thromboembolic disorders, but deep vein thrombosis is also a concern.

CVAs are time-sensitive events caused by either bleeding or, more commonly, a clot obstructing blood flow to the brain [86]. If a CVA is suspected, a CT scan and/or CT angiography of the head should be performed promptly. The traditional treatment is the systemic administration of thrombolytic medications such as tissue plasminogen activase (Alteplase). Particularly in the postpartum population, bleeding is a significant concern, especially in postcesarean patients. Catheter-directed therapy is available in areas with access to neuro-interventional procedures. Localized infusion of thrombolytics at the site of the clot or removal of the clot through thrombectomy carries less bleeding risk than systemic infusion of thrombolytics but are not as widely available [68]. Prompt recognition of CVA symptoms provides the best possible opportunity for transport to a facility where neuro-intervention is available. Patients receiving thrombolytics should be carefully monitored for signs of bleeding, and most notably intracranial bleeding [68]. There are several considerations with the selection of systemic or catheter-directed therapies, particularly timing, bleeding risk, and availability. Systemic administration of thrombolytic medications is the fastest method but also carries the most bleeding risk. Catheter-directed therapies are not available everywhere and also take extra time to begin infusion, but carry a lower bleeding risk [59].

It is also possible to have thromboembolic issues in areas of the brain other than the cerebrum. As an example, cerebellar stroke does not present with the traditional stroke symptoms, instead presenting with jerky and uncoordinated movements [67]. Other medical issues such as migraine may present similarly to traditional strokes.

Outside of pregnancy, women have a unique risk regarding thromboembolism, contraception. Oral contraceptives, particularly combined hormonal methods, increase the risk for stroke and thromboembolic events [71].

16.9.1.7 Hypotension

Hypotension in the obstetrical setting is most likely for two reasons: regional anesthesia and hemorrhage. These are not the only reasons for hypotension, issues such as cardiogenic shock from cardiomyopathy, or spontaneous coronary artery disease. Primarily, hypotension during pregnancy, particularly in the intrapartum setting, is treated with crystalloid fluid bolus [13]. It is a standard practice to preload with a bolus of fluids prior to administration of epidural or spinal anesthesia. This increases the intravascular volume ahead of the vasodilatory effects of the regional anesthesia reducing the occurrence of hypotension. In many cases, this is not adequate and pharmacologic agents are needed to temporarily maintain normotension [13]. Ephedrine is the most common drug used for this, but there is not a consensus on dosage. Phenylephrine is also used to provide a boost in blood pressure, and some data show that phenylephrine may have less fetal impact than ephedrine. There is also not a consensus on how significant a drop in blood pressure must occur before administering a pharmacological agent. Symptomatic hypotension should be treated. Recognizing that intermittent auscultation or intermittent electronic fetal monitoring is safe, use of regional anesthesia necessitates continuous EFM to assess for perfusion issues related to potential hypotension and medication interactions.

Many of the medications used to treat hypotension are transmitted through the placenta to the fetus. However, it is important to realize that significant maternal hypotension adversely impacts the fetus. The fetal impact of these medications is secondary to the need to ensure adequate placental perfusion. If a mother requires ongoing pharmacological therapy to treat hypotension, immediate delivery should be considered.

16.9.1.8 Pharmacology for Advanced Cardiac Life Support

There are not many significant differences pharmacologically in ACLS for pregnancy. In the 2010 American Heart Association guidelines on ACLS, it does state that "drug administration during ACLS should adhere to the standard adult guidelines without concern for teratogenicity" [32]. Subsequent updates have not addressed this guidance differently. Amiodarone is the most concerning medication for fetal effects which may include fetal bradycardia and arrhythmia, as well as hypothyroidism. Severe maternal cardiovascular events are situations where, without intervention, fetal death is likely. Fetal bradycardia, arrhythmia, and hypothyroidism can all be managed clinically; the damage from fetal hypoxia related to inadequate perfusion in utero is not easily managed.

The foundation of ACLS for cardiac arrest is strong Basic Cardiac Life Support (BLS) [32,75]. There are some different fundamentals for BLS in pregnant patients. A primary consideration is the compression of the inferior vena cava by a gravid uterus. This has traditionally been accomplished by tilting the mother's pelvis to allow. It can take a significant amount of tilt, >30°, to relieve this compression. This can significantly impact the quality of chest compressions. Another strategy involves manual uterine displacement [75].

Perimortem Cesarean Delivery (PMCD) is another consideration that should be considered promptly. Contrary to its name, PMCD is not simply a decision to give up on efforts to save the mother and focus efforts on saving the baby. Statistically, PMCD increases the fetus' odds of survival, but it can also increase the chances of maternal survival [47].

It is essential to have standardized procedures. Maternal cardiac arrest is a relatively uncommon event, and maternal health providers are not as likely to be experienced in this as physicians, advanced practice providers, nurses, and other healthcare personnel working in critical care areas such as emergency and cardiology. Practice makes perfect. Most ACLS and BLS require renewal every 2 years. It is evident that ACLS skills require frequent exposure and practice. Departments should incorporate frequent emergency drills that include ACLS skills to provide staff with the familiarity and confidence to function in a real emergency [38].

16.9.1.9 Congenital heart disease in the adult

Significant congenital heart disease (CHD) affects around 1% of births in the United States and 25% of those are classified as critical. Over the past decades, the procedures and management options for CHD have led to a point where patients who likely would not have survived childhood 50–60 years ago can now not only consider pregnancy, but in many cases have a strong likelihood of a healthy pregnancy [58,69]. All patients with CHD need to be counseled on family planning options. Prevention of unplanned pregnancy can be a life-saving event for patients with ACHD. It is also important to note that even patients with significant physical or mental impairments can become pregnant and are a population at high risk for sexual abuse, and patients with CHD can have psychological trauma from their experienced [5].

Pregnancy in a patient with ACHD requires a multidisciplinary approach including congenital heart providers and maternal–fetal medicine specialists. Preconception planning is important for ACHD patients [56]. Management decisions and choices should be highly individualized based on the patient's specific needs. Long-acting reversible contraception methods, if not contraindicated, are extremely effective in prevention of unwanted pregnancy. A concern with contraception, particularly combined hormonal methods, is the increased risk for clotting-related issues. It is also important to note that even in patients of the same age with identical CHD, depending on the location of their childhood repair(s), they could have very different postrepair anatomy. A great example of this are patients with transposition of the great vessels. There was a period of time where patients could have received either a Mustard or Senning procedure (atrial swap) or a Jatene (arterial swap) [50].

Each ACHD patient has unique cardiovascular pharmacological needs that draw on all the medications discussed earlier in this chapter. They also require individualized therapy. Some critical considerations for ACHD pharmacology are the need for anticoagulation. Mechanical valves in the ACHD population are not as prevalent as they once were, but coumadin is the preferred choice for anticoagulation of mechanical heart valves [30]. This is complicated by the fact that coumadin has potentially teratogenic effects. This can be minimized by avoiding use from conception through the first trimester and using heparin instead. Though the evidence is largely based on small population studies and on expert opinion, some providers are prescribing coumadin in the first trimester. Recommendations favor a shared decision-making model where patients can choose to favor maternal health (coumadin through first trimester) or fetal health [26].

16.9.1.10 Cardiovascular effects of noncardiovascular medications

Many common drugs have cardiovascular side effects. One of the more common is QT-Prolongation, which can lead to sudden cardiac arrest. Medications used in obstetrical practice such as ondansetron, which are commonly prescribed for treatment of nausea and vomiting, such as that occurring with hyperemesis gravidarum or azithromycin, commonly prescribed for both respiratory and sexually transmitted infections, can cause QT-Prolongation [87]. Pitocin can also cause QT-Prolongation or exacerbate existing long QT [11]. A challenge for obstetrical providers is that many of these medications are commonly used in our clinical setting and many patients have never had an ECG, so it is possible that they could have long QT syndrome. Females are at an increased risk to have QT-Prolongation [76]. It is common to expect this effect in medications such as antiarrhythmics and other cardiovascular medications, but noncardiovascular medications are frequently culprits.

Not specifically pregnancy related, but certain chemotherapy agents have cardiotoxicity. In the case of breast cancer, the heart, being in close proximity to breast tissue, can be exposed to significant amounts of radiation which can have adverse effects [63]. Cardio-oncology is an emerging area of cardiovascular medicine that is addressing these issues, and consultation with a cardio-oncology provider is warranted for a patient with a prior history of cancer [16].

References

[1] Abalos E, Duley L, Steyn D. Antihypertensive drug therapy for mild to moderate hypertension during pregnancy. Cochrane Database Syst Rev 2014;(2). https://doi.org/10.1002/14651858.CD002252.pub3.

[2] ACOG practice bulletin no. 212: pregnancy and heart disease. Obstet Gynecol 2019;133(5). Retrieved from: https://journals.lww.com/greenjournal/Fulltext/2019/05000/ACOG_Practice_Bulletin_No__212__Pregnancy_and.40.aspx.

[3] Amaral LM, Wallace K, Owens M, LaMarca B. Pathophysiology and current clinical management of preeclampsia. Curr Hypertens Rep 2017;19(8). https://doi.org/10.1007/s11906-017-0757-7. 61-61.

[4] Amsterdam EA, Wenger NK, Brindis RG, Casey DE, Ganiats TG, Holmes DR, et al. 2014 AHA/ACC guideline for the management of patients with Non−ST-elevation acute coronary syndromes. J Am Coll Cardiol 2014;64(24):e139−228. https://doi.org/10.1016/j.jacc.2014.09.017.

[5] Andonian C, Beckmann J, Biber S, Ewert P, Freilinger S, Kaemmerer H, et al. Current research status on the psychological situation of adults with congenital heart disease. Cardiovasc Diagn Ther 2018;8(6):799−804. https://doi.org/10.21037/cdt.2018.12.06.

[6] Bateman BT, Patorno E, Desai RJ, Seely EW, Mogun H, Dejene SZ, et al. Angiotensin-converting enzyme inhibitors and the risk of congenital malformations. Obstet Gynecol 2017;129(1):174−84. https://doi.org/10.1097/AOG.0000000000001775.

[7] Bello N, Rendon ISH, Arany Z. The relationship between pre-eclampsia and peripartum cardiomyopathy. 2013. https://doi.org/10.1016/j.jacc.2013.08.717.

[8] Beyer KH. Chlorothiazide. Br J Clin Pharmacol 1982;13(1):15−24. https://doi.org/10.1111/j.1365-2125.1982.tb01332.x.

[9] Bibbins-Domingo K, Pletcher MJ, Lin F, Vittinghoff E, Gardin JM, Arynchyn A, et al. Racial differences in incident heart failure among young adults. N Engl J Med 2009;360(12):1179−90. https://doi.org/10.1056/NEJMoa0807265.

[10] Blackburn S. Maternal, fetal, & neonatal physiology: a clinical perspective. 5th ed. St. Louis, MO: Elsevier; 2018.

[11] Bodi I, Sorge J, Castiglione A, Glatz SM, Wuelfers EM, Franke G, et al. Postpartum hormones oxytocin and prolactin cause pro-arrhythmic prolongation of cardiac repolarization in long QT syndrome type 2. EP Europace 2019;21(7):1126−38. https://doi.org/10.1093/europace/euz037.

[12] Brubaker S, Long B, Koyfman A. Alternative treatment options for atrioventricular-nodal-reentry tachycardia: an emergency medicine review. J Emerg Med 2018;54(2):198−206. https://doi.org/10.1016/j.jemermed.2017.10.003.

[13] Butterworth J, Mackney D, Wasnick J, editors. Morgan & mikhail's clinical anesthesiology. 6th ed. New York, New York: McGraw-Hill Education; 2018.

[14] Cain MA, Salemi JL, Tanner JP, Kirby RS, Salihu HM, Louis JM. Pregnancy as a window to future health: maternal placental syndromes and short-term cardiovascular outcomes. Am J Obstet Gynecol 2016;215(4):484.e1–484.e14. https://doi.org/10.1016/j.ajog.2016.05.047.

[15] California Quality Maternal Care Collaborative. Improving health care response to cardiovascular disease in pregnancy and postpartum. 2017. Retrieved from: https://www.cmqcc.org/resource/improving-health-care-response-cardiovascular-disease-pregnancy-and-postpartum.

[16] Campia U, Moslehi JJ, Amiri-Kordestani L, Barac A, Beckman JA, Chism DD, et al. Cardio-oncology: vascular and metabolic perspectives: a scientific statement from the American Heart Association. Circulation 2019;139(13):e579–602. https://doi.org/10.1161/CIR.0000000000000641.

[17] Centers for Disease Control. Pregnancy mortality surveillance system. 2020. Retrieved from: https://www.cdc.gov/reproductivehealth/maternal-mortality/pregnancy-mortality-surveillance-system.htm.

[18] Chen C, Wei J, AlBadri A, Zarrini P, Bairey Merz CN. Coronary microvascular dysfunction: epidemiology, pathogenesis, prognosis, diagnosis, risk factors and therapy. Circ J 2017;81(1):3–11. https://doi.org/10.1253/circj.CJ-16-1002.

[19] Christodoulidis G, Vittorio TJ, Fudim M, Lerakis S, Kosmas CE. Inflammation in coronary artery disease. Cardiol Rev 2014;22(6). Retrieved from: https://journals.lww.com/cardiologyinreview/Fulltext/2014/11000/Inflammation_in_Coronary_Artery_Disease.4.aspx.

[20] Cooper WO, Hernandez-Diaz S, Arbogast PG, Dudley JA, Dyer S, Gideon PS, et al. Major congenital malformations after first-trimester exposure to ACE inhibitors. N Engl J Med 2006;354(23):2443–51. https://doi.org/10.1056/NEJMoa055202.

[21] Cuker A, Burnett A, Triller D, Crowther M, Ansell J, Van Cott EM, et al. Reversal of direct oral anticoagulants: guidance from the anticoagulation forum. Am J Hematol 2019;94(6):697–709. https://doi.org/10.1002/ajh.25475.

[22] Davis Melinda B, Walsh MN. Cardio-obstetrics. Circ Cardiovasc Qual & Outcomes 2019;12(2):e005417. https://doi.org/10.1161/CIRCOUTCOMES.118.005417.

[23] Davis M, Duvernoy C. Peripartum cardiomyopathy: current knowledge and future directions. Women's Health 2015;11(4):565–73. https://doi.org/10.2217/WHE.15.15.

[24] De Santis M, De Luca C, Mappa I, Cesari E, Mazza A, Quattrocchi T, Caruso A. Clopidogrel treatment during pregnancy: a case report and a review of literature. Intern Med 2011;50(16):1769–73. https://doi.org/10.2169/internalmedicine.50.5294.

[25] Doumas M, Boutari C, Viigimaa M. Arterial hypertension and erectile dysfunction: an under-recognized duo. E-J Cardiovasc Pract 2016;14(4).

[26] D'Souza R, Ostro J, Shah PS, Silversides CK, Malinowski A, Murphy KE, et al. Anticoagulation for pregnant women with mechanical heart valves: a systematic review and meta-analysis. Eur Heart J 2017;38(19):1509–16. https://doi.org/10.1093/eurheartj/ehx032.

[27] Duley L, Meher S, Jones L. Drugs for treatment of very high blood pressure during pregnancy. Cochrane Database Syst Rev 2013;7. https://doi.org/10.1002/14651858.CD001449.pub3.

[28] East JM, Cserti-Gazdewich C, Granton JT. Heparin-induced thrombocytopenia in the critically ill patient. Chest 2018;154(3):678–90. https://doi.org/10.1016/j.chest.2017.11.039.

[29] Ebrahim S, Taylor F, Ward K, Beswick A, Burke M, Davey Smith G. Multiple risk factor interventions for primary prevention of coronary heart disease. Cochrane Database Syst Rev 2011;1. https://doi.org/10.1002/14651858.CD001561.pub3.

[30] Elkayam U, Goland S, Pieper PG, Silversides CK. High-risk cardiac disease in pregnancy: part I. 2016. https://doi.org/10.1016/j.jacc.2016.05.048.

[31] Elkayam U, Schäfer A, Chieffo A, Lansky A, Hall S, Arany Z, Grines C. Use of impella heart pump for management of women with peripartum cardiogenic shock. Clin Cardiol 2019;42(10):974−81. https://doi.org/10.1002/clc.23249.

[32] Field John M, Hazinski MF, Sayre Michael R, Leon C, Schexnayder Stephen M, Robin H, et al. Part 1: executive summary advanced cardiac life support. Circulation 2010;122(18):S640−56. https://doi.org/10.1161/CIRCULATIONAHA.110.970889.

[33] Fowler K, Schafer D, Sica M, Pogasic D, Gardner K, Szczepanski S, et al. Peripartum cardiomyopathy (PPCM): interdisciplinary coordination for a complex patient population. Heart & Lung J Acute Crit Care 2017;46(3):212−3. https://doi-org.frontier.idm.oclc.org/10.1016/j.hrtlng.2017.04.015.

[34] Fuster V, Harrington R, Narula J, Eapen Z, editors. Hurst's the heart. 14th ed. New York: McGraw-Hill Education; 2017.

[35] Garcia T, Holtz N. 12-lead ECG: the art of interpretation. Burlington, MA: Jones & Bartlett; 2013.

[36] Gauthier C, Sèze-Goismier C, Rozec B. Beta 3-adrenoceptors in the cardiovascular system. Clin Hemorheol Microcirc 2007;37:193−204.

[37] Gentry MB, Dias JK, Luis A, Patel R, Thornton J, Reed GL. African-American women have a higher risk for developing peripartum cardiomyopathy. 2010. https://doi.org/10.1016/j.jacc.2009.09.043.

[38] Green M, Rider C, Ratcliff D, Woodring BC. Developing a systematic approach to obstetric emergencies. J Obstet Gynecol Neonatal Nurs 2015;44(5):677−82. https://doi.org/10.1111/1552-6909.12729.

[39] Honigberg MC, Zekavat SM, Aragam K, Klarin D, Bhatt DL, Scott NS, et al. Long-term cardiovascular risk in women with hypertension during pregnancy. J Am Coll Cardiol 2019;74(22). https://doi.org/10.1016/j.jacc.2019.09.052. 2743-2744-2754.

[40] Honigberg MC, Elkayam U, Rajagopalan N, Modi K, Briller JE, Drazner MH, et al. Electrocardiographic findings in peripartum cardiomyopathy. Clin Cardiol 2019b; 42(5):524−9. https://doi.org/10.1002/clc.23171.

[41] Immordino L, Connolly S, Crijns H, Roy D, Capucci A, Radzik D, et al. Effects of dronedarone started rapidly after amiodarone discontinuation. Clin Cardiol 2013;36(2): 88−95. https://doi.org/10.1002/clc.22090.

[42] Irizarry O, Levine L, Lewey J. Comparison of clinical characteristics and outcomes of peripartum cardiomyopathy between African American and Non−African American women. JAMA Cardiol 2017;2(11):1256−60. https://doi.org/10.1001/jamacardio.2017.3574.

[43] James PA, Oparil S, Carter BL, Cushman WC, Dennison-Himmelfarb C, Handler J, et al. 2014 evidence-based guideline for the management of high blood pressure in adults: report from the panel members appointed to the eighth joint national committee (JNC 8). JAMA 2014;311(5):507−20. https://doi.org/10.1001/jama.2013.284427.

[44] Janke AT, McNaughton CD, Brody AM, Welch RD, Levy PD. Trends in the incidence of hypertensive emergencies in US emergency departments from 2006 to 2013. J Am Heart Assoc 2016;5(12):e004511. https://doi.org/10.1161/JAHA.116.004511.

[45] Jneid H, Addison D, Bhatt DL, Fonarow GC, Gokak S, Grady KL, et al. AHA/ACC clinical performance and quality measures for adults with ST-elevation and non—ST-elevation myocardial infarction: a report of the American College of Cardiology/American Heart Association task force on performance measures. 2017. p. 2017. https://doi.org/10.1016/j.jacc.2017.06.032.

[46] John AS, Gurley F, Schaff HV, Warnes CA, Phillips SD, Arendt KW, et al. Cardiopulmonary bypass during pregnancy. Ann Thorac Surg 2011;91(4):1191—6. https://doi.org/10.1016/j.athoracsur.2010.11.037.

[47] Katz VL. Perimortem cesarean delivery: its role in maternal mortality. 2012. https://doi.org/10.1053/j.semperi.2011.09.013.

[48] Katzung B, editor. Basic and clinical pharmacology. 14th ed. New York, New York: McGraw-HIll Education; 2018.

[49] Keegan P, Lisko JC, Kamioka N, Maidman S, Binongo JN, Wei J, et al. Nurse led sedation: the clinical and echocardiographic outcomes of the 5-year emory experience. Struct Heart 2020. https://doi.org/10.1080/24748706.2020.1773591.

[50] Kirzner J, Pirmohamed A, Ginns J, Singh HS. Long-term management of the arterial switch patient. Curr Cardiol Rep 2018;20(8):68. https://doi.org/10.1007/s11886-018-1012-9.

[51] Kristanto W, Chan P, Chen Elaine BC, Chan WX. Not all heart failure post pregnancy is due to peripartum cardiomyopathy. JACC 2016. https://doi.org.frontier.idm.oclc.org/10.1016/S0735-1097(16)31055-5.

[52] Kumar A, Rabah R, Hung O, Eshtehardi P, Hosseini H, Sabbak N, et al. Results from the microvascular assessment of ranolazine in non-obstructive atherosclerosis (marina): a double-blinded randomized controlled trial. J Am Coll Cardiol 2018; 71(11 Suppl.):A169. https://doi.org/10.1016/S0735-1097(18)30710-1.

[53] Laurent S. Antihypertensive drugs. 2017. https://doi.org/10.1016/j.phrs.2017.07.026.

[54] Leathersich SJ, Vogel JP, Tran TS, Hofmeyr GJ. Acute tocolysis for uterine tachysystole or suspected fetal distress. Cochrane Database Syst Rev 2018;7(7). https://doi.org/10.1002/14651858.CD009770.pub2. CD009770-CD009770.

[55] Lebrun S, Bond RM. Spontaneous coronary artery dissection (SCAD): the underdiagnosed cardiac condition that plagues women. 2018. https://doi.org/10.1016/j.tcm.2017.12.004.

[56] Lindley KJ, Madden T, Cahill AG, Ludbrook PA, Billadello JJ. Contraceptive use and unintended pregnancy in women with congenital heart disease. Obstet Gynecol 2015; 126(2). Retrieved from: https://journals.lww.com/greenjournal/Fulltext/2015/08000/Contraceptive_Use_and_Unintended_Pregnancy_in.21.aspx.

[57] Mahmoud AN, Taduru SS, Mentias A, Mahtta D, Barakat AF, Saad M, et al. Trends of incidence, clinical presentation, and in-hospital mortality among Women with acute myocardial Infarction with or without spontaneous coronary artery dissection: a population-based analysisdoi. 2018. https://doi.org/10.1016/j.jcin.2017.08.016.

[58] Marelli A, Miller SP, Marino BS, Jefferson AL, Newburger JW. Brain in congenital heart disease across the lifespan: the cumulative burden of injury. Circulation 2016; 133(20):1951—62. https://doi.org/10.1161/CIRCULATIONAHA.115.019881.

[59] Martillotti G, Boehlen F, Robert-Ebadi H, Jastrow N, Righini M, Blondon M. Treatment options for severe pulmonary embolism during pregnancy and the postpartum period: a systematic review. J Thromb Haemostasis 2017;15(10):1942—50. https://doi.org/10.1111/jth.13802.

[60] McCance K, Huether S. In: Brashers V, Rote N, editors. Pathophysiology: the biological basis for disease in adults and children. 7th ed. St. Louis, MO: Elsevier; 2014.

[61] McLean K, Cushman M. Venous thromboembolism and stroke in pregnancy. Hematology Am Soc Hematol Educ Program 2016;2016(1):243–50. https://doi.org/10.1182/asheducation-2016.1.243.

[62] Mehta LS, Beckie TM, DeVon HA, Grines CL, Krumholz HM, Johnson MN, et al. Acute myocardial infarction in women. Circulation 2016;133(9):916–47. https://doi.org/10.1161/CIR.0000000000000351.

[63] Mehta LS, Watson KE, Barac A, Beckie TM, Bittner V, Cruz-Flores S, et al. Cardiovascular disease and breast cancer: where these entities intersect: a scientific statement from the American Heart Association. Circulation 2018;137(8):e30–66. https://doi.org/10.1161/CIR.0000000000000556.

[64] O'Callaghan KM, Hennessy Ã, Malvisi L, Kiely M. Central haemodynamics in normal pregnancy: a prospective longitudinal study. J Hypertens 2018;36(10). Retrieved from: https://journals.lww.com/jhypertension/Fulltext/2018/10000/Central_haemodynamics_in_normal_pregnancy__a.10.aspx.

[65] Pasupathy S, Tavella R, Beltrame JF. The what, when, who, why, how and where of myocardial infarction with non-obstructive coronary arteries (MINOCA). Circ J 2016;80(1):11–6. https://doi.org/10.1253/circj.CJ-15-1096.

[66] Pepine CJ, Ferdinand KC, Shaw LJ, Light-McGroary KA, Shah RU, Gulati M, et al. Emergence of nonobstructive coronary artery disease. J Am Coll Cardiol 2015;66(17):1918–33. https://doi.org/10.1016/j.jacc.2015.08.876.

[67] Perloff MD, Patel NS, Kase CS, Oza AU, Voetsch B, Romero JR. Cerebellar stroke presenting with isolated dizziness: brain MRI in 136 patients. Am J Emerg Med 2017;35(11):1724–9. https://doi.org/10.1016/j.ajem.2017.06.034.

[68] Powers William J, Derdeyn Colin P, José B, Coffey Christopher S, Hoh Brian L, Jauch EC, et al. 2015 American Heart Association/American stroke Association focused update of the 2013 guidelines for the early management of patients with acute ischemic stroke regarding endovascular treatment. Stroke 2015;46(10):3020–35. https://doi.org/10.1161/STR.0000000000000074.

[69] Ramage K, Grabowska K, Silversides C, Quan H, Metcalfe A. Association of adult congenital heart disease with pregnancy, maternal, and neonatal outcomes. JAMA Netw Open 2019;2(5). https://doi.org/10.1001/jamanetworkopen.2019.3667. e193667-e193667.

[70] Regitz-Zagrosek V, Roos-Hesselink J, Bauersachs J, Blomström-Lundqvist C, Cífková R, De Bonis M, et al. 2018 ESC guidelines for the management of cardiovascular diseases during pregnancy: the task force for the management of cardiovascular diseases during pregnancy of the european society of cardiology (ESC). Eur Heart J 2018;39(34):3165–241. https://doi.org/10.1093/eurheartj/ehy340.

[71] Roach RE, Helmerhorst FM, Lijfering WM, Stijnen T, Algra A, Dekkers OM. Combined oral contraceptives: the risk of myocardial infarction and ischemic stroke. Cochrane Database Syst Rev 2015;8. https://doi.org/10.1002/14651858.CD011054.pub2.

[72] Salvetti M, Paini A, Bertacchini F, Aggiusti C, Stassaldi D, Verzeri L, et al. Therapeutic approach to hypertensive emergencies: hemorrhagic stroke. High Blood Pres Cardiovasc Prev 2018;25(2):191–5. https://doi.org/10.1007/s40292-018-0262-3.

[73] Shah R, Rao SV, Latham SB, Kandzari DE. Efficacy and safety of drug-eluting stents optimized for biocompatibility vs bare-metal stents with a single month of dual anti-platelet therapy: a meta-analysis. JAMA Cardiol 2018;3(11):1050−9. https://doi.org/10.1001/jamacardio.2018.3551.

[74] Sharma KJ, Greene N, Kilpatrick SJ. Oral labetalol compared to oral nifedipine for postpartum hypertension: a randomized controlled trial. Hypertens Pregnancy 2017; 36(1):44−7. https://doi.org/10.1080/10641955.2016.1231317.

[75] Soskin PN, Yu J. Resuscitation of the pregnant patient. Emerg Med Clin North Am; Obstet & Gynecol Emerg 2019;37(2):351−63. https://doi.org/10.1016/j.emc.2019.01.011.

[76] Trinkley KE, Lee Page R, Lien H, Yamanouye K, Tisdale JE. QT interval prolongation and the risk of torsades de pointes: essentials for clinicians. Curr Med Res Opin 2013; 29(12):1719−26. https://doi.org/10.1185/03007995.2013.840568.

[77] Tweet MS, Hayes SN, Codsi E, Gulati R, Rose CH, Best PJM. Spontaneous coronary artery dissection associated with pregnancy. 2017. https://doi.org/10.1016/j.jacc.2017.05.055.

[78] Tweet MS, Miller VM, Hayes SN. The evidence on estrogen, progesterone, and spon-taneous coronary artery dissection. JAMA Cardiol 2019;4(5):403−4. https://doi.org/10.1001/jamacardio.2019.0774.

[79] Vogel JP, Nardin JM, Dowswell T, West HM, Oladapo OT. Combination of tocolytic agents for inhibiting preterm labour. Cochrane Database Syst Rev 2014;7. https://doi.org/10.1002/14651858.CD006169.pub2.

[80] Webster LM, Conti-Ramsden F, Seed PT, Webb AJ, Nelson-Piercy C, Chappell LC. Impact of antihypertensive treatment on maternal and perinatal outcomes in pregnancy complicated by chronic hypertension: a systematic review and meta-analysis. J Am Heart Assoc 2017;6(5):e005526. https://doi.org/10.1161/JAHA.117.005526.

[81] Wild R, Weedin EA, Wilson D. Dyslipidemia in pregnancy. 2015. https://doi.org/10.1016/j.ccl.2015.01.002.

[82] Williams B, Mancia G, Spiering W, Agabiti Rosei E, Azizi M, Burnier M, et al. 2018 ESC/ESH guidelines for the management of arterial hypertension: the task force for the management of arterial hypertension of the European Society of Cardiology (ESC) and the European Society of Hypertension (ESH). Eur Heart J 2018;39(33): 3021−104. https://doi.org/10.1093/eurheartj/ehy339.

[83] Wright JM, Page RL, Field ME. Antiarrhythmic drugs in pregnancy. Expet Rev Car-diovasc Ther 2015;13(12):1433−44. https://doi.org/10.1586/14779072.2015.1107476.

[84] Wu P, Randula H, Kwok CS, Aswin B, Kotronias RA, Claire R, et al. Preeclampsia and future cardiovascular health. Circ: Cardiovasc Qual & Outcomes 2017;10(2):e003497. https://doi.org/10.1161/CIRCOUTCOMES.116.003497.

[85] Gestational hypertension and preeclampsia: ACOG practice bulletin, number 222. Obstet Gynecol 2020;135(6). Retrieved from: https://journals.lww.com/greenjournal/Fulltext/2020/06000/Gestational_Hypertension_and_Preeclampsia__ACOG.46.aspx.

[86] Lappin Julia M, Shane D, Johan D, Sharlene K, Michael F. Fatal stroke in pregnancy and the puerperium. Stroke 2018;49(12):3050−3. https://doi.org/10.1161/STROKEAHA.118.023274.

[87] Roden DM. Predicting drug-induced QT prolongation and torsades de pointes. J Physiol 2016;594(9):2459−68. https://doi.org/10.1113/JP270526.

[88] Georgiopoulos G, Tsiachris D, Kordalis A, Kontogiannis C, Spartalis M, Pietri P, et al. Pharmacotherapeutic strategies for atrial fibrillation in pregnancy. Expet Opin Pharmacother 2019;20(13):1625—36. https://doi.org/10.1080/14656566.2019.1621290.

[89] Arany Z, Elkayam U. Peripartum cardiomyopathy. Circulation 2016;133(14): 1397—409. https://doi.org/10.1161/CIRCULATIONAHA.115.020491.

[90] Whelton Paul K, Carey Robert M, Aronow Wilbert S, Casey Donald E, Collins Karen J, Dennison HC, et al. 2017 ACC/AHA/AAPA/ABC/ACPM/AGS/APhA/ ASH/ASPC/NMA/PCNA guideline for the prevention, detection, evaluation, and management of high blood pressure in adults: a report of the American College of Cardiology/American Heart Association task force on clinical practice guidelines. Hypertension 2018;71(6):e13—115. https://doi.org/10.1161/HYP.0000000000000065.

[91] Sliwa K, Petrie MC, Hilfiker-Kleiner D, et al. Long-term prognosis, subsequent pregnancy, contraception and overall management of peripartum cardiomyopathy: Practical guidance paper from the heart failure association of the european society of cardiology study group on peripartum cardiomyopathy. Eur J Heart Fail 2018;20(6): 951—62. https://doi-org.proxy.lib.umich.edu/10.1002/ejhf.1178. https://doi-org.proxy. lib.umich.edu/10.1002/ejhf.1178.

[92] Thurber C, Dugas LR, Ocobock C, Carlson B, Speakman JR, Pontzer H. Extreme events reveal an alimentary limit on sustained maximal human energy expenditure. Sci Adv 2019;5(6). https://doi.org/10.1126/sciadv.aaw0341. eaaw0341.

[93] Carrick D, Haig C, Maznyczka AM, et al. Hypertension, microvascular pathology, and prognosis after an acute myocardial infarction. Hypertension (Dallas, Tex.: 1979). 2018;72(3):720-730. https://www-ncbi-nlm-nih-gov.proxy.lib.umich.edu/pubmed/3001 2869; https://www-ncbi-nlm-nih-gov.proxy.lib.umich.edu/pmc/articles/PMC6080885/. doi: 10.1161/HYPERTENSIONAHA.117.10786.

[94] Jameson J, Kasper D, Longo D, Fauci A, Hauser S, Loscalzo J, editors. Harrison's Principles of Internal Medicine. 20th ed. New York, NY: McGraw-Hill Education; 2018.

[95] Mann SJ. Redefining beta-blocker use in hypertension: selecting the right beta-blocker and the right patient. J Am Soc Hypertens 2017;11(1):54—65. https://doi-org.proxy.lib. umich.edu/10.1016/j.jash.2016.11.007.

[96] Allahdadi KJ, Tostes RCA, Webb RC. Female sexual dysfunction: Therapeutic options and experimental challenges. Cardiovasc Hematol Agents Med Chem 2009;7(4): 260—9. https://doi.org/10.2174/187152509789541882. https://pubmed.ncbi.nlm.nih. gov/19538161. https://www-ncbi-nlm-nih-gov.proxy.lib.umich.edu/pmc/articles/PMC 3008577/.

[97] Davies JE, Sen S, Dehbi H, et al. Use of the instantaneous wave-free ratio or fractional flow reserve in PCI. N Engl J Med 2017;376(19):1824—34. https://doi.org/10.1056/ NEJMoa1700445. https://doi-org.proxy.lib.umich.edu/10.1056/NEJMoa1700445.

[98] Feinberg J, Nielsen EE, Greenhalgh J, et al. Drug-eluting stents versus bare-metal stents for acute coronary syndrome. Cochrane Database Syst Rev 2017;8(8). https:// doi.org/10.1002/14651858. CD012481-CD012481, https://pubmed.ncbi.nlm.nih.gov/ 28832903. https://www-ncbi-nlm-nih-gov.proxy.lib.umich.edu/pmc/articles/PMC648 3499/. CD012481.pub2.

[99] Giustino G, Harari R, Baber U, et al. Long-term safety and efficacy of new-generation drug-eluting stents in women with acute myocardial infarction: from the women in innovation and drug-eluting stents (WIN-DES) collaboration. JAMA cardiology 2017;2(8):855−62. https://doi.org/10.1001/jamacardio.2017.1978. https://pubmed. ncbi.nlm.nih.gov/28658478. https://www-ncbi-nlm-nih-gov.proxy.lib.umich.edu/pmc/ articles/PMC5710588/.

[100] Titterington JS, Hung OY, Wenger NK. Microvascular angina: an update on diagnosis and treatment. Future Cardiol 2015;11(2):229−42. https://doi.org/10.2217/fca.14.79. https://doi-org.proxy.lib.umich.edu/10.2217/fca.14.79.

[101] D'Souza R, Ostro J, Shah PS, et al. Anticoagulation for pregnant women with mechanical heart valves: a systematic review and meta-analysis. Eur Heart J 2017;38(19): 1509−16. https://doi.org/10.1093/eurheartj/ehx032. https://pubmed.ncbi.nlm.nih. gov/28329059. https://www-ncbi-nlm-nih-gov.proxy.lib.umich.edu/pmc/articles/PMC 5429939/.

Antidepressants in pregnancy

17

Janelle Komorowski

Department of Nurse-midwifery, Frontier Nursing University, Versailles, KY, United States

17.1 Introduction

Depression is common among women during pregnancy, and although pregnancy is a time of increased health care utilization, it is likely as many as 66% of women affected during pregnancy are neither identified nor treated [1,2]. In an effort to accurately estimate the number of pregnant women with depressive disorders, Haight et al. (2019) examined US public databases to identify women admitted to inpatient facilities for the purpose of childbirth, who also had an ICD-9-CM diagnosis code for a depressive disorder as described in the *Diagnostic and Statistical Manual of Mental Disorders*, fifth Edition. In 2008, 4.1 women per 1000 had a diagnosis of depression; the rate increased to 28.7 per 1000 women in 2015 [1]. Adding to the challenges of identifying depressive disorders during pregnancy is the fact that changes in appetite, sleep habits, energy level, and libido are normal symptoms during pregnancy, but may also be symptoms of depression [3]. Women may avoid disclosing their feelings of depression for fear the baby may be removed from the mother's care [4].

The size, complexity, and frequently inconsistent nature of the literature regarding the safety of psychotropic medications in pregnancy are daunting; consequently, many primary healthcare providers are reluctant to manage psychiatric illness during pregnancy. Untreated maternal depression may be associated with significant morbidity or even mortality for the mother—infant dyad [5], and both psychiatric illness and psychotropic medication must be conceptualized as agents of fetal exposure [6]. Prescribing psychiatric medication to pregnant women requires a complex risk—benefit calculus that balances the risks of untreated psychiatric illness to mother and fetus with the potential risks of medication use during pregnancy. This process ideally includes shared decision-making between the patient and psychiatric, obstetric, and primary care providers. However, significant shortages and uneven distribution of qualified behavioral health providers have resulted in many primary care providers being forced to assume sole management of treatment for depression during pregnancy [7]. All health care providers who care for women during pregnancy need to be prepared to assess, diagnose, and treat the woman with depression in pregnancy. The goal of this chapter is to provide an overview of the management of depression during pregnancy and to summarize the most relevant issues impacting clinical decision-making.

Symptoms of depression include depressed mood or anhedonia for at least a 2-week period, accompanied by symptoms that include changes in sleep, appetite, energy, concentration, psycho-motor activity, feelings of guilt or worthlessness, and/or suicidal ideation [8]. Diagnosis of depression in pregnant women is complicated by the similarity of normal symptoms of pregnancy to symptoms of depression; consequently, the presence of affective symptoms such as feelings of guilt or worthlessness, anhedonia, and thoughts of suicide may more strongly support a diagnosis of depression in pregnant women. Risk factors for developing perinatal depression encompass elements of a woman's genetics, hormonal/reproductive history, current stressors, and life experiences. Biologic factors that have consistently been associated with increased risk include a past history of depression or premenstrual dysphoric disorder and a family history of depression. Psychosocial factors, including stressful life events and lack of perceived social support, have consistently been found to predict perinatal depression [9].

17.2 Effects of untreated perinatal depression on women and children

Untreated perinatal depression is associated with significant morbidity for mother–infant dyad via adverse obstetric outcomes related to poor maternal health, inadequate prenatal care, and postpartum depression [6]. Poor nutrition, increased number of exposures to medications or herbal remedies, increased alcohol and tobacco use, and decreased compliance with prenatal care have been consistently associated with untreated psychiatric illness during pregnancy [6,9]. Data regarding specific adverse obstetric outcomes resulting from untreated depression during pregnancy are inconsistent. Miscarriage, fetal growth effects (low birth weight and intrauterine growth restriction), and preterm delivery have all been associated with untreated maternal depression. The strongest association appears to be with preterm birth; however, because of methodological limitations of the available data, it is not currently possible to draw definitive conclusions regarding associations between untreated maternal depression and these adverse reproductive outcomes [6,10–12].

In addition to the potential negative impact on pregnancy outcomes, perinatal depression is associated with increased irritability, decreased attentiveness, and decreased facial expressions in neonates. Children and adolescents born to depressed mothers are at risk for delayed cognitive and language development, lower IQ, and increased prevalence of psychiatric and emotional problems [13–20]. Depression that begins during pregnancy frequently continues or worsens after delivery [21].

17.3 Approach to treatment

Current guidelines created by a joint task force of the American Psychiatric Association (APA) and the American College of Obstetricians and Gynecologists (ACOG) recommend individual or group therapy as an initial treatment approach for pregnant women with mild to moderate depression [21]. Additional nonpharmacologic interventions that may be recommended to women with mild depression include improved nutrition, exercise; eliminating nicotine, caffeine, and alcohol from the diet; good sleep hygiene; and reducing stressors and using relaxation techniques, support groups, and light therapy [33].

For women who are unable to access or have not responded to nonpharmacologic interventions, who are experiencing an episode of moderate to severe depression during pregnancy, and/or who have a history of recurrent severe depression or suicidal ideation, initiation or maintenance of psychiatric medications is likely indicated [21].

It is ideal to evaluate women with a history of psychiatric illness prior to pregnancy in order to generate an individualized treatment plan. However, since nearly 50% of pregnancies in US women ages 15−44 are unplanned, preconception evaluation is often not feasible in practice [22]. Discontinuation of antidepressants during pregnancy is common and is associated with significant increase in relapse. In one large study, women who stopped antidepressants were five times as likely to have a relapse during pregnancy as women who continued their medication [9]. Frequently, patient and physician concerns about potential teratogenesis or other negative neonatal outcomes overshadow consideration of the risks associated with untreated maternal psychiatric illness. This decision-making process is complicated by several factors, including varying fetal risks at different stages of gestation, inadequacy of the US Food and Drug Administration (FDA) medication categorization system, and limitations of currently available data regarding the safety of antidepressants in pregnancy [23].

The approach to prescribing antidepressants in pregnancy can be guided by several general principles. The goal of treatment is remission of depressive symptoms, as inadequately treated depression subjects the fetus to risks associated with maternal illness and medication exposure. Choosing a medication with an established safety profile and a proven history of efficacy in the patient maximizes the potential for symptom response and minimizes potential risks to the fetus. One medication at higher dose is preferred to multiple medications at lower doses in order to decrease the total number of fetal exposures; pregnant women should receive the minimal effective dose of a single antidepressant [21,24].

Antidepressant dose requirements may increase across gestation as a consequence of induction of cytochrome enzymes 3A4 and 2D6 that increase drug metabolism in the second half of pregnancy [21,23,24]. Although limited literature suggests levels of both tricyclic antidepressants (TCAs) and selective serotonin reuptake inhibitors (SSRIs) decrease in many women in late pregnancy, there is wide interpersonal variability in the pharmacokinetic changes of these medications across gestation. Currently, there are no evidence-based guidelines for altered dosing or therapeutic monitoring of antidepressants during pregnancy [12]. Considering the possibility of increased antidepressant metabolism during pregnancy, women must be monitored closely for the re-emergence of depressive symptoms, especially during the third trimester. The possibility that some women may require higher doses of antidepressants in late pregnancy contradicts the clinical approach that advocates tapering antidepressants prior to delivery in hopes of mitigating potential adverse neonatal effects of medication use. Tapering antidepressants proximal to delivery has not been shown to decrease the potential risk of neonatal complications associated with medication use in late pregnancy [25]. Discontinuing antidepressants has been associated with significant increase in relapse of depressive symptoms, and currently, neither the APA nor ACOG recommends tapering antidepressants prior to delivery [11,19,21].

In addition to periodic assessment of antidepressant dose requirements across gestation, optimal management of perinatal mood and anxiety disorders includes recognizing the potential for postpartum illness. Women who are not already engaged in psychotherapy should be provided with referrals to begin depression-focused psychotherapy, specifically cognitive behavioral therapy (CBT) or interpersonal psychotherapy (IPT), both of which have been well studied for perinatal depression [25–27]. Supportive dynamic psychotherapy has been less well studied in pregnancy but is a reasonable approach if CBT and IPT are not available [21]. In addition to specific considerations regarding antidepressant use in pregnancy, prescribers should be familiar with current practice guidelines for the treatment of depression in general. There is no specific antidepressant that is better than another, and the choice of medication should be based on side effect profile, safety, tolerability, and previous response to medication in the individual patient [28]. Antidepressants should be started at low dose and titrated over time to effectiveness; the speed of the titration depends upon the severity of associated side effects. Frequently, patients require 4–8 weeks of antidepressant treatment prior to experiencing moderate symptom reduction. Once remission of depression has been achieved, patients with fewer than three prior depressive episodes should be continued on antidepressants for a minimum of 4–9 months prior to considering discontinuation. Patients with three or more episodes of major depression may require maintenance antidepressant treatment indefinitely [28]. Tapering antidepressants slowly over at least 2 weeks decreases both the risk of relapse of depressive illness and the severity of antidepressant discontinuation syndrome (flu-like symptoms, paresthesias, and insomnia) which is associated more strongly with SSRIs with short half-lives [18,28]. Decisions regarding tapering and discontinuation should be made in consultation with prescribing clinicians, if applicable, and patients should be monitored to assess for re-emergence of depressive symptoms.

17.4 Potential risks of selective serotonin reuptake inhibitor use during pregnancy

Due to their efficacy, tolerability, and safety profile, SSRIs are currently among the first-line pharmacologic treatments of major depression, and recent data suggest that up to 13% of US pregnancies have antidepressant exposure [29]. All SSRIs indeed, all psychotropic medications, cross the placenta and are excreted in breast milk [11]. The reproductive safety of SSRIs in pregnancy has been extensively studied. However, the data are often contradictory and limited by several factors, including the lack of randomized controlled trials, small sample sizes and limited power of many studies, the absence of information about disease state of the mother, and the failure to control for multiple confounding variables that impact reproductive outcomes [21]. Currently available data in the major domains of reproductive toxicity will be summarized here.

17.4.1 Obstetric outcomes

Similar to untreated depression during pregnancy, miscarriage, fetal growth effects, and preterm delivery have all been inconsistently associated with SSRI use during pregnancy [21]. The APA and ACOG treatment guideline report states there is not enough evidence to establish an association between SSRI use in early pregnancy and miscarriage [11,21]. There appears to be adequate evidence to support a true association between low birth weight and SSRI use in pregnancy; however, there is not enough evidence to support causality, and the impact of the underlying disorder and other confounders must be considered [21]. Finally, a growing literature supporting an association between preterm delivery and SSRI use in pregnancy is emerging, including at least one study that attempts to control for maternal depression [30]. Studies that do identify an association between preterm delivery and SSRI use in pregnancy tend to find a small effect size, with decrease in gestational age of less than or equal to 1 week [30]. The literature about whether observed adverse obstetric outcomes are related to antidepressant treatment or to depressive illness itself is often inconclusive, and research that adequately controls for underlying disease state is necessary to either support or refute these associations [29].

17.4.2 Congenital malformations

A large body of evidence supports the conclusion that SSRIs as a group are not associated with increased risk of major congenital anomalies [3,21,23,30]. There is some evidence that individual SSRIs may be associated with very low risk of minor malformations; however, this finding is not widely replicated [31]. Specific concern over paroxetine use and increased risk of congenital cardiac malformations emerged in 2005 when GlaxoSmithKline reported a 1.5–2-fold increase in atrial and ventricular septal defects in infants exposed to paroxetine in the first trimester. This finding prompted a change in the medication's FDA pregnancy rating from C to D and generated the current recommendation that paroxetine should be avoided during the first trimester of pregnancy and in women contemplating pregnancy. In 2016, a large meta-analysis and systematic review of studies published between 1966 and 2016 found that paroxetine is associated with an increased risk of cardiac malformations [31]. Avoiding first-trimester fetal exposure to paroxetine and considering fetal echocardiography in exposed cases is recommended [3,11,21,30].

In summary, the overwhelming convergence of data suggests that the absolute risk of congenital malformations associated with SSRI use during early pregnancy is small; consequently, SSRIs are not considered to be teratogenic [3,11,21].

17.4.3 Persistent pulmonary hypertension of the newborn

Persistent pulmonary hypertension of the newborn (PPHN) is a clinical syndrome characterized by failure of the normal fetal-to-neonatal circulatory transition causing right-to-left shunting of blood through the ductus arteriosus and foramen ovale and subsequent neonatal hypoxia. PPHN is a rare condition: baseline population rates are 1—2 infants/1000 live births. In December 2011, the FDA released a drug safety communication concluding that there is currently insufficient evidence to support a potential link between SSRI use in pregnancy and PPHN and recommending that prescribers continue to treat depression in pregnancy according to their current clinical practice.

A 2019 meta-analysis of the link between maternal SSRI use and PPHN found SSRI use during pregnancy was associated with an increased likelihood of PPHN. The clinical significance is uncertain since the absolute risk difference is 0.6/1000 live births. The study's authors suggest that the risk of untreated perinatal depression and associated adverse outcomes may outweigh the risk of continued use of SSRIs during pregnancy [31]. In summary, the absolute risk of PPHN remains quite low and there is currently no evidence that tapering SSRIs proximal to delivery decreases this potential risk.

17.4.4 Neonatal adaptation syndrome

Exposure to SSRIs in late pregnancy has also been associated with transient neonatal distress, including tachypnea, jitteriness, poor muscle tone, weak cry, and irritability. Withdrawal symptoms have been extensively investigated for many years in pregnant women with substance use disorders. Some prescription drugs have also been reported to be associated with such events in neonates. Their clinical presentation is variable and usually includes several signs and symptoms, ranging from behavioral abnormalities to neurological impairments. For this reason, these effects are usually defined as a syndrome, which has been termed "neonatal abstinence syndrome," [6] "neonatal withdrawal syndrome," [7] "neonatal adaptation syndrome (NAS)," [8] or even "neonatal behavioral syndrome," [9] depending on the putative mechanism. Convertino et al. (2016) argue for "neonatal abstinence syndrome" as the preferred term to describe withdrawal symptoms in the neonate, as opposed to other symptoms which can be explained as lingering effects of medication taken by the mother during pregnancy [34]. NAS lasts from several hours to 2 weeks post-delivery. It occurs in roughly 15%—30% of infants of mothers who used SSRIs in late pregnancy. Symptoms are generally mild, transient, and managed by supportive care in special care nurseries or specialized rooming-in care [11,21,32].

Symptoms have been reported with all SSRIs, but the highest reported rates for this syndrome occur with fluoxetine and paroxetine [11,21,32]. It is unclear if these symptoms represent neonatal serotonin toxicity, a discontinuation phenomenon, or are the result of some as-yet undiscovered mechanism, and tapering antidepressants toward the end of pregnancy has not been shown to decrease neonatal symptoms [31]. Future studies examining potential impact of SSRI exposure on neonates must control for the impact of maternal psychiatric illness, as behavioral symptoms such as irritability and decreased attentiveness have also been strongly associated with poorly treated maternal depression [21].

17.4.5 Neurodevelopmental outcomes

The impact of prenatal antidepressant exposure on long-term cognitive, behavioral, and motor outcomes in exposed children has not been extensively investigated. Despite a general paucity of information, the available data are largely reassuring. The majority of studies show no difference in measures of intelligence, language development, or behavior between children exposed to antidepressants in utero and unexposed controls. Larger, well-designed studies with increased length of follow-up are required to either support or refute associations between in utero exposure to SSRIs and negative neurodevelopmental outcomes [32,33].

17.5 Potential risks of non-SSRI antidepressant use during pregnancy

Non-SSRI antidepressants include bupropion, duloxetine, mirtazapine, nefazodone, trazodone, and venlafaxine, and as a group, they have been much less well studied than the SSRIs. Currently available data do not suggest increased risk of adverse obstetric outcomes, major congenital malformations, or PPHN with non-SSRI antidepressants in pregnancy. A syndrome of poor neonatal adaptation similar to that attributed to SSRIs has been consistently documented in infants born to mothers who have used non-SSRI antidepressants in late pregnancy, and virtually, no information exists on long-term neurocognitive outcomes in exposed children [11,21,33]. This general lack of negative findings should be interpreted with caution as it currently reflects a paucity of data as opposed to a true absence of risk. In general, non-SSRI antidepressants should not be considered first-line agents for treatment of depression during pregnancy unless there is a compelling clinical reason to use them instead of medications with more established safety profiles. Such indications may include established history of efficacy in an individual patient, lack of response or inability to tolerate SSRIs, fetal exposure to non-SSRI antidepressants in early pregnancy, or patient preference.

17.6 Potential risks of older antidepressant use during pregnancy

TCAs, the mainstay of treatment for depression prior to the introduction of SSRIs in the late 1980s, have been well studied in pregnancy; due to their side effect profile and lethality potential in overdose, they are no longer considered a first-line treatment for depression. Similar to the SSRIs, there are conflicting data regarding potential association with obstetric complications like low birth weight and preterm delivery, while most studies reveal no association with increased rates of congenital malformations [11,21,33]. The use of TCAs in late pregnancy has been associated with transient neonatal toxicity and withdrawal symptoms including jitteriness, tachycardia, mild respiratory distress, hypertonia, and irritability; currently, there is no evidence of negative long-term neurobehavioral sequelae [11,21,33]. Monoamine oxidase inhibitors are infrequently used in modern clinical practice due to their severe side effect profile; they are essentially contraindicated during pregnancy due to increased rate of congenital anomalies in animal studies and the possibility of precipitating a hypertensive crisis if tocolytic medications are required to postpone labor.

17.7 Anxiety

Anxiety disorders such as generalized anxiety, panic disorder, obsessive compulsive disorder, and posttraumatic stress disorder may exist independently of, or comorbid with, depressive illness. A detailed discussion of anxiety disorders during pregnancy is beyond the scope of this chapter; however, the approach to management of anxiety during pregnancy is similar to that of depression and SSRIs are currently considered a first-line treatment for anxiety spectrum illness.

17.8 Summary

Depression during pregnancy is associated with significant risks for women and infants, and the goal of treatment should be remission. Ideal management of depressed pregnant women includes maximization of nonpsychopharmacologic treatments such as psychotherapy, diet and exercise, light therapy, and support groups. Utilization of antidepressant medication is indicated for pregnant women with moderate to severe depressive symptoms and for women with mild to moderate depression whose symptoms are unimproved with nonpsychopharmacologic treatments. Optimal patient care includes an individualized treatment approach that balances the potential maternal and fetal risks of untreated depression with the potential risks of antidepressant exposure. Avoiding polypharmacy, using the lowest effective dose of a medication with a history of efficacy in the individual patient, and monitoring patient response over time are strategies that may mitigate potential risks of antidepressant use or untreated depression during pregnancy.

References

[1] Lyell DJ, Chambers AS, Steidtmann D, Tsai E, Caughey AB, Wong A, Manber R. Antenatal identification of major depressive disorder: a cohort study. Am J Obstet Gynecol 2012;207(6). 506.el-6.

[2] Haight SC, Byatt N, Moore Simas TA, Robbins CL, KO JY. Recorded diagnoses of depression during hospitalizations in the United States, 2000 2015. Obstet Gynecol 2019;133(6):1216–23. https://doi.org/10.1097/AOG.0000000000003291.

[3] The American College of obstetricians and gynecologists committee opinion no. 630. Screening for perinatal depression. Obstet Gynecol 2015;125(5):1268–71. https://doi.org/10.1097/01.AOG.0000465192.34779.de.

[4] National Institute for Health and Care Excellence (NICE). Antenatal and postnatal mental health: clinical management and service guidance. NICE clinical guideline 192. 2014. http://www.nice.org.uk/guidance/cg192.

[5] Pearlstein T. Depression during pregnancy. Best Pract Res Clin Obstet Gynaecol 2015; 29:754.

[6] Grigoriadis S, VonderPorten EH, Mamisashvili L, et al. The impact of maternal depression during pregnancy on perinatal outcomes: a systematic review and meta-analysis. J Clin Psychiatr 2013;74(4):E321–41. https://doi.org/10.4088/JCP.12R07968.

[7] Health Resources and Services Administration, Health Workforce. Behavioral health workforce projections, 2016–2030. Retrieved from: https://bhw.hrsa.gov/sites/default/files/bhw/health-workforce analysis/research/projections/Behavioral-Health-Workforce-Projections.pdf.

[8] American Psychiatric Association. Diagnostic and statistical manual of mental disorders: diagnostic and statistical manual of mental disorders. 5th ed. Arlington, VA: American Psychiatric Association; 2013.

[9] Vigod SN, Wilson CA, Howard LM. Depression in pregnancy. BMJ Clin Res Ed 2016; 352:1547. https://doi.org/10.1136/bmj/k1547.

[10] ACOG Practice Bulletin. Use of psychiatric medications during pregnancy and lactation. Obstet Gynecol 2008;111(4):1001–20.

[11] Molenaar NM, Kamperman AM, Boyce P, Bergink V. Guidelines on treatment of perinatal depression with antidepressants: an international review. Aust NZJ Psychiat 2018; 52(4):320–7. https://doi.org/10.1177/0004867418762057.

[12] Maarcus S, Lopez JF, McDonough S, et al. Depressive symptoms during pregnancy: impact on neuroendocrine and neonatal outcomes. Infant Behav Dev 2011;34:26.

[13] Field T, Diego MA, Dieter J, et al. Depressed withdrawn and intrusive mothers' effects on their fetuses and neonates. Infant Behav Dev 2001;24:27.

[14] Salisbury AL, O'Grady KE, Battle CL, et al. The roles of maternal depression, serotonin reuptake inhibitor treatment, and concomitant benzodiazepine use on infant neurobehavioral functioning over the first postnatal month. Am J Psychiatr 2016;173:147.

[15] Lundy BL, Jones NA, Field T, , et alLundy BL, Jones NA, Field T, et al. Prenatal depression effects on neonates. Infant Behav Dev 1999;22:119.

[16] Salisbury AL, Wisner KL, Pearlstein T, et al. Newborn neurobehavioral patterns are differentially related to prenatal maternal major depressive disorder and serotonin reuptake inhibitor treatment. Depress Anxiety 2011;28:1008.

[17] Field T, Diego M, Hernandez-Reif M, et al. Sleep disturbances in depressed pregnant women and their newborns. Infant Behav Dev 2007;30:127.

[18] Diego MA, Field T, Hernandez-Reif M. Prepartum, postpartum and chronic depression effects on neonatal behavior. Infant Behav Dev 2005;28:155.

[19] Santucci AK, Singer LT, Wisniewski SR, et al. Impact of prenatal exposure to serotonin reuptake inhibitors or maternal major depressive disorder on infant developmental outcomes. J Clin Psychiatr 2014;75:1088.

[20] Aris-Meijer J, Bockting C, Stolk R, et al. What if pregnancy is not seventh heaven? The influence of specific life events during pregnancy and delivery on the transition of antenatal into postpartum anxiety and depression. Int J Environ Res Publ Health 2019; 16(16):2851. https://doi.org/10.3390/ijerph16162851.

[21] Yonkers KA, Wisner KL, Stewart DE, et al. The management of depression during pregnancy: a report from the American Psychiatric Association and the American College of Obstetricians and Gynecologists. Obstet Gynecol 2009;114(3):703—13. https://doi.org/10.1097/AOG.0b013e3181ba0632.

[22] Cohen LS, Altshuler LL, Harlow BL, Nonacs R, Newport DJ, Viguera AC, et al. Relapse of major depression during pregnancy in women who maintain or discontinue antidepressant treatment. J Am Med Assoc 2006;295(5):499—507.

[23] Chaudron LH. Complex challenges in treating depression during pregnancy. Am J Psychiatr 2013;170:12—20.

[24] Westin AA, Brekke M, Molden E, Skogvoll E, Spigset O. Selective serotonin reuptake inhibitors and venlafaxine in pregnancy: changes in drug disposition. PLoS One 2017; 12(7):e0181082. https://doi.org/10.1371/journal.pone.0181082. pmid:28708853.

[25] Stuart S, Koleva H. Psychological treatments for perinatal depression. Best Pract Res Clin Obstet Gynaecol 2014;28(1):61—70. https://doi.org/10.1016/j.bpobgyn.2013.09.004.

[26] Work Group on Major Depressive Disorder. Practice guidelines for the treatment of patients with major depressive disorder. Am J Psychiatr 2010;167(10):S9—118.

[27] Keks N, Hope J, Keogh S. Switching and stopping antidepressants. Aust Prescr 2016; 39(3):76—83. https://doi.org/10.18773/austprescr.2016.039.

[28] Wilson E, Lader M. A review of the management of antidepressant discontinuation symptoms. Ther Adv Psychopharmacol 2015;5(6):357—68. https://doi.org/10.1177/2045125315612334.

[29] Bérard A, Iessa N, Chaabane S, Muanda FT, Boukhris T, Zhao JP. The risk of major cardiac malformations associated with paroxetine use during the first trimester of pregnancy: a systematic review and meta-analysis. Br J Clin Pharmacol 2016;81(4): 589—604. https://doi.org/10.1111/bcp.12849.

[30] US Food and Drug Administration. reportFDA Drug Safety Communication: selective serotonin reuptake inhibitor (SSRI) antidepressant use during pregnancy and reports of a rare heart and lung condition in newborn babies. Retrieved from: https://www.fda.gov/drugs/drug-safety-and-availability/fda drug-safety-communication-selective-serotonin-reuptake-inhibitor-ssri antidepressant-use-during.

[31] Ornoy A, Koren G. SSRIs and SNRIS (SRI) in pregnancy: effects on the course of pregnancy and the offspring: how far are we from having all the answers? Int J Mol Sci 2019;20(10):2370. https://doi.org/10.3390/ijms20102370.

[32] Gentile S. Untreated depression during pregnancy: short and long-term effects in offspring. A systematic review. Neuroscience 2017;342:154—66.

[33] Wichman CL, Stern TA. Diagnosing and treating depression during pregnancy. Prim Care Compan CNS Disord 2015;17(2). https://doi.org/10.4088/PCC.15f01776.

[34] Convertino I, Sansone AC, Marino A, Galiulo MT, Mantarro S, Antonioli L, et al. Neonatal adaptation issues after maternal exposure to prescription drugs: withdrawal syndromes and residual pharmacological effects: an international journal of medical toxicology and drug experience. Drug Saf 2016;39(10):903−24. https://doi.org/10.1007/s40264-016-0435-8.

Further reading

[1] Guttmacher Institute. Unintended pregnancy in the United States. 2019. Retrieved from: https://www.guttmacher.org/fact-sheet/unintended pregnancy-united-states.

[2] Warburton W, Hertzman C, Oberlander TF. A register study of the impact of stopping third trimester selective serotonin reuptake inhibitor exposure on neonatal health. Acta Psychiatr Scand 2010;121(6):471−9.

[3] Cooper WO, Willy ME, Pont SJ, Ray WA. Increasing use of antidepressants in pregnancy. Am J Obstet Gynecol 2007;196(544):el−5.

[4] Mitchell J, Goodman. J. Comparative effects of antidepressant medications and untreated major depression on pregnancy outcomes: a systematic review. Arch Womens Ment Health 2018;21:505.

[5] Prady SL, Hanlon I, Fraser LK, Mikocka-Walus A. A systematic review of maternal antidepressant use in pregnancy and short- and long-term offspring's outcomes. Arch Womens Ment Health 2018;21(2):127−40. https://doi.org/10.1007/s00737-017-0780-3.

[6] Creeley CE, Denton LK. Use of prescribed psychotropics during pregnancy: a systematic review of pregnancy, neonatal, and childhood outcomes. Brain Sci 2019;9(9):235. https://doi.org/10.3390/brainsci9090235.

Uterotonics and tocolytics

Jeffrey S. Fouche-Camargo

School of Health Sciences, Georgia Gwinnett College, Lawrenceville, GA, United States

18.1 Introduction

The uterus has two major components: the cervix and the corpus. The uterine cervix comprises the external os, the internal os, and the cervical canal that connects them. The corpus comprises the uterine fundus and the main uterine body. Anatomically, there are four layers of the uterus. The outermost layer, the perimetrium, is serosal in nature and is analogous to the peritoneum. Beneath the serosal layer lies the parametrium, a layer of connective tissue connecting the uterus to the other tissues of the pelvis. The myometrium lies beneath these outer layers and is primarily composed of smooth muscle tissue. The innermost layer is the endometrium composed of glandular epithelial tissue.

While each layer serves an important function in pregnancy and parturition, it is the myometrium that is of primary concern during parturition. The uterine myocytes are capable of significant enlargement during pregnancy to accommodate the growing fetus. Although there are multiple factors that trigger the beginning of labor (some of which remain unknown), one factor is activation of stretch receptors within the myometrium that trigger regular uterine contractions. During normal labor contractions, the fundus serves as the pacemaker for the contractions and sends electrical impulses throughout the myometrium causing coordinated contraction of the myocytes.

Obstetric providers often need to alter uterine contraction activity in the care of pregnant women. Medications that induce or augment uterine contraction are known as uterotonics, while medications that reduce or arrest uterine contractions are known as tocolytics. Uterotonic medications are also used to ripen or prepare the cervix for dilation and to effect uterine contractions to control uterine bleeding. It should be noted that the use of most of these uterine medications is not FDA approved and is considered off-label usage. There is, however, considerable evidence to support their clinical use.

18.2 Uterotonics

Uterotonics are by far the most common drugs administered on any labor and delivery suite. Clinically, they are used primarily for induction or augmentation of labor and to prevent and/or control postpartum hemorrhage. All agents in this category cause uterine contraction, but each does so through a different pathway. It is important to have a working knowledge of each medication, as each can cause as much harm as good (Table 18.1).

18.2.1 Oxytocin

Oxytocin is a polypeptide composed of nine amino acids. Endogenous oxytocin is primarily produced by the hypothalamus and is stored and released from the posterior pituitary gland (neurohypophysis). Oxytocin has multiple functions, mostly related to sexuality (orgasm), reproduction (uterine contractions), and lactation (milk ejection). It also has a role in social bonding and mood regulation.

Synthetic exogenous oxytocin is bioidentical to its natural endogenous analog. As a uterotonic medication, it is currently approved for medically indicated labor induction (i.e., premature rupture of membranes, diabetes, hypertension, preeclampsia, etc.), labor augmentation, and as an adjunctive therapy in the management of an incomplete or inevitable abortion. Additionally, oxytocin is a first-line agent for the treatment of postpartum hemorrhage secondary to uterine atony or subinvolution.

Oxytocin stimulates uterine contractions by increasing intracellular calcium. In the uterus, oxytocin binds to the oxytocin receptors located on the myometrial cell membrane and stimulates phospholipase C (Fig. 18.1).

This leads to increased production of inositol triphosphate which acts to mobilize intracellular calcium by promoting release from the sarcoplasmic reticulum. Binding to the oxytocin receptor also induces an influx of extracellular calcium through nonselective, cation channels on the myometrial cell membrane. Intracellular calcium then binds with calmodulin to form the calcium−calmodulin complex. This complex activates myosin light-chain kinase (MLCK), the key regulator of smooth muscle contractility. MLCK phosphorylates myosin which in turn binds actin, initiating myometrial smooth muscle contraction [1].

Because of the potential for significant harm to pregnant women and their fetuses, oxytocin is listed as a "high-alert" medication by the Institute for Safe Medication Practices [2]. Mismanagement of oxytocin often results in litigation against physicians, nurses, and midwives. In is incumbent upon providers, therefore, to have an understanding of the pharmacokinetics of oxytocin and published clinical practice guidelines. Despite extensive information on the pharmacokinetics of oxytocin, there is considerable disagreement about optimal dosing regiments of oxytocin for induction and augmentation of labor [3−6]. Oxytocin has an onset of action within 3−5 min and a half-life of 10−12 min. Steady state (the point where the plasma concentration is stable such that the full effect of that concentration of the medication will be observed) is not achieved until 30−60 min, which corresponds to 3−5 half-lives [2]. Response to exogenous oxytocin administration is highly variable [5]. A rare but serious maternal side effect is water intoxication secondary to the antidiuretic properties of oxytocin. This condition has been reported in women who received oxytocin in D5 water and/or high-dose protocols (>20 milliunits/min)

Table 18.1 Uterotonics.

Medication	Clinical indication	Route	Dose	Frequency	Considerations
Oxytocin (Pitocin®)	Induction/ augmentation of labor	Intravenous	Low-dose regimen: Start at 0.5–2 milliunits/min	Increase by 1–2 milliunits/min every 15–40 min, maximum dose 20 –40 milliunits/min	Titrate to maternal response and fetal tolerance. Goal is 2–5 contractions in 10 min
			High-dose regimen: Start at 6 milliunits/min	Increase by 3–6 mU/min every 15 –40 min, maximum dose 40 mU/min	Titrate to maternal response and fetal tolerance. Goal is 2–5 contractions in 10 min
	Postpartum hemorrhage	Intravenous	Prophylactic: 10–20 units in 1 L isotonic solution; run 500 mL over 30 min, then 125 mL/h for 3.5 h Treatment: 40 units in 1 L isotonic solution; infuse rapidly until bleeding is controlled, then titrate to maintain uterine tone	Continuous	Observe for signs of water intoxication with rapid infusion of large amount of oxytocin
		Intramuscular	10 units (thigh, gluteal, or myometrial)	Once	
Methylergonovine (Methergine®)	Postpartum hemorrhage	Intramuscular	0.2 mg	Can repeat dose every 2–4 h, maximum 5 doses	Avoid in women with uncontrolled HTN. Use in women with preeclampsia or HTN should only be considered if benefits outweigh risk
		Oral	0.2 mg	Can repeat dose every 6–8 h for 2 –3 days (maximum 7 days)	

Continued

Table 18.1 Uterotonics.—*cont'd*

Medication	Clinical indication	Route	Dose	Frequency	Considerations
Carboprost – PGF2α (Hemabate®)	Postpartum hemorrhage	Intramuscular	250 mcg	Can repeat dose every 15–90 min (maximum 8 doses or 2 mg)	Avoid in patients with asthma or pulmonary disease, can cause bronchoconstriction Administer antidiarrheal medication
Misoprostol – PGE1 (Cytotec®)[a]	Cervical ripening/labor induction	Oral or vaginal	25 mcg	Can repeat dose of 25–50 mcg every 3–6 h	Hold dose if more than 2 contractions in 10 min Oxytocin can be started 4 h after last dose
	Postpartum hemorrhage	Rectal	800–1000 mcg	Single dose	
Dinoprostone – PGE2 (Cervidil®)	Cervical ripening/labor induction	Vaginal insert	1 insert contains 10 mg	Continual release for 12 h	If cervical ripening not achieved after 12 h, may repeat Oxytocin can be started 30 –60 min following removal Caution in patients with asthma or glaucoma
Dinoprostone – PGE2 (Prepidil®)	Cervical ripening/labor induction	Vaginal (cervical canal)	0.5 mg	Single dose	If cervical ripening not achieved after 6 h, may repeat Oxytocin can be started 6 h after last dose Caution in patients with asthma or glaucoma
Dinoprostone – PGE2 (Prostin®)	Postpartum hemorrhage	Rectal or vaginal	20 mg	Single dose	Caution in patients with asthma or glaucoma

[a] *Misoprostol for cervical ripening/labor induction and for postpartum hemorrhage is an off-label use.*

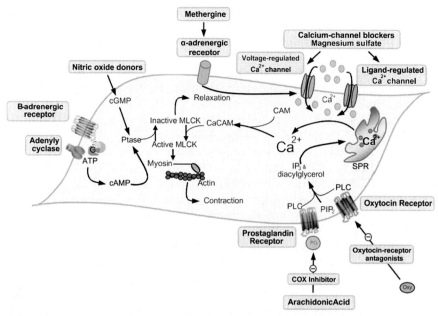

FIGURE 18.1

Contractant and relaxant pathways of a myometrial cell. *CaCAM*, calcium—calmodulin complex; *CAM*, calmodulin; *IP3*, inositol triphosphate; *MLCK*, myosin light-chain kinase; *Oxy*, oxytocin; *Pg*, prostaglandin; *PIP2*, phosphatidylinositol 4,5-biphosphate; *PLC*, phospholipase C; *Ptase*, phosphate kinase; *SPR*, sarcoplasmic reticulum.

for prolonged periods of time. To avoid this, it is recommended that oxytocin be administered with an isotonic solution, and strict intake and output should be monitored.

The primary risk to the fetus is interruption in oxygen delivery from the placenta. For this reason, patients receiving oxytocin for induction or augmentation of labor should be placed on continuous electronic fetal and uterine monitoring by a competent registered nurse and obstetric provider. Unless there are other contraindications, patients may be monitoring continuously with reliable telemetry-based fetal and uterine monitoring.

Dosing regimens are categorized as either high dose or low dose. High-dose regimens usually begin with a dose of 6 milliunits/min, with incremental increases of 1—6 milliunits/min every 15—40 min, and a maximum dose of 40 milliunits/min [7]. Low-dose regimens usually begin with a dose of 0.5—1 milliunits/min, with incremental increases of 1—2 milliunits/min every 15—40 min, and a maximum dose 20—40 milliunits/min [7]. A Cochrane systematic review concluded that high-dose regimens do not increase the rate of vaginal delivery within 24 h, do not decrease total time in labor, do not increase cesarean section rates, but they do result in increased rates of uterine tachysystole [4]. Additionally, a large retrospective study concluded that there were no significant differences in neonatal outcomes or cesarean section rates between patients that received high-dose versus low-dose regimens, but the study did not make conclusions about the rate of uterine tachysystole [6]. In conclusion, there are not any significant advantages for high-dose regimens. General knowledge about medication dosing is to use the lowest effective dose for the shortest duration possible to achieve the desired outcomes. For these reasons, the author recommends using low-dose dosing regimens.

Prolonged exposure to exogenous oxytocin results in desensitization of oxytocin receptors [8]. The receptors are downregulated, and by 4 h, around half of the receptors are no longer exerting an effect when bound to oxytocin. This downregulation of oxytocin receptors may result in dysfunctional labor patterns and paradoxically prolong labor as well as increase risk for postpartum hemorrhage [5,8].

Oxytocin is also used as an adjunctive therapy for incomplete, inevitable, and elective abortions in the first and second trimester but is less effective than other methods using mifepristone and/or misoprostol [9].

Oxytocin is a first-line medication for preventing and controlling postpartum hemorrhage. Usual dosing for postpartum hemorrhage prophylaxis is 10–20 units in 1000 mL of isotonic solution. An initial bolus of 500 mL is given over 30 min, then reduced to 125 mL/h for the next 3.5 h. Alternatively, 10 units may be administered IM [10,11]. For the treatment of postpartum hemorrhage, 40 units of oxytocin mixed in 1000 mL of isotonic solution should be infused rapidly until bleeding is controlled, then titrated to maintain uterine tone [12].

18.2.2 Methylergonovine

Methylergonovine, a semisynthetic ergot alkaloid, is a potent uterotonic that increases the force and frequency of uterine contractions at low doses. At higher doses, methylergonovine can increase basal uterine tone and cause uterine tetany. In obstetrics, methylergonovine is indicated for the treatment of postpartum hemorrhage secondary to uterine atony or subinvolution [13].

The uterotonic properties of ergot alkaloids have been known for centuries. Their use as a labor stimulant was first described by Adam Louicer in 1582 [14]. Although the uterine effects of ergots were discovered hundreds of years ago, the exact mechanism by which methylergonovine causes myometrial contraction is not known. Ergot alkaloids are known to cause vasoconstriction, uterine contractions, and stimulation of central dopamine receptors.

Ergots have been shown to bind alpha adrenergic, serotonin, and dopamine D1 receptors. It is likely that methylergonovine specifically interacts with alpha adrenergic receptors on the myometrial cell (Fig. 18.1). This interaction alters transmembrane calcium channel activity, causing an influx of calcium into the myometrial cell and activation of the contraction cascade [14].

After oral administration or intramuscular injection, methylergonovine is rapidly absorbed and distributed throughout the plasma and extracellular fluid. Approximately 25% more medication is absorbed via the intramuscular route compared to oral [14]. Methylergonovine is metabolized by the liver and excreted in the urine. The half-life of methylergonovine is 3.4 h (1.5−12.7 h) when administered intramuscularly [14].

In the case of postpartum hemorrhage, the preferred dose and route of methylergonovine administration is 0.2 mg intramuscularly every 2−4 h, for a maximum of five doses. It can also be directly injected into the uterus; however, one should be careful to avoid intravascular administration as this has been reported to result in acute coronary vasospasm and/or myocardial infarction [15]. Alternatively, the medication can be administered orally at a dose of 0.2 mg every 6−8 h for 2−3 days (maximum of 7 days).

Methylergonovine should be avoided by those who are pregnant, those with uncontrolled hypertension, and those with sensitivity to the drug. Methergine use in postpartum women with preeclampsia should only be considered if the benefits outweigh the risks. Common side effects include nausea, vomiting, hyper- or hypotension, and headache. Patients should be monitored closely for any adverse side effects after administration of the drug.

18.2.3 Prostaglandins

Prostaglandins are potent uterotonics with utility in several circumstances in obstetrics including facilitation of second trimester abortion, cervical ripening, labor induction, and the treatment of postpartum hemorrhage. The prostaglandins used in obstetrics include prostaglandin E2 (PGE2) (dinoprostone), prostaglandin E1 (PGE1) (misoprostol), and prostaglandin F2α (PGF2α) (carboprost).

The prostaglandins used in obstetric practice are synthetic analogs of endogenous prostaglandins which are cyclic, unsaturated fatty acids. Prostaglandins are grouped into subtypes (A,B,C,D,E,F,G,H,I,J,K) according to the chemical substitution on the pentane ring. All prostaglandins are excreted by the kidneys, so their use in the presence of renal insufficiency warrants caution. All of the prostaglandin preparations have common side effects: abdominal pain, diarrhea, nausea, vomiting, headache, paresthesias, fever, and shivering. They all may have the potential to increase or decrease systolic blood pressure. Therefore, patients should be closely monitored when administering any prostaglandin.

Prostaglandins are most commonly used to ripen and prepare the uterine cervix for labor. Prostaglandins promote the softening and distensibility of the cervix which often leads to early cervical effacement and dilatation. Prostaglandins cause uterine contractions by altering membrane permeability and increasing intracellular calcium. They promote the formation of gap junctions, facilitating transmission of signals throughout the myometrium. Additionally, they upregulate the expression of oxytocin receptors in the uterus which in turn promotes contractility.

18.2.3.1 PGE2—dinoprostone

PGE2, or dinoprostone, is available as a sustained-release vaginal insert (Cervidil) or as a gel (Prepidil), both of which are the only FDA-approved medications for cervical ripening. Both must be refrigerated for storage. The sustained-release vaginal insert is much more commonly used. Cervidil is encased in a Dacron polyester pouch with an attached string to allow for quick removal. Once placed in posterior vaginal fornix, it releases dinoprostone at a rate of approximately 0.3 mg/h [16]. Because the medication is released continually, continuous electronic fetal monitoring (EFM) should be implemented. If EFM telemetry is available, patients may ambulate 2 h after initial insertion [16,17]. It is not recommended to use dinoprostone in patients with a previous uterine scar [16,17]. The insert should be removed once cervical ripening has been achieved, or by 12 h, whichever occurs first [16,17]. If cervical ripening has not been achieved after 12 h, a repeat dose may be started [16]. Once cervical ripening has been achieved, oxytocin can be initiated following 30−60 min after removal of the insert [17]. Uterine tachysystole is the most common side effect [17]. In the event of uterine tachysystole, the insert can be quickly removed by grasping the string and pulling the insert out of the vagina. Prepidil is supplied as a prefilled syringe containing 0.5 mg of dinoprostone [18]. It is administered into the cervical canal. The patient should remain recumbent for 15−30 min following administration to avoid leakage from the cervical canal [18]. After 6 h, if cervical ripening has been achieved, it is acceptable to begin oxytocin infusion. If cervical ripening has not been achieved, an additional dose may be administered [18]. Continuous EFM should be initiated for at least 2 h following administration. If the patient is not in labor, it is reasonable to switch to intermittent EFM after 2 h [18]. Both preparations should be used with caution in patients with a history of glaucoma or childhood asthma [16,18].

Dinoprostone is also available in 20 mg immediate-release rectal or vaginal suppositories for the treatment of postpartum hemorrhage [12].

18.2.3.2 PGE1—misoprostol

PGE1, or misoprostol, is available as 100 mcg or 200 mcg tablets. It is used in obstetrics for cervical ripening, induction of labor, as a part of medical abortion, and for the treatment of postpartum hemorrhage. All of these uses are off-label as misoprostol is FDA approved for the treatment of peptic ulcers. When used according to published clinical guidelines [7,17], the most common side effect is uterine tachysystole. It is contraindicated in patients with prior uterine scars [7,17]. The recommended starting dose for cervical ripening is 25 mcg [7,17]. It should be noted, however, that the tablets are unscored. Unscored tablets may not have the active ingredient uniformly distributed through the tablet. Repeat dosing can be 25−50 mcg every 3−6 h as long as the patient is not having more than two contractions in 10 min and there is a category I fetal heart rate tracing [7,17]. Continuous EFM is indicated. Once cervical ripening has been achieved, oxytocin can be administered as long as at least 4 h have passed since the last dose [7,17].

Misoprostol is also used with or without mifepristone to induce abortion medically. There are multiple well-studied protocols available, and the reader is referred to those for more information about the use of misoprostol for this indication.

Misoprostol is well studied in the treatment of postpartum hemorrhage [12]. It is often used as a second-line medication following oxytocin. The recommended dose is 800–1000 mcg rectally [12].

18.2.3.3 PGF2α—carboprost

PGF2α, or carboprost, is FDA approved for the treatment of severe postpartum hemorrhage. It is available in 250 mcg preparations to be administered IM. Carboprost should not be administered to patients with a history of asthma or significant pulmonary disease because of the potential for acute bronchospasm. It must be refrigerated when stored. Dosing is 250 mcg IM (including direct injection into the uterine muscle) every 15–90 min to a max dose of 2 mg [12]. Of all the prostaglandin preparations, carboprost causes the most severe diarrhea. It is recommended that patients be advised of this unsettling side effect and be given antidiarrheal medications concurrently.

18.2.4 Uterotonics summary

- All of these medications have extensive side effect profiles and the potential for maternal and/or fetal toxicity. Thus, a good understanding of their administration and dosing is essential for safe and effective use.
- In general, this class of medications works to promote myometrial contraction by increasing intracellular calcium concentrations.
- Oxytocin increases intracellular calcium via the phospholipase C/IP3 pathway.
- Methylergonovine is thought to bind to alpha adrenergic receptors on the myometrial cell and alter transmembrane calcium channel activity, resulting in calcium influx.
- Prostaglandins not only increase intracellular calcium by altering transmembrane permeability but they also promote gap junction formation and upregulate expression of oxytocin receptors.

18.3 Tocolytics

Preterm birth is a leading cause of neonatal morbidity and mortality worldwide. There are several pathogenic processes that can trigger uterine contractions and cervical dilation with subsequent delivery of the preterm neonate. The goal of tocolysis is to arrest uterine contractions and prolong pregnancy to allow for administration of steroids, administration of prophylactic antibiotics, and possibly transport to a tertiary care center. Available treatments are intended to arrest uterine contractility and are not necessarily geared toward the underlying pathogenic process initiating labor. It is important to acknowledge that studies evaluating tocolytics are limited and difficult to analyze secondary to significant bias and inherent design flaws. Additionally, there is a paucity of placebo-controlled trials assessing the efficacy of these medications. Thus, the literature is somewhat limited regarding optimal tocolytic therapy and current protocols are based on the best available evidence. Presently, no agent is FDA approved for this indication and all are used off-label (Table 18.2).

18.3.1 Magnesium sulfate

Magnesium sulfate was first used as a tocolytic in the 1960s after it was shown to reduce uterine contractility both in vitro and in vivo [19]. Magnesium acts via extracellular and intracellular mechanisms to decrease intracellular calcium concentrations, thereby preventing the contractile response [20]. The most recent literature on the use of magnesium sulfate is highly variable on its efficacy and recommendations for use [21–25]. Even when different authors examined the same studies, different conclusions were reached. In the United States, the use of magnesium sulfate for acute tocolysis is still accepted [21]. Magnesium sulfate has an additional indication for threatened preterm birth at less than 32 weeks gestation: fetal neuroprotection [21]. When used for tocolysis, it is recommended not to exceed 48 h of administration [21]. Magnesium sulfate is usually administered with a loading dose of 4–6 g over 20–30 min, followed by a maintenance dose of 2 g/h. To prevent dosing errors, the loading dose should be administered from a separate premixed bag with the prescribed dose. Magnesium sulfate must be administered via an infusion pump and requires close observation, particularly during the loading dose. The most common side effects include flushing, nausea, headache, generalized muscle weakness, and diplopia. The patient must be monitored for signs of magnesium toxicity: absent deep tendon reflexes, respiratory depression, pulmonary edema, cardiac arrythmias, and cardiopulmonary arrest. Magnesium sulfate is excreted via the kidneys, so careful intake and output monitoring is indicated. In the presence of renal impairment, the likelihood of magnesium toxicity is increased. The antidote for magnesium toxicity is calcium gluconate, which should be readily available. Magnesium sulfate is contraindicated in patients with myasthenia gravis.

18.3.2 β-Adrenergic receptor agonists

β-Adrenergic receptor agonists (β-sympathomimetics) have been studied extensively in several randomized controlled trials with comparisons to both placebo and other tocolytics and have been used clinically since the 1970s. A 2014 Cochrane systematic review concluded that these medications are better than placebo at delaying birth for at least 2 days [26]. Two additional reviews concluded that β-sympathomimetics are useful in delaying birth for up to 48 h [22,25]. Another review concluded, however, that these medications should no longer be used for tocolysis because there are safer efficacious options available [23].

β-Adrenergic receptor agonists work to arrest uterine contractions by binding β2-adrenergic receptors on the myometrial cell (Fig. 18.1). This interaction leads to increased levels of cyclic AMP which activates protein kinase. Protein kinase inactivates MLCK thus preventing uterine contractility.

Table 18.2 Tocolytics.

Medication	Clinical indication	Route	Dose	Frequency	Considerations
Magnesium sulfate	Acute tocolysis	Intravenous	Loading: 4–6 g over 20–30 min Maintenance: 2 g/h	Continuous	Use is inconclusive. ACOG still recommends. Also used for fetal neuroprotection at <32 weeks Also used as seizure prophylaxis in preeclampsia Contraindicated in patients with myasthenia gravis
Terbutaline	Acute tocolysis	Subcutaneous	250 mcg	Every 20–30 min up to 4 doses or until tocolysis is achieved	May repeat a dose every 3 –4 h for 24–48 h Hold dose if maternal HR > 120 Avoid in patients with cardiac disease Caution in diabetic patients
Nifedipine (Procardia®)	Acute tocolysis	Oral	ACOG: 30 mg, then 10 –20 mg q 4–6 h NICE: 20 mg, then 10 –20 mg 3–4 times/day	See dose information	Only administer immediate-release preparations. Only administer orally. Use with caution in patients concomitantly receiving magnesium sulfate
Indomethacin	Acute tocolysis	Oral	50–100 mg	Every 4–6 h up to 48 h	Restrict to use in patients <32 weeks Check AFI prior to administration
Atosiban[a]	Acute tocolysis	Intravenous	6.75 mg bolus followed by 300 mcg/min infusion for 3 h	100 mcg/hour for up to 45 h	Not available in the United Sates
Nitroglycerin	Acute uterine or cervical relaxation	Intravenous	100–200 mcg	Can consider repeating dose after 1–4 min if inadequate response	Monitor for hypotension and uterine atony

[a] Medication is not approved for use in the United States.

Among the β-adrenergic-receptor agonists, ritodrine and terbutaline have been the two medications most commonly used for labor inhibition. Historically, ritodrine was the only medication ever to receive FDA approval for uterine tocolysis. However, this medication was voluntarily removed from the US market by the manufacturer after cases of maternal death were reported in the setting of ritodrine-induced pulmonary edema. Currently, the only β-adrenergic receptor agonist used in the United States for uterine tocolysis is terbutaline. Recently, the FDA issued a black box warning regarding the use of terbutaline for tocolysis. The warning states that oral terbutaline should not be used for the prevention or treatment of preterm labor because it has not been shown to be effective and has the potential for serious maternal heart problems and death. Injectable terbutaline should not be used for the prevention or prolonged treatment (>48−72 h) of preterm labor because of similar safety concerns [27].

Typically, terbutaline is administered for acute tocolysis intrapartum in the setting uterine tachysystole [28]. Additionally, it can be used for uterine relaxation prior to external cephalic version and/or maternal/fetal surgery.

For preterm labor tocolysis, 250 mcg of terbutaline can be administered subcutaneously every 20−30 min up to four doses or until tocolysis is achieved. A dose of 250 mcg may then be repeated every 3−4 h for 24−48 h depending on uterine activity and maternal hemodynamic response. For acute tocolysis in the setting of uterine tachysystole with associated fetal heart rate changes, a dose of 250 mcg subcutaneous or 125 mcg intravenous can be administered. The medication should be held if the maternal heart rate is > 120 beats per minute. The medication is rapidly absorbed with the onset of action typically occurring within 5−15 min after subcutaneous dosing. It is faster with intravenous administration. The half-life of the medication in pregnancy is 3.7 h. The majority of the medication is eliminated unchanged via the kidney.

This medication has an extensive side effect profile including the following: tachycardia, flushing, nervousness, dizziness, hyperglycemia, hypokalemia, and hyperthyroidism. More serious side effects including cardiac arrhythmia, hypo-/hypertension, pulmonary edema/acute respiratory distress syndrome, and myocardial ischemia/infarction have been reported with an incidence of 0.3%−5%. Maternal death has been reported in the setting of long-term use (injectable or oral use) [27]. Care should be taken when administering terbutaline to women with diabetes because it stimulates the release of glucagon. Terbutaline should be avoided in pregnant women with either preexisting or pregnancy-related cardiac disease.

18.3.3 Calcium channel blockers

Calcium channel blockers are commonly used as first-line agents for acute tocolysis. Calcium channel blockers work to relax smooth muscle by directly blocking entry of calcium ions into the myometrial cell and through prevention of intracellular calcium release from the sarcoplasmic reticulum (Fig. 18.1). Calcium is necessary for MLCK-mediated phosphorylation. In the absence of calcium, MLCK is inactivated resulting in myometrial relaxation.

Nifedipine is the most common calcium channel blocker used for acute tocolysis. A recent systematic review concluded that calcium channel blockers are the preferred tocolytic because they offered the greatest benefit with the least complications [22]. These conclusions are also supported in another review which concluded nifedipine is superior to β-Adrenergic receptor agonists in regards to efficacy and safety [23]. Nifedipine is not effective for prolonged tocolysis. Nifedipine has a half-life of 2−3 h with a maximum plasma concentration after a 10-mg tablet of 30−60 min [23].

While the optimal dosing for nifedipine has not been established, there are two primary regimens used in clinical practice and supported by published clinical guidelines. The 2016 ACOG guidelines recommend 30 mg nifedipine initially, then 10−20 mg every 4−6 h [29]. The 2015 National Institute for Health and Care Excellence guidelines recommend an initial 20 mg oral dose, followed by 10−20 mg three to four times daily, depending on uterine activity [30]. Only oral administration of the immediate-release form of the medication should be used. Sustained-release forms and sublingual administration have been associated with serious maternal and fetal complications [23].

Common side effects include hypotension, flushing, nausea, headache, dizziness, anxiety, cough, and dyspnea. Thus, patients should be counseled and advised to monitor for symptoms. Additionally, maternal blood pressure should be monitored closely as acute hypotension can result in fetal heart rate changes and lead to maternal syncope. In the case of concurrent or recent administration of magnesium sulfate, increased surveillance for maternal complications is necessary [29].

18.3.4 Cyclooxygenase inhibitors

Cyclooxygenase (COX) inhibitors are used as a second-line tocolytic. They are most commonly used in conjunction with other tocolytics. COX inhibitors prevent the conversion of arachidonic acid to prostaglandin. Prostaglandins have a significant role in the labor process by stimulating myometrial gap junction formation and by increasing the intracellular calcium levels. Thus, COX inhibitors work to inhibit labor through the prevention of prostaglandin formation (Fig. 18.1). The most common COX inhibitor used for tocolysis is indomethacin. Indomethacin is typically administered as a loading dose of 50−100 mg orally, followed by 25−50 mg orally every 4−6 h up to 48 h. Its use should be restricted to patients with an estimated gestational age of <32 weeks [22,23]. Oral indomethacin is rapidly absorbed and distributed systemically in the plasma with 99% being protein bound. The half-life of the medication is approximately 4.5 h. It is eliminated via renal and biliary excretion.

Although recent reviews have had conflicting conclusions [23], it remains a widely used tocolytic. Other than maternal GI upset (which can be ameliorated with H2 antagonists), the primary concern with using indomethacin as a tocolytic is its fetal effects. Indomethacin readily crosses the placenta. In utero, it can cause premature closure of the fetal ductus arteriosus and oligohydramnios. Neither of these complications has been reported in the setting of short-term tocolysis ($\leq$48 h) prior to 32 weeks' gestation [22,23]. Providers should check an AFI prior to administration. There is limited evidence that suggests an increased risk of necrotizing enterocolitis and intraventricular hemorrhage, but the study is limited by its design of not isolating patients that only received indomethacin [31]. Additionally, the medication should be discontinued if delivery becomes imminent. Although there are conflicting recommendations on its use, ACOG continues to recommend indomethacin when used as suggested [29].

18.3.5 Oxytocin receptor antagonists (atosiban)

Atosiban is not available for use in the United States. It is currently used throughout Europe for acute tocolysis. The drug itself is a selective oxytocin—vasopressin receptor antagonist that competitively inhibits oxytocin from binding to its receptors in the myometrium and decidua (Fig. 18.1). Several trials have compared atosiban to placebo or other tocolytics with conflicting reports on efficacy [23]. The Rath review did conclude that atosiban had the fewest complications of any tocolytic and should be considered as a first-line tocolytic in mothers with cardiovascular disease [23]. One randomized controlled trial carried out in the United States reported a trend toward higher rates of fetal death in women treated with atosiban [32]. These results may have been confounded by infection and extreme prematurity; however, an association with atosiban could not be excluded. Thus, the United States FDA denied approval of atosiban for tocolysis secondary to safety concerns. In Europe, however, clinical studies have not demonstrated these complications and remains widely used in clinical practice [23].

18.3.6 Nitric oxide donors

Nitric oxide is a potent vasodilator and smooth muscle relaxant produced by a variety of cells. Nitric oxide relaxes smooth muscle via interaction with guanylyl cyclase (Fig. 18.1). This interaction increases guanosine monophosphate (cGMP), which in turn inactivates MLCK leading to smooth muscle relaxation.

Nitroglycerin (NG) is most commonly used for acute uterine relaxation in the setting of uterine inversion or to facilitate external cephalic version, fetal delivery at the time of c-section, uterine relaxation for fetal surgery, and/or to relieve fetal head entrapment with vaginal breech delivery [33]. It has been shown to be an effective uterine/cervical relaxant when administered at a dose of 100—200 mcg IV [33]. The half-life of NG is very short at 1—4 min. Common side effects include hypotension, flushing, and headache. One may encounter uterine atony after administration; thus, uterotonics should be readily available. Its use as a routine tocolytic is not recommended nor supported by multiple reviews [23].

18.3.7 **Tocolytics summary**

- There is an overwhelming abundance of data regarding tocolytics; however, the studies are often flawed and their results are difficult to interpret and implement in clinical practice.
- It is important to choose a tocolytic based on efficacy and safety, and the choice at times will be patient and situation specific (i.e. not administering indomethacin to a patient greater than 32 weeks' gestation or adjusting the nifedipine dose for a patient with mild hypotension).
- It is important to remember appropriate fetal surveillance when indicated, especially with indomethacin administration.

References

[1] Arias F. Pharmacology of oxytocin and prostaglandins. Clin Obstet Gynecol 2000;43: 455—68.

[2] Clark S, Simpson K, Knox E, Garite T. Oxytocin: new perspectives on an old drug. Am J Obstet Gynecol 2009;200:35e1—6.

[3] Bostanci E, Kilicci C, Ozkaya E, Abide Yayla C, Eroglu M. Continuous oxytocin versus intermittent oxytocin for induction of labor: a randomized study. J Matern Fetal Neonatal Med 2018:1—6.

[4] Budden A, Chen LJ, Henry A. High-dose versus low-dose oxytocin infusion regimens for induction of labour at term. Cochrane Database Syst Rev 2014:CD009701.

[5] Page K, McCool WF, Guidera M. Examination of the pharmacology of oxytocin and clinical guidelines for use in labor. J Midwifery Wom Health 2017;62:425—33.

[6] Prichard N, Lindquist A, Hiscock R, Ruff S, Tong S, Brownfoot FC. High-dose compared with low-dose oxytocin for induction of labour of nulliparous women at term. J Matern Fetal Neonatal Med 2019;32:362—8.

[7] American College of Obstetricians and Gynecologists. ACOG practice bulletin No. 107: induction of labor. Obstet Gynecol 2009;114:386—97.

[8] Robinson C, Schuman R, Zhang P, Young R. Oxytocin-induced desensitization of the oxytocin receptor. Am J Obstet Gynecol 2003;188:496—502.

[9] Borgatta L, Kapp N. Clinical guidelines. Labor induction abortion in the second trimester. Contraception 2011;84:4—18.

[10] Evensen A, Anderson JM, Fontaine P. Postpartum hemorrhage: prevention and treatment. Am Fam Physician 2017;95:442—9.

[11] Association of Women's Health Obstetric and Neonatal Nurses. AWHONN practice brief No. 2: oxytocin administration for management of third stage of labor. J Obstet Gynecol Neonatal Nurs 2015;44:161—3.

[12] Harvey C, Dildy GA. Obstetric hemorrhage. Washington, DC: Association of Women's Health, Obstetric and Neonatal Nurses; 2012.

[13] Methergine. 2012. Available from: https://www.accessdata.fda.gov/drugsatfda_docs/nda/2012/006035Orig1S078.pdf.

[14] deGroot A, van Dongen P, Vree T, Hekster Y, van Roosmalen J. Ergot alkaloids. current status and review of clinical pharmacology and therapeutic use compared with other oxytocics in obstetrics and gynaecology. Drugs 1998;56:523—35.

[15] Bateman BT, Huybrechts KF, Hernandez-Diaz S, Liu J, Ecker JL, Avorn J. Methylergonovine maleate and the risk of myocardial ischemia and infarction. Am J Obstet Gynecol 2013;209:459e1—459e13.

[16] Cervidil. Ferring Pharmaceuticals; 2015. Available from: https://www.cervidil.com/hcp/.

[17] Simpson KR. Cervical ripening and labor induction and augmentation. 4th ed. Washington, DC: Association of Women's Health, Obstetric and Neonatal Nurses; 2013.

[18] Prepidil. Pfizer; 2019. Available from: http://labeling.pfizer.com/ShowLabeling.aspx?id=675.

[19] Kumar D, Zourlas P, Barnes A. In vitro and in vivo effects of magnesium sulfate on human uterine contractility. Am J Obstet Gynecol 1963;86:1036—40.

[20] Fomin V, Gibbs S, Vanam R, Morimiya A, Hurd W. Effect of magnesium sulfate on contractile force and intracellular calcium concentration in pregnant human myometrium. Am J Obstet Gynecol 2006;194:1384—90.

[21] American College of Obstetricians and Gynecologists. Committee opinion No. 652: magnesium sulfate use in obstetrics. Obstet Gynecol 2016;127. e52—3.

[22] Hanley M, Sayres L, Reiff ES, Wood A, Grotegut CA, Kuller JA. Tocolysis: a review of the literature. Obstet Gynecol Surv 2019;74:50—5.

[23] Rath W, Kehl S. Acute tocolysis - a critical analysis of evidence-based data. Geburtshilfe Frauenheilkd 2018;78:1245—55.

[24] Yoneda S, Yoneda N, Fukuta K, et al. In which preterm labor-patients is intravenous maintenance tocolysis effective? J Obstet Gynaecol Res 2018;44:397—407.

[25] Younger JD, Reitman E, Gallos G. Tocolysis: present and future treatment options. Semin Perinatol 2017;41:493—504.

[26] Neilson J, West H, Dowswell T. Betamimetics for inhibiting preterm labour. Cochrane Database Syst Rev 2014:CD004352.

[27] New warnings against use of terbutaline to treat preterm labor. 2011. Available from: https://www.fda.gov/Drugs/DrugSafety/ucm243539.htm.

[28] Leathersich SJ, Vogel JP, Tran TS, Hofmeyr GJ. Acute tocolysis for uterine tachysystole or suspected fetal distress. Cochrane Database Syst Rev 2018;7:CD009770.

[29] American College of Obstetricians and Gynecologists. Practice bulletin No. 171: management of preterm labor. Obstet Gynecol 2016;128:e155—64.

[30] Preterm labour and birth. NICE guideline [NG25]. 2015. Available from: http://www.nice.org.uk/guidance/ng25.

[31] Vermillion S, Scardo J, Lashus A, et al. The effect of indomethacin tocolysis on fetal ductus arteriosus constriction with advancing gestational age. Am J Obstet Gynecol 1997:256—9.

[32] Romero R, Sibai B, Sanchez-Ramos L, et al. An oxytocin receptor antagonist (atosiban) in the treatment of preterm labor: a randomized, double-blind, placebo-controlled trial with tocolytic rescue. Am J Obstet Gynecol 2000;182:1173—83.

[33] Axemo P, Xin F, Lindberg B, Ulmsten U, Wessen A. Intravenous nitroglycerin for rapid uterine relaxation. Acta Obstet Gynecol Scand 1998;77:50—3.

Antenatal thyroid disease and pharmacotherapy in pregnancy

19

Shannon M. Clark, Luis A. Monsivais

Department of ObGyn, Division of Maternal-Fetal Medicine, University of Texas Medical Branch-Galveston, Galveston, TX, United States

19.1 Thyroid function and physiology in pregnancy

In pregnancy, abnormalities of the thyroid gland can be easily overlooked due to the normal physiologic changes of pregnancy often mimicking disturbances of thyroid gland function. As a result, basic knowledge of thyroid gland function and the changes the thyroid gland undergoes during the course of pregnancy are essential. Regulation of the thyroid gland and its hormones is controlled through an endocrine feedback loop that includes the hypothalamus and anterior pituitary [1]. The hypothalamus initiates this feedback loop with the release of thyrotropin-releasing hormone, which in turn regulates the release of thyroid-stimulating hormone (TSH) from thyrotrope cells in the anterior pituitary. TSH then prompts the release of thyroid hormones T4 and T3 from the thyroid gland. Abnormal production of T4 and T3 occurs with hyperthyroidism and hypothyroidism in the pregnant patient, with various etiologies accounting for the observed abnormal levels (see Table 19.1).

The physiologic changes of normal pregnancy affect thyroid function in numerous ways. The thyroid gland itself increases in size and can be newly palpable on physical examination. This increase in size is due to an increase in thyroid volume, the formation of new thyroid nodules, and/or increased iodine turnover [2,3]. In fact, the maternal thyroid volume is 30% larger in the third trimester than in the first trimester [4]. Although the formation of thyroid nodules can occur during pregnancy, any palpable nodule should be evaluated with an ultrasound of the thyroid gland [1]. Overall, these changes normally occur without any significant change in thyroid hormone levels, but physical examination of the thyroid gland during pregnancy is important on entry to prenatal care, especially if the patient is exhibiting potential signs or symptoms of thyroid gland dysfunction (see Table 19.2).

The observed increase in iodine turnover and subsequent depletion of the maternal iodine pool is predominantly the result of a reduction in serum iodine due to fetal use of maternal iodine and increased maternal renal clearance of iodine, which also causes an increase in thyroid gland size in 15% of pregnant women [5–7]. As pregnancy progresses, maternal renal clearance of iodine increases due to an increase in renal blood flow and glomerular filtration rate, which further

Table 19.1 Maternal thyroid function testing and associated physiologic alterations in normal pregnancy.

Increased	Decreased	No change
Thyroid-binding globulin (TBG)	TSH	Free T3 (FT3)
Total T3 (TT3)	Plasma iodide	Free T4 (FT4)
Total T4 (TT4)	Hepatic clearance	
Thyroid gland size		
hCG		
Albumin		

Table 19.2 Maternal signs and symptoms of hyperthyroidism and hypothyroidism.

Hyperthyroidism	Hypothyroidism
Nervousness	Fatigue
Tremors	Constipation
Tachycardia	Cold intolerance
Frequent stools	Muscle cramps
Excessive sweating	Weight gain
Heat intolerance	Edema
Weight loss	Dry skin
Goiter	Hair loss
Insomnia	Prolonged relaxation phase of reflexes
Palpitations	
Hypertension	
Lid lag and lid retraction	
Localized or pretibial myxedema	

increases iodine clearance [8]. The American Thyroid Association (ATA) recommends a daily allowance of iodine of 150 mcg for nonpregnant adults, 220—250 mcg in pregnant women, and 250—290 mcg in breastfeeding women. As a result, women should take multivitamins containing 150 mcg of iodine daily in the form of potassium iodine during the preconception period, pregnancy, and lactation [9—11].

The physiologic changes of thyroid gland function, particularly during the first trimester of pregnancy, are well documented. TSH and human chorionic gonadotropin (hCG) are glycoproteins that share similar alpha subunits. This similarity between the alpha subunits results in negative feedback on the pituitary by hCG and decreased TSH production [6,9,11,12]. As hCG levels continue to rise during the first trimester, TSH levels decline by approximately 20%—50% reaching a maximal decrease at 8—14 weeks' gestation [6,13,14]. In fact, TSH levels may decrease below the lower limit of normal in up to 20% of women with little clinical

Table 19.3 Maternal thyroid disease and relation to TSH and FT4.

	TSH	FT4
Subclinical hyperthyroidism (or GTT)	Decreased	Normal to high normal
Hyperthyroidism	Decreased	Increased
Subclinical hypothyroidism	Increased	Normal to low normal
Hypothyroidism	Increased	Decreased

consequence [12]. As a result of this decrease in TSH, the levels of FT4 and FT3 may slightly increase and even reach high-normal levels. The observed changes in TSH, FT4, and FT3 are referred to as transient subclinical hyperthyroidism or gestational transient thyrotoxicosis (GTT). GTT affects 1%−5% of pregnant women and typically does not require treatment since it is not due to intrinsic thyroid disease [1,15−17]. In the second and third trimesters, TSH levels will start to rise due to the increased renal clearance of iodine and placental degradation of thyroid hormone, and a decrease in FT4 and FT3 levels back into normal range will follow [1] (see Table 19.3).

Although circulating T4 and T3 are predominantly bound (>99%) to the carrier proteins TBG and albumin, it is the free hormone (<1%) that is biologically active. During pregnancy, serum TBG levels increase 2−3-fold due to increased TBG synthesis through the effects of increased estrogen and decreased hepatic clearance [6,11,12,18,19]. Increased TBG leads to a rise in TT4 and TT3 concentrations by approximately 50% starting at 6 weeks of gestation without significantly altering FT4 and FT3 concentrations [1,7,20−22]. In addition, the thyrotrophic effect of hCG likely further contributes to the increase in TT4 and TT3 concentrations [23].

Since FT4 and FT3 are the biologically active hormones, unaltered levels of FT4 and FT3 ideally allow the pregnant patient to remain euthyroid during this time. Although there can be a transient rise in FT4 during the first trimester due to increasing levels of hCG and its thyrotropic effect, TSH will start to increase in the latter trimesters resulting in a fall in FT4 as previously mentioned [24]. Overall, the FT4 levels should remain within normal to high-normal range, and FT3 levels will parallel that of FT4 and remain in the normal reference range as well [24] (see Table 19.1).

19.2 Hyperthyroidism in pregnancy

Hyperthyroidism occurs in 0.2% of pregnant women, or 1 in every 1000−2000 pregnancies [9,20,25,26]. The causes of hyperthyroidism are multiple and include autoimmune disease, nodular goiter, solitary toxic adenoma, gestational trophoblastic disease, subacute and lymphocytic thyroiditis, and tumors of the pituitary gland or ovary [12].

Graves' disease is the most common cause in pregnancy, occurring in 85%—95% of all pregnant patients with hyperthyroidism [12,27]. It is an autoimmune disease caused by autoantibodies that activate the TSH receptor and stimulate the thyroid to produce an excessive amount of thyroid hormone [1,19]. TSH (thyrotropin) receptor antibodies (TRAb) can be stimulating, blocking, or neutral. The thyroid-stimulating antibodies (TSAb) cause hyperthyroidism, while the thyroid-blocking antibodies (TBAb) cause hypothyroidism. The receptor assays that measure TSH receptor—binding inhibitory immunoglobulins measure antibodies that block binding of TSH to an in vitro TSH receptor preparation and do not differentiate between TSAb and TBAb [28,29]. These TRAb cause thyroid hyperfunction and thyroid gland hypertrophy, although there is no correlation between levels of antibody activity and disease severity [12]. Of note, Graves' disease may also be caused by TSH receptor—blocking antibodies as well.

TRAb are measurable in around 95% of patients with active Graves' hyperthyroidism [11]. Furthermore, elevated TRAb levels carry a prognostic value for fetal and neonatal thyrotoxicosis as TRAb can cross the placenta resulting in neonatal thyrotoxicosis in 1%—5% of neonates of mothers with Graves' disease [14,30]. If high titers persist in the third trimester, fetal or neonatal hyperthyroidism is more likely to develop [11,31]. Such a complication is more likely if maternal Graves' disease has been difficult to control or there has been a delay in diagnosis [7,11]. Once the diagnosis of hyperthyroidism is established, consideration for evaluation of TRAb levels in early pregnancy and again in the third trimester to assess for the potential of neonatal disease is recommended by some [11,30]. The ATA recommends evaluation of TRAb since levels greater than >5 IU/L, or 3 times the upper level of normal in the latter half of pregnancy, predicted neonatal hyperthyroidism with 100% sensitivity and 43% specificity [32] (see Table 19.4).

As previously discussed, GTT can occur in the first trimester of pregnancy due to the cross-reactivity of the alpha subunits of TSH and hCG. During this period of gestation, differentiating between GTT and true Graves' disease is important as the former is expected to resolve spontaneously without intervention and the latter requires therapeutic intervention. The symptoms specific to hyperthyroidism should help to confirm the diagnosis of intrinsic thyroid disease versus normal physiologic changes of pregnancy (see Table 19.2).

Table 19.4 Maternal thyroid antibodies and neonatal thyroid gland effects.

Hyperthyroidism	Hypothyroidism
TSH receptor antibodies (TRAbs):	Thyroglobulin antibodies (TgAbs):
(Can be activating (TSI) or blocking (TBII))	Do not affect fetal thyroid gland function
Thyroid-stimulating antibodies (TSAbs)-Can cause neonatal thyrotoxicosis	Thyroid peroxidase antibodies (TPOAbs):
Thyroid-blocking antibodies (TBAbs)-Can cause hypothyroidism or transient neonatal hypothyroidism	Do not affect fetal thyroid gland function

In the first trimester, if the TSH is suppressed, FT4 is elevated, and the patient is symptomatic, the diagnosis of overt hyperthyroidism should be established. Laboratory assays of TRAb will likely be abnormal and are not necessary to make a diagnosis. If the TSH is suppressed, FT4 is normal to high normal, and the patient is symptomatic, laboratory assays of TRAb should be considered to help differentiate between a diagnosis of hyperthyroidism or GTT [30]. If TRAb are normal, the diagnosis is GTT or subclinical hyperthyroidism. If elevated levels of TRAb exist, the diagnosis of hyperthyroidism is confirmed.

Once again, GTT (suppressed TSH and normal-high normal FT4) is the diagnosis if there are no TRAb, thyroid nodules, goiter, or orbitopathy present, and there is no prior maternal history of Graves' disease [23,30]. Once the diagnosis of GTT is confirmed, the patient can be reassured that symptoms and laboratory abnormalities will resolve without intervention. Of note, the increase in hCG that is associated with GTT is also a contributor to the development of hyperemesis gravidarum (HG), which is the more severe form of nausea and vomiting in pregnancy (NVP) typically seen in the first trimester. HG is defined as persistent nausea and vomiting resulting in greater than 5% weight loss, ketonuria, dehydration, and electrolyte imbalance [17,22,30]. Abnormal thyroid function tests similar to that observed in GTT, including elevated FT4 into the high-normal range and suppressed or undetectable TSH, are found in about 60% of women with HG with levels typically normalizing after 16–20 weeks [17,33]. Finally, newly diagnosed cases of overt hyperthyroidism can present with HG or NVP, making thyroid function testing essential. In this scenario, once therapy is initiated, symptoms resolve with successful treatment of the disease [7].

Uncontrolled or poorly controlled hyperthyroidism in pregnancy has significant maternal and fetal/neonatal effects. Maternal complications include insufficient weight gain, heart failure, preeclampsia, and thyroid storm, a true medical emergency that may be precipitated by labor and delivery, infection, or preeclampsia. When considering the fetus, there is an increase in fetal loss, low birth weight, preterm labor, and congenital malformations [11,16,34,35]. As stated earlier, the neonate can be affected by the transplacental transfer of TRAb [16,36,37]. Furthermore, the fetus may also develop tachycardia and goiter in utero due to the presence of these antibodies, and in severe cases cardiac failure and fetal hydrops. There is not a general consensus on whether to routinely follow TRAb in a patient with Graves' disease. However, if the patient is poorly controlled, continues to be symptomatic, or is noncompliant with treatment, evaluation of TRAb should be considered. The 2017 guidelines of the ATA lists specific indications for ordering TRAb in pregnancy and recommends repeat testing at weeks 18–22 of pregnancy if the maternal TRAb concentration is elevated in early pregnancy or if treatment with antithyroid drugs (ATDs) is indicated [11]. However, such rigorous use of TRAb testing in maternal thyroid disease has not been recommended by the American College of Obstetricians and Gynecologists (ACOG).

19.3 Pharmacotherapy with thionamides in pregnancy

Once a diagnosis of hyperthyroidism is made, prompt initiation of treatment with thionamides is recommended. Thionamides inhibit thyroid hormone synthesis by interfering with thyroid peroxidase—mediated iodination of tyrosine residues in thyroglobulin, an important step in the synthesis of T4 and T3 [38]. Propylthiouracil (PTU) and methimazole (MMI) are the mainstays of treatment in pregnancy. PTU has historically been used more commonly in the United States because it was believed that PTU crossed the placenta to a lesser degree than MMI due to the increased protein binding of PTU, therefore decreasing the chance of fetal hypothyroidism and anomalies. However, in 2009, the U.S. Food and Drug Administration (FDA) issued a safety alert on PTU-associated hepatotoxicity. This was based on 32 reports of PTU liver toxicity in the FDA's event reporting system compared with five reports of liver toxicity for MMI during a period when PTU was the preferred treatment for hyperthyroidism in the United States [9]. On the other hand, MMI has been associated with aplasia cutis, a fetal scalp defect, and "MMI embryopathy," which is characterized by facial abnormalities and choanal atresia, growth restriction, developmental abnormalities, and esophageal atresia/tracheoesophageal fistula when used in the first trimester [16,39,40]. Clinicians can limit the potential adverse outcomes associated with thionamides by applying a trimester-specific ATD prescribing strategy consisting of PTU in the first trimester followed by MMI beginning in the second trimester and continuing postpartum. This strategy allows the clinician to balance the risk of rare events like PTU hepatotoxicity and MMI embryopathy [9,19]. The goal is treatment with the lowest possible thionamide dose needed to maintain free T4 levels slightly above or in the high-normal range, regardless of TSH levels, while adequately controlling the signs and symptoms of hyperthyroidism [9]. In addition, this strategy aims to best avoid fetal hypothyroidism, goiter, and abnormal brain development that could result from the transplacental passage of thionamides [11,12,41].

MMI can be given once daily because it has a longer duration of action than PTU. The oral dosing regimen of MMI is typically started at 10—15 mg a day and adjusted accordingly, with the maximum dose being 40 mg a day. As symptoms improve, a maintenance dose of 5—15 mg a day is usually sufficient. Because of its shorter half-life, less thyroidal tissue concentration, and decreased maximal concentration when compared to MMI, PTU requires twice daily to three times daily dosing in pregnancy. PTU is started at 100—150 mg every 8—12 h up to a maximum dose of 600—800 mg a day [26,40,42]. A maintenance dose of 50—150 mg a day is ideal. If a patient requires more than 300 mg a day, dosing every 4—6 h is recommended [43]. Monitoring of thyroid function tests (TSH, FT4, and FT3) every 4 weeks is recommended after initiation of therapy in the mildly symptomatic patient. This can be decreased to every 6 weeks once the patient is euthyroid.

Although information on the effectiveness of PTU versus MMI in the treatment of hyperthyroidism in pregnancy is limited, studies thus far have shown that they are equally effective. In a retrospective cohort study by Wing et al. examining the maternal and fetal outcomes of 185 patients treated for hyperthyroidism with PTU or MMI, both drugs were found to be equally effective, with similar rates of normalization of thyroid hormone levels [44]. Finally, the pharmacokinetics of PTU and MMI do not appear to differ significantly in the pregnant and nonpregnant patient in the limited number of studies addressing this issue.

Therapy with PTU and MMI can be started at moderate doses in order to bring the disease under control more quickly, i.e., in cases with a large goiter or significant symptoms. MMI can be started at 20–30 mg a day in divided doses and PTU can be started at 100 mg three times daily for a period of 2–3 days, with tapering once symptoms are under control. Treatment with PTU and MMI may take 6–8 weeks to see a change both clinically and in laboratory assessments. After initiation of therapy with higher doses, thyroid function tests (TSH and FT4) should be evaluated in 2 weeks followed by levels every 4–6 weeks depending on response to therapy. When monitoring response to therapy, normalization of FT4 precedes that of FT3 making FT4 a better indicator for the adjustment of medication dosage [45]. However, maternal TSH may remain suppressed for weeks to months following normalization of FT4 [30]. Monitoring of maternal thyroid function frequently during pregnancy is important in order to avoid overtreatment and the potential development of fetal hypothyroidism and goiter, especially when starting at a higher dose [30]. Approximately, 25% of cases of transient neonatal hypothyroidism can be attributed to treatment of maternal hyperthyroidism with thionamides, which can cause neuropsychological damage in severe cases when the fetus is overtreated [46].

Although maternal Graves' disease is associated with the passage of TRAb across the placenta to the fetus, whether or not to check antibody levels during pregnancy is debated, as mentioned previously. In those patients who enter pregnancy with a history of Graves' disease, but who have no active disease and do not need treatment, neonatal hyperthyroidism may still occur [24]. As a result, it is argued that TRAb should be monitored, and if the level is high, the fetus should be evaluated early in gestation and again at 32–36 weeks of pregnancy. If there is a detectable level of TRAb at 32–36 weeks, evaluation of the neonate for hyperthyroidism is warranted [11,24]. If the patient enters pregnancy already on adequate treatment and is asymptomatic, there is usually no need to measure TRAb as clinical and laboratory maternal thyroid function gives a reliable estimate of fetal thyroid status and the risk of neonatal hyperthyroidism is very low in these cases [24]. Whether or not TRAb are followed, serial sonograms and fetal heart rate monitoring to assess the fetus for tachycardia, goiter, and growth are recommended during the course of the pregnancy [47].

The occurrence of minor and major side effects with the use of thionamides does not appear to change in frequency in pregnancy. Minor side effects occur in approximately 3%–5% of patients and include the development of a papular urticarial rash, pruritus, joint pain, headache, nausea, and hair loss [11,43,48,49]. These side effects can often be managed conservatively with antihistamines, by switching therapy, or stopping treatment [38]. However, if arthralgias develop, this may indicate the

Table 19.5 Maternal side effects with thionamides

Minor (5% of patients)	Major
Papular urticarial rash	Arthralgias — severe transient migratory polyarthritis, or "antithyroid arthritis syndrome"
Pruritus	Drug fever
Joint pain	Bronchospasm
Headache	Agranulocytosis — 0.35% (more common with PTU)[a]
Nausea	Hepatotoxicity — 0.1%—0.2%[a]
Hair loss	Vasculitis — "lupus-like" syndrome[a]

[a] More Common with PTU.

development of severe transient migratory polyarthritis, or "antithyroid arthritis syndrome," and discontinuation of thionamide therapy is recommended [38].

The more major side effects include drug fever, bronchospasm, agranulocytosis, hepatotoxicity, and vasculitis, which includes a lupus-like syndrome [12,50,51]. Agranulocytosis, believed to be autoimmune mediated, occurs in approximately 0.35% of patients taking thionamides and 0.1% of patients taking PTU and is considered a major side effect [12,52]. It has been associated with higher doses of MMI, but is not related to any particular dosage of PTU.

Agranulocytosis is a contraindication to further thionamide therapy [12]. A baseline white blood cell count should be obtained prior to starting therapy, and if fever and sore throat develop, agranulocytosis should be suspected and therapy immediately stopped. Hepatotoxicity, in the form of allergic hepatitis followed by hepatocellular injury, is reported to occur in 0.1%—0.2% of patients and is more common with PTU [48]. Vasculitis, which is considered to be autoimmune mediated as in agranulocytosis, is also a major side effect and is more common with PTU than MMI (see Table 19.5).

19.4 Hypothyroidism in pregnancy

Hypothyroidism occurs in 2—10 per 1000 pregnancies [9]. Universal screening for thyroid disease in pregnancy is not recommended because identification and treatment of maternal subclinical hypothyroidism has not been shown to result in improvement of neurocognitive function in offspring [9]. The percentage of pregnant women with an abnormal TSH that have autoimmune thyroiditis (AITD) is 40%—60% compared to a prevalence of 7%—11% of antibody-positive nonpregnant women in the same age range [53]. In pregnant women, TSH is the primary screening test for thyroid disease and should be obtained in high-risk women, i.e., those with other autoimmune diseases (i.e., diabetes), thyroid nodules, goiter, exposure to radiation, or personal or strong family history of thyroid disease

[1,9]. Of note, women can have a firm painless goiter and be euthyroid initially during pregnancy, but then become hypothyroid as the pregnancy progresses [12]. As a result, rescreening can be considered.

The most common cause of hypothyroidism in pregnancy is a primary thyroid abnormality known as Hashimoto's thyroiditis, or chronic AITD, which is caused by the presence of thyroid antibodies [23]. In this disorder, titers of antithyroglobulin antibodies (TgAb) are elevated in 50%−70% of patients and almost all patients have antithyroid peroxidase antibodies (TPOAb) present as well [54]. TPOAb are also found in 10% of euthyroid women in early pregnancy and are associated with the subsequent development of hypothyroidism during pregnancy [55]. Although TgAb and TPOAb are known to cross the placenta during the last trimester, they do not negatively affect fetal thyroid function [23]. Conversely, TBAb also cross the placenta, and if the patient has a high titer of these antibodies, the fetus is at risk for hypothyroidism or transient neonatal hypothyroidism [56,57] (see Table 19.4).

The signs and symptoms of hypothyroidism are similar in the nonpregnant and pregnant patient, but some symptoms are considered to be a normal response to the hypermetabolic state of pregnancy [53]. Symptoms include modest weight gain, lethargy, decrease in exercise capacity, intolerance to cold, constipation, hoarseness, hair loss, dry skin, goiter, or delayed relaxation of the deep tendon reexes [9,12] (see Table 19.2). A combination of these symptoms may be seen with overt hypothyroidism or symptoms may be subtle and thus attributed to the normal physiologic changes of pregnancy. If hypothyroidism is suspected at any point during pregnancy, serum TSH and FT4 should be measured.

Overt hypothyroidism has elevated concentrations of TSH and low concentrations of FT4 (see Table 19.3). The ATA guidelines in 2017 advocate for the use of population-based trimester−specific references ranges for serum TSH during pregnancy based on a typical population for whom care is provided. References ranges should be defined by healthy, TPOAb-negative pregnant woman with optimal iodine intake and without thyroid illness. An upper reference limit of normal of 4.0 mIU/L for TSH is typically used. This was proposed due to recent studies which have shown that pregnancy can cause only a modest reduction in the upper reference limits [17]. As an alternative, the guidelines set forth by ACOG in 2015 for TSH may be used: first trimester 0.1−2.5 mIU/L; second trimester 0.2−3.0 mIU/L; and third trimester 0.3−3.0 mIU/L [9]. Measurement of thyroid antibodies, TgAb and TPOAb, can be obtained to aid in the diagnosis especially when TSH and FT4 levels are not fitting the typical pattern for hypothyroidism. Finally, as mentioned above, the presence of TPOAb and a normal to high-normal TSH level at the beginning of pregnancy has been shown to correlate positively with the risk of developing hypothyroidism in pregnancy [9,30]. As a result, if the decision is made not to initiate treatment, monitoring with TSH and FT4 during pregnancy is recommended.

Subclinical hypothyroidism (elevated TSH and normal to low-normal FT4) occurs in up to 2.5% of pregnancies, with a majority of patients being asymptomatic [9,14,19]. The decision whether to treat these patients has been controversial

[9,11,19,58]. It is well established that normal maternal thyroid function is essential for normal fetal brain and neurologic development [47]. It was previously thought that treatment with thyroid hormone replacement in this setting is not harmful and in fact was likely advantageous for the patient and fetus [59—62]. However, recent studies have suggested that treatment of subclinical hypothyroidism with levothyroxine (LT4) replacement and/or elevated FT4 (even in the subclinical hyperthyroid range) in pregnancy is associated with preeclampsia, small for gestational age fetus, preterm delivery, gestational diabetes, and lower IQ [63]. ACOG does not recommend treatment of pregnant women with subclinical hypothyroidism or testing for TPOAb status [9]. However, the ATA 2017 guidelines differ from ACOG recommendations and base treatment of subclinical hypothyroidism on TSH level and TPOAb status. Treatment is recommended for TPOAb-positive women with TSH greater than the pregnancy-specific reference range (see above) and TPOAb-negative women with TSH greater than 10 mUI/L [11]. A recent randomized control trial showed no difference in neurodevelopmental outcomes in children whose mothers received treatment for subclinical hypothyroidism [64].

The same trial also showed no significant effect of thyroxine treatment on pregnancy and neonatal outcomes [64]. In another study, treatment of euthyroid, TPOAb-positive women with LT4 did not result in significant differences in pregnancy outcomes (pregnancy loss, preterm birth, or neonatal outcomes) compared to placebo [65].

Although the most common cause of hypothyroidism worldwide is iodine deficiency, it is typically not a cause in the United States due to dietary iodine supplementation [12]. It is well established that the transplacental passage of maternal T4 is necessary for fetal brain development during the first trimester as the fetal thyroid has yet to develop and start producing its own thyroid hormones. As a result, lack of maternal iodine during the first trimester may lead to impaired fetal neurological development. Furthermore, if there is inadequate iodine substrate for the fetal thyroid gland to use once it has developed, the fetus is unable to synthesize its own thyroid hormones [12]. In fact, during the second trimester, when there is development of the fetal brain, fetal thyroxine is derived almost exclusively from the mother [53,66]. If a woman enters pregnancy with low iodine levels, the available iodine can decrease even further due to the increased renal clearance of iodine and the fetal—placental unit competing for available iodine [67,68].

Severe iodine deficiency during the first trimester causes cretinism, with infants developing severe mental retardation, deafness, muteness, and pyramidal symptoms [12]. Other causes of maternal hypothyroidism include history of radioactive iodine treatment for Graves' disease or thyroidectomy, subacute viral thyroiditis, suppurative thyroiditis, and hypothyroidism secondary to pituitary disease [12,69]. Some drugs, i.e., ferrous sucralfate, sucralfate, carbamazepine, phenytoin, and rifampin, can also depress thyroid function causing symptomatic hypothyroidism.

There are significant consequences of unrecognized or undertreated hypothyroidism in pregnancy. In general, there is an association between hypothyroidism and decreased fertility which is primarily due to ovulatory disturbances attributed to modified levels of gonadotropin, estradiol, testosterone, and sex hormone—binding globulin [11,53,70]. When a hypothyroid woman does become pregnant, there is an increased rate of miscarriage, anemia, postpartum hemorrhage, preeclampsia, placental abruption, growth restriction, prematurity and stillbirth, neonatal respiratory distress, and impaired neurologic development of the fetus [12,71].

The presence of thyroid antibodies in the maternal circulation is associated with a two- to threefold increased risk for preterm delivery and lower birth weight [11,72]. In addition, the presence of circulating thyroid antibodies in the maternal circulation is associated with an increased rate of early spontaneous abortions in both the overt hypothyroid patient and in the hypothyroid patient who is now euthyroid [19,73,74]. As a result, the presence of thyroid immunity represents an independent marker of an at-risk pregnancy [19,53]. Finally, because diabetes and thyroid disorders are both autoimmune conditions, monitoring the hypothyroid patient for the development of diabetes is important.

19.5 Pharmacotherapy with levothyroxine in pregnancy

Treatment with thyroid hormone replacement should be initiated once the diagnosis of hypothyroidism is made so that potential adverse obstetrical outcomes, especially abnormal fetal neurodevelopment, can be minimized. LT4 is the drug of choice for thyroid hormone replacement therapy in pregnancy [9,11]. Synthetic LT4 is a levo isomer of thyroxine with identical activity to the endogenous hormone [75]. It has a long half-life (6—7 days), thus allowing once daily dosing [76]. LT4 is converted to T3 supplying active hormone in the maternal circulation, with T3 concentrations rising much later than T4 concentrations due to the time needed for conversion of T4 to T3 [75,76].

The initial dose is typically 1—2 mcg/kg/day, or between 100 and 150 mcg a day, with dosage adjustments every 4 weeks to keep the TSH at the lower end of normal [9,11,12]. Monitoring of thyroid function is accomplished through routine measurement of maternal serum TSH and making LT4 dosage adjustments in 25—50 mcg increments until TSH values become normal [9]. Another approach consists of doubling the LT4 dose for 2 days a week which equates to a 30% increase once a patient finds out they are pregnant [77].

If the patient is newly diagnosed in pregnancy and she is symptomatic and with significantly abnormal thyroid function testing, treatment with LT4 may be initiated at a dose that is 2—3 times the estimated maintenance dose for a period of 2—3 days [53]. This approach should allow for rapid normalization of the T4 pool and circulating T4 levels, and euthyroidism can be achieved more quickly [53]. In this scenario, TSH and FT4 should be evaluated 2 weeks after initiation of therapy rather than 4 weeks. As the pregnancy progresses, it is not uncommon for T4 requirements to increase due to increased maternal demand and the decreased maternal intestinal absorption that is associated with prenatal iron replacement therapy [12]. As a result, patients should be instructed to take their iron and thyroxine at least 4 h apart to minimize the effect of the decreased intestinal absorption. Other medications that might affect the absorption of LT4 include aluminum hydroxide, dietary fiber, calcium carbonate, calcium citrate, cholestyramine, and colesevelam [78].

Women who enter pregnancy on LT4 will often require an increase in dosage as early as the fifth week of gestation in order to stay euthyroid [30,79,80]. Ideally, this should be accomplished before the onset of pregnancy, but the patient can immediately increase her prepregnancy maintenance dose once pregnancy is diagnosed. The dose of LT4 may need to be increased even further as the pregnancy progresses. This is due to the estrogen-dependent increase in serum TBG concentration, increased placental production of Type II and III deiodinases that degrade T4, and increased tissue volume of distribution, which all contribute to the decrease in serum maternal T4 [6,9,11,81,82]. Typically, a 40%−50% increase in dosage (50−100 mcg a day) is necessary in 75%−85% of patients, and this increase should occur in the first trimester in order to minimize the morbidities associated with undertreatment of maternal hypothyroidism [9,24,30,80,83,84]. Women with a history of radioiodine ablation for hyperthyroidism tend to need a more significant increase in LT4 dosage, whereas women with AITD typically need a smaller increase in dosage [53].

19.6 Summary

To date, much is known about thyroid and maternal physiology and how they interplay during the course of the gestation. However, the physiologic changes of pregnancy can not only make the diagnosis of maternal thyroid disease difficult, but make appropriate pharmacotherapy more challenging as well. Adequate treatment of hyperthyroidism and hypothyroidism is necessary not only to treat the mother but also to allow for normal fetal neurodevelopment. Management of hyperthyroidism in pregnancy can be maximized by limiting the adverse outcomes associated with thionamides by applying a trimester-specific ATD strategy; PTU in the first trimester followed by MMI beginning in the second trimester and continued postpartum. When considering hypothyroidism, early initiation of treatment for overt disease is key. There is still continued debate on whether treatment of subclinical hypothyroidism is beneficial for the fetus. ACOG recommendation is for no treatment, while ATA guidelines recommend treatment in certain scenarios. More research into the benefits of treatment is warranted in order to establish a more robust recommendation on the treatment of subclinical hypothyroidism in obstetrical patients.

References

[1] Spitzer TLB. What the obstetrician/gynecologist should know about thyroid disorders. Obstet Gynecol Surv 2011;65:779−85.

[2] Kung AWC, Chau MT, Lao TT, Tam SC, Low LC. The effect of pregnancy on thyroid nodule formation. J Clin Endocrinol Metab 2002;87:1010–4.

[3] Davies TF, Cobin R. Thyroid disease in pregnancy and the postpartum period. Mt Sinai J Med 1985;52:59–77.

[4] Fister P, et al. Thyroid volume changes during pregnancy and after delivery in an iodine-sufficient republic of Slovenia. Euro J Obstetr Gynecol Reproduct Biol 2009;145(1): 45–8. https://doi.org/10.1016/j.ejogrb.2009.03.022.

[5] Ferris TF. Renal disease. In: Burrow GN, Ferris TF, editors. Medical complications during pregnancy. Philadelphia: WB Saunders; 1988.

[6] Burrow GN, Fischer DA, Larsen PR. Maternal and fetal thyroid function. N Engl J Med 1994;331:1072–8.

[7] Wang KW, Sum CF. Management of thyroid disease in pregnancy. Singap Med J 1989; 30:476–8.

[8] Poppe K, Velkeniers B, Glinoer D. Thyroid disease and female reproduction. Clin Endocrinol 2007;66:309–21.

[9] American college of Obstetricians and Gynecologists. ACOG practice bulletin on thyroid disease in pregnancy. Am Fam Phys 2002;65(10). pp. 2158, 2161–2162.

[10] American Thyroid Association. American Thyroid Association (ATA) issues statement on the potential risks of excess iodine ingestion and exposure. American Thyroid Association; 2013. https://www.thyroid.org/american-thyroid-association-ata-issues-statement-on-the-potential-risks-of-excess-iodine-ingestion-and-exposure/.

[11] Alexander EK, et al. 2017 guidelines of the American Thyroid Association for the diagnosis and management of thyroid disease during pregnancy and the postpartum. Thyroid 2017;27(3):315–89. https://doi.org/10.1089/thy.2016.0457.

[12] Neale D, Burrow G. Thyroid disease in pregnancy. Obstet Gynecol Clin 2004;31: 893–905.

[13] Glinoer D. What happens to the normal thyroid during pregnancy? Thyroid 1999;9: 631–5.

[14] Lazarus JH. Thyroid function in pregnancy. Br Med Bull 2011;97:137–48.

[15] Glinoer D, De Nayer P, Robyn C, Lejeune B, Kinthaert J, Meuris S. Serum levels of intact human chorionic gonadotropin (HCG) and its free alpha and beta subunits, in relation to maternal thyroid stimulation during normal pregnancy. J Endocrinol Invest 1993;16:881–8.

[16] Nguyen CT, et al. Graves' hyperthyroidism in pregnancy: a clinical review. Clin Diab Endocrinol 2018;4(1). https://doi.org/10.1186/s40842-018-0054-7.

[17] Goldman AM, Mestman JH. Transient non-autoimmune hyperthyroidism of early pregnancy. J Thyroid Res 2011;2011. https://doi.org/10.4061/2011/142413.

[18] Ain KB, Mori Y, Refetoff S. Reduced clearance of thyroxine-binding globulin (TBG) with increased sialylation: a mechanism for estrogen-induced elevation of serum TBG concentration. J Clin Endocrinol Metab 1987;65:689–96.

[19] Korevaar TIM, et al. Thyroid disease in pregnancy: new insights in diagnosis and clinical management. Nat Rev Endocrinol 2017;13(10):610–22. https://doi.org/10.1038/nrendo.2017.93.

[20] Demers LM. Thyroid disease: pathophysiology and diagnosis. Clin Lab Med 2004;24: 19–28.

[21] Seth J, Beckett G. Diagnosis of hyperthyroidism: the newer biochemical tests. Clin Endocrinol Metabol 1985;14:373–96.

[22] Pearce EN. Thyroid disorders during pregnancy and postpartum. Best Pract Res Clin Obstet Gynaecol 2015. https://doi.org/10.1016/j.bpobgyn.2015.04.007.

[23] Sack J. Thyroid function in pregnancy—maternal—fetal relationship in health and disease. Pediatr Endocrinol Rev 2003;1:170—6.

[24] Lazarus JH. Thyroid disorders associated with pregnancy. Treat Endocrinol 2005;4: 31—41.

[25] Nader S. Thyroid disease and other endocrine disorders in pregnancy. Obstet Gynecol Clin N Am 2004;31:257—85.

[26] Mandel SJ, Cooper DS. The use of antithyroid drugs in pregnancy and lacta- tion. J Clin Endocrinol Metab 2001;86(6):2354—9.

[27] Marx H, Amin P, Lazarus JH. Hyperthyroidism and pregnancy. BMJ 2008;22:663—7.

[28] Kamath C, et al. "The role of thyrotrophin receptor antibody assays in Graves' disease. J Thyroid Res 2012;2012. https://doi.org/10.1155/2012/525936.

[29] Michalek M, Krzysztof, et al. TSH receptor autoantibodies. Autoimmun Rev 2009;9(2): 113—6. https://doi.org/10.1016/j.autrev.2009.03.012.

[30] Chen YT, Khoo DHC. Thyroid disease in pregnancy. Ann Acad Med Singapore 2002; 31:296—302.

[31] McGregor AM, Hall R, Richards C. Autoimmune thyroid disease and pregnancy. Br Med J 1984;288:1780—1.

[32] Abeillon-Du Payrat J, et al. Predictive value of maternal second-generation thyroid-binding inhibitory immunoglobulin assay for neonatal autoimmune hyperthyroidism. Eur J Endocrinol 2014;171(4):451—60. https://doi.org/10.1530/EJE-14-0254.

[33] Goodwin TM, Montoro M, Mestman JH. Transient hyperthyroidism and hyperemesis gravidarum: clinical aspects. Am J Obstet Gynecol 1992;167:648—52.

[34] Momotani N, Ito K, Hamada N, Ban Y, Nishikawa Y, Mimura T. Maternal hyperthyroid-ism and congenital malformation in the offspring. Clin Endocrinol 1984;21:81—7.

[35] Mestman JH. Hyperthyroidism in pregnancy. Clin Obstet Gynecol 1997;40:45—64.

[36] McKenzie JM, Zakarija M. Fetal and neonatal hyperthyroidism and hypo- thyroidism due to maternal TSH receptor antibodies. Thyroid 1992;2(2):155—9.

[37] Weetman AP. Graves' disease. N Engl J Med 2000;343:1236—48.

[38] Cooper DS. Antithyroid drugs. N Engl J Med 2005;352(9):905—17.

[39] Di Gianantonio E, Schaeffer C, Mastroiacovo PP, Counot MP, Benedicenti F, Reuvers M, et al. Adverse effects of prenatal methimazole exposure. Teratology 2001;64:262—6.

[40] Takaya K, et al. Antithyroid arthritis syndrome: a case report and review of the literature. Intern Med 2016;55(24):3627—33. https://doi.org/10.2169/internalmedicine.55.7379.

[41] Azizi F, Amouzegar A. Management of hyperthyroidism during pregnancy and lactation. Eur J Endocrinol 2011;164:871—6.

[42] Mestman J. Hyperthyroidism in pregnancy. Baillieres Best Pract Res Clin Endocrinol Metab 2004;18(2):267—88.

[43] Farwell AP, Braverman LE. Thyroid and antithyroid drugs. In: Hardman JG, Limbird LE, editors. Goodman and gilman's the pharmacological basis of therapeutics. 10th ed. New York: McGraw-Hill; 2001. p. 1563—96.

[44] Wing DA, Millar LK, Koonings PP, Montoro MN, Mestman JH. A comparison of pro-pylthiouracil versus methimazole in the treatment of hyperthyroidism in pregnancy. Am J Obstet Gynecol 1994;170(1):90—5.

[45] Mestman JH. Hyperthyroidism in pregnancy. Endocrinol Metab Clin N Am 1998;27: 127—49.

[46] Momotani N, Noh JY, Ishikawa N, Ito K. Effects of propylthiouracil and methimazole on fetal thyroid status in mothers with Graves' hyperthyroidism. J Clin Endocrinol Metab 1997;82(11):3633−6.

[47] Lao TT. Thyroid disorders in pregnancy. Curr Opin Obstet Gynecol 2005;17:123−7.

[48] Cooper DS. The side effects of antithyroid drugs. Endocrinologist 1999;9:457−76.

[49] Jansson R, Dahlbeg PA, Winsa B. The postpartum period constitutes an important risk for development of clinical Graves' disease in young women. Acta Endocrinol 1987; 116:321−5.

[50] Cooper DS. Which anti-thyroid drug. Am J Med 1986;80:1165−8.

[51] Meyer-Gessner M, Benker G, Lederbogen S, Olbricht T, Reinwein D. Antithyroid drug-induced agranulocytosis: clinical experience with ten patients treated at one institution and review of the literature. J Endocrinol Invest 1994;17(1):29−36.

[52] Tajiri J, Noguchi S. Antithyroid drug-induced agranulocytosis: special reference to normal white blood cell count agranulocytosis. Thyroid 2004;14:459−62.

[53] Glinoer D. Management of hypo- and hyperthyroidism during pregnancy. Growth Hormone IGF Res 2003;13:S45−54.

[54] Weetman AP, McGregor AM. Autoimmune thyroid disease: further developments in our understanding. Endocr Rev 1994;15:788−830.

[55] Mandel SJ. Hypothyroidism and chronic autoimmune thyroiditis in the pregnant state: maternal aspects. Best Pract Res Clin Endocrinol Metabol 2004;18:213−4.

[56] Brown RS, Bellisario RL, Botero D, Fournier L, Abrams CA, Cowger ML, et al. Incidence of transient congenital hypothyroidism due to maternal thyrotropin receptor blocking antibodies in over one million babies. J Clin Endocrinol Metab 1996;81: 1147−51.

[57] Matsuura N, Konishi J, Harada S, Yuri K, Fujieda K, Kasagi K, et al. The prediction of thyroid function in infants born to mothers with thyroiditis. Endocrinol Jpn 1989;36: 865−71.

[58] Klein RZ, Haddow JE, Faixt JD, Brown RS, Hermos RJ, Pulkkinen A, et al. Prevalence of thyroid deficiency in pregnant women. Clin Endocrinol 1991;35:41−6.

[59] Glinoer D. The systematic screening and management of hypothyroidism and hyperthyroidism in pregnancy. Trends Endocrinol Metab 1998;9:403−11.

[60] Glinoer D, Rihai M, Grun JP, Kinthaert J. Risk of subclinical hypothyroidism in pregnant women with autoimmune thyroid disorders. J Clin Endocrinol Metab 1994;79: 197−204.

[61] Wasserstrum N, Anania CA. Perinatal consequences of maternal hypothyroidism in early pregnancy and inadequate replacement. Clin Endocrinol 1995;42:353−8.

[62] Haddow JE, Palomaki GE, Allan WC, Williams JR, Knight GJ, Gagnon J, et al. Maternal thyroid deficiency during pregnancy and subsequent neuropsychological development of the child. N Engl J Med 1999;341:549−55.

[63] Yamamoto Y, Jennifer M, et al. Impact of levothyroxine therapy on obstetric, neonatal and childhood outcomes in women with subclinical hypothyroidism diagnosed in pregnancy: a systematic review and meta-analysis of randomised controlled trials. BMJ Open 2018;8(9):e022837. https://doi.org/10.1136/bmjopen-2018-022837.

[64] Casey BM, et al. Treatment of subclinical hypothyroidism or hypothyroxinemia in pregnancy. N Engl J Med 2017;376(9):815−25. https://doi.org/10.1056/NEJMoa1606205.

[65] Dhillon-Smith RK, et al. Levothyroxine in women with thyroid peroxidase antibodies before conception. N Engl J Med 2019;380(14):1316−25. https://doi.org/10.1056/NEJMoa1812537.

[66] Vulsma T, Gons MH, de Vijlder JJM. Maternal—fetal transfer of thyroxine in congenital hypothyroidism due to a total organification defect in thyroid agenesis. N Engl J Med 1989;321:13—6.

[67] Aboul-Khair SA, Crooks J, Turnball AC, Hytten FE. The physiological changes in thyroid function during pregnancy. Clin Sci 1964;27:195—207.

[68] Fisher DA. Maternal—fetal thyroid function in pregnancy. Clin Perinatol 1983;10: 615—26.

[69] Okosieme O, Marx H, Lazarus JH. Medical management of thyroid dysfunction in pregnancy and the postpartum. Expet Opin Pharmacother 2008;9:2281—93.

[70] Redmond GP. Thyroid dysfunction and women's reproductive health. Thyroid 2004; 14(Suppl. 1):S5—15.

[71] Idris I, Srinivasan R, Simm A, Page RC. Maternal hypothyroidism in early and late gestation: effects on neonatal and obstetric outcome. Clin Endocrinol 2005;63:560—5.

[72] Gartner R. Thyroid diseases in pregnancy. Curr Opin Obstet Gynecol 2009;21:501—7.

[73] Prummel MF, Wiersinga WM. Thyroid autoimmunity and miscarriage. Eur J Endocrinol 2004;150:751—5.

[74] Glinoer D. Editorial: miscarriage in women with positive anti-TPO antibodies: is thyroxine the answer? J Endocrinol Metab 2006;91:2500—1.

[75] Mandel SJ, Brent GA, Larsen PR. Levothyroxine therapy in patients with thyroid disease. Ann Intern Med 1993;119:492—502.

[76] Bach-Huynh TG, Jonklaas J. Thyroid medications in pregnancy. Ther Drug Monit 2006; 28:431—41.

[77] Okosieme OE, et al. Preconception management of thyroid dysfunction. Clin Endocrinol 2018;89(3):269—79. https://doi.org/10.1111/cen.13731.

[78] Colucci P, et al. A review of the pharmacokinetics of levothyroxine for the treatment of hypothyroidism. Eur Endocrinol 2010;9(1):40. https://doi.org/10.17925/ EE.2013.09.01.40.

[79] Shah MS, Davies TF, Stagnaro-Green A. The thyroid during pregnancy: a physiological and pathological stress test. Minerva Endocrinol 2003;28:233—45.

[80] Alexander EK, Marqusee E, Lawrence J, Jarolim P, Fischer GA, Larsen PR. Timing and magnitude of increases in levothyroxine requirements during preg- nancy in women with hypothyroidism. N Engl J Med 2004;351:241—9.

[81] Frantz CR, Dagogo-Jack S, Ladenson JH, Gronowski AM. Thyroid function during pregnancy. Clin Chem 1999;45:2250—8.

[82] Mestman J, Goodwin TM, Montoro MM. Thyroid disorders of pregnancy. Endocrinol Metab Clin N Am 1995;24:41—71.

[83] Glinoer D. The regulation of thyroid function in pregnancy: pathways of endocrine adaptation from physiology to pathology. Endocr Rev 1997;18:404—33.

[84] Kaplan MM. Management of thyroxine therapy during pregnancy. Endocr Pract 1996;2: 281—6.

Further reading

[1] ACOG Practice Bulletin No. 37. Thyroid disease in pregnancy. Int J Gynaecol Obstet 2002;79(2):171—80.

[2] Gardner DF, Cruishank DP, Hays PM, Cooper DS. Pharmacology of propylthiouracil (PTU) in pregnant hyperthyroid women: correlation of maternal PTU concentrations with cord serum thyroid function tests. J Clin Endocrinol Metab 1986;62(1):217—20.

[3] Mortimer RH, Cannell GR, Addison RS, Johnson LP, Roberts MS, Bernus I. Methimazole and propylthiouracil equally cross the perfused human term placental lobule. J Clin Endocrinol Metab 1997;82(9):3099—102.

[4] Chen C-H, Xirasagar S, Lin C-C, Wang L-H, Kou YR, Lin H-C. Risk of adverse perinatal outcomes with antithyroid treatment during pregnancy: a nationwide population-based study. BJOG 2011;118:1365—73.

[5] Pop VJ, de Vries E, van Baar AL, Waelkens JJ, de Rooy HA, Horsten M, et al. Maternal thyroid peroxidase antibodies during pregnancy a marker of impaired child development. J Clin Endocrinol Metab 1995;80:3561—6.

[6] Pop VJ, Kuijpens JL, van Baar AL, Verkerk G, van Son MM, de Vijlder JJ, et al. Low maternal free thyroxine concentrations during early pregnancy are associated with impaired psychomotor development in early infancy. Clin Endocrinol 1999;50:149—55.

[7] Andersen S, Bruun NH, Pedersen KM, Laurberg P. Biologic variation is important for interpretation of thyroid function tests. Thyroid 2003;13:1069—78.

[8] Pop VJ, Brouwers EP, Vader HL, Vulsma T, van Baar AL, de Vijlder JJ. Maternal hypothyroxinemia during early pregnancy and subsequent child development: a 3-year follow-up study. Clin Endocrinol 2003;59:282—8.

[9] Casey BM, Dashe JS, Wells CE, McIntire DD, Byrd W, Leveno KJ, et al. Subclinical hypothyroidism and pregnancy outcomes. Obstet Gynecol 2005;105:239—45.

[10] ACOG Committee Opinion No. 381. Subclinical hypothyroidism in pregnancy. Obstet Gynecol 2007;110:959—60.

[11] Maraka S, et al. Thyroid hormone treatment among pregnant women with subclinical hypothyroidism: US national assessment. BMJ 2017;356. https://doi.org/10.1136/bmj.i6865.

Management of dermatological conditions in pregnancy

20

Carmen V. Harrison

School of Nursing, Simmons University, Boston, MA, United States

20.1 Introduction

Every system in the body undergoes drastic changes during pregnancy, including the integumentary system. These dermatological changes are a result of varying factors, such as alterations in collagen formation, increase in sebaceous and eccrine gland secretion, shifts in hormone production, and increased circulatory blood volume [1]. This can lead to the development of new or worsening of current dermatological conditions during pregnancy. While these conditions are oftentimes minor and resolve after pregnancy, some can be of significant concern for the woman during the antepartum period [1]. This may prompt the pregnant woman to seek treatment from the health care provider, who will need to utilize sound clinical judgment on how to safely manage dermatological conditions during pregnancy and the postpartum period. Overall, management can be addressed with one of four approaches: (1) delay treatment until after pregnancy; (2) consider nonpharmacologic alternatives; (3) judiciously prescribe medications; or (4) discontinue breastfeeding during the postpartum period and prescribe accordingly.

Even when considering one of the before mentioned approaches, the clinical decision regarding medication use during pregnancy is hazed by the paucity of randomized clinical trials that include pregnant women. Furthermore, the new Federal Drug Administration (FDA) Pregnancy Category that replaced the previous A, B, C, D, and X system in 2015 has been faced with criticism for being confusing when it comes to interpreting medication safety and fetal risk assessment [2]. This is especially alarming since findings from a large, prospective cohort study of nulliparous women suggested that more than 90% of the study participants took at least one medication while pregnant [3]. Therefore, it is imperative that guidance be provided to health care providers with regards to the practice of prescribing medications to patients who are pregnant or breastfeeding. The choice to take medications should be a joint decision between the patient and health care provider [4].

The purpose of this chapter is to provide direction for health care providers who are faced with the dilemma of prescribing medications for managing dermatological conditions for patients during the antepartum and postpartum periods. Although a plethora of conditions impacting the integumentary system during pregnancy exists, this chapter will focus on managing the most common alterations. These include acne, psoriasis, dermatoses, bacterial infections, viral infections, fungal infections, and parasitic infections. When describing medication safety risk for the pregnant patient, the FDA categorical method will be utilized.

20.2 Acne

Acne is a common dermatological condition that can vary from mild comedones to severe inflammation and scarring [5]. The pregnancy state can exacerbate clinical manifestations of acne. The basis for deciding to treat acne during pregnancy and the postpartum period is based on the severity of the condition. However, prescribing medications for acne can be perplexing since there are a limited number of safe pharmacologic choices available for patients who are pregnant or breastfeeding [5].

20.2.1 Topical agents

Because of their low systemic absorption, topical medications should be the initial line of treatment when managing mild to moderate acne during pregnancy and lactation. Meredith and Ormerod [5] described several considerations that should be taken into account with the use of topical agents, such as the "amount of agent applied; surface area of application; length of application time; frequency of application; application to broken skin/erosions; choice of vehicle used; and thickness of stratum corneum" (p. 353).

Although antibacterial agents, such as erythromycin (category B) 1%−3% in petroleum jelly once daily, clindamycin (B) 1% once daily, and metronidazole (category B) 0.75%, may be prescribed, monotherapy with topical antibacterial medications is of concern due to the problem of antibiotic resistance [5]. Another concern exists regarding the use of topical metronidazole among pregnant women since animal studies have suggested a link between oral metronidazole and carcinogenicity with no adequate studies of pregnant women to support its use [6]. Therefore, topical metronidazole should be regarded as an alternative to topical erythromycin and clindamycin when treating acne in pregnancy. Topical metronidazole should be avoided altogether for lactating women due to its secretion in breast milk, having comparable concentration levels to plasma levels with oral use [6]. Limited data exist regarding the use of topical dapsone (category C) and nadifloxacin (category N) by pregnant and lactating women.

Comedolytics, such as azelaic acid (category B) and benzoyl peroxide 2.5% (category C), are considered safe in pregnancy and lactation due to their low systemic absorption. In fact, findings from a study estimated that the systemic absorption of topical benzoyl peroxide is approximately 5% [7]. Topical benzoyl peroxide is also a popular pharmacologic agent in managing acne because it possesses some antiinflammatory properties.

Another class of medications used to treat comedones of mild to moderate acne is topical retinoids, such as tretinoin (category C), isotretinoin (category C), tazarotene (category X), and adapalene (category C). Tazarotene has been assigned an FDA category X; thereby, it is contraindicated in pregnancy. Conflicting reports exist regarding the safe use of topical retinoids among pregnant women. Several reports have suggested a correlation between topical tretinoin and congenital birth defects, such as cardiac anomalies, diaphragmatic hernia, and ear and limb malformations, in the neonates of women who used these agents during early pregnancy [8–11]. On the contrary, findings from a case control study did not suggest an increased risk for birth defects among infants exposed to topical tretinoin from maternal use [12]. Furthermore, findings from a prospective observational study comparing women who were exposed to topical retinoid in the first trimester of pregnancy to a control group of pregnant women indicated no statistically significant difference in neonatal birth defects among these two groups [13]. On the other hand, when assessing the safety of adapalene use in pregnancy, an association between this medication and anophthalmia has been suggested [14]. Even the manufacturers of topical retinoids caution their use in pregnancy.

Since data regarding the excretion levels of tazarotene into breast milk are unknown, it is not recommended for use by lactating women. Tretinoin and adapalene have low levels of systemic absorption. Therefore, they are regarded as being safe for use in women who are breastfeeding.

20.2.2 Oral agents

For women who have acne unresponsive to topical agents, oral medications may be considered. One category of medications used for systemic treatment is antibiotics. However, caution regarding antibiotic resistance holds true for oral antibiotics, as with topical antibiotic agents. With the exception of early pregnancy, erythromycin (category B) 400 mg every 8 h before meals is the oral antibiotic of choice in helping to manage acne. When prescribing erythromycin for this indication, it recommended that it be combined with a topical agent, if possible, to address concerns regarding antibiotic resistance [15]. Another concern pertains to the use of erythromycin estolate, which should not be used in pregnancy due to risks of maternal hepatotoxicity [16]. Azithromycin (category B) with varying dosing regimens may be another option, but there are less data supporting its safe use in pregnancy when compared to erythromycin [5]. Another choice may be amoxicillin (category B) 250–500 mg twice daily alone or in combination with another agent, although data support that its use in early pregnancy may increase the risk for oral clefts [17].

Trimethoprim (category C) use in early pregnancy has been associated with spontaneous abortions [18], fetal cardiovascular defects, oral clefts, and urinary tract anomalies in women who did not take a folic acid supplement [19]. Therefore, trimethoprim/sulfamethoxazole 160/800 mg twice a day should only be prescribed if other options are lacking and the benefits outweigh the risks. Moreover, sulfonamides can remain in the neonatal circulation in the first few days following birth if maternal ingestion of the drug takes place near term [20]. This can lead to the development of jaundice, hemolytic anemia, hyperbilirubinemia, and theoretically, kernicterus in the newborn. As a result, this drug should not be administered to pregnant women near the end of their pregnancies.

Tetracycline (category D) should be avoided altogether in pregnancy due to embryo and fetal toxicity, including staining of deciduous teeth and impaired skeletal development [20]. If fetal exposure to this medication takes place after the 20th week of pregnancy, the deciduous teeth become yellow and progressively darken because tetracycline binds to calcium orthophosphate, subsequently becoming actively deposited in teeth and bones [20]. The effects on the fetal skeletal bone are considered reversible, but it can retard growth of the fibula in premature infants [21]. Studies have also suggested its use in pregnancy can cause acute fatty metamorphosis of the liver in the pregnant woman [20].

Oral retinoids are a popular choice for managing acne in the nonpregnant patient. Due to its severe teratogenic effects, isotretinoin (category X) is contraindicated for use in pregnancy. Isotretinoin has been linked to fetal craniofacial, cardiac, central nervous system, and thymus and parathyroid gland malformations [22]. Manufacturers of the drug advise women to avoid pregnancy 1 month before, during, and 1 month after taking isotretinoin and that women must use two different forms of contraception during this time [23]. Prescribers of isotretinoin in the United States are required to participate in the iPledge [24] program, a computer-based risk management system designed to prevent use by pregnant women. Oral retinoids are not recommended for use during the lactating period.

20.3 Psoriasis

Psoriasis is an autoimmune disease characterized by thick, pruritic, scaly plaques on the skin. The increased estrogen levels that occur during pregnancy are thought to lead to an immune tolerant state, resulting in an improvement of these symptoms for many pregnant women [25]. Results of a study examining pregnant women with psoriasis found 55% demonstrated improvement, 21% had no change, and 23% experienced worsening of symptoms during pregnancy [25]. For pregnant women who do require treatment, pharmacologic management can be challenging for the prescriber.

20.3.1 Topical agents

In general, topical agents, such as moisturizers, calcipotriene (category C), and low-to-moderate-potency corticosteroids (category C), are the first line of treatment to manage localized psoriasis for pregnant and breastfeeding women [26]. A study assessing the outcomes of pregnant women exposed to topical corticosteroids found no increased risk of low birth weight infants, fetal anomalies, or preterm birth [27]. However, more potent topical corticosteroids applied to a large body surface area have similar effects as systemic oral preparations and should be used with caution by pregnant women [28]. Calcipotriene (category C), a synthetic derivative of vitamin D3, is considered a safe topical agent for use by pregnant women [29,30]. Another option is topical tacrolimus (category C), a calcineurin inhibitor that is primarily effective as a local agent in treating psoriasis in the facial or intertriginous areas [31]. Results of animal studies have indicated no reports of teratogenicity associated with topical tacrolimus [20]. Other topical agents, such as crude coal tar (category C) and tazarotene (category X), should not be used during pregnancy since teratogenic risks are seemingly unknown [26].

The second-line treatment option for managing psoriasis in pregnancy is both narrow and broadband ultraviolet B phototherapy, which can be used alone or in combination with topical agents [26]. Since penetration of the ultraviolet light is limited to the maternal skin, this is considered safe for the fetus and breastfeeding newborn [26]. However, decreased maternal folic acid levels have been associated with repeated exposure to broadband ultraviolet B with recommendations for folic acid monitoring by the prescriber [32]. Psoralen and ultraviolet A light should not be used in pregnancy due to associated mutagenic properties [33].

20.4 Oral agents

If psoriasis is persistent or worsens during pregnancy, systemic treatment may be warranted. Cyclosporine (category C) 2.5–5 mg/kg/day is considered the initial oral agent of choice [34]. The drug passively crosses the placental blood barrier resulting in 10%–50% of the maternal plasma concentration and lacks mutagenic or teratogenic properties [34]. Contrary to its acceptable use in pregnancy, oral cyclosporine should be avoided in lactating women since it possesses immunosuppressive characteristics, potentially impacting the breastfed newborn [35].

Oral corticosteroids, such as prednisone (category D), prednisolone (category D), or methylprednisolone (category C), are not used in the treatment of common psoriasis in pregnancy due to reports indicating an association with their use and gastroesophageal reflux, low birth weight, intrauterine growth restriction, and oral clefts among neonates exposed in utero [36–39]. Although a metaanalysis failed to find an increased risk for serious fetal anomalies, the authors raised concern with using oral corticosteroids during the first trimester of pregnancy [38]. These medications may be used by lactating women with a recommended 3–4 h interval from ingestion to a breastfeeding episode [26].

Mycophenolate mofetil (category D) has been associated with congenital anomalies and first trimester spontaneous abortion; thereby, should not be used by pregnant women or those attempting to conceive [40]. Similarly, methotrexate (category X) and acitretin (category X) should be avoided by pregnant and lactating women. Methotrexate is an abortifacient with mutagenic and teratogenic properties, such as anencephaly, cleft palate, and ear and skeletal malformations, and should not be used by women or men for 3 months prior to conception [34]. Due to storage in adipose tissue, stricter guidelines are used for acitretin by which pregnancy should be avoided up to 3 years after discontinuing treatment due to risks for severe fetal anomalies, such as craniofacial, ear, thymus, central nervous system, and cardiovascular system malformations [41].

Biologic agents, such as etanercept (category B), infliximab (category B), and adalimumab (category B), are becoming an increasingly popular choice in treating psoriasis. However, severely limited data on their use in pregnancy make prescribing to the pregnant and lactation populations somewhat perplexing. The majority of studies examining the administration of these medications to pregnant women are from their use in managing irritable bowel syndrome and rheumatoid arthritis [42]. One report indicated that newborns exposed to infliximab and adalimumab in utero had significantly higher concentrations of these drugs when compared to their mothers, with levels still detectable during the first 2–7 months of life [43]. While the placental transfer of etanercept to the fetus is much lower [44], there has been a case report of a neonate who developed VACTERL syndrome while exposed to etanercept in utero [45]. This condition, which causes vertebral anomalies, anal atresia, cardiac anomalies, tracheoesophageal fistula, esophageal atresia, renal anomalies, and limb anomalies, was also observed in animal studies involving etanercept [26]. Moreover, a study involving 41 women who took etanercept or infliximab while pregnant found 59% of their newborns displayed at least one clinical manifestation of VACTERL syndrome [46]. A case of partial VACTERL association was also reported in an infant whose mother took adalimumab while pregnant [47,48]. It is noteworthy that there have been no other reported anomalies in newborns exposed to etanercept in utero [48,49]. A comparison of women who took infliximab while pregnant also noted no increased risk of fetal or neonatal anomalies [50]. The potential for immunosuppression in the newborn exposed to biologic agents is also of concern, especially after an infant who was exposed to infliximab in utero died from disseminated bacillus Calmette-Guerin infection after being vaccinated [51].

Due to the low levels of etanercept and infliximab in breast milk, evidence supports their safe use by breastfeeding women [52]. Although evidence seemingly supports the use of these biologic agents in pregnant and nursing women, due to the lack of long-term and rigorous studies, it makes arriving at a definitive conclusion regarding their safe use difficult to determine. Further lacking are empirical data on the use of newer biologic agents, such as ustekinumab, secukinumab, and ixekizumab, with pregnant and lactating women [42].

20.5 Dermatoses

Dermatologic conditions that only occur in pregnancy and the immediate post-partum period are referred to as dermatoses of pregnancy. In 2006, these conditions were reclassified by Ambros-Rudolph, Mullegger, Vaughan-Jones, Kerl, and Black to include four conditions: (1) pemphigoid gestationis (PG); (2) polymorphic eruption of pregnancy (PEP); (3) intrahepatic cholestasis of pregnancy (ICP); and (4) atopic eruption of pregnancy (AEP) [53]. While there are vast differences among these conditions, the underlying commonality is the intense pruritus associated with these dermatoses. Therefore, the hallmark treatment includes the use of antihistamines since they are considered the first line of treatment in managing pruritus associated with dermatological conditions during pregnancy [54].

Systemic antihistamines are classified as first generation and second generation, with the primary difference being that first-generation antihistamines, such as chlorpheniramine (category B), diphenhydramine (category B), dexchlorpheniramine (category B), and hydroxyzine (category C), have sedating effects, while second-generation antihistamines, such as loratadine (category B), cetirizine (category B), fexofenadine (category C), and azelastine (category C), do not [54]. This impact on the central nervous system should be taken into consideration by prescribers since it may pose a safety risk and interfere with the patient's quality of life by producing long-lasting sedative effects associated with first-generation oral antihistamines [55]. Even so, when prescribing a first-generation oral antihistamine, the prescriber should educate the patient to take this medication prior to sleeping.

However, more empirical data exist assessing the use of first-generation antihistamines, likely because they have been used longer when compared to newer, second-generation antihistamines. A metaanalysis of 24 studies with more than 200,000 pregnant women who took an oral first-generation antihistamine during the first trimester of their pregnancies discovered no increased fetal or maternal risk [56]. Moreover, this result was corroborated by the findings of several studies [57–59]. Nonetheless, because oral diphenhydramine has been associated with retinopathy of prematurity, formerly known as retrolental fibroplasia, it should be avoided during the last 2 weeks of pregnancy [20]. It should also not be used during this time frame because it may cause withdrawal symptoms, such as irritability and difficulty feeding, in newborns exposed to this medication in utero [60]. Additionally, high doses of diphenhydramine can cause uterine contractions, resulting in premature births [60]. Another first-generation antihistamine, hydroxyzine, should not be taken in the first trimester of pregnancy due to its association with fetal anomalies [60].

First-generation systemic antihistamines are not recommended for use by lactating women primarily due to the lack of supporting evidence [20]. It is recognized that these drugs may lead to drowsiness and lethargy in the breast-fed newborn [60]. It has also been proposed that first-generation oral antihistamines may cause decreased maternal milk production due to their impact on dopamine secretion [60].

With regards to second-generation antihistamines, systemic loratadine and cetirizine are considered safe during the second and third trimesters of pregnancy and lactation [60]. Initial concerns regarding the risk of hypospadias in newborns exposed to maternal oral use of loratadine in utero were refuted by the Centers for Disease Control and Prevention after assessing data from the National Birth Defects Prevention Study [61]. As with first-generation antihistamines, these second-generation medications should not be taken in large doses near the time of delivery [60].

20.5.1 Pemphigoid gestationis

PG is a rare, autoimmune condition that is most commonly seen late in pregnancy [53]. Although classic clinical manifestations of this condition are blister-like lesions, resembling the herpes simplex virus (HSV), it is not related to HSV [53]. Instead, these pruritic lesions typically start on the umbilical area and then spread to the trunk and extremities. PG is of concern because it can pose adverse effects to the fetus, leading to premature birth and low birth weight [62]. Management during pregnancy is aimed at relieving the associated itching and inflammation with the use of oral antihistamines, such as diphenhydramine (category B) or hydroxyzine (category C) 25−50 mg at night or topical corticosteroids, such as hydrocortisone acetate 1% (category C) for mild cases [62]. Severe conditions may require the administration of oral corticosteroids, weighing the risks and benefits of such use, as well as considering the dose and duration. There have been reports of rare cases of PG unresponsive to the before mentioned treatments that resolved with the administration of cyclosporine [63,64].

20.5.2 Polymorphic eruption of pregnancy

PEP was formerly referred to as pruritic urticarial papules and plaques of pregnancy [53]. Classic symptoms of PEP are intense pruritus and inflammation that begins within the abdominal striae. A report suggested that an estimated 1 in 160 pregnant women develop this condition, which most commonly occurs in the third trimester of pregnancy and immediate postpartum period [65]. Although this condition is self-limiting, relief of the pruritus and inflammation may be achieved with oral antihistamines, such as diphenhydramine (category B) or hydroxyzine (category C) 25−50 mg at night or topical corticosteroids, such as hydrocortisone acetate 1% (category C).

20.5.3 Intrahepatic cholestasis of pregnancy

Formerly known as pruritus gravidarum, ICP is a disorder of the liver that leads to an alteration in the excretion of bile salts that deposit on the skin, causing pruritus [53]. Most pregnant women with ICP initially report itching on the soles of the feet and palms of the hands that then spreads to the abdomen, back, and face [62]. Increased serum bile acid concentrations are also commonly observed [62]. There have been reports of preterm birth, fetal distress, and intrauterine fetal demise thought to be related to ICP [65]. Typically, oral antihistamines, such as diphenhydramine (category B) or hydroxyzine (category C) 25−50 mg at night, are used to effectively manage the pruritus. In severe cases, ursodeoxycholic acid (category B) 500 mg twice daily or 300 mg three times a day, with a maximum dose of 15−20 mg/kg/day may be prescribed to relieve pruritus, decrease total bile acid, help normalize liver function levels, and assist in achieving optimal pregnancy outcomes [66]. A metaanalysis of solely randomized control trials was conducted in an attempt to meticulously analyze the effects and safe use of ursodeoxycholic acid in patients diagnosed with ICP [67]. Findings suggested that not only is ursodeoxycholic acid effective in helping to alleviate pruritus and improve liver function in patients with ICP, it also serves to protect the overall health and well-being of the pregnant woman and fetus [67].

20.5.4 **Atopic eruption of pregnancy**

AEP includes eczema, prurigo, and pruritic folliculitis [53]. This is reportedly the most common dermatosis of pregnancy and can present any time during gestation [65]. Classic symptoms of AEP include intensely pruritic skin eruptions on the face, neck, chest, trunk, and extremities [62]. Oatmeal baths and emollients may provide some relief [62]. Topical antipruritics, such as 1% menthol in aqueous cream (category N), calamine in aqueous cream (category N), hydrocortisone acetate 1% (category C), and oral diphenhydramine (category B) or hydroxyzine (category C) 25–50 mg at night, may also be used [62]. In some cases, ultraviolet B phototherapy can help to relieve the associated symptoms and rarely will a short course of oral corticosteroids be needed, assessing the risks and benefits of their use [65].

20.6 **Bacterial infections**
20.6.1 **Topical agents**

Selecting a topical agent over an oral agent to treat a bacterial dermatological condition is primarily based on the severity of the condition, with an oral agent being the first choice for a widespread infection. The recommendations for administering topical antibacterial agents to pregnant women follow many of the same principles as oral agents. Topical erythromycin (category B) is considered the first-line option for this route of administration in a short term dose of 0.5–2 g in petroleum jelly of 50–100 mg daily. Other options include bacitracin (category C), although data on use by pregnant women are limited, or mupirocin (category C). According to the manufacturer of mupirocin, findings of reproduction studies on rats and rabbits indicated no fetal toxicity [68]. The concern for the development of bacterial resistance should be taken into account when prescribing a topical antibacterial agent.

20.6.2 **Oral agents**

Options for prescribing an oral antibiotic to treat bacterial skin infections in pregnancy include erythromycin (category B), penicillins (category B), cephalosporins (category B), and azithromycin (category B). Erythromycin should not be used in early pregnancy and erythromycin estolate should not be used at all during pregnancy [16]. First-line treatment consists of erythromycin 400 mg every 8 h or a penicillin, such as ampicillin 250–500 mg every 6 h or amoxicillin 250–500 mg every 8 h or 500–875 mg every 12 h, depending on the type and severity of the infection being treated. As previously mentioned (see Section 20.2), amoxicillin should not be prescribed to women early in their pregnancies due to the potential risk of oral cleft development [17]. Penicillin G is commonly prescribed to pregnant women to treat a variety of conditions [20]. Intramuscular (IM) or intravenous (IV) penicillin G may be prescribed in varying doses of 1,200,000–6,000,000 UI/day every 4–6 h to treat bacteria causing dermatologic conditions in pregnancy. Both erythromycin and penicillin are safe for use by lactating women [20].

Cephalosporins, such as cephalexin 500 mg every 6–12 h or cefaclor 250–500 mg every 8 h, may also be prescribed. If the IM or IV route is preferred, ceftriaxone 1–2 g may be administered to pregnant women with relative safety. Findings from most studies involving pregnant women who took a cephalosporin support its safe use. However, results of a Michigan Medicaid surveillance study suggested some association between cephalosporins taken early in pregnancy to congenital anomalies [20]. Recommendations are to postpone prescribing cephalosporins to pregnant women until after the first trimester. If the first-line treatment cannot be prescribed, another substitute is azithromycin 250–500 mg daily.

Due to the variety of safer options, clarithromycin (category C) or dirithromycin (category C) should not be prescribed to pregnant women. Because of the risk for damage to the tendons, muscles, joints, nerves, and central nervous system of the fetus, maternal use of fluoroquinolones, such as ciprofloxacin (category C), norfloxacin (category C), or levofloxacin (category C), should also be avoided [20]. The risks of fetal and maternal exposure to tetracycline (category D) have been previously discussed (see Section 20.2). As with other conditions, the clinical use of tetracycline to treat bacterial skin infections in pregnant women should not be implemented. Sulfonamides also hold the same prescribing recommendations, as previously described (see Section 20.2).

20.7 Viral infections

20.7.1 Topical agents

Chemical or ablative methods for treating viral infections in pregnancy may be considered a safer option when compared to pharmacologic agents. With regards to human papilloma virus (HPV), cryotherapy or electrodesiccation can be used to treat genital warts associated with the virus. The provider may also apply a solution of 80%–90% of trichloracetic acid or bichloracetic acid to small genital warts. Imiquimod (category B) cream in strengths of 3.75% every night or 5% nightly three times a week for up to 16 weeks is a patient-applied agent that may be used in nonpregnant individuals. Limited human data of use by pregnant women exist, but because of this paucity of evidence, imiquimod is not recommended for use by this population. It is considered compatible with breastfeeding [20]. Due to the risk of toxicity, patient-applied podofilox (podophyllotoxin) (category C) or provider-applied podophyllin resin (category X) should not be used by lactating or pregnant women [20].

20.7.2 Oral agents

For pregnant and lactating women, who develop a viral infection, such as the HSV, acyclovir (category B) is considered first-line management with a regimen of 200 mg every 4 hours (maximum 1 g per day). Other antivirals, such as famciclovir (category B) and valacyclovir (category B), should be reserved as alternative options. A large retrospective cohort study of pregnant women in Denmark, who took an antiviral during pregnancy, was analyzed with results revealing no significant increase in congenital anomalies among the newborns exposed to acyclovir, famciclovir, or valacyclovir in utero [69]. However, because more women used acyclovir than the other two antivirals, the researchers support the use of acyclovir as the first line treatment [69]. Another viral infection to consider is HPV. A retrospective cohort study of women who received a quadrivalent HPV vaccination during pregnancy analyzed pregnancy outcomes, such as spontaneous abortion, stillbirth, major congenital anomaly, small for gestational age, low birth weight, and preterm birth with results suggesting no significant increase in these adverse outcomes among the women who were vaccinated during pregnancy [70]. Nonetheless, due to the limited data, current recommendations are to avoid the administration of an HPV vaccine to pregnant women.

20.8 Fungal infections

20.8.1 Topical agents

Due to miniscule percutaneous absorption, topical antifungals are considered a safer alternative than oral agents. However, they should not be used to treat large areas of fungal infected skin. First-line options for topical antifungal agents include varying doses of nystatin (category C) twice daily, clotrimazole (category B) twice daily, and miconazole (category C) twice daily. Numerous reports of pregnant women taking these medications to treat dermatological infections indicated no teratogenic or embryotoxic effects [20]. Even though human studies on their use during breastfeeding are lacking, they are seemingly safe for use by lactating women [20]. Other choices for topical antifungal agents include econazole (category C) 1−2 times daily and bifonazole (category C) daily.

20.8.2 Oral agents

Amphotericin B (category B) IV is regarded as the drug of choice for pregnant women with severe, widespread fungal skin infections [20,71]. There have been no reports of harm to the embryo or fetus when exposed in utero [20]. Although data are limited regarding the use of amphotericin B by women who are breastfeeding, it is presumed safe during this period [20]. Due to the paucity of data investigating the use of oral terbinafine by pregnant women, the current recommendation is to delay treatment with this medication until after the pregnancy, if at all possible [20]. It is also recommended that terbinafine not be used by women who are breastfeeding for two primary reasons. First, there are limited data on the use of terbinafine by lactating women [20]. Secondly, the duration of treatment is typically 6−12 weeks, which would mean long-term exposure of the infant to this medication when consuming the maternal breast milk [20].

Although there are a variety of other antifungal oral agents that may be used to treat skin infections in nonpregnant individuals, such as griseofulvin (category C), ketoconazole (category C), fluconazole (category C), and itraconazole (category C), these medications are contraindicated during pregnancy. Findings from animal studies involving the use of griseofulvin resulted in the drug regarded as being tumorigenic, embryotoxic, and teratogenic [20]. A report published by the FDA described a potential correlation between griseofulvin taken in early pregnancy and two sets of conjoined twins [72]. Even though a subsequent report refuted this association [73], griseofulvin remains on the list of contraindicated medications for use by pregnant and lactating women due to the limited evidence supporting its use [20].

Teratogenic and embryotoxic effects leading to syndactyly and oligodactyly have been noted with high doses (80 mg/kg/day) of ketoconazole [20]. Reports have also suggested oral ketoconazole can lead to the inhibition of androgen synthesis, abnormal progesterone secretion, and sexual ambiguity in the male fetus [74]. Concerns also exist with high doses of fluconazole and itraconazole by pregnant women. Continuous oral doses of 400 mg daily or more of fluconazole taken by pregnant women during the first trimester are considered teratogenic, leading to fetal anomalies of the head, face, long bones, and heart [75]. Contrarily, small or short-term doses of fluconazole prescribed to the mother during the first trimester of pregnancy have indicated no adverse effects to the fetus [76−79]. Likewise, small, short-term doses of itraconazole of 50−800 mg taken during the first trimester yielded no fetal anomalies [80], while animal studies involving higher doses suggested different outcomes [20]. Reports of the use of fluconazole by lactating women suggested no risk to the newborn, but due to the lack of human studies on itraconazole, this medication cannot be considered nontoxic to the breastfeeding infant [20].

20.9 Parasitic infections

20.9.1 Topical agents

The first-line topical treatment of scabies for pregnant and lactating women is permethrin (category B) 5% cream thoroughly massaged into the skin from the neck to the feet, left on for 8−14 h, and then washed off the skin by bathing or showering. Typically, one application will suffice unless live mites remain after 7−14 days of the initial treatment. The recommended treatment for pregnant and lactating women with pediculosis is permethrin (category B) 1% lotion applied to clean, dry hair and scalp until fully saturated by paying attention to application behind the ears and nape of the neck, leaving on for 10 min, rinsing with water, and then combing out the nits and eggs. This may be repeated in 7 days if nits remain. Although human research is limited, existing human data and animal research indicate a lack of toxicity to the embryo or fetus [20]. Due to the small amount of systemic absorption and high rate of metabolism of permethrin, it is considered compatible with breastfeeding [20].

Alternative treatments of scabies for pregnant women include benzyl benzoate (category C) 25% lotion or malathion (category B) 0.5% lotion, though both are considered less effective when compared to permethrin 5% cream [20]. Benzyl benzoate is not commercially available in the United States or Canada because toxicities associated with its metabolite, benzyl alcohol, were thought to be related to neonatal fatalities of preterm infants when used in cleansing central vein catheters [81]. Reports regarding the use of benzyl benzoate by lactating women are lacking, but topical application of the drug is thought to be safe. Malathion is also considered safe for breastfeeding and pregnant women, though the aqueous solution should be used over the alcoholic-based solution [82]. When used to treat scabies, both benzyl benzoate and malathion should be applied to the skin, left on for 24 h, and then washed with soap and water. For severe cases, the process may need to be repeated in 7 days following the initial application. Benzyl benzoate may also be used to treat lice by thoroughly applying the lotion to clean, dry hair and the scalp, leaving on for 12−24 h, cleansing with shampoo and water, drying with a towel, and then using a comb to remove nits and eggs. This may be repeated in 7 days if infestation persists. The same process may be followed when using malathion lotion to treat pediculosis, although it is left on for 8−12 h.

Crotamiton (category C) 10% lotion may be considered an alternative treatment for managing scabies in pregnant women, but caution should be taken due to the lack of research supporting its safe use [83]. Ivermectin (category C) 0.5% topical lotion is available for the treatment of pediculosis and a 1% strength can be used as an alternative treatment of scabies, but this is not recommended for use by pregnant women due to the lack of supporting empirical evidence.

20.9.2 Oral agents

Both animal and human studies have investigated the use of oral ivermectin (category C) in pregnancy. Results of animal studies involving high doses of ivermectin indicated teratogenicity [20]. Although significant differences were not found in a study comparing the pregnancy outcomes of women exposed to ivermectin during pregnancy to those who were not exposed [84], oral ivermectin is not recommended for use by pregnant women to treat scabies or pediculosis. Due to low concentrations of ivermectin found in breast milk, the drug is regarded as being compatible with breastfeeding [20].

Oral mebendazole (category C) may be used by women after the first trimester of pregnancy and while breastfeeding to treat infections caused by *Ascaris lumbricoides* (roundworms), *Ancylostoma duodenale* (hookworms), *Enterobius vermicularis* (pinworms), and *Trichuris trichiura* (whipworms) [20]. Albendazole (category C) is categorized as a broad-spectrum anthelmintic that is contraindicated for use in the first trimester of pregnancy [85]. A report indicated no adverse pregnancy outcomes in 61 pregnant women who were exposed to oral albendazole in the second trimester of their pregnancies [86]. A study examining the use of albendazole by lactating women suggested low concentrations of the drug, labeling it as compatible with breastfeeding [87]. Thiabendazole (category C) is another anthelmintic but is considered contraindicated in pregnancy due to a lack of human studies [88].

20.10 Dermatological wounds

Pregnant women may experience dermatological wounds, requiring the use of local antiseptics or analgesics. Alcohol-based solutions, such as ethanol (category C) or isopropanol (category N), are considered first-line options when disinfecting a wound. Another option that may be used is topical chlorhexidine (category B). Agents that contain iodine, such as povidone-iodine 10% aqueous solution (category D), should not be used in pregnancy due to the risk for maternal skin absorption which can effect fetal thyroid function [89].

Lidocaine (category B) and EMLA (lidocaine 2.5% and prilocaine 2.5%) (category B) creams are regarded as safe agents for providing local analgesia for pregnant women [90]. Alternative options are mepivacaine (category C) or bupivacaine (category C). Although it is recommended that cosmetic procedures be delayed until after pregnancy, these local analgesics may provide pain relief for pregnant women undergoing excisions, skin biopsies, or wound care.

References

[1] Bartling SJ, Zito PM. Dermatologic changes in pregnancy. Int J Childbirth Educ 2016; 31(2):38—40.

[2] Pernia S, DeMaagd G. The new pregnancy and lactation labeling rule. Pharm Therapeut 2016;41(11):713—5.

[3] Haas DM, Marsh DJ, Dang DT, Parker CB, Wing DA, Simhan HN, et al. Prescription and other medication use in pregnancy. Obstetr Gynecol 2018;131(5):789—98. Available from: https://europepmc.org/articles/pmc5912972#R24.

[4] Lynch MM, Amoozegar JB, McClure EM, Squiers LB, Broussard CS, Lind JN, et al. Improving safe use of medications during pregnancy: the roles of patients, physicians, and pharmacists. Qual Health Res 2017;27(13):2071—80. https://doi.org/10.1177/1049732317732027.

[5] Meredith FM, Ormerod AD. The management of acne vulgaris in pregnancy. Am J Dermatol 2013;14(5):351—8. https://doi.org/10.1007/s40257-103-0041-9.

[6] Prasco. Our products. Metronidazole. 2019. Available from: http://www.prasco.com/our-products-desktop.html.

[7] Yeung NS, Beasley JN, Maibach HI. Benzoyl peroxide: percutaneous penetration and metabolic disposition. J Am Acad Dermatol 1981;4(1):31—7.

[8] Camera G, Pregliasco P. Ear malformation in baby born to mother using tretinoin cream. Lancet 1992;339(8794):687. https://doi.org/10.1016/0140-6736(92)90854-V.

[9] Lipson AH, Collins C, Webster W. Multiple congenital defects associated with maternal use of topical tretinoin. Lancet 1993;341(8856):1352—3. https://doi.org/10.1016/0140-6736(93)90868-H.

[10] Navarre-Belhassen C, Blanchet P, Hillaire-Buys D, Sarda P, Blayac JP. Multiple congenital malformations associated with topical tretinoin. Ann Pharmacother 1998; 32(4):505−6. https://doi.org/10.1345/aph.17138.

[11] Selcen D, Seidman S, Nigro MA. Otocerebral anomalies associated with topical tretinoin use. Brain Dev 2000;22(4):218−20. https://doi.org/10.1016/S0387-7604(00) 00104-2.

[12] Jick SS, Terris BZ, Jick H. First trimester topical tretinoin and congenital disorders. Lancet 1993;341(8854):1181−2. https://doi.org/10.1016/0140-6736(93)91004-6.

[13] Panchaud P, Csajka C, Merlob P, Schaefer C, Berlin M, De Santis M, Vial T, Ieri A, Malm H, Eleftheriou G, Stahl B, Rousso P, Winterfeld U, Rothuizen LE, Buclin T. Pregnancy outcome following exposure to topical retinoids: a multicenter prospective study. J Clin Pharmacol 2012;52(12):1844−51. https://doi.org/10.1177/0091270011429566.

[14] Autret E, Berjot M, Jonville-Bera AP, Aubry MC, Moraine C. Anophthalmia and agenesis of optic chiasma associated with adapalene gel in early pregnancy. Lancet 1997; 350(9074):339. https://doi.org/10.1016/S0140-6736(05)63390-9.

[15] Thiboutot D, Gollnick H, Bettoli V, Dreno B, Kang S, Leyden JJ, et al. New insights into the management of acne: an update from the Global Alliance to improve outcomes in acne group. J Am Acad Dermatol 2009;60(5 Suppl.):S1−50. https://doi.org/10.1016/j.jaad.2009.01.019.

[16] Shafia S, Chandluri P, Ganpisetti R, Swami PA. Erythromycin use as broad spectrum antibiotic. World J Pharmaceut Med Res 2016;2(6). Available from: https://www.researchgate.net/profile/Aravinda_Swami/publication/309175100_ERYTHROMYCIN_USE_AS_BROAD_SPECTRUM_ANTIBIOTIC/links/58026b0c08ae6c2449f7faff.pdf.

[17] Lin KJ, Mitchell AA, Yau WP, Louik C, Hernandez-Diaz S. Maternal exposure to amoxicillin and the risk of oral clefts. Epidemiology 2012;23(5):699−705. https://doi.org/10.1097/EDE.0b013e318258cb05.

[18] Andersen JT, Petersen M, Jimenez-Solem E, Broedbaek K, Andersen EW, Andersen NL, et al. Trimethoprim use in early pregnancy and the risk of miscarriage: a register-based nationwide cohort study. Epidemiol Infect 2013;141(8):1749−55. https://doi.org/10.1017/S0950268812002178.

[19] Hernandez-Diaz S, Werler MM, Walker AM, Mitchell AA. Folic acid antagonists during pregnancy and the risk of birth defects. N Engl J Med 2000;343(22):1608−14.

[20] Briggs GG, Freeman RK, Towers CV, Forinash AB. Drugs in pregnancy and lactation. 11th ed. Philadelphia, PA: Wolters Kluwer Health; 2017.

[21] Cohlan SQ, Bevelander G, Tiamsic T. Growth inhibition of prematures receiving tetracycline: a clinical and laboratory investigation of tetracycline-induced bone fluorescence. Am J Disab Child 1963;105(5):453−61. https://doi.org/10.1001/archpedi.1963.02080040455005.

[22] Lammer EJ, Chen DT, Hoar RM, Agnish ND, Benke PJ, Braun JT, et al. Retinoic acid embryopathy. N Engl J Med 1985;313(14):837−41. https://doi.org/10.1056/NEJM198510033131401.

[23] Sun Pharmaceutical Industries. Absorica. 2019. Available from: https://absorica.com/.

[24] iPledge. Prescriber information. 2016. Available from: https://www.ipledgeprogram.com/iPledgeUI/prInfo.u.

[25] Murase JE, Chan KK, Garite TJ, Cooper DM, Weinstein GD. Hormonal effect on psoriasis in pregnancy and postpartum. Arch Dermatol 2005;141(5):601−6. https://doi.org/10.1001/archderm.141.5.601.

[26] Bae YS, Van Voorhees AS, Hsu S, Korman NJ, Lebwohl MG, Young M, et al. Review of treatment options for psoriasis in pregnant or lactating women: from the Medical Board of the National Psoriasis Foundation. J Am Acad Dermatol 2012;67(3):459−77. https://doi.org/10.1016/j.jaad.2011.07.039.

[27] Mygind H, Thulstrup AM, Pedersen L, Larsen H. Risk of intrauterine growth retardation, malformations and other birth outcomes in children after topical use of corticosteroid in pregnancy. Acta Obstet Gynecol Scand 2002;81(3):234−9. https://doi.org/10.1034/j.1600-0412.2002.810308.x.

[28] Chi CC, Kirtschig G, Aberer W, Gabbud JP, Lipozenčić J, Kárpáti S, et al. Evidence-based (S3) guideline on topical corticosteroids in pregnancy. Br J Dermatol 2011;165(5):943−52. https://doi.org/10.1111/j.1365-2133.2011.10513.x.

[29] Tauscher AE, Fleischer AB, Phelps KC, Feldman SR. Psoriasis and pregnancy. J Cutan Med Surg 2002;6(6):561−70.

[30] Lebwohl M. A clinician's paradigm in the treatment of psoriasis. J Am Acad Dermatol 2005;53(1S):S59−69.

[31] Malecic N, Young H. Tacrolimus for the management of psoriasis: clinical utility and place in therapy. Psoriasis Targets Ther 2016;6:153−63. https://doi.org/10.2147/PTT.S101233.

[32] Park KK, Murase JE. Narrowband UV-B phototherapy during pregnancy and folic acid depletion. Arch Dermatol 2012;148(1):132−3. https://doi.org/10.1001/archdermatol.2011.1614.

[33] Stern RS, Lange R. Outcomes of pregnancies among women and partners of men with a history of exposure to methoxsalen photochemotherapy (PUVA) for the treatment of psoriasis. Arch Dermatol 1991;127(3):347−50.

[34] Vena GA, Cassano N, Bellia G, Colombo D. Psoriasis in pregnancy: challenges and solutions. Psoriasis Targets Ther 2015;15(5):83−95. https://doi.org/10.2147/PTT.S82975.

[35] Ryan C, Amor KT, Menter A. The use of cyclosporine in dermatology: Part II. J Am Acad Dermatol 2010;63(6):949−72. https://doi.org/10.1016/j.jaad.2010.02.062.

[36] Chin SO, Brodsky NL, Bhandari V. Antenatal steroid use is associated with increased gastroesophageal reflux in neonates. Am J Perinatol Rep 2003;20(4):205−13.

[37] Gur C, Diav-Citrin O, Schechtman S, Arnon J, Ornoy A. Pregnancy outcome after first trimester exposure to corticosteroids: a prospective controlled study. Reprod Toxicol 2004;18(1):93−101.

[38] Park WL, Mazzotta P, Pastuszak A, Moretti ME, Beique L, Hunnisett L, et al. Birth defects after maternal exposure to corticosteroids: prospective cohort study and meta-analysis of epidemiological studies. Teratology 2000;62(6):385−92.

[39] Wapner RJ, Sorokin Y, Mele L, Johnson F, Dudley DJ, Spong CY, et al. Long-term outcomes after repeat doses of antenatal corticosteroids. N Engl J Med 2007;357(12):1190−8.

[40] Hoeltzenbein M, Elefant E, Vial T, Finkel-Pekarsky V, Stephens S, Clementi M, et al. Teratogenicity of mycophenolate confirmed in a prospective study of the European network of teratology information services. Am J Med Genet 2012;158A(3):588−96. https://doi.org/10.1002/ajmg.a.35223.

[41] Lam J, Polifka JE, Dohil MA. Safety of dermatologic drugs used in pregnant patients with psoriasis and other inflammatory skin diseases. J Am Acad Dermatol 2008;59(2):295−315. https://doi.org/10.1016/j.jaad.2008.03.018.

[42] Porter ML, Lockwood SJ, Kimball AB. Update on biologic safety for patients with psoriasis during pregnancy. Int J Women Dermatol 2017;3(1):21−5. https://doi.org/10.1016/j.ijwd.2016.12.003.

[43] Østensen M, Förger F. How safe are anti-rheumatic drugs during pregnancy? Curr Opin Pharmacol 2013;13(3):470−5. https://doi.org/10.1016/j.coph.2013.03.004.

[44] Martin PL, Sachs C, Imai N, Tsusaki H, Oneda S, Jiao Q, Treacy G. Development in the cynomolgus macaque following administration of ustekinumab, a human anti-IL-12/23p40 monoclonal antibody, during pregnancy and lactation. Birth Defects Res Part B Dev Reproductive Toxicol 2010;89(5):351−63. https://doi.org/10.1002/bdrb.20250.

[45] Carter JD, Valeriano J, Vasey FB. Tumor necrosis factor-alpha inhibition and VATER association: a causal relationship. J Rheumatol 2006;33(5):1014−7.

[46] Carter JD, Ladhani A, Ricca LR, Valeriano J, Vasey FB. A safety assessment of tumor necrosis factor antagonists during pregnancy: a review of the Food and Drug Administration database. J Rheumatol 2009;36(3):635−41. https://doi.org/10.3899/jrheum.080545.

[47] Mishkin DS, Van Deinse W, Becker JM, Farraye FA. Successful use of adalimumab (Humira) for Crohn's disease in pregnancy. Inflamm Bowel Dis 2006;12(8):827−8. https://doi.org/10.1097/00054725-200608000-00020.

[48] Rump JA, Schönborn H. Conception and course of eight pregnancies in five women on TNF blocker etanercept treatment. Zeitschr Rheumatol 2010;69(10):903−9. https://doi.org/10.1007/s00393-010-0652-y.

[49] Berthelot JM, De Bandt M, Goupille P, Solau-Gervais E, Liote F, Goeb V, et al. Exposition to anti-TNF drugs during pregnancy: outcome of 15 cases and review of the literature. Joint Bone Spine 2009;76(1):28−34. https://doi.org/10.1016/j.jbspin.2008.04.016.

[50] Katz JA, Antoini C, Keenan GF, Smith DE, Jacobs SJ, Lichtenstein GR. Outcome of pregnancy in women receiving infliximab for the treatment of Crohn's disease and rheumatoid arthritis. Am J Gastroenterol 2004;99(12):2385−92.

[51] Cheent K, Nolan J, Shariq S, Kiho L, Pal A, Arnold J. Case report: fatal case of disseminated BCG infection in an infant born to a mother taking infliximab for Crohn's disease. J Crohn Colit 2010;4(5):603−5. https://doi.org/10.1016/j.crohns.2010.05.001.

[52] Kane S, Ford J, Cohen R, Wagner C. Absence of infliximab in infants and breast milk from nursing mothers receiving therapy for Crohn's disease before and after delivery. J Clin Gastroenterol 2009;43(7):613−6. https://doi.org/10.1097/MCG.0b013e31817f9367.

[53] Ambros-Rudolph CM, Mullegger RR, Vaughan-Jones SA, Kerl H, Black MM. The specific dermatoses of pregnancy revisited and reclassified: results of a retrospective two-center study on 505 pregnant patients. J Am Acad Dermatol 2006;54(3):395−404.

[54] Kar S, Krishnan A, Preetha K, Mohankar A. A review of antihistamines used during pregnancy. J Pharmacol Pharmacother 2012;3(2):105−8. https://doi.org/10.4103/0976-500X.95503.

[55] Casale TB, Blaiss MS, Gelfand E, Gilmore T, Harvey PD, Hindmarch I, et al. First do no harm: managing antihistamine impairment in patients with allergic rhinitis. J Allergy Clin Immunol 2003;111(5):S835−42. https://doi.org/10.1067/mai.2003.1550.

[56] Seto A, Einarson T, Koren G. Pregnancy outcome following first trimester exposure to antihistamines: meta-analysis. Am J Perinatol 1997;14(3):119−24.

[57] Gilboa SM, Strickland MJ, Olshan AF, Werler MM, Correa A. Use of antihistamine medications during early pregnancy and isolated major malformations. Birth Defects Res Part A Clin Mol Teratol 2009;85(2):137−50. https://doi.org/10.1002/bdra.20513.

[58] Stephansson O, Granath F, Svensson T, Haglund B, Ekbom A, Kieler H. Drug use during pregnancy in Sweden - assessed by the prescribed drug register and the medical birth register. Clin Epidemiol 2011;3:43–50. https://doi.org/10.2147/CLEP.S16305.

[59] Weber-Schoendorfer C, Schaefer C. The safety of cetirizine during pregnancy. A prospective observational cohort study. Reprod Toxicol 2008;26(1):19–23. https://doi.org/10.1016/j.reprotox.2008.05.053.

[60] Brzezińska-Wcisło L, Zbiciak-Nylec M, Wcisło-Dziadecka D, Salwowska N. Pregnancy: a therapeutic dilemma. Adv Dermatol Allergol 2017;34(5):433–8. https://doi.org/10.5114/ada.2017.71108.

[61] Centers for Disease Control and Prevention [CDC]. Evaluation of an association between loratadine and hypospadias – United States, 1997–2001. Morb Mortal Wkly Rep 2004;53(10):219–21. Available from: https://www.cdc.gov/mmwr/preview/mmwrhtml/mm5310a5.htm.

[62] Maharajan A, Aye C, Ratnavel R, Burova E. Skin eruptions specific to pregnancy: an overview. Obstet Gynaecol 2013;15(4):233–40. https://doi.org/10.1111/tog.12051.

[63] Huilaja L, Mäkikallio K, Hannula-Jouppi K, Väkevä L, Höök-Nikanne J, Tasanen K. Cyclosporine treatment in severe gestational pemphigoid. Acta Derm Venereol 2015; 95(5):593–5. https://doi.org/10.2340/00015555-2032.

[64] Özdemir O, Atalay CR, Asgarova V, Ilgin BU. A resistant case of pemphigus gestations successfully treated with cyclosporine. Intervent Med Appl Sci 2016;8(1):20–2. https://doi.org/10.1556/1646.8.2016.1.3.

[65] Ambros-Rudolph CM. Dermatoses of pregnancy – clues to diagnosis, fetal risk and therapy. Ann Dermatol 2011;23(3):265–75. https://doi.org/10.5021/ad.2011.23.3.265.

[66] Zhang Y, Lu L, Victor DW, Xin Y, Xuan S. Ursodeoxycholic acid and S-adenosylmethionine for the treatment of intrahepatic cholestasis of pregnancy: a meta-analysis. Hepat Month 2016;16(8):e38558. https://doi.org/10.5812/hepatmon.38558.

[67] Kong X, Kong Y, Zhang F, Wang T, Yan J. Evaluating the effectiveness and safety of ursodeoxycholic acid in treatment of intrahepatic cholestasis of pregnancy: a meta-analysis (a prisma-compliant study). Medicine 2016;95(40):e4949.

[68] GlaxoSmithKline. Bactroban. 2015. Available from: https://www.gsksource.com/pharma/content/dam/GlaxoSmithKline/US/en/Prescribing_Information/Bactroban_Ointment/pdf/BACTROBAN-OINTMENT-PI-PIL.PDF.

[69] Pasternak B, Hviid A. Use of acyclovir, valacyclovir, and famciclovir in the first trimester of pregnancy and the risk of birth defects. J Am Med Assoc 2010;304(8): 859–66.

[70] Scheller NM, Pasternak B, Mølgaard-Nielsen D, Svanström H, Hvidd A. Quadrivalent HPV vaccination and the risk of adverse pregnancy outcomes. N Engl J Med 2017; 376(13):1223–33. https://doi.org/10.1056/NEJMoa1612296.

[71] Pilmis B, Jullien V, Sobel J, Lecuit M, Lortholary O, Charlier C. Antifungal drugs during pregnancy: an updated review. J Antimicrob Chemother 2015;70(1):14–22. https://doi.org/10.1093/jac/dku355.

[72] Rosa FW, Hernandez C, Carlo WA. Griseofulvin teratology, including two thoracopagus conjoined twins. Lancet 1987;329(8525):171. https://doi.org/10.1016/S0140-6736(87)92015-0.

[73] Knudsen LB. No association between griseofulvin and conjoined twinning. Lancet 1987;2(8567):1097. https://doi.org/10.1016/s0140-6736(87)91533-9.

[74] Malka I, Ziv M. Safety of common medications for treating dermatology disorders in pregnant women. Curr Dermatol Rep 2013;2(4):249−57.

[75] Lopez-Rangel E, Van Allen MI. Prenatal exposure to fluconazole: an identifiable dysmorphic phenotype. Birth Defects Res Part A Clin Mol Teratol 2005;73(11):919−23.

[76] Jick SS. Pregnancy outcomes after maternal exposure to fluconazole. Pharmacotherapy 1999;19(2):221−2.

[77] Mastroiacovo P, Mazzone T, Botto LD, Serafini MA, Finardi A, Caramelli L, Fusco D. Prospective assessment of pregnancy outcomes after first-trimester exposure to fluconazole. Am J Obstet Gynecol 1996;175(6):1645−50.

[78] Mølgaard-Nielsen D, Pasternak B, Hviid A. Use of oral fluconazole during pregnancy and the risk of birth defects. N Engl J Med 2013;369(9):830−9.

[79] Nørgaard M, Pedersen L, Gislum M, Erichsen R, Søgaard KK, Schønheyder HC, Sørensen HT. Maternal use of fluconazole and risk of congenital malformations: a Danish population-based cohort study. J Antimicrob Chemother 2008;62(1):172−6. https://doi.org/10.1093/jac/dkn157.

[80] Bar-Oz B, Moretti ME, Bishai R, Mareels G, Van Tittleboom T, Verspeelt J, Koren G. Pregnancy outcome after in utero exposure to itraconazole: a prospective cohort study. Am J Obstet Gynecol 2000;183(3):617−20.

[81] Hall CM, Milligan DW, Berrington J. Probable adverse reaction to a pharmaceutical excipient. Fetal and Neonatal Edition Arch Dis Childh 2004;89(2):F184. https://doi.org/10.1136/adc.2002.024927.

[82] Patel VM, Clark Lambert W, Schwartz RA. Safety of topical medications for scabies and lice in pregnancy. Indian J Dermatol 2016;61(6):583−7. https://doi.org/10.4103/0019-5154.193659.

[83] Murase JE, Heller MM, Butler DC. Safety of dermatologic medications in pregnancy and lactation: Part I. Pregnancy. J Am Acad Dermatol 2014;70(3):e401−14. https://doi.org/10.1016/j.jaad.2013.09.010.

[84] Pacque M, Munoz B, Poetschke G, Foose J, Greene BM, Taylor HR. Pregnancy outcome after inadvertent ivermectin treatment during community-based distribution. Lancet 1990;336(8729):1486−9.

[85] de Silva N, Guyatt H, Bundy D. Anthelmintics: a comparative review of their pharmacology. Drugs 1997;53(5):769−88.

[86] Torlesse H, Hodges M. Anthelmintic treatment and haemoglobin concentrations during pregnancy. Lancet 2000;356(9235):1083.

[87] Abdel-Tawab AM, Bradley M, Ghazaly EA, Horton J, El-Setouhy M. Albendazole and its metabolites in the breast milk of lactating women following a single oral dose of albendazole. Br J Clin Pharmacol 2009;68(5):737−42. https://doi.org/10.1111/j.1365-2125.2009.03524.x.

[88] Roth MM, Solovan C. Dermatological medications and local therapeutics. In: Mattison DR, editor. Clinical pharmacology in pregnancy; 2013. p. 358.

[89] Tyler KH, Zirwas MJ. Pregnancy and dermatologic therapy. J Am Acad Dermatol 2013;68(4):663−71. https://doi.org/10.1016/j.jaad.2012.09.034.

[90] Richards KA, Stasko T. Dermatologic surgery and the pregnant patient. Dermatol Surg 2002;28(3):248−56. https://doi.org/10.1046/j.1524-4725.2002.01177.x.

Herbs and alternative remedies

Henry M. Hess

Emeritus Professor of Obstetrics and Gynecology, University of Rochester School of Medicine, Rochester, NY

Pregnancy can be an ideal time to use herbal and alternative remedies. Herbs are often mild preparations of natural compounds that can be just perfect for some of the discomforts and illnesses during pregnancy. Several studies have shown that as many as 50% or more of women will choose herbs and alternative remedies as therapies during pregnancy [1–5].

Although herbal therapies have been used for centuries, herbs are complex mixtures of many compounds, and some have potentially significant negative effects for both the pregnant woman and the fetus. In the companion book *Drugs during Pregnancy and Lactation*, third edition, edited by Schaefer, Peters, and Miller [2], we focused on the safety of herbs during pregnancy and counseled health care providers that the use of some herbs during pregnancy can have significant risks depending on the herb, the purity of the preparation, and the timing of use during pregnancy. In this chapter, we have focused on the herbs and alternative remedies that are potentially safe and efficacious for many conditions during pregnancy. Using the best available up-to-date scientific evidence, evidence based and traditional, we have listed and categorized herbs, supplements, and other alternative remedies that are potentially safe and efficacious for many of the common medical conditions and discomforts that occur during pregnancy.

For herbs and supplements, we have listed forms and dosage. It is important to recognize that herbs are extracts of plants or plant roots, and they therefore contain numerous compounds. This is very different to a pharmaceutical preparation, which is usually a single active ingredient. Different forms of herbal preparations will have different compounds and concentrations depending on how the plant or plant root is extracted. Herbal preparations are usually available in the following forms: teas or infusions (hot water extracts of dried herbs), capsules, dried extracts, and tinctures (alcohol extracts of dried herbs). The most common forms of herbs used in pregnancy are teas or infusions. These usually have the lowest concentration, contain the least amount of compounds, and therefore are the safest. Capsules and dried extracts are the next most commonly used. Tinctures should be avoided during pregnancy because of their higher concentrations as well as the use of alcohol as a carrier.

A very important difference between the use of herbs or supplements and a pharmaceutical preparation is the integrity and purity of the specific herb or supplement

Clinical Pharmacology During Pregnancy. https://doi.org/10.1016/B978-0-12-818902-3.00017-8

preparation [2]. Herbs and supplements are often produced in other countries where lead and other impurities can be a problem. There is no Food and Drug Administration oversight of these products, so it is extremely important that patients as well as providers find guidance on product selection from sources such as ConsumerLab.com [6]. ConsumerLab.com independently and periodically evaluates individual products for purity and integrity. We strongly recommend frequent evaluation of the integrity of the individual preparation. Patients and providers should also be aware of potential herb–drug interactions with all herbal and alternative remedies [7].

We also have discussed the use of hypnosis and meditation as alternative remedies for many of the common discomforts and illnesses in pregnancy and delivery, where otherwise medications might be needed.

21.1 Herbal teas frequently used during pregnancy

The herbs most frequently used during pregnancy are teas or infusions. Some herbal teas have specific indications; others are used by patients as general health tonics. Although there are minimal clinical trials available, and minimal evidence-based proof of safety and efficacy in terms of Western medical standards, herbal teas have been used for centuries and are regarded as safe and efficacious during pregnancy. It is the general recommendation [2] that consumption of herbal teas be limited to two cups per day during pregnancy. This is similar to the safety data regarding coffee. The safety is unknown when used at higher levels. The following herbal teas are frequently and safely used during pregnancy [2,4,8,9]:

- Red raspberry leaf — Relief of nausea, increase in milk production, increase in uterine tone, and ease of labor pains. There is some controversy over the use of red raspberry leaf in the first trimester, primarily because of concern of stimulating the uterine tone and potentially causing miscarriage. Use in the second and third trimester is generally considered safe. In a small study, red raspberry leaf, when used to induce and shorten labor, has been associated with increased cesarean delivery [7].
- Peppermint — Nausea and flatulence. Tea is the most common. Enteric-coated tablets (187 mg three times a day maximum) are also used. Peppermint may cause gastroesophageal refiux.
- Chamomile (German) — Gastrointestinal irritation, insomnia, and joint irritation. Potentially significant herb–drug interactions have been reported when used together with drugs with sedative properties [7,10].
- Dandelion — A mild diuretic, and to nourish the liver; known for high amounts of vitamins A and C, and the elements of iron, calcium, and potassium, as well as other trace elements.
- Alfalfa — General pregnancy tonic; a source of high levels of vitamins A, D, B, and K, minerals, and digestive enzymes; thought to reduce the risk of postpartum hemorrhage.
- Oat and oat straw — Sources of calcium and magnesium; helps to relieve anxiety, restlessness, insomnia, and irritable skin.

- Nettle leaf — Traditional pregnancy tonic; source of high amounts of vitamins A, C, K, calcium, potassium, and iron. NB: nettle root is different from nettle leaf; it is used for inducing abortions and is otherwise not safe in pregnancy.
- Slippery elm bark — Nausea, heartburn, and vaginal irritations.

21.2 Essential oils used as aromatherapy during pregnancy

Some essential oils are frequently used as aromatherapy during pregnancy, and the ones described below are considered to be safe and efficacious during pregnancy based on traditional and historic use. They should always be used carefully, in well-diluted form, and in an aromatherapy diffuser. They should not be ingested. Such essential oils and their uses are listed below [2,4,8]:

- Chamomile — Respiratory tract disorders.
- Tangerine — Antispasmodic, decongestant, and general relaxant.
- Grapefruit — Stimulant and antidepressant.
- Geranium — Dermatitis, hormone imbalances, mood dysfunction, and viral infections.
- Rose — Astringent, used for mild inflammation of the oral and pharyngeal mucosa.
- Jasmine — Stimulant, antidepressant, and anxiety.
- Ylang-ylang — Antispasmodic, cardiac arrhythmias, anxiety, antidepressant, hair loss, and intestinal problems.
- Lavender — Loss of appetite, nervousness, and insomnia.

21.3 Herbs used as capsules or dried extracts
21.3.1 Ginger

- Nausea and vomiting of pregnancy. Dose: 250 mg 3—4 times per day.
- Ginger is the herb with the most evidence-based data showing efficacy and safety in pregnancy. When used at 250 mg 3—4 times a day, it is considered safe and effective for nausea and vomiting of pregnancy, as well as hyperemesis gravidarum [1—5,8,11]. Most of the antiemetic activity is believed to be due to the constituent 6-gingerol which acts directly in the gastrointestinal tract. The constituent galanolactone also acts on 5-HT3 receptors in the ileum, which are the same receptors affected by some prescription antiemetics. Ginger's antiemetic activity may also involve the central nervous system, where the constituents 6-shogaol and galanolactone act on serotonin receptors [5]. The continual use of ginger throughout pregnancy has been associated with a nonsignificant increase in the incidence of stillbirth and a significant decrease in gestational age at delivery [12]. Ginger has also been identified as a source of potentially significant herb—drug interactions with insulin, metformin, and nifedipine, medicines commonly used during pregnancy [13].

21.3.2 **Cranberry**

- Prevention and treatment of urinary tract infection. Dose: 300–400 mg 3 times a day. Can cause gastrointestinal upset.
- Cranberry is one of the most commonly used herbs during pregnancy, primarily for the prevention and treatment of urinary tract infections. Although there is a long history of the safe and efficacious use of cranberry during pregnancy, there are very little evidence-based data [1,4,5,8,14]. The literature does suggest that cranberry capsules may be more efficacious than cranberry juice. Studies on the pharmacology of cranberry show that the proanthocyanidins in cranberry interfere with bacterial adherence to the urinary tract epithelial cells [5].

21.3.3 **Echinacea**

- Prevention and treatment of upper respiratory tract infections, vaginitis, and herpes simplex virus. Dose: 900 mg of dried root or equivalent 3 times a day.
- There is a long history of safe and efficacious use of *Echinacea* in pregnancy [1–5,8,15,16]. Two scientific studies are frequently cited as evidence-based studies showing its safety in pregnancy [5,17]. The efficacy is based on tradition, not evidence based. *Echinacea* is known to inhibit the influenza virus and the herpes simplex I and II viruses. It has been shown to increase the proliferation of phagocytes in the spleen and bone marrow, stimulate monocytes, increase the number of polymorphonuclear leukocytes and promote their adherence to the endothelial cells, and activate macrophages [5].

21.3.4 **St. John's wort**

- Treatment of mild to moderate depression, anxiety, and seasonal affective disorder. Dose: 300 mg 3 times daily, of a standardized extract.
- Although there is minimal evidence-based medicine of its safety or efficacy in pregnancy, St. John's wort is considered safe in pregnancy by the German Commission E, the American Herbal Products Association, and much traditional literature [1–5,8,15,16]. It is very commonly used in pregnancy for mild to moderate depression. Studies have shown that St. John's wort acts as an SSRI (selective serotonin reuptake inhibitor), and inhibits the reuptake of serotonin, norepinephrine, and dopamine. Also of significance is that the hypericin in St. John's wort induces some of the cytochrome P450 enzymes and may interfere with the metabolism of other drugs similarly metabolized [5,8]. St. John's wort can cause photosensitization, so caution must be exercised, and patients advised [8].

21.3.5 **Valerian**

- Treatment of anxiety and insomnia. Dose: 2–3 g of crude herb as a capsule or tea at bedtime.
- Valerian root is also very commonly used in pregnancy, but there is lack of any evidence-based medicine showing either its efficacy or safety. Some scientific

publications as well as the World Health Organization [8] suggest caution in the use of valerian during pregnancy because its safety has not been clinically established. However, the German Commission E [2,8,15] and the *Botanical Safety Handbook* [16], as well as several articles and books, support the use of valerian during pregnancy and generally conclude that occasional use is safe and efficacious when used in the dose described above. Valerian has sedative, anxiolytic, antidepressant, anticonvulsant, hypotensive, and antispasmodic effects. The major constituents, valerenic acid and kessyl glycol, are known to cause sedation in animals. Valerenic acid may inhibit the enzyme system responsible for the catabolism of gamma-aminobutyric acid (GABA), thereby increasing GABA concentrations and decreasing central nervous activity [5].

21.3.6 Milk thistle/silymarin

■ Treatment for intrahepatic cholestasis of pregnancy, alcoholic and nonalcoholic liver cirrhosis, chronic and acute viral hepatitis, drug-induced liver toxicity, and fatty degeneration of the liver. Dose: 400 mg of standard silymarin extract in 2—3 divided doses per day. Recommended to be used in the second and third trimester of pregnancy only [5,18—20].

■ There are many references in the natural and herbal literature to the use of milk thistle in pregnancy for liver dysfunctions and for enhancement of milk production [5]. There are also concerns and warnings about possible significant side effects and insufficient evidence-based studies to recommend milk thistle in pregnancy. However, the few evidence-based studies do support the safety and efficacy for use of this herb for specific situations described above. In four studies, no evidence of adverse effects was reported in the mothers and offspring [5,19,20]. There are no reports of estrogenic effects on the fetus, a potential concern because the constituents of milk thistle are flavonolignans [5]. There have been many suggestions as to the mechanism of action, but silybin has been shown to stimulate RNA polymerase A and DNA synthesis, increasing the regenerative capacity of the liver. Silymarin, the active constituent, is thought to competitively bind some toxins and act as a free radical scavenger [5]. Clinically, regular consumption of milk thistle has been shown to reduce elevated liver enzymes [5].

21.3.7 Senna

■ Treatment of constipation. Dose: 10—60 mg at bedtime for a maximum of 10 days, in the second and third trimester [2,3,5,21].

■ The use of senna in pregnancy is very controversial because senna is a member of the anthraquinone laxatives group, thought to be contraindicated in pregnancy because overstimulation of the bowel or bladder has the potential to irritate/stimulate the uterus, potentially causing premature labor, or even miscarriage in the first trimester [2]. The *Compendium on Herbal Safety* offered the opinion that senna should be avoided during pregnancy [2,5]. However, there are no reports in the literature showing senna to be contraindicated during pregnancy.

A review article has reported that senna would appear to be the stimulant laxative of choice during pregnancy, probably because of the poor intestinal absorption of senna compared to the other anthraquinone laxatives [5,21]. Traditional use has shown that with careful use, senna may be used in the second and third trimester with minimal risk. There are no studies showing a risk in the first trimester either, but avoidance of use in the first trimester is recommended based on the potential for senna to be an abortifacient [22]. The literature reports that sennosides irritate the lining of the large intestine, causing its contraction and evacuation. Sennosides A and B also induce fluid secretion from the colon, softening the stool, and may also induce prostaglandins for more effective contractions of the colon. The laxative effect occurs 8–12 h after administration, although sometimes up to 24 h can be required. It is important not to overuse senna in pregnancy. Diarrhea, fluid loss, and electrolyte imbalance, as well as habituation, have been reported [5].

21.3.8 Horse chestnut

- Chronic venous insufficiency — 300 mg twice daily of Venostasin (reg)retard (240–290 mg of horse chestnut seed extract, standardized to 50 mg escin). NB: Do not use unprocessed raw horse chestnut preparations. These can be very toxic and lethal when ingested in adults [5,23].
- Oral horse chestnut has been shown in the literature to significantly reduce leg edema and varicose veins and chronic venous insufficiency when taken orally [5,8,23]. While oral horse chestnut has been found very useful, caution is advised when recommending this herb to a pregnant woman, as there is minimal evidence-based study of efficacy or safety in pregnancy. However, there is a randomized placebo-controlled trial of 52 women with symptomatic leg edema attributed to pregnancy-induced venous insufficiency where improvements were found with horse chestnut, and the authors did not observe any serious adverse effects after 2 weeks [5,23].

21.4 Herbal topical preparations used in pregnancy

21.4.1 Aloe vera gel

- Treatment of skin burns. Topical use only [2,4,8,15].
- There is a long history of safe and efficacious topical use of aloe vera gel during pregnancy, but no evidence-based studies.

21.4.2 Horse chestnut

- Treatment of severe hemorrhoids in pregnancy. Topical 2% gel (escin) 2–4 times a day [5,24].
- The few studies done have shown safe and efficacious use, particularly with severe hemorrhoids in pregnancy.

21.4.3 **Almond oil**

Topical use of almond oil during the third trimester to avoid stretch marks is associated with preterm birth and is not recommended. It is speculated that continuous rubbing of the belly might stimulate myometrial contractions or that the components of almond oil might act as prostaglandin precursors [7,25].

21.5 **Nonherbal supplements used in pregnancy**

21.5.1 **Fish oils**

- Support for the development of a healthy mother and baby—including prevention of colds in infants of treated mothers, support for the heart, immune system, inflammatory response, the development and maintenance of the brain, eyes, and central nervous system. Dose: 300−400 mg DHA (docosahexaenoic acid) and 100−220 mg of EPA (eicosapentaenoic acid) daily. The freshness of the oil is important because rancid fish oils have an extremely unpleasant odor and also may not be as effective [5,6].
- Omega 3s have been found to be essential for both neurological and early visual development of the baby. Research has confirmed that adding omega 3s to the diet of pregnant women has a positive effect on visual and cognitive development of the child. Studies also have shown that higher consumption may reduce the risk of allergies in the fetus, may help to prevent preterm labor and delivery, lower the risk of preeclampsia, may increase birth weight, and may decrease the incidence of maternal and postpartum depression [5,6]. Omega 3s are a family of long-chain polyunsaturated fatty acids that are essential nutrients for health and development. They are not synthesized by the human body, and must be obtained through diet or supplementation. The typical American diet is greatly lacking in omega 3s. The two most beneficial omega 3s are EPA and DHA, and they work together in the body [6].
- Because of the potential for contamination of fish oils by mercury and other potential contaminants, the use of purified fish oils is essential [6]. Flaxseed is not a substitute for fish oils in pregnancy, as flaxseed constituents have potential estrogenic properties [2,5].

21.5.2 **Probiotics**

- Prevention and treatment of vaginal infections (yeast vaginitis and bacterial vaginosis). Dose: At least 4 billion organisms daily, with at least 1 billion each of *Lactobacillus*, *Bifidobacterium*, and *Saccharomyces* [5,6,9].
- May prevent preterm labor in the third trimester when caused by these infections. Maintains digestive systems in the face of pregnancy-related problems, eases diarrhea, constipation, and hemorrhoids, as well as boosting the immune system. Studies have also shown that babies and toddlers up to 2 years old were 40% less likely to suffer eczema/atopic dermatitis when mothers took probiotics. Limited studies have also shown that probiotics may help limit excessive weight gain in pregnancy.

21.6 Herbs used to induce labor

In the traditional literature [26,27], there are herbs and herbal mixtures reportedly used to induce labor. According to the recent literature [5,26], many midwives in the United States and elsewhere in the world use herbal mixtures to induce labor. There is no evidence-based literature establishing the safety or efficacy of the herbs used, but there exists some literature expressing concern regarding significant risks and bad outcomes. Currently, there simply is not enough evidence of safety to recommend these treatments for this indication.

21.7 Acupuncture and acupressure therapy in pregnancy

There is a significant amount of evidence-based medicine in the literature regarding the use, efficacy, and safety of acupuncture and acupressure therapy in pregnancy [1,28].

The practice of acupuncture and acupressure dates back 5000 years. Acupuncture is based on a belief that a vital energy called "qi" (chee) flows through the body along pathways called meridians. Along these meridians, there are some 2000 acupuncture points where the thin needles (or pressure) are inserted to relieve symptoms, cure the disease, and restore balance.

In pregnancy, both the mother and infant benefit. Acupuncture has been used successfully in pregnancy for maintenance of health, treatment for preexisting medical issues, and treatment of pregnancy-related issues (including psychological issues, physical problems, fatigue, morning sickness, heartburn, constipation, hemorrhoids, back pain and sciatica, edema, carpal tunnel syndrome, and rhinitis of pregnancy). Acupressure is popular for relief of nausea and vomiting in pregnancy. It has also been successfully used to assist with versions in breech presentations and for pain analgesia in labor. Acupuncture has also been found efficacious for many postpartum disorders such as fatigue, postpartum vaginal discharge, postpartum depression, mastitis, insufficient or excessive lactation, and postoperative healing. A trained and experienced acupuncturist understands and knows the target points for the needle insertions during pregnancy and for specifically related pregnancy problems. Efficacy rates are significant, and there are no known risks. Acupuncture (and acupressure) may be very useful for pregnancy-related situations where otherwise a medication may be necessary.

21.8 Meditation and hypnosis in pregnancy

Meditation [29] and hypnotherapy [22] are excellent natural therapies for managing health during pregnancy, including the discomforts of pregnancy and labor and delivery as well as prevention of illnesses and management of illnesses. Used for centuries, there are recent and long-term evidence-based studies showing their efficacy and safety. These modalities, like other natural therapies, are becoming very popular with pregnant and postpartum women. The internet has several sites as well as CD products making it easier for patients to learn about and practice mindfulness meditation and self-hypnosis.

Mindful meditation and hypnosis have many similarities. Hypnosis is a slightly deeper process where it is easier for suggestions to be incorporated by the subconscious. Hypnosis has been used for pregnancy-related symptoms including labor and delivery and has become particularly popular since the 1930s. Evidence-based data show that hypnosis in particular helps with an easier and less painful labor. For mindful meditation during pregnancy, studies have shown that it decreases stress and produces endorphins which reduce physical pain. It has also been shown to increase the production of dehydroepiandrosterone (DHEA), which stimulates the production of T and B lymphocytes, supporting the immune system. DHEA has also been linked to decreasing sadness and depression, both before and after birth. Studies have also shown that the meditation increases the level of melatonin, supporting the immune system and increasing the quality of sleep and improved mood. Endorphins are similarly increased, which have a strong pain relieving effect in preparation for childbirth. Studies also show that mindfulness meditation can be very effective in lowering blood pressure and heart rate, potentially lowering the risk of preeclampsia.

References

[1] Fugh-Berman A, Kronenberg F. Complementary and Alternative Medicine (CAM) in reproductive-age women: a review of randomized controlled trials. Reprod Toxicol 2003;17:137—52.

[2] Hess HM, Miller RK. Herbs during pregnancy. In: Schaefer C, Peters P, Miller RK, editors. Drugs during pregnancy and lactation. 3rd ed. San Diego, CA: Academic Press; 2015. p. 511—25.

[3] Holst L, Wright D, Haavick S, Nordeng H. Safety and efficacy of herbal remedies in obstetrics, review and clinical implications. Midwifery 2011;27:80—6.

[4] Low Dog T, Micozzi MS. Women's health in complementary and integrative medicine: clinical guide. Oxford: Elsevier; 2005.

[5] Mills E, Dugoua JJ, Perri D, Koren G. Herbal medicines in pregnancy & lactation. An evidence-based approach. Boca Raton, FL: Taylor and Francis; 2006.

[6] https://www.consumerlab.com.

[7] Munoz Balbontin Y, Stewart D, Shetty A, Fitton C, McLay J. Herbal medicinal product use during pregnancy and the postnatal period. A systematic review. Obstet Gynecol 2019;133:920—32.

[8] Blumenthal M, editor. The ABC clinical guide to herbs. New York, NY: Thieme Medical Publishing; 2003.

[9] Dugoua JJ, Machado M, Xu Z, Chen X, Koren G, Einarson TR. Probiotic safety in pregnancy: a systematic review and meta-analysis of randomized controlled trials of *Lactobacillus*, *Bifidobacterium*, and *Saccharomyces* spp. J Obstet Gynaecol Can 2009;31(6):542—52.

[10] Nordeng H, Bayne K, Havnen GC, Paulsen BS. Use of herbal drugs during pregnancy among 600 Norwegian women in relation to concurrent use of conventional drugs and pregnancy outcome. Compl Ther Clin Pract 2011;17:147–51.

[11] Fischer-Rasmussen W, Kojer SK, Dahl C, Asping U. Ginger treatment of hyperemesis gravidarum. Eur J Obstet Gynecol Reprod Biol 1990;38:19–24.

[12] Choi JS, Han JY, Ahn HK, Lee SW, Koong MK, Veluzquez-Armenta EY, et al. Assessment of fetal and neonatal outcomes in the offspring of women who have been treated with dried ginger for a variety of illnesses during pregnancy. J Obstet Gynaecol 2015; 35:125–30.

[13] McLay J, Izzati N, Pallivalapilla A, Shetty A, Pande B, Rore C, et al. Pregnancy, prescription medicines and the potential of herb-drug interactions: a cross-sectional survey. BMC Compl Alternative Med 2017;17:543.

[14] Wing DA, Rumney PJ, Preslicka CW, Chung JH. Daily cranberry juice for the prevention of asymptomatic bacteriuria in pregnancy: a randomized, controlled pilot study. J Urol 2008;180:367–1372.

[15] Thomson H, editor. Physician's desk reference for herbal medicines. 4th ed. Montvale, NJ: Thomson Reuters Publishing; 2007.

[16] McGuffin M, Hobb C, Upton R, Goldberg P. American herbal products association's botanical safety Handbook. Boca Raton, FL: CRC Press; 1998.

[17] Gallo M, Koren G. Can herbal remedies be used safely during pregnancy? Focus on Echinacea. Can Fam Physician 2001;47:1727–8.

[18] Giannola C, Buogo F, Forestiere G. A two-center study on the effects of silymarin in pregnant women and adult patients with so-called minor hepatic insufficiency. Clin Therapeut 1998;114:129–35.

[19] Reys H. The spectrum of liver and gastrointestinal disease seen in cholestasis of pregnancy. Gastrointestinal Clin North Am 1992;21:905–21.

[20] Reyes H, Simon FR. Intrahepatic cholestasis of pregnancy. An estrogen-related disease. Semin Liver Dis 1993;13:289–301.

[21] Gattuso JM, Kamm MA. Adverse effects of drugs used in the management of constipation and diarrhea. Drug Saf 1994;10:47–65.

[22] Harms RW. Hypnobirthing: how does it work? Mayo Clin April 14, 2011. http://www./mayoclinic.com/health/hypnobirthing/AN02138.

[23] Steiner M. Untersuchungen Zur Odemvermindernden und O demportektiven Wirking von ro Kastanienoamenextrakt. Phlebol Prookto 1990;19:239–42.

[24] Damianov L, Katsarova M. Our experience in using the preparation Proctosedyl from the Roussel firm in pregnant women with hemorrhoids. Akush Ginekol 1993;32:71.

[25] Facchinetti F, Pedrielli G, Benoni G, Joppi M, Verlato G, Dante G, et al. Herbal supplements in pregnancy: unexpected results from a multicenter study. Human Reprod 2012; 27:3161–7.

[26] McFarlin BL, Gibson MH, O'Rear J, Harmon P. A national survey of herbal preparation use by nurse-midwives for labor stimulation. J Nurse Midwifery 1999;44:205–16.

[27] Weed S. Wise women herbal for the childbearing year. Woodstock, NY: Ash Tree Publishing; 1986.

[28] Carlsson CP. Manual acupuncture reduces hyperemesis gravidarum: a placebo controlled, randomized, single-blind, crossover study. Pain Sympt Manag 2000;41: 273–9.

[29] Murphy M, Donovan S. The physical and psychological effects of meditation: a review of contemporary research with a comprehensive bibliography. 1931–1996. 2nd ed. San Francisco CA: Institute of Noetic Sciences Press; 1997.

Further reading

[1] Park J, Sohn Y, White A, Lee H. The safety of acupuncture in pregnancy: a systematic review. Acupunct Med 2014;32(3):257–66.

[2] Soliday E, Betts D. Treating pain in pregnancy with acupuncture: observational Study results from a file clinic in New Zealand. J Acupunct Merid Stud 2018;11:25–30.

Envenomations and antivenom during pregnancy

22

Maria P. Ramirez-Cruz[1], William F. Rayburn[2], Steven A. Seifert[3,4]

[1]*Department of Obstetrics and Gynecology, University of New Mexico School of Medicine, Albuquerque, NM, United States;* [2]*Obstetrics and Gynecology, University of New Mexico School of Medicine, Albuquerque, NM, United States;* [3]*Department of Emergency Medicine, University of New Mexico School of Medicine, Albuquerque, NM, United States;* [4]*Medical, New Mexico Poison and Drug Information Center, Clinical Toxicology, Albuquerque, NM, United States*

22.1 General principles about envenomation

Envenomation is the exposure to a poison or toxin resulting from a bite or sting from an animal. The medically important venomous animals consist of several major categories: snakes, spiders, scorpions, hymenoptera (bees, wasps, and ants), and marine animals (some fish and cnidarians, such as jellyfish, anemones, and corals). Information about a bite or sting is often obtained secondhand from patients or primary caregivers, and additional exposures may go unreported.

US poison control centers assist in the assessment and management of envenomations. The national database (National Poison Data System) is a source of demographic and clinical data regarding such cases, although it is subject to a number of limitations; the database does not include all envenomations, as there is no mandatory reporting requirement, and the source of information on clinical effects and treatments is secondhand, often incomplete, and variably documented [1]. Shown in Table 22.1 are the 3555 exposures to the most common venomous animals in pregnancy from 2009 to 2018 as reported to US poison control centers. A retrospective observational study of the American Association of Poison Control Centers (AAPCC) between 2009 and 2018 revealed most venomous animal exposures in pregnancy had no effects or minor effects, there were no maternal deaths, and three fetal demises were reported following snake envenomations, although a direct correlation could not be drawn. This same study documented an increased likelihood of antivenom administration in pregnant patients with rattlesnake (85.0% vs. 58.9%) and black widow envenomations (4.8% vs. 2.2%) and decreased use of antihistamines in scorpion and hymenoptera stings [2].

Symptoms from an envenomation often produce a characteristic reaction, depending on the venomous animal involved, which may be the same as in the nonpregnant patient, or may be more pronounced during pregnancy due to physiologic circulatory changes. For example, black widow envenomation may produce

Clinical Pharmacology During Pregnancy. https://doi.org/10.1016/B978-0-12-818902-3.00011-7

Table 22.1 Cases of venomous animal exposures in pregnancy, 2009—18. American association of poison control centers database, NPDS.

Envenomation	Common name	Cases
Caterpillars		**96**
Centipedes/millipedes		**127**
Hymenoptera		**333**
	Ant/fire ant	35
	Bee/wasp/hornet	298
Marine		**47**
	Fish	19
	Jellyfish	27
	Unknown	1
Scorpion		**2097**
Spider		**664**
	Black widow	145
	Brown recluse	90
	Other	429
Snake		**191**
	Unidentified	89
	Copperhead	69
	Rattlesnake	20
	Cottonmouth	10
	Coral	3

Numbers in bold represent total number of cases reported in literature for each type of envenomation

hypertension, tachycardia, sweating, and other signs of adrenergic excess in both the pregnant and nonpregnant patient [3]. Scorpion stings can have a wide range of outcomes, from localized pain and swelling to fatal neuromuscular or cardiotoxic effects. In pregnancy, pelvic pain has been reported [4] with animal studies showing increase in frequency and amplitude of contractions mediated by kinins [5].

Pharmacologic therapy of envenomations is directed at symptomatic and supportive care, as well as specific therapy, if available and appropriately indicated. In general, symptomatic and supportive drugs are used sparingly and at the lowest effective doses in order to avoid confounding clinical assessment [6]. The need for tetanus toxoid should be assessed and administered to people at risk of tetanus regardless of pregnancy status. The current American College of Obstetricians and Gynecologists recommendations include administering the Tdap vaccine between 27 and 36 weeks during every pregnancy. However, it is appropriate to administer the vaccine outside of this window during extenuating circumstances such as wound management for infection prevention [7].

Routine use of antibiotics (e.g., dicloxacillin, cefazolin, and metronidazole) after envenomation is questionable unless signs suggestive of infection are present [8], which is unlikely to be seen prior to 24—48 h after a bite or sting. There is no evidence in support of the administration of prophylactic antibiotics, even in snake envenomation, with its extensive tissue injury effects, unless tissue necrosis occurs. Any short-term course of standard antibiotics is presumed to be safe during pregnancy.

Any decision to use a specific antidotal therapy—antivenom—must take into account the potential for allergic reactions, either Type 1 (anaphylaxis or anaphylactoid) or Type 3 (serum sickness) and the risk—benefit assessment in pregnancy includes the potential for adverse effects on the fetus. Antivenoms, currently available for some snake, spider, and scorpion envenomations, are generally indicated when there is (1) evidence of systemic envenomation (e.g., neurotoxicity, coagulopathy, rhabdomyolysis, persistent hypotension, or renal failure) or (2) severe local envenomation effects; for example, extensive local tissue injury in snakebite [9,10]. Antivenoms have not been specifically evaluated in pregnant patients, but despite limited evidence, long experience and observation have not demonstrated any particular risks. Antidotes should be used when there is a clear maternal indication to decrease the morbidity and mortality associated with envenomation [9] and, in general, the management which is most beneficial to the mother will provide the best outcome for the pregnancy. Consultation with a poison center and its medical toxicologist or other clinician with expertise in managing envenomations is recommended when treating an envenomated pregnant patient. The poison center can also be helpful in locating and obtaining antivenom for unusual or nonnative (exotic) species, which may not be stocked routinely at a hospital pharmacy.

Pregnancy tests are recommended for any woman of reproductive age who is envenomated. Other laboratory studies are guided by the usual assessment of any particular envenomation. Additional serum testing (electrolytes, coagulation tests, liver enzymes, etc.) may be needed depending upon the scenario and clinical course. As an example, it is standard to obtain a complete blood count, platelets, and coagulation studies with certain Crotalinae [WU3] (rattlesnake, copperhead, and cottonmouth) snakebites.

Concerns about pregnancy, or obvious pregnancy-related risks or effects, may prompt providers to observe envenomated patients longer in an emergency department, or to admit them to the hospital for monitoring or additional treatment. There are little data on pregnancy outcomes in most envenomations. Some studies and reports of high rates of fetal loss in other parts of the world may be secondary to venomous animals with higher degrees of maternal or fetal toxicity or may be secondary to a lack of appropriate medical care in their native environments. In the United States, there are few reports of adverse pregnancy outcomes with envenomations, other than when there is significant maternal toxicity. Regardless, before discharge from a health facility, patients should be coherent, tolerate oral intake, have no progression of symptoms, and any pain should be adequately controlled with oral analgesics. Pregnant patients should have no pregnancy-related risks, and appropriate discharge instructions and follow-up care should be given. More long-term evaluations of individual cases are encouraged to better characterize the long-term results of specific envenomations in pregnancy and to determine any additional strategies other than standard therapies.

22.2 Snake bites

The World Health Organization reports there is evidence that 4.5—5.4 million people a year are bitten by snakes, 1.8—2.7 million of them develop clinical illness, and the death toll could range from 81,000 to 138,000 [11]. There are five major families of venomous snakes: Atractaspididae, Colubridae, Elapidae, Hydrophiidae, and Viperidae. In the United States, Viperidae are represented by three genera and over 30 species of the subfamily Crotalinae (rattlesnakes, copperheads, and cottonmouths) and two genera and three species of one elapid (family: Elapidae), the coral snake.

Crotalinae generally produce a syndrome characterized by local tissue injury, which may include necrosis and hematologic toxicity, including thrombocytopenia, hypofibrinogenemia, and other coagulation abnormalities. There may be systemic effects, such as nausea and diaphoresis or hypotension and, rarely, neurotoxicity such as muscle fasciculation or weakness, that usually do not result in respiratory compromise. The coral snake generally does not produce significant local tissue effects and primarily produces neurotoxicity, which can include respiratory arrest. In other parts of the world, elapids may produce significant local tissue injury, rhabdomyolysis, renal injury, or other effects [12].

Knowledge about the toxicity profiles of local snake species is vital. Expert advice should be sought managing a snake envenomation in a pregnant patient if the envenomation is unfamiliar to the clinician or severe or unusual effects occur. Snakes vary widely in appearance, and identification is rarely possible by the clinician. A digital photo taken at a safe distance may be useful. In places where numerous genera or species overlap, and species-specific antivenom is available, such as Australia, venom detection kits can be useful in determining the appropriate monovalent antivenom [13]. If there is doubt about the snake's identity, treatment should be administered for an unidentified snake bite.

22.2.1 Management during pregnancy

Initial first aid is directed at reducing spread of the venom and expediting transfer to an appropriate medical center [14,15]. The patient should be removed from the snake's territory, kept warm and at rest, and be reassured. The injured part should be immobilized in a functional position below the level of the heart. As with nonpregnant adults, ongoing management is largely supportive but may be accompanied with significant allergic phenomena. Investigations into venom removal devices do not show additional benefit and are therefore not recommended [15]. Use of antivenom for systemic or severe local envenomation warrants consideration of corticosteroids, beforehand. Corticosteroids are often used with early and late allergic reactions. We do not use skin tests, whether or not included with an antivenom or included in the package insert. These have been shown to be insufficiently sensitive or specific to be useful and only exposes the patient to the source animal's protein.

Prolonged corticosteroids are associated with delayed fetal growth in humans [16]. These medications increase oral clefting in experimental animals, yet are less likely to do so in humans [17,18]. None of the antivenoms in use in the United States require pretreatment with corticosteroids, epinephrine, or antihistamines. For a global audience, premedication, especially with epinephrine, is appropriate when either antivenom is associated with high rates of allergic reactions or the management of acute allergic reactions is problematic due to limited staff or facilities [13]. Injection of epinephrine in experimental animals interferes with embryo development, possibly through hemodynamic effects and decreased uterine perfusion [19]. Human studies on inhaled beta-sympathomimetics during pregnancy have not suggested an increased risk of birth defects [20].

Snake envenomations during pregnancy may be accompanied by blood coagulation abnormalities, so prolonged monitoring in the hospital is understandable [20–23]. We recommend a minimum of 8 h of fetal heart rate (FHR) monitoring if the pregnancy is at a viable stage (usually beginning at 24 weeks) [22]. Reports of decreased fetal movements and fetal death a few days after clinically significant envenomations suggest ongoing outpatient surveillance with daily FHR monitoring for up to 1 week may be helpful in identifying pregnancies at risk for an adverse outcome [24,25].

22.2.2 Reports during pregnancy

Several reports about snake bites during pregnancy have revealed normal outcomes, even when antivenom was necessary [21,26,27]. Case reports support management according to the same guidelines used in nonpregnant patients with snake envenomations [28,29]. Adverse pregnancy effects may be due largely to maternal illness. For example, there are case reports of placental abruptions associated with a maternal hypercoagulable state following snake bite [25,30]. In another report, death of a gravid woman after a snakebite was believed to be associated with supine hypotension from aortocaval compression rather than entirely from the venom itself [31]. A third case involved a woman bitten by a pit viper at 10 weeks' gestation [24]. Although the woman recovered from systemic symptoms, a fetal demise was confirmed 1 week later on ultrasound examination.

In a letter to the editor from Sri Lanka in 1985, indirect evidence of placental transfer was described with adverse fetal effects in the absence of maternal symptoms [32]. Four cases of maternal snakebites were reported in which fetal movements were perceived as being less or became absent before or in the absence of maternal illness. In three of those cases, where bites occurred at 32–36 weeks' gestation, the fetuses survived and were delivered alive at term. In the fourth case, of unspecified gestational age, fatal maternal illness developed, although not until after fetal movement had slowed. The fetus was stillborn the day before the mother's death, after the onset of maternal signs and symptoms of illness.

A 2010 report from Nepal described a 33-week pregnant woman who was bitten by a green tree viper [33]. She developed vaginal bleeding, anemia, and severe abnormalities in her coagulation profile. Her fetus was dead when she presented for care. After correction of the coagulation profile, labor was induced and she subsequently recovered. In 2019, two case reports of North American rattlesnake envenomation revealed recurrent coagulopathy of pregnant women in the first trimester, requiring readmission and retreatment with Crotalidae Polyvalent Immune Fab [34]. A 1992 review of 50 cases of North American Crotalinae snakebites during pregnancy in the United States reported a 10% maternal mortality rate and a 43% fetal demise rate [22]. However, this was prior to the introduction of the current Fab and F(ab')2 antivenoms. A 2002 series of 39 snake-envenomated pregnant women had a fetal loss rate of 30% [12]. A more recent 2010 literature review reported a rate of fetal loss around 20% and maternal mortality rate of 4%–5%. This same review reported only two fetal demises and no maternal deaths from US native species [35].

AAPCC database reported 191 snake envenomations between 2009 and 18 with no difference in regards to outcome codes between pregnant and nonpregnant patients. There was an increased likelihood of antivenom administration in pregnancy with rattlesnake exposures, no adverse reactions to antivenom, no maternal deaths, and three fetal losses following snake bites, although a direct correlation cannot be extrapolated [2].

22.3 Spider bites

Spider bites are rare medical events, since only a handful of species cause difficulties in humans. Very few species have muscles powerful enough to penetrate human skin, and most of those spiders bite humans only in rare circumstances. Furthermore, the venom of most spiders has little or no effect. The most likely to inflict significant bites in humans are *Latrodectus* ("widow") spiders and *Loxosceles* species ("recluse") spiders. A spider bite usually presents acutely as a localized solitary papule, pustule, or wheal. Systemic symptoms can accompany some envenomations. Allergic reactions typically result from contact with spiders.

Widow venom contains α-latrotoxin, which provokes a massive presynaptic release of acetylcholine, dopamine, norepinephrine, epinephrine, and glutamate. After a bite, the wound site may become painful, erythematous, and edematous and can have a classic appearance of isolated diaphoresis within an area of central clearing. Neuromuscular symptoms, including severe muscle pain and cramping, usually occur within an hour. Increased autonomic functions leading to tachycardia, tachypnea, and hypertension are also associated and are often correlated with increased pain. Some patients may progress to systemic manifestations (latrodectism) with symptoms including diffuse muscle rigidity and cramping, tenderness, and burning around the bite, truncal and abdominal tenderness, nausea, and vomiting [36].

Bites from *Loxosceles* spiders are customarily necrotic. Their venom contains hyaluronidase and sphingomyelinase D enzymes that along with platelet aggregation and neutrophil activity exacerbate necrosis. Local manifestations of the bite include edema, inflammation, hemorrhage, damage to the vessel wall, thrombosis, and necrosis [37]. Systemic loxoscelism can include acute renal failure, rhabdomyolysis, intravascular hemolysis, and coagulopathy [38] although very few cases and no associated mortalities have been reported in pregnancy. Given extensive differential diagnosis for skin necrosis, and low prevalence of spider bites, the diagnosis of loxoscelism syndrome should be considered only when a spider is caught in the act of biting or otherwise reliably associated with a lesion [39].

Most patients' reports of spider bites are unreliable unless directly witnessed and retrieved for identification. Those who did not clearly witness the bite should be presumed to have some other disorder, and the finding of multiple skin lesions essentially excludes the diagnosis of spider bite. Papules and pustules should be carefully unroofed and cultured to identify infectious causes. Common infections that could be mistaken for spider bites include staphylococcal and streptococcal infections, a skin lesion of early Lyme disease, and atypical presentations of herpes zoster or herpes simplex.

22.3.1 Management during pregnancy

Most patients who sustain a spider bite require only topical therapy (clean with mild soap and water; apply cold, not frozen, packs; and elevate affected body parts). Patients with moderate to severe envenomations, such as those from widow spiders as characterized by severe local symptoms or the presence of regional or systemic symptoms, require supportive care and monitoring for complications. Oral analgesia, parenteral benzodiazepines, and tetanus toxoid may be used safely during pregnancy in the short term [40].

Early surgical excision or debridement is not recommended for patients with *Loxosceles* spider bites that have a dusky center or other signs of developing necrosis. Only antivenom is helpful following a *Loxosceles* envenomation. It is produced by the Instituto Butantan (Brazil) but is not available in the United States. There are reports of approximately 1000 pregnant women who have been treated with dapsone without adverse effect [41—43] although no benefit has been shown. Those reviews and case reports were not specifically designed to study possible reproductive effects of dapsone, however, and dosage and timing of dapsone use were not always clear. Some cases of hemolytic anemia have occurred in mothers and their offspring after exposure to dapsone, both during gestation and while breastfeeding [44].

Mortality from widow bites is low, although envenomation can cause significant pain and require hospitalization [45]. Antivenom reduces the pain and the need for hospitalization, especially when other therapies are unsuccessful [46]. Several widow spider antivenoms are commercially available, although there is sufficient chemical similarity among widow venoms that all widow antivenoms provide some degree of relief. Representative symptoms in which antivenom therapy may be valuable include the following: severe and persistent local pain or muscle cramping, significant pain or diaphoresis extending beyond the immediate site of the bite, alterations in vital signs, difficulty breathing, and nausea and vomiting.

22.3.2 Reports during pregnancy

Black widow spider envenomation is a rare occurrence in pregnant women, and short-term outcomes appear to be favorable [47]. A systematic review revealed four case reports and an observational case series between 1979 and 2011 was found [48,49]. Most common symptoms reported included local erythema, spasms, abdominal cramps, muscle rigidity, hypertension, and anxiety. In only one case, the onset of labor was attributed to the bite and this resolved after antivenom administration [49]. A large observational study based on a review of the AAPCC database from 2000 to 2007 showed 12,640 human black widow spider envenomations, 3194 (25.3%) involved women of reproductive age, and 97 were pregnant [46]. Comparing pregnant with nonpregnant women, there were no significant differences in recommended or administered treatments. A significantly higher percentage of pregnant than nonpregnant patients were treated at a health care facility where they were either released (36.1% vs. 19.9%, $P < .001$) or admitted (13.4% vs. 4.0%, $P < .001$). There were no documented immediate pregnancy losses in that series. Similarly, a review of the AAPCC database from 2009 to 2018 revealed 145 black widow envenomations with no difference in outcomes between pregnant and nonpregnant patients although cases in pregnancy were more likely to receive antivenom treatment [2].

There have been six reported cases of *Loxosceles* (recluse) spider bites in pregnant women. Although the victims were apparently in considerable discomfort, pregnancy outcomes were favorable in all instances [50–52]. We have been unable to locate any reference about the use of *Loxosceles* antivenom, currently not available in the United States, during pregnancy.

22.3.3 Scorpion stings

Scorpion envenomations have been shown to cause pregnancy complications including stillbirth, miscarriage, and preterm birth in some parts of the world [4,53]. However, the extent of adverse effects depends on individual species' cytotoxic, neurotoxic, and hemolytic effects which are not usually a significant problem in the North America region. Stings from *Centruroides sculpturatus* found primarily in northern Mexico and the southwestern United States (e.g., Arizona, New Mexico, western Texas, southeastern California, and near Lake Mead, Nevada) primarily cause localized effects but have the potential to develop neurotoxic symptoms. The tubercle at the base of the stinger of its lobster-like body is helpful in differentiating this highly neurotoxic scorpion from other species.

Envenomations involve injection of a scorpion toxin protein which acts as a neurotoxin. In neuronal membranes, these toxins cause incomplete inactivation of sodium channels which lead to membrane hyperexcitability and consequent repetitive uncontrolled firing of axons [30]. Enhanced release of neurotransmitters at synapses and the neuromuscular junction leads to excessive neuromuscular activity and autonomic dysfunction. In most cases, localized pain and paresthesia represent the extent of symptoms from the envenomation. In some instances, overstimulation of the parasympathetic nervous system may cause systemic neurotoxic effects such as wild flailing and jerking motions of the extremities, visual disturbances, and fasciculations of the tongue [54].

After *C. sculpturatus* envenomation, symptoms typically begin immediately, progress to maximum severity within 5 h, and improve within 9–30 h without antivenom therapy. Local pain and paresthesias occur at the sting site. The puncture wound may be too small to be observed initially, and local inflammation does not occur customarily. However, the sting site is usually very tender to touch. Symptoms often radiate proximally up the affected extremity but may present in remote sites as generalized paresthesias. Rarely, envenomations produce cranial nerves (e.g., roving eye movements) or somatic skeletal neuromuscular dysfunction (e.g., uncoordinated respiratory activity), which may lead to respiratory insufficiency.

22.3.4 Management during pregnancy

Most scorpion stings result in mild envenomations. Management would be the same during pregnancy by cleansing of the sting site, using oral medications (e.g., ibuprofen 10 mg/kg; maximum single dose 800 mg), and administering tetanus prophylaxis. An increased risk of miscarriage was reported with use of ibuprofen or naproxen particularly near the time of conception, but a reanalysis of the data weakened the association [55]. Some, though not all, epidemiology studies have suggested that use of nonsteroidal antiinflammatory drugs, including ibuprofen, during pregnancy may increase the risk of cardiac defects and gastroschisis. Multidosing, especially, during late pregnancy, is likely best to avoid due to concerns about premature ductal closure [56].

Pregnant patients should be observed for about 4 h to ensure that there is no further progression. Those with rare but significant systemic symptoms, including restlessness, muscular fasciculation, hypersalivation, or cranial nerve palsies, require immediate supportive interventions. Airway management, including frequent suctioning of oral secretions or endotracheal intubation, may be indicated in patients with pulmonary edema accompanied by hypoxemia or significant difficulties maintaining airway patency. Maintaining adequate maternal oxygenation is of major importance to the fetus. Close monitoring for and treatment of myocardial ischemia is also warranted in patients with severe symptoms. Short-term treatments during pregnancy may include intravenous fentanyl (1 mcg/kg) for pain, and intravenous benzodiazepines (lorazepam or continuous midazolam infusion) may be given for sedation and to treat muscle spasticity.

Anascorp, an antivenom effective against *C. sculpturatus* envenomation, is primarily used in children (https://www.fda.gov/vaccines-blood-biologics/approved-blood-products/anascorp). Pain and systemic symptoms usually resolve or are significantly decreased within 4 h [82]. However, there are reports of its use in adults, which includes one pregnant woman [83].

22.3.5 Reports during pregnancy

A 2016 review reported five published papers with a total of 27 cases [54]. The majority of patients recovered with only minimal intervention. There was one C-section performed for diagnosis of eclampsia attributed to a scorpion sting, and one fetal death was observed at 6 weeks postenvenomation. A retrospective case series of 24 pregnant women in Taiwan and 11 cases in Turkey showed supportive therapy was adequate in treating scorpion envenomations without need for antivenom. A more recent review of Poison Control Center data from 2009 to 2018 revealed 2097 cases of scorpion stings in the United States with a higher proportion of envenomations determined to have minor effects when compared to nonpregnant reproductive age women. There were no maternal or fetal deaths observed [2].

Evidence regarding the natural history and treatment of scorpion envenomations in pregnancy is derived from animal data [57−59]. Investigations in gravid rodents have revealed mixed results. Turkish investigators reported that pregnant rats treated with venom from the scorpion *Androctonus amoreuxi* had an elevated incidence of fetal resorption, ossification defects, and reduced weight [57]. Use of radiolabeled venom indicated only a small fraction (0.08−0.331/0) was detected in fetuses or placenta [57].

A single subcutaneous injection in pregnant rats with venom from the scorpion *Tityus serrulatus* at 0.3 or 1 mcg/kg on gestation day 5 or 10 did not produce adverse effects on the offspring [58]. Pregnant rats exposed to *Tityus bahiensis* venom at doses not toxic to the dame bore offspring with alterations in the time to achieve developmental milestones [59].

The 5-hydroxytryptamine in some scorpion venoms may act as a uterine stimulant and induce abortion [5,60]. There are also anecdotal reports about pregnant women treated with antivenom without adverse fetal effects [54,61]. We have been unable to locate any additional references on possible adverse reproductive or lactation effects from these agents.

A 2017 report of Anascorp use in three adults included a woman who was 23 weeks pregnant. She obtained relief of her symptoms within 1 h and was discharged home after 4 h of observation, without apparent adverse effects [83].

22.3.6 Hymenoptera

Hymenoptera of clinical relevance include winged insects such as bees, wasps, hornets, and yellowjackets, as well as wingless insects such as imported fire ants. Stings related to these hymenoptera involve the injection of venom, which is almost always acutely painful and noticed by the patient. Although most stings require only symptomatic relief for acute pain, anaphylactic hypersensitivity occurs in 0.3%−3% of patients with a venom allergy and can be the most severe side effect of hymenoptera envenomation [62]. Anaphylaxis and maternal hypoxia can lead to placenta vasoconstriction and uterine contractions, and are a known cause of fetal abnormalities, premature labor, and consequently maternal morbidity or even mortality [63]. This risk can be mitigated with the use of venom immunotherapy (VIT) which has been shown to be safe when continued during pregnancy [64,65].

22.3.7 Winged hymenoptera

Exposure to the venom of winged hymenoptera is common. Depending on the climate, more than half of the general adult population remember receiving a hymenoptera sting at least once from the Apidae family (honey bees and bumblebees) or the Vespidae family (yellowjackets and wasps). The venom of winged hymenoptera consists of 95% aqueous proteins, which are the substrate in human hypersensitivity reactions [66].

In the setting of hymenoptera venom allergy (HVA), the stings of the Apidae and the Vespidae families can result in life-threatening anaphylaxis, and the most severe reactions can be refractory to single or multiple doses of epinephrine [67,68]. HVA is an IgE-mediated disease. Its clinical manifestations result from the degradation of mast cells or basophils, triggered by the binding of allergens to specific IgE on the surface of these cells.

In the HVA setting, sequelae of stings range from large local reactions at the sting site to life-threatening anaphylaxis [69]. Initial management of the winged hymenoptera sting should include removal of foreign bodies such as the detached aculeus or "stinger," and application of cold compresses. Uncomplicated local reactions should resolve within hours. Large local reactions may be treated with oral prednisone and antihistamines. Rarely, the stings of the winged hymenoptera can result in life-threatening anaphylaxis, and the most severe reactions can be refractory to single or multiple doses of epinephrine.

22.3.8 Imported fire ants

Imported fire ants are aggressive venomous insects found in the southern half of the United States from Florida to California. These ants have been known to attack in large numbers when a nest is disturbed and when food availability is scarce. Strong mandibles and an aculeus on the mandible allow the ant to powerfully inject venom, rotate, and inject several more times.

The stings of imported fire ants create an immediate burning sensation appropriate for their name. Their venom consists primarily of alkaloid compounds with hemolytic and cytotoxic properties. The small amount of aqueous proteins is responsible for systemic reactions and anaphylaxis, while the alkaloid component is likely only relevant to humans in cases of mass attacks with numerous stings.

Initial management of this sting includes measures similar to treatment of winged hymenoptera stings. Often a sterile pustule, which is pathognomonic for an imported fire ant sting, develops along with an intense pruritus. Topical steroids and antihistamines are appropriate, and the pustule should be left intact to prevent infection.

22.3.9 Management during pregnancy

In the pregnant patient, as in the general population, the primary concern after hymenoptera venom exposure is identification and treatment of life-threatening anaphylaxis. In this setting, optimization of maternal cardiopulmonary status is of primary concern. Standard treatment for signs of anaphylaxis (widespread hives, wheezing, airway compromise, or altered mental status) should be administered, including early administration of intramuscular epinephrine in the anterolateral aspect of the thigh [70]. We recommend trendelenburg/left lateral recumbent positioning, which may be especially important as poor cardiac return has been suggested as the final step in anaphylactic deaths [71]. An anaphylactic death during pregnancy has been attributed presumably due to uterine compression of venous return [72].

Immunotherapy for venom allergy for prevention of future reactions in previously stung patients with large local or systemic reactions has been available for over 30 years and is highly effective [73]. Initiation of VIT in pregnancy is generally avoided by allergists due to a lack of safety data, though limited reports of use in pregnancy do not suggest an increased risk of adverse outcomes. As such, pregnant women may be allowed to continue VIT if initiated prior to pregnancy [74]. Care should be taken to monitor for signs of preterm labor in this group, because uterine contractions have been reported during or after VIT in several case reports [75]. Victims of hymenoptera envenomation who develop systemic reactions or severe local reactions should be referred upon discharge to an immunologist for evaluation and possible treatment with immunotherapy.

22.3.10 Reports during pregnancy

Few case reports of hymenoptera envenomation are in the obstetric literature and predictably focus on clinically significant events such as anaphylaxis. It is unknown if pregnancy makes systemic reactions to hymenoptera venom more or less likely. Unfavorable outcomes are most likely to be reported, and fetal effects of envenomations are speculative.

A case report from Croatia described a multigravida who presented at 27 weeks' gestation with anaphylaxis after a wasp sting. The authors note that delivery occurred at 35 weeks despite tocolysis and a cerclage and attribute the delivery to a "post anaphylactic reaction." The child developed normally after the delivery [76].

Another adverse outcome was reported in association with anaphylaxis after a bee sting. A 31-year-old was stung at 30 weeks' gestation and developed severe anaphylaxis. Subsequently, the fetus was noted to have an increased biparietal diameter and decreased movement. Spontaneous preterm labor occurred at 35 weeks, and the infant was noted to be cyanotic and hypotonic. The infant died at 64 days, and an autopsy demonstrated cystic cavitation of the white matter consistent with hypoxic injury. Infantile encephalomalacia was attributed to maternal anaphylaxis after bee envenomation [77].

A case from the United Arab Emirates linked placental abruption and intrauterine death with an ant sting. A 21-year-old woman at 40 weeks' gestation presented with dyspnea and swelling after a Samsun ant sting. She was treated for anaphylaxis, then developed vaginal bleeding 16 h later. On ultrasound, a placental separation and fetal demise were diagnosed. A retroplacental clot was confirmed at delivery [72].

22.4 Jellyfish

Jellyfish are responsible for more exposures as well as more severe sequelae than any other source of marine envenomation. Jellyfish stings are common in both warm and cold coastal waters of the United States and Australia. Although there are over 100 species of jellyfish known to cause human envenomations, the most clinically relevant species include *Chironex fleckeri*, *Carukia barnesi*, and the Portuguese man-of-war.

The mechanism of injury in jellyfish stings starts with skin-to-tentacle contact, which allows transfer of multiple venomous capsules called nematocysts. The nematocysts discharge rapidly on contact, allowing intradermal injection of proteinaceous toxins. The subsequent local and potentially systemic reactions range from minor nuisance to myocardial injury or Irukandji syndrome, a life-threatening cascade of multisystem organ failure due to systemic hypersensitivity.

If a jellyfish sting is suspected or confirmed, symptom relief and observation are usually the only necessary treatment [78]. Tentacles and nematocysts should be removed with a plastic object such as a credit card and washed with seawater. Vigorous rubbing and immersion in cold freshwater should be avoided due to the potential to trigger nematocyst discharge. Immersion in water heated to 110–113°F and treatment of affected areas with acetic acid (household vinegar) have both been shown to be beneficial.

Severe jellyfish stings with systemic effects require immediate medical care and possibly antivenom administration [79]. In Australia, major box jellyfish (*C. fleckeri*) stings have caused more than 70 known deaths. Large tentacle exposure can produce cardiotoxic, neurotoxic, dermonecrotic, and hemolytic effects [80]. *C. barnesi*, found in Australia, Hawaii, and Florida, can cause a hypersensitivity reaction marked by myocardial injury and pulmonary edema known as Irukandji syndrome. Sheep serum antivenom and magnesium sulfate may play a role for patients with cardiogenic shock, pulmonary edema, or deteriorating critical condition [81].

A delayed hypersensitivity reaction can occur 7–14 days after jellyfish envenomation. Symptoms can include papules, urticaria, and an erythematous welt in the shape of the jellyfish tentacles. Antihistamines and topical corticosteroids are recommended. Resolution is expected within 10 days, although some reactions can be refractory.

22.4.1 Management during pregnancy

We recommend steps to limit jellyfish exposure during pregnancy. Protective clothing and commercially available Safe Sea lotion have been shown to reduce sting frequency. Pregnant women with a small-area sting and mild, strictly local symptoms do not require medical attention other than tentacle removal, seawater and vinegar application, and topical management of any symptoms.

Any sign of systemic reaction should be taken seriously and would include inpatient evaluation or prolonged observation. If cardiopulmonary compromise is present or suspected, supportive intervention should be initiated as with a nonpregnant patient. Sheep serum antivenom may be considered in severe cases with life-threatening processes such as airway compromise or cardiovascular collapse if maternal benefit would be expected [78]. Magnesium sulfate adjuvant therapy is commonly used for other obstetric conditions and is considered to be safe.

22.4.2 Reports during pregnancy

Only one case report of serious jellyfish envenomation was found in the obstetric literature. This case involved a 20-year-old woman at 34 weeks' gestation in Australia [80]. She was stung by the box jellyfish *C. fleckeri*, began screaming in pain, and then experienced pallor and altered mental status. A park official reported that she developed apnea and cyanosis. He doused the tentacles and stings with methylated spirits and began cardiopulmonary resuscitation (CPR) with expired air. A nurse was summoned, who also happened to be pregnant at 37 weeks. She also observed cyanosis and performed CPR, which led to spontaneous ventilation. In doing so, the gravid nurse suffered stings from adherent tentacles. The original victim was transported by ambulance to a hospital, and antivenom was administered within 30 min of the envenomation. She recovered and was discharged from hospital after 4 days. Both pregnant women subsequently delivered healthy term infants.

22.5 Antivenom use during pregnancy

Most reports of antivenom use during pregnancy are anecdotal. The most reported experience has been with snake bites, and observations from limited case reports are reassuring. Reproduction studies regarding the crotalid antivenom have not been reported in animals. Black widow spider antivenom was not associated with apparent adverse effects beyond those inherent to the antidote. While there are limited long-term evaluations of children whose mothers were administered black widow spider antivenom, it appears to be a reasonable therapy if indicated after clinical evaluation.

Current evidence indicates that antivenom is effective and may significantly reduce the duration of suffering and hospitalization. Antivenoms should be considered when envenomations seriously threatens a pregnancy or have the potential to cause long-term effects and are unresponsive to other therapies. Consideration should be given for the following moderate to severe symptoms: severe and persistent local pain or muscle cramping, significant pain or diaphoresis extending beyond the immediate site of the bite, alterations in vital signs, difficulty breathing, nausea and vomiting, and potential limb-threatening effects. Consultation with a medical toxicologist or other physician with experience in managing various envenomations is recommended before any antivenom administration. Several antivenoms may be commercially available, and toxicologists can be helpful in ordering the antivenom which may not be at the hospital pharmacy.

Frequencies of allergic reactions and delayed serum sickness-like reactions from antivenom are presumed to be similar regardless of pregnancy. Allergic reactions should be managed by immediately stopping intravenous infusion of the antivenom (if applicable) and treating symptoms appropriately. Before administering any antivenom, medications and equipment for the treatment of anaphylaxis should be immediately available, including intravenous fluids, epinephrine, and intubation equipment. Delayed serum sickness-like reactions are unlikely. However, any patient receiving antivenom should be informed about possible symptoms suggestive of serum sickness (rashes, pruritus, arthralgia, and fever) and advised to seek medical care if such symptoms develop.

Thimerosal (merthiolate; thiomersal) is an antiinfective and preservative that has been used as an additive in many biologics, vaccines, and antivenom. There are insufficient data to make a causal connection between thimerosal and any increased risk for birth defects in exposed offspring [82]. Epidemiologic studies have not demonstrated a causal relationship between thimerosal and autism or autism spectrum disorders. The manufacturer cautions that the thimerosal (0.11 mg of mercury per vial) may be associated with mercury-related toxicities, including neurologic and renal toxicities in the fetus and very young children [82]. The amount of mercury in a typical dose would not otherwise be likely to produce fetal harm.

22.6 **Conclusions**

Envenomations from snake or spider bites or from scorpion, hymenoptera, or jellyfish stings likely occur with similar frequencies among reproductive-aged women regardless of pregnancy. Although adults appear to be envenomated more often, children are more likely to develop severe illness. Furthermore, any adverse outcomes may not result directly from the venom in the fetal circulation but indirectly from maternal illness or from placental compromise. For these reasons, more prolonged or more frequent monitoring of both the patient and her fetus is justified. The same fundamental principles of conservative and drug therapy apply when someone is pregnant. Very limited experience with antivenom therapy suggests that it is well tolerated during pregnancy with standard precautions. Prospective evaluations of individual cases that require prolonged monitoring or hospitalization, especially with antivenom administration, would permit a clearer understanding of long-term pregnancy outcomes.

References

[1] Cases of envenomation in pregnancy, 2009—2018. American association of poison control centers database. Accessed July 2019.

[2] Ramirez-Cruz MP, Smolinske SC, Warrick BJ, Rayburn WF, Seifert SA. Envenomations during pregnancy reported to the national poison data system. 2009-2018, 168. Toxicon; 2020. p. 78—82.

[3] Vetter RS, Isbister GK. Medical aspects of spider bites. Annu Rev Entomol 2008;53:409—29.

[4] Ben Nasr H, Hammami TS, Sahnoun Z, Rebai T, Bouaziz M, Kassis M, et al. Scorpion envenomation symptoms in pregnant women. J Venom Anim Toxins Incl Trop Dis 2007;13:94—102. http://www.scielo.br/scielo.php?script=sci_arttext&pid=S1678-91992007000100007.

[5] Osman OH, Ismail M, El-Asmar MF, Ibrahim SA. Effect on the rat uterus on the venom from the scorpion Leiurus quinquestriatus. Toxicon 1972;10:363—6.

[6] Kroger AT, Atkinson WL, Marcuse EK, Pickering LK. Advisory committee on immunization practices (ACIP) centers for disease control and prevention (CDC). General recommendations on immunization: recommendations of the advisory committee on immunization practices (ACIP). MMWR Recomm Rep 2006;55(RR-15):1—48.

[7] American College of Obstetricians and Gynecologists. Update on immunization and pregnancy: tetanus, diphtheria, and pertussis vaccination. Obstet Gynecol 2017;130:e153—7. Committee Opinion No. 718.

[8] Kularasiri SA, Kumarasiri PV, Pushpakumara SK, Dissanayaka WP, Ariyasena H, Gawarammana IB, et al. Routine antibiotic therapy in the management of the local inflammatoryswelling in venomous snakebites: results of a placebo- controlled study. Ceylon Med J 2005;50:151—5.

[9] Bailey B. Are the teratogenic risks associated with antidotes used in the acute management of poisoned pregnant women? Birth Defects Res (Part A) 2003;67:133—40.

[10] Cheng AC, Winkel KD. Antivenom efficacy, safety and availability: measuring smoke. Med J Aust 2004;180:5—6.

[11] World Health Organization. Prevalence of snakebite envenoming. https://www.who.int/snakebites/epidemiology/en/.

[12] Gold BS, Dart RC, Barish RA. Bites of venomous snakes. N Engl J Med 2002;347:347—56.

[13] Sutherland SK. Antivenom use in Australia. Premedication, adverse reactions and the use of envenom detection kits. Med J Aust 1992;157:734—9.

[14] Cheng AC, Currie BJK. Venomous snakebites worldwide with a focus on the Australia-Pacific region: current management and controversies. J Intensive Care Med 2004;19:259—69.

[15] Principles of snakebite management worldwide. UpToDate; 2011. www.uptodate.com.

[16] Pirson Y, Van Lierde M, Ghysen J, Squifflet JP, Alexandre GP, van Ypersele de Strihou C. Retardation of fetal growth in patients receiving immunosuppres- sive therapy. N Engl J Med 1985;313:328.

[17] Pinsky L, DiGeorge AM. Cleft palate in the mouse: a teratogenic index of glu- cocorticoid potency. Science 1965;147:402—3.

[18] Carmichael SL, Shaw GM, Ma C, Werler MM, Rasmussen SA, Lammer EJ. Maternal corticosteroid use and orofacial clefts. Am J Obstet Gynecol 2007;197:e1—7. 585.

[19] Norris MC, Grieco W, Arkoosh VA. Does continuous intravenous infusion of low-concentration epinephrine impair uterine blood flow in pregnant ewes? Reg Anesth 1995;20(3):206—11.

[20] Schatz M, Zeiger RS, Harden KM, Hoffman CP, Forsythe AB, Chilingar LM, et al. The safety of inhaled (beta)-agonist bronchodilators during pregnancy. J Allergy Clin Immunol 1988;82:686—95.

[21] Kravitz J, Gerardo CJ. Copperhead snake bite treated with crotalidae polyva- lent immune fab(ovine) antivenom in third trimester pregnancy. Clin Toxicol 2006;44(3): 353—4.

[22] Dunnihoo DR, Rust BM, Wise RB, Brooks GG, Otterson WN. Snake bite poisoning in pregnancy: a review of the literature. J Reprod Med 1992;37:653—8.

[23] LaMonica GE, Selfert SA, Rayburn WF. Rattlesnake bites in pregnant women. J Reprod Med 2010;55(11—12):520—2.

[24] Nasu K, Sueda T, Miyakawa I. Intrauterine fetal death caused by pit viper venom poisoning in early pregnancy. Gynecol Obstet Invest 2004;57(2):114—6.

[25] Hanprasertpong J, Hanprasertpong T. Abruptio placentae and fetal death following a Malayanpit viper bite. J Obstet Gynaecol Res 2008;34(2):258—61.

[26] Habib AG, Abubakar SB, Abubakar IS, Larnyang S, Durfa N, Nasidi A, et al. Envenoming after carpet viper (*Echis ocellatus*) bite during pregnancy: timely use of effective antivenom improves maternal and fetal outcomes. Trop Med Int Health 2008;13(9): 1172—5.

[27] Duru M, Helvaci M, Peker E, Dolapcioglu K, Kaya E. Reptile bite in pregnancy. Hum Exp Toxicol 2008;27(12):931—2.

[28] Vikrant S, Parashar A. Case report: snakebite -induced acute kidney injury: report of a successful outcome during pregnancy. Am J Trop Med Hyg 2017;96:885—6. Ghosh N, Henderson J, Kim H, Ancar F. Rattlesnake Envenomation in the Third Trimester of Pregnancy. Obstet & Gyneco. 2018; 132(3).

[29] Zugaib M, de Barros AC, Bittar RE, Burdmann EA, Neme B. Abruptio placentae following snake bite. Am J Obstet Gynecol 1985;151:754—5.

[30] Sutherland SK, Duncan AW, Tibballs J. Death from a snake bite associated with the supine hypotensive syndrome of pregnancy. Med J Aust 1982;2:238—9.

[31] James RF. Snake bite in pregnancy (letter). Lancet 1985;2:731.

[32] Pant HP, Poudel R, D'souza V. Intrauterine death following green tree viper bite presenting as antepartum hemorrhage. Int J Obstet Anesth 2010;19(1):102—3.

[33] Moore EC, Porter LM, Ruha AM. Rattlesnake venom-induced recurrent coagulopathy in first trimester pregnant women—two cases. Toxicon 2019;163:8—11.

[34] Langley RL. Snakebite during pregnancy: a literature review. Wilderness Environ Med 2010;21(1):54—60.

[35] Williams M, Anderson J, Nappe TM. Black widow spider toxicity [Updated 2020 Apr 22]. In: StatPearls [internet]. Treasure Island (FL): StatPearls Publishing; January, 2020. Available from: https://www.ncbi.nlm.nih.gov/books/NBK499987/.

[36] Rahmani F, Khojasteh SMB, Bakhtavr HE, Rahmani F, Nia KS, Faridaalaee G. Poisonous spiders: bites, symptoms, and treatment; an educational review. Emergency 2014;2(2):54—8.

[37] Malaque C, Santoro ML, Cardoso JLC, et al. Clinical picture and laboratorial evaluation in human loxoscelism. Toxicon;58(8):664—671.

[38] Bennett RG, Vetter RS. An approach to spider bites. Erroneous attribution of dermone-crotic lesions to brown recluse or hobo spider bites in Canada. Can Fam Physic 2004; 50(8):1098.

[39] Vetter RS, Swanson DL, White J, White J. Management of widow spider bites. In: Post T, editor. UpToDate. Waltham, MA: UpToDate; 2020. www.uptodate.com. [Accessed 8 August 2020].

[40] Kahn G. Dapsone is safe during pregnancy. J Am Acad Dermatol 1985;13:838−9.

[41] Lyde CB. Pregnancy in patients with Hansen disease. Arch Dermatol 1997;133:623−7.

[42] Brabin BJ, Eggelte TA, Parise M, Verhoeff F. Dapsone therapy for malaria during pregnancy:maternal and fetal outcomes. Drug Saf 2004;27:633−48.

[43] Sanders SW, Zone JJ, Flotz RL, Tolman KG, Rollins DE. Haemolytic anemia induced by dapsone transmitted through breast milk. Ann Intern Med 1982;90:465−6.

[44] Scalzone JM, Wells SL. Lactrodectus mactans (black widow spider) envenomation: an unusual cause for abdominal pain in pregnancy. Obstet Gynecol 1994;83:830−1.

[45] Wolfe MD, Myers O, Caravati EM, Rayburn WF, Seifert SA. Black widow spider envenomation in pregnancy. J Matern Fetal Neonatal Med 2011;24(1):122−6.

[46] Handel CC, Izquierdo LA, Curet LB. Black widow spiders (Latrodectus mac- tans) bite during pregnancy. West J Med 1994;160:261−2.

[47] Clark RF, Wethern-Kestner S, Vance MV, Gerkin R. Clinical presentation and treatment of black widow spider envenomation: a review of 163 cases. Ann Emerg Med 1992;21: 782−7.

[48] Troiano G, Bagnoli A, Nante N. Venomous bites during pregnancy: the black widow spider (*Latrodectus mactans*). Toxin Rev 2019;38(3):171−5.

[49] Sherman RP. Black widow spider (*Latrodectus mactans*) envenomation in a term pregnancy. Curr Surg 2000;57(4):346−8.

[50] Anderson PC. Loxoscelism threatening pregnancy: five cases. Am J Obstet Gynecol 1991;165:1454−6.

[51] Elgabalawi E. Loxoscelism in a pregnant woman. Eur J Dermatol 2009;19(3):289.

[52] Najafian M, Ghorbani A, Zargar M, Baradaran M, Baradaran N. Scorpion stings in pregnancy: an analysis of outcomes in 66 envenomed pregnant patients in Iran. J Venom Anim Toxins Incl Trop Dis 2020;26.

[53] Shah N, Martens MG. Scorpion envenomation in pregnancy. Med J 2016;109(6): 338−41.

[54] Nielsen GL, Sorensen HT, Larsen H, Pedersen L. Risk of adverse birth outcome and miscarriage in pregnant users of non-steroidal anti-inflammatory drugs; population basedo bservational study and case−control study. BMJ 2001;322:266−70.

[55] Ofori B, Oraichi D, Blais L, Rey E, Berard A. Risk of congenital anomalies in pregnant users of non-steroidal anti-infiammatory drugs: a nested case− control study. Birth Defects Res B DevReprod Toxicol 2006;77:268−79.

[56] LoVecchio F, Welch S, Klemens J, Curry SC, Thomas R. Incidence of immediate and delayed hypersensitivity to Centruroides antivenom. Ann Emerg Med 1999;34:615.

[57] Dorce AL, Bellot RG, Dorce VA, Nencioni AL. Effects of prenatal exposure to *Tityus Bahiensis* scorpion venom on rat offspring development. Reprod Toxicol 2009;28(3): 365−70.

[58] Cruttenden K, Nencioni ALA, Bernardi MM, Dorce VAC. Reproductive toxic effects of Tityus serrulatus scorpion venom in rats. Reprod Toxicol 2008;25:497−503.

[59] Marei ZA, Ibrahim SA. Stimulation of rat uterus by venom from the scorpion *L. quinquestriatus*. Toxicon 1979;17:251—8.

[60] Langley RL. A review of venomous animal bites and stings in pregnant patients. WildernessEnviron Med 2004;15:207—15.

[61] Bilo BM, Bonifazi F. Epidemiology of insect-venom anaphylaxis. Curr Opin Allergy Clin Immunol 2008;8:330—7.

[62] Oykhman P, Kim HL, Ellis AK. Allergen immunotherapy in pregnancy. Allergy Asthma Clin Immunol 2015;11:31.

[63] Pałgan K, Żbikowska-Götz M, Chrzaniecka E, Bartuzi Z. Venom immunotherapy and pregnancy. Postepy Dermatologii I Alergologii 2018;35(1):90—2.

[64] Bilò MB, Cichocka-Jarosz E, Pumphrey R, et al. Self-medication of anaphylactic reactions due to hymenoptera stings — an EAACI task force consensus statement. Allergy 2016;71:931—43.

[65] Antonicelli L, Bilò MB, Bonifazi F. Epidemiology of hymenoptera allergy. Curr Opin Allergy Clin Immunol 2002;2:341—6.

[66] Baer H, Liu TY, Anderson MC, Blum M, Schmid WH, James FJ. Protein components of fire antvenom (*Solenopsis invicta*). Toxicon 1979;17:397—405.

[67] Hunt KJ, Valentine MD, Sobotka AK, Benton AW, Amodio FJ, Lichtenstein LM. A controlled trial of immunotherapy in insect hypersensitivity. N Engl J Med 1978; 299:157—61.

[68] Smith PL, Kagey-Sobotka A, Bleecker ER, et al. Physiologic manifestations of human anaphylaxis. J Clin Invest 1980;66:1072—80.

[69] Severino M, Bonadonna P, Passalacqua G. Large local reactions from stinging insects: from epidemiology to management. Curr Opin Allergy Clin Immunol 2009;9(4): 334—7.

[70] Brown SG. Cardiovascular aspects of anaphylaxis: implication for treatment and diagnosis. Curr Opin Allergy Clin Immunol 2005;5:359—64.

[71] Rizk D, Mensah-Brown E, Lukic M. Placental abruption and intrauterine death following an ant sting. Int J Gynaecol Obstet 1998;63(1):71—2.

[72] La Shell MS, Calabria CW, Quinn JM. Imported fire ant field reaction and immunotherapy safety characteristics: the IFACS study. J Allergy Clin Immunol 2010;125(6): 1294—9.

[73] Golden DB. Insect sting anaphylaxis. Immunol Allergy Clin 2007;27(2):261—72. vii.

[74] Schwartz HJ, Golden DB, Lockey RF. Venom immunotherapy in the Hymenoptera-allergic pregnant patient. J Allergy Clin Immunol 1990;85(4):709—12.

[75] Habek D, Cerkez-Habek J, Jalsovec D. Anaphylactic shock in response to wasp sting in pregnancy. Zentralbl Gynakoi 2000;122(7):393.

[76] Erasmus BW, Wilson J. Infantile multicystic encephalomalacia after maternal bee sting anaphylaxis during pregnancy. Arch Dis Child 1982;57:785—7.

[77] Lopez EA, Weisman RS, Bernstein J. A prospective study of the acute therapy of jellyfishenvenomations. J Toxicol Clin Toxicol 2000;38:513.

[78] Currie BJ. Marine antivenoms. J Toxicol Clin Toxicol 2003;41:301—8.

[79] Currie BJ, Jacups SP. Prospective study of Chironex fleckeri and other box jellyfish stings in the"Top End" of Australia's Northern Territory. Med J Aust 2005;183:631—6.

[80] Corkeron MA. Magnesium infusion to treat Irukandji syndrome. Med J Aust 2003;178: 411.

[81] Thimerosal in vaccines. 2009. Last online update July 1, http://www.fda.gov/cber/vaccine/thimfaq.

[82] Boyer L, Theodorou A, Berg R, Mallie J. Antivenom for critically ill children with neurotoxicity from scorpion stings. N Engl J Med 2009;14;360(20):2090−8.

[83] Hurst N, Lipe D, Karpen S, Patanwala A, Taylor A, Boesen K, Shirazi F. Centruroides sculpturatus envenomation in three adult patients requiring treatment treatment with antivenom. Clin Toxicol 2017;56(4):294−6.

Gastrointestinal disorders

Megan Lutz, Sumona Saha

University of Wisconsin School of Medicine and Public Health, Department of Medicine, Madison, WI, United States

23.1 Gastroesophageal reflux disease

Gastroesophageal reflux disease (GERD), most commonly manifested as heartburn, is estimated to affect 40%−85% of pregnant women [1]. Risk factors for GERD in pregnancy include increasing gestational age, parity, and a history of heartburn [2]. In addition to heartburn, pregnant women may experience other GERD-related symptoms such as regurgitation and epigastric pain. Less likely manifestations of GERD include chest pain, hoarseness, sore throat, chronic cough, and asthma [3].

The pathophysiology of GERD is believed to be multifactorial. Decreased resting lower esophageal sphincter (LES) pressure due to the effects of estrogen and progesterone are thought to be important contributors to gestational GERD along with decreased sensitivity of the LES to physiologic stimuli [4]. Other proposed factors include decreased esophageal peristalsis, esophageal dysmotility, and delayed gastric emptying due to hormonal and mechanical changes [5].

Most patients have a benign disease course, with only a few experiencing GERD-related complications such as gastrointestinal (GI) bleeding or stricture formation. In general, symptoms begin at the end of the first trimester, worsen through the remainder of pregnancy, and then resolve promptly after delivery. Diagnosis is made based on symptoms, and more invasive measures such as endoscopy and esophageal pH studies are generally not indicated. Barium studies such as esophagrams should be avoided in pregnancy due to the risks of radiation exposure to the fetus.

23.1.1 Treatment

23.1.1.1 Therapeutic lifestyle modifications

Treatment of GERD in pregnancy should follow a "step-up" approach. Treatment should begin with therapeutic lifestyle modifications including strict abstinence from tobacco and alcohol and avoiding late-night meals, recumbency after eating, and trigger foods (e.g., spicy or sour foods, carbonated beverages, coffee, and chocolate). Eating several small meals throughout the day, elevating the head of the bed by 6 inches, and sleeping on the left side may provide additional benefit [6].

Clinical Pharmacology During Pregnancy. https://doi.org/10.1016/B978-0-12-818902-3.00016-6

In addition, medications known to provoke GERD such as anticholinergics, sedatives, theophylline, prostaglandins, and calcium channel blockers should be discontinued, when possible. It is estimated that 25% of patients with uncomplicated GERD have symptom resolution after making these modifications [7].

23.1.2 Antacids

For patients who fail to respond to conservative measures, antacids and alginic acid constitute first-line pharmacologic therapy. Aluminum, magnesium, and calcium-based antacids are generally considered safe in pregnancy. Calcium-based antacids have the added benefit of increasing calcium intake which has been associated with the prevention of preeclampsia [8].

Patients taking antacids, however, should be aware of the possibility of aluminum-containing antacids causing constipation and magnesium-containing antacids causing diarrhea [9]. Furthermore, magnesium-containing antacids should be avoided later in pregnancy, due to their ability to arrest labor and precipitate seizures. Magnesium trisilicate has potentially teratogenic properties in high doses and should be avoided throughout pregnancy [1]. Also patients on iron should be advised not to take iron and antacids together in order to maximize iron absorption by an acidic gastric pH. Sodium bicarbonate should not be taken due to the risk of metabolic alkalosis and fluid overload in the mother and fetus [10].

Alginic acid is considered effective and fast acting in most pregnant patients. Although it has not been studied extensively, it should be safe because it is not absorbed systemically. An open-label trial reported "very good" or "good" symptom relief in the majority of women taking alginic acid within 10 min [11].

23.1.3 Sucralfate

Sucralfate is an aluminum salt of a sulfated disaccharide. As it is poorly absorbed from the GI tract, it acts mainly as a local mucosal protectant. Sucralfate has been shown in a randomized controlled trial in pregnancy to provide greater relief from heartburn and regurgitation than lifestyle and dietary modifications alone [12].

23.1.4 Promotility agents

Metoclopramide is a prokinetic, dopamine antagonist which may be useful in the treatment of GERD by increasing LES pressure, improving esophageal acid clearance, and promoting gastric emptying. Use of metoclopramide is often limited by its poor tolerability and the risk for extrapyramidal side effects. Due to the rare risk of tardive dyskinesia, a black-box warning was issued in 2009. The risk of tardive dyskinesia increases with high dose or long-term use of the drug (use greater than 3 months) and continues even after the drug has been discontinued. It has been reported that the risk of tardive dyskinesia is likely <1% [12].

23.1.5 H_2-receptor antagonists

The H_2-receptor antagonists (H_2-RAs) form the next tier of therapy. H_2-RAs are considered safe in pregnancy. A 2009 metaanalysis by Gill et al. (with data from 2398 H_2-RA exposed pregnancies and 119,892 unexposed controls) found no increased risk of fetal malformations with the use of H_2-RAs in pregnancy [13]. No increased risks for spontaneous abortions, preterm delivery, and small for gestational age were found either.

Despite the longstanding availability of H_2-RAs, only ranitidine, studied at a dose of 150 mg twice daily, has been shown in a randomized, double-blind trial to be efficacious in pregnancy [14]. However, due to the detection of low levels of N-nitrosodimethylamine (NDMA), a probable human carcinogen, in 2020, the FDA requested all manufacturers withdraw all prescription and over-the-counter ranitidine formulations from the market [15]. Cimetidine is likely equally effective; however, due to the antiandrogenic effects seen in animals and nonpregnant humans, some authors advise against its use in pregnancy [15,16]. Although it appears to be safe, famotidine carries fewer safety data in pregnancy. Nizatidine is approved for use in pregnancy; however, studies in some animal models have reported abortions, fewer live fetuses, and low fetal weights with high dose exposure [17]; it is a less preferred option among the H_2-RAs [18]. Furthermore, liquid and capsule formulations have recently been voluntary recalled by their manufacturer due to the detection of NDMA [19].

23.1.6 Proton pump inhibitors

Proton pump inhibitors (PPIs) are typically reserved for patients with severe symptoms refractory to lifestyle modification and the older generation medications. Previous animal studies suggested concern with omeprazole; however, a growing amount of data supports the safety of PPIs during pregnancy.

In the same 2009 metaanalysis which examined H_2-RAs, there was no statistically significant difference found in rates of major malformations, spontaneous abortions, or preterm delivery with first-trimester use of PPIs in 1530 PPI-exposed versus 133,410 nonexposed controls [20].

A Danish cohort study examining 840,968 live births, of which 5082 were exposed to a PPI between 4 weeks before conception and the end of the first trimester, did find a minor difference in abnormalities in the newborns of exposed (3.2%) and nonexposed (2.6%) women (adjusted prevalence odds ratio, 1.23; 95% CI, 1.05−1.44) [19]. The risk of birth defects, however, was not significantly increased in secondary analyses of exposure to individual PPIs during the first trimester.

Thus, based on the available data, PPI use in pregnancy does appear to be safe with anecdotal data favoring lansoprazole [21]. First trimester exposure, however, should be avoided when possible due to the possible increased risk for fetal malformations. While most patients can be effectively treated with once-a-day dosing, some may need to be dosed twice daily. The various medical therapies for GERD are summarized in Table 23.1.

Table 23.1 Medications for gastroesophageal reflux disease.

Drug		Recommendations in pregnancy c	Recommendations in lactation
Antacids	Calcium based	Safe	Compatible
	Magnesium based	Avoid in late pregnancy as may arrest labor and precipitate seizures; can cause diarrhea.	Avoid magnesium trisilicate
	Aluminum based	Can cause constipation and possibly fetal neurotoxicity	
	Alginic acid	Safe	
	Sodium bicarbonate	Contraindicated due to risk for maternal fluid overload and metabolic alkalosis	
Sucralfate		Safe	Compatible
Metoclopramide		Avoid long-term, high-dose use due to risk for tardive dyskinesia	Limited human data: potential toxicity
H_2-receptor antagonists	Ranitidine	Not advised due to contamination with NMDA	Not advised
	Cimetidine	May have antiandrogenic properties	Compatible
	Famotidine	Probably safe	Compatible
	Nizatidine	Not advised due to contamination with NMDA	Not advised
	Omeprazole	Reserve for refractory patients; avoid first trimester use	Not recommended
Proton pump inhibitors	Lansoprazole Pantoprazole Rabeprazole Esomeprazole		

NMDA, *N nitrosodimethylamine*.

23.2 Peptic ulcer disease

Older studies suggest the incidence of peptic ulcer disease (PUD) is decreased in pregnancy [22]. The reported incidence rate of 0.005% is likely an underestimate, however, due to the underreporting of symptoms by patients and the reluctance to perform endoscopy during pregnancy by physicians. Risk factors for PUD in pregnancy include smoking, nonsteroidal antiinflammatory drug use, alcoholism, genetic predisposition, gastritis, *Helicobacter pylori* infection, and advanced maternal age [22].

23.2.1 Treatment

H$_2$-RAs constitute first-line therapy for PUD in pregnancy. In patients who remain symptomatic, PPIs should be used. These drug classes are covered in detail in Section 23.1. Patients found to have *H. pylori* infection during their work-up should generally be treated for this after pregnancy and lactation have been completed.

The most common treatment regimen is triple therapy with a 10-day course of twice daily PPI, amoxicillin, and clarithromycin. For patients who are penicillin allergic or have resistant infection, quadruple therapy with twice daily PPI, metronidazole, bismuth, and tetracycline is used. In the rare case when treatment is warranted during pregnancy, tetracycline and bismuth should not be used. Bismuth is discussed below, while the antibiotics used to treat *H. pylori* are discussed in Section 23.6 and summarized in Table 23.3.

23.2.1.1 Bismuth subsalicylate

Bismuth subsalicylate is hydrolyzed in the GI tract into organic bismuth salts which are poorly absorbed and salicylates which are readily absorbed. Although bismuth has not been reported to cause fetal abnormalities in humans, chronic administration of bismuth tartrate in animal studies has been associated with poor outcomes [23]. Furthermore, chronic ingestion of salicylates during pregnancy may lead to fetal malformations, premature closure of the ductus arteriosus in utero, and intrauterine growth retardation [21]. Thus, bismuth subsalicylate should not be used in pregnancy or lactation.

23.2.1.2 Pancreatitis

Acute pancreatitis in pregnancy is most commonly caused by gallstones [24]. It generally resolves with supportive care including aggressive hydration, analgesia, and early enteral nutrition as tolerated. Unfortunately, biliary pancreatitis has an exceptionally high recurrence rate in pregnancy [25] and early cholecystectomy should be discussed [26]. Occasionally, patients require treatment with antimicrobials for infected pancreatic necrosis. Use of agents known to penetrate pancreatic necrosis such as metronidazole or meropenem should be considered in this setting. These antibiotics are discussed in Section 23.6 and summarized in Table 23.3.

Chronic pancreatitis is often the result of alcohol abuse. Patients should be monitored for malabsorption. Pancreatic enzymes supplement endogenous enzyme production. They are likely safe in pregnancy; however, due to limited safety data, they should be avoided if nonessential.

23.2.1.3 Irritable bowel syndrome

Irritable bowel syndrome (IBS) is a group of functional bowel disorders in which abdominal discomfort or pain is associated with defecation or a change in bowel habits [27]. Patients typically report abdominal pain, bloating, constipation, or diarrhea. Despite the prevalence of IBS among women [28], few large studies of pregnant women with IBS have been conducted [29]. One recent study using the United Kingdom General Practice Research database found a higher risk of miscarriage and ectopic pregnancy in women with IBS [30]. Whether there is a causal link between IBS and these adverse outcomes or whether confounding by a comorbidity such as pelvic inflammatory disease accounts for these results is not known. Below is a discussion of the most common symptoms of IBS including recommendations for treatment in pregnancy.

23.3 Constipation

Constipation is one of the most frequently encountered GI disorders in pregnancy [31]. It is estimated to affect up to 40% of pregnant women [32]. Low frequency of stools (<3 per week), hard stools, and/or difficulties on evacuation of feces have been suggested to be good clinical criteria for constipation in pregnancy [33]. The pathophysiology of constipation in pregnancy is multifactorial. Decreased colonic motility due to the effect of progesterone, poor oral intake of food and fluid due to nausea and vomiting, psychological stress, iron supplementation, thyroid disease, gestational diabetes, and mechanical pressure on the rectosigmoid colon by the gravid uterus may all contribute to its development [34].

23.3.1 Treatment

23.3.1.1 Conservative treatment

The initial management of constipation in pregnancy includes patient education and reassurance about normal bowel function in pregnancy. In addition, patients should increase their physical activity, gain better control of pelvic floor musculature using Kegel exercises, and schedule defecation after meals to take advantage of the gastrocolic reflex. Patients should also avoid constipating foods such as those containing iron and calcium and increase their fluid and fiber intake [35].

23.3.1.2 Stool-bulking agents

Stool-bulking agents such as methylcellulose, psyllium, and unprocessed bran are the preferred first-line therapy in pregnancy as they are not systemically absorbed and thus considered safe for the developing fetus and the neonate during lactation. Stool-bulking agents soften stool and increase stool volume by drawing water into the GI tract. A recent Cochrane review found clear evidence of the effectiveness of fiber supplements on the frequency of defecation (OR 0.18, 95% CI 0.05−0.67) and softening of stools, although notes that these agents may take several days to take full effect [36].

23.3.1.3 Hyperosmotic agents

Hyperosmotic agents increase osmolar tension, thereby causing an increase in water secretion into the gut lumen. These include saline osmotics (magnesium and sodium salts), saccharated osmotics (lactulose, sorbitol), and polyethylene glycol (PEG). Saline osmotic laxatives such as magnesium citrate, magnesium hydroxide, and sodium phosphate work rapidly, but only provide short-term, intermittent relief and are not advisable for daily use [37]. In addition, magnesium citrate and magnesium hydroxide can cause sodium retention in the mother and thus they are contraindicated in patients with renal and cardiac disease. Their general side effect profile includes GI upset, hypotension, and hypermagnesemia [38].

Lactulose and sorbitol have not been associated with fetal malformations in animal models; however, human studies are lacking. Both agents can be given either orally or rectally in similar doses. Side effects of these agents include abdominal pain, flatulence, and electrolyte imbalances [38].

PEG is the preferred treatment of the American Gastroenterological Association for chronic constipation in pregnancy [39]. It is generally very well tolerated.

23.3.1.4 Stimulant laxatives

Stimulant laxatives directly stimulate colonic smooth muscle and/or interfere with water and sodium reabsorption. Derivatives of diphenylmethane phenolphthalein (bisacodyl), the anthraquinones (sennosides, aloe, dantron, and cascara), and castor oil are drugs in this category. Stimulant laxatives have been found to be more effective than stool-bulking agents for constipation in pregnancy (OR 0.30, 95% CI 0.14–0.61) in randomized trials; however, they also carry more side effects [36]. In a study of 236 newborns exposed to phenolphthalein during the first trimester, no increased risk for congenital defects was found [40].

Bisacodyl is available in oral and suppository form. Bisacodyl should not be taken within an hour of consuming calcium-containing compounds as it can cause early medication release and gastric irritation. The most common side effects are electrolyte and fluid imbalance, abdominal pain, nausea, and vomiting. Senna was not found to be associated with a higher risk for congenital abnormalities or adverse birth outcomes [41]. It is considered acceptable for short-term use [37]. Adverse effects include abdominal cramps, diarrhea, nausea, and vomiting. Dantron is a sennoside which has been associated with congenital malformations [40,42]. It should not be used in pregnancy.

Castor oil works quickly; however, it is contraindicated in pregnancy as it may induce uterine contractions [10].

23.3.1.5 Emollient laxatives

Docusate sodium is widely used to treat constipation in pregnancy; however, studies on efficacy in pregnancy are lacking. It is a nonionic surfactant that allows for the penetration of intestinal fluids into the fecal mass, thereby creating softer stools.

Mineral oil use is associated with decreased maternal absorption of fat-soluble vitamins including vitamin K and increased risk for neonatal hypoprothrombinemia and hemorrhage [43]. It is contraindicated in pregnancy.

23.3.1.6 Prokinetic agents

Lubiprostone is a chloride channel activator which increases intestinal fluid secretion. As there are no data currently on its safety in pregnant women, it is not recommended for use in pregnancy.

Linaclotide is a guanylate cyclase-C agonist which is involved in intestinal fluid secretion as well as gut afferent nerve modulation. It is thus commonly used in constipation predominant IBS. Linaclotide is minimally absorbed from the gut; however, there is insufficient data regarding its use in pregnant women [44].

Prucalopride is a highly selective serotonin 5-HT4 receptor agonist which was recently FDA approved for the treatment of chronic constipation [45]. Its main effect is to stimulate colonic motility. Due to insufficient data, its use is not advised during pregnancy.

23.4 Diarrhea

The prevalence of diarrhea in pregnancy has not been firmly established. One study found that 34% of pregnant women reported more frequent bowel movements [46]. Prostaglandins, via their ability to stimulate smooth muscle, increase GI tract motility, and increases in intestinal secretion of water and electrolytes have been implicated in the pathophysiology of diarrhea in pregnancy. As in the treatment of constipation, treatment of diarrhea in pregnancy should begin with dietary modification. Reduction of fats and dairy products may be particularly helpful. Therapeutic options for patients with persistent diarrhea are discussed below.

23.4.1 Treatment

When pharmacologic therapy of diarrhea in pregnancy is required due to severe symptoms, most clinicians recommend small amounts of loperamide. Loperamide is a peripherally acting opiate receptor agonist which increases intestinal water and electrolyte absorption, decreases intestinal transit, and strengthens anal sphincter tone [47]. Data on this commonly used over-the-counter agent are limited and conflicting. Loperamide was not found to increase the rate of congenital defects in women with first trimester use; however, it was associated with lower birth weights in 20% of exposed infants [48]. Diphenoxylate with atropine has been found to have teratogenic effects in animals and humans and therefore is not recommended in pregnancy [49].

Cholestyramine, colesevelam, and colestipol are a bile acid sequestrant that can be used to treat diarrhea. As these agents interfere with the absorption of fat-soluble vitamins including vitamin K, they may lead to maternal coagulopathy.

Due to the addition of bismuth subsalicylate to Kaopectate in 2003, Kaopectate should be avoided in pregnancy. Bismuth subsalicylate is discussed further in Section 23.2.

Alosetron is a 5-HT$_3$ receptor antagonist approved for the treatment of diarrhea-predominant IBS. Use of alosetron is restricted due to concerns over ischemic colitis [50]. Use in pregnancy should be avoided.

23.5 Abdominal pain

23.5.1 Tricyclic antidepressants

Amitriptyline, desipramine, nortriptyline, and imipramine are tricyclic antidepressants (TCAs) which in low doses are helpful for the treatment of IBS. Although withdrawal symptoms have been reported in neonates exposed to TCAs in utero, a joint study of several European teratology information services on the effect of antidepressants during pregnancy found them to be safe [51,52]. Nevertheless, currently, these drugs are only recommended for use in pregnancy in women with severe GI symptoms of IBS, and when needed, amitriptyline is preferred [53].

23.5.2 Selective serotonin reuptake inhibitors

The selective serotonin reuptake inhibitors (SSRIs) are also frequently used in the treatment of IBS and have been deemed safe in pregnancy [54]. Use of paroxetine should be avoided, however, due to the potential risk of fetal heart defects, newborn persistent pulmonary hypertension, and other negative effects [55]. As with TCAs, use of SSRIs for the treatment of IBS in pregnancy should be limited to those women with severe symptoms.

23.5.3 Antispasmodics

Antispasmodics are used to treat abdominal pain in IBS. Dicyclomine has been associated with congenital malformations when used in combination with the antihistamine doxylamine; however, findings of teratogenicity have not been consistent [56]. Hyoscyamine has not been well studied in pregnancy. Routine use in pregnancy is not recommended.

The medications used to treat IBS are summarized in Table 23.2.

23.6 Gastrointestinal infections

Acute diarrhea is usually the result of viral or bacterial infections that are self-limited, and thus do not require specific treatment. Other GI infections that may occur during pregnancy are cholecystitis, cholangitis, and appendicitis. The most commonly used antibiotics for the treatment of GI infections are discussed below.

23.6.1 Amoxicillin

Amoxicillin is used in the treatment of *H. pylori*. It is considered safe in pregnancy. Using a prescription database, a population-based study of amoxicillin exposure in pregnancy and pregnancy outcomes did not find any increased risk of fetal malformation or other adverse event [57].

23.6.1.1 Clarithromycin

Clarithromycin has been associated with an increased rate of cardiovascular anomalies, cleft palate, and embryonic loss in animal reproductive studies. In a prospective study of clarithromycin in pregnancy, no significant differences were found between exposed and unexposed groups in the rates of major and minor malformations; however, spontaneous abortion rates in the exposed group were significantly higher [58]. Based on these data, some experts recommend delaying use until after the first trimester or until pregnancy had been completed [59].

Table 23.2 Medications used to treat irritable bowel syndrome.

	Drug	FDA pregnancy category	Recommendations in pregnancy	Recommendations in lactation
Stool-bulking agents	Methylcellulose Unprocessed bran	NA	Increase dose gradually to avoid bloating; take with fluid	Safe Psyllium
Hyperosmotic agents	Magnesium citrate	C	Safe but not advisable for daily use; contraindicated in patients with renal and cardiac disease as can cause maternal sodium retention	Compatible
	Magnesium hydroxide	NA	Safe but not advisable for daily use; contraindicated in patients with renal and cardiac disease	
	Sodium phosphate	C	Safe but not advisable for daily use	Safety unknown
	Polyethylene glycol	C	Preferred laxative in pregnancy	Low risk
	Sorbitol	C	Probably safe	
	Lactulose	B	Probably safe	
Stimulant laxatives	Bisacodyl	C	Should not be taken within 1 h of calcium-containing compounds as can cause early medication release and gastric irritation	May cause colic in breast-fed infants
	Senna	C	Acceptable for short-term use	May cause diarrhea in breast-fed infants
	Dantron		Contraindicated due to increased risk for malformations	
	Castor oil	X	Contraindicated as may induce uterine contractions	Possibly unsafe
Emollient laxatives	Docusate	C	Limited efficacy data in pregnancy	Compatible
	Mineral oil	X	Contraindicated due to decreased maternal absorption of fat-soluble vitamins and risk for neonatal hypoprothrombinemia and hemorrhage	Possibly unsafe

	Drug	Category	Comment	Safety
	Prucalopride		Not recommended due to limited safety data	Safety unknown
	Lubiprostone	C	Not recommended due to absence of safety data	Limited human data; probably compatible
	Loperamide	B	Preferred antidiarrheal in pregnancy	Limited human data; potential toxicity
	Diphenoxylate/atropine	C	Not recommended due to possible teratogenicity	
	Cholestyramine, colesevelam, and colestipol	C	Interferes with the absorption of fat-soluble vitamins and may lead to maternal coagulopathy	
	Kaopectate	C	Not safe due to bismuth component	No human data; probably compatible
Tricyclic antidepressants	Amitriptyline	C	Limit use to patients with severe symptoms	Limited human data
	Nortriptyline	D		
	Desipramine	C		
	Imipramine	D		
Selective serotonin reuptake inhibitors		Generally category C; paroxetine (D)	Generally safe; avoid use of paroxetine; limit use to patients with severe symptoms	Limited human data; potential toxicity
Antispasmodics	Dicyclomine	B	Not recommended for routine use due to limited safety data	Limited human data; potential toxicity
	Hyoscyamine	C		No human data; probably compatible

NA, *not applicable.*

23.6.1.2 Tetracycline

Tetracycline when given in the second trimester has been associated with staining of newborn teeth [60]. It has also been associated with maternal fatty liver and jaundice [61]. Thus, use of tetracycline is not recommended in pregnancy or during lactation.

23.6.1.3 Metronidazole

Metronidazole is used to treat amebiasis, giardiasis, and other intraabdominal infections. Multiple studies have suggested that metronidazole use in pregnancy is safe [62–64].

23.6.1.4 Fluoroquinolones

Fluoroquinolone antibiotics (ciprofloxacin, levofloxacin, and norfloxacin) bind to fetal cartilage and may cause arthropathies in children. First trimester exposure in 200 women, however, was not found to increase the risk for major malformations when compared to matched controls; however, the rate of therapeutic abortion was higher in the fluoroquinolone group [65]. Long-term use of the fluoroquinolones is not advised in pregnancy.

23.6.1.5 Rifaximin

Rifaximin is a nonabsorbable antibiotic that is FDA approved for treatment of traveler's diarrhea and hepatic encephalopathy. It is also used in the treatment of some forms of IBS. There have been reports of teratogenic effects in rifaximin-treated animal models; however, human data are lacking.

23.6.1.6 Amphotericin and imipenem

Amphotericin is not associated with an increased risk for congenital malformations and is the preferred antifungal during pregnancy. There is limited safety data for imipenem in pregnancy. Because of changes in the pharmacokinetics of imipenem during pregnancy, caution should be applied to dosing.

23.6.1.7 Trimethoprim-sulfamethoxazole

Trimethoprim-sulfamethoxazole (TMP/SMX) should be avoided in pregnancy because of the antifolate properties of trimethoprim and the potential for sulfamethoxazole to cause kernicterus. Cardiovascular defects, in particular, have been reported with TMP/SMX use in pregnancy [66,67].

23.6.1.8 Vancomycin

Vancomycin is used first line in the treatment of *C. difficile* colitis. When given orally, systemic absorption is low. It is considered low risk in pregnancy.

23.7 Inflammatory bowel disease

The inflammatory bowel diseases (IBDs) are chronic, idiopathic, and inflammatory conditions of the GI tract. The two main subtypes of IBD are Crohn's disease and ulcerative colitis (UC). Since women with IBD are often diagnosed during the reproductive years, medication safety during pregnancy and lactation are important concerns.

Physicians counseling women about IBD medication safety in pregnancy must first understand that pregnant women with Crohn's disease and UC have higher rates of such complications of pregnancy such as preterm birth, miscarriage, small for gestational age, and cesarean section, and that the greatest risk of complication occurs in the context of active disease [68,69]. Stopping medications before or during pregnancy significantly increases the risk for flare within 1 year. Thus, in general, women should be advised to continue their medications during pregnancy.

23.7.1 Treatment

23.7.1.1 Aminosalicylates

Most aminosalicylates are considered low risk in pregnancy. A population-based study did not find a significant increase in the prevalence of congenital abnormalities in infants exposed to sulfasalazine in utero [70]. However, as sulfasalazine inhibits folate metabolism and can increase the risk for neural tube defects, it should be given with 2 mg daily of supplemental folate. Unlike with other sulfonamides, bilirubin displacement, and therefore kernicterus, does not occur in sulfasalazine-exposed infants.

Prospective studies have found mesalamine to be safe in pregnancy [71]. Side effects of mesalamine include GI intolerance, headache, rash, and (rarely) pancreatitis and interstitial nephritis.

23.7.1.2 Antibiotics

Prolonged antibiotics for the primary treatment of IBD are generally avoided during pregnancy. Patients with abdominal abscesses, phlegmons, impending perforation, fulminant colitis, or pouchitis may, however, require them. The antibiotics used most commonly in IBD are ciprofloxacin, metronidazole, and rifaximin. They are covered in Section 23.6 and summarized in Table 23.3.

23.7.1.3 Corticosteroids

Corticosteroids have been used extensively for the treatment of various inflammatory conditions in pregnancy. Although there have been reports of an increased risk of oral clefts, especially with first trimester exposure [72], other studies suggest minimal teratogenicity [73]. Corticosteroids should not be used as maintenance therapy in pregnancy due to the increased risk of infant infection, preterm birth, and gestational diabetes. However, if needed for a flare, corticosteroids should not be withheld.

A small retrospective review of patients with IBD on the corticosteroid budesonide during pregnancy did not demonstrate an increased risk for congenital malformations or other adverse outcome [74]. It is probably safe in pregnancy.

Table 23.3 Medications used to treat gastrointestinal infections.

Drug	FDA pregnancy recommendations in category	Pregnancy	Recommendations in lactation
Amoxicillin	B	Safe	Compatible
Clarithromycin	C	Avoid first trimester and/or delay use until after delivery as may increase risk for fetal loss	No human data; probably compatible
Tetracycline	D	Not recommended due to staining of newborn teeth and risk for maternal fatty liver and jaundice	Compatible
Metronidazole	B	Safe	Safe
Fluoroquinolones	C	Avoid long-term use as bind to fetal cartilage and may cause arthropathy in children	Limited human data; probably compatible
Amphotericin	C	Preferred antifungal in pregnancy	
Imipenem	C	Dose adjust in pregnancy	
Rifaximin	C	Probably safe as nonabsorbed	No human data; probably compatible
Trimethoprim-sulfamethoxazole	C	Not safe due to antifolate properties; risk for kernicterus	Compatible
Vancomycin	C	Probably safe when given orally due to low systemic absorption	Limited human data; probably compatible

23.7.1.4 Thiopurines

The thiopurines azathioprine and 6-mercaptopurine (6-MP) are used as maintenance therapy in patients with moderate IBD and in combination with antitumor necrosis factor alpha (anti-TNFα) agents in moderate to severe disease. Although animal studies have demonstrated teratogenicity, studies on their use in pregnancy in the transplant setting have not confirmed an increased risk of fetal malformations [75]. In addition, a study of pregnant women with IBD on thiopurines did not find any increase in preterm delivery, spontaneous abortion, congenital abnormalities, or childhood cancer [76]. Human fetuses are likely protected from the potential harmful effects of the thiopurines during organogenesis as they lack the enzyme inosinate pyrophosphorylase which is required to convert the thiopurines to their active metabolites. Thus, most experts agree that the benefits of continuing these drugs in pregnancy when being used as monotherapy outweigh their potential risks [40]. When used in combination with a biologic, consideration should be given to discontinuing the thiopurine in pregnancy to decrease risk of infection in the newborn [77]. It should be noted, however, that an increased risk of infection in babies born to mothers on combination therapy has not been consistently shown and thus the decision to stop the thiopurine must be individualized and based on the indication for combination therapy and the patient's IBD severity [78,79]. Side effects of the thiopurines include pancreatitis, bone marrow suppression, and pancreatitis thus starting azathioprine or 6-MP during pregnancy is not advised.

23.7.1.5 Methotrexate
Methotrexate is used for moderate Crohn's disease or in combination with anti-TNFα agents to reduce antidrug antibody formation. Methotrexate is a known teratogen and an abortifacient. It should be used with extreme caution in women of reproductive age and discontinued for at least 3 months prior to conception.

23.7.1.6 Biologics
Four anti-TNFα agents are FDA approved for the treatment of IBD: infliximab, adalimumab, golimumab, and certolizumab pegol. These drugs neutralize membrane-bound and soluble TNFα, thereby decreasing inflammation. Additional biologic agents approved to treat Crohn's disease and UC include the antiintegrins, vedolizumab, and natalizumab, as well as the IL12−23 inhibitor, ustekinumab. Infliximab and adalimumab have the greatest amount of available data in pregnancy and have not been found to be teratogenic or associated with miscarriage [80,81]. They also have not been associated with infections in the first year of life for infants exposed in utero [82,83].

All biologic agents (with the exception of certolizumab pegol) are actively transported across the placenta with increasing rates of transfer in the latter half of pregnancy. Therapy should not be interrupted; however, timing of the biologic agent should be adjusted such that drug levels will be at a trough at time of delivery. Certolizumab pegol may be continued without modification of administration schedule.

23.7.1.7 Tofacitinib
Tofacitinib is a small molecule, orally administered Janus Kinase inhibitor, which is approved for the treatment of UC. It remains unknown whether this newer agent is safe in pregnancy and thus should generally be avoided, especially in the third trimester. The half-life of tofacitinib is only approximately 3.2 h [84] and therefore attempting conception after a week washout period appears to be safe.

The medications used to treat IBD are summarized in Table 23.4.

Table 23.4 Medications used to treat inflammatory bowel disease.

Drug		Recommendations for pregnancy	Recommendations for lactation
Mesalamine		Low risk	Limited human data; potential diarrhea in breast-fed infants
Sulfasalazine		Interferes with folate metabolism; give with 2 mg of folate	Limited human data; potential diarrhea in breast-fed infants
Corticosteroids		Infant infection, preterm birth, and gestational diabetes	Compatible
Azathioprine/6-mercaptopurine		Probably safe for continued use in pregnancy; avoid starting de novo in pregnancy	Not recommended
Immunomodulators	Methotrexate	Contraindicated due to teratogenicity; stop 6 months prior to conception	Contraindicated
	Infliximab	Low risk; dose adjust all but certolizumab in third trimester	Compatible
	Adalimumab		
	Biologics		
	Golimumab		
	Certolizumab pegol		
	Vedolizumab		
	Gastrointestinal disorders		
	Ustekinumab		
	Tofacitinib	Contraindicated	Not compatible

Liver diseases in pregnancy

23.8 Hepatitis B

Women are often first identified as being Hepatitis B virus (HBV) positive during routine prenatal screening which in the United States is universal. The effect of chronic HBV on pregnancy is not well known; however, the risk of progression to chronic hepatitis B is inversely related to age and thus preventing vertical transmission in utero and peripartum is essential.

Women newly diagnosed with chronic HBV during pregnancy should undergo staging of their disease in order to determine the need for therapy. Given the invasiveness of liver biopsy, the need for medical therapy in pregnancy is usually based on HBV serologic markers, hepatitis B DNA levels, aminotransferases, and noninvasive imaging (e.g., right upper quadrant ultrasound) [85]. In hepatitis B, e antigen (HBeAg) positive pregnant women with HBV DNA levels greater than 20,000 international units/mL or evidence of cirrhosis, treatment should be initiated. Generally, if HBV DNA is > 2000 international units/mL and ALT>2 times the upper limit of normal in the setting of negative HBeAg, treatment should also be initiated (as in nonpregnant women). If the liver disease is mild (i.e., ALT between two and five times the upper limit), postponing treatment until after delivery and continuing lab monitoring every 3 months can be considered [86].

In addition, experts recommend measuring HBV DNA viral load in the third trimester and considering initiation of therapy in the third trimester if the viral load is high to decrease the risk of intrauterine fetal infection [87].

Women on HBV therapy who become pregnant should continue treatment if there is significant liver disease, as withdrawing medication can prompt a flare which can be detrimental to both mother and fetus [88].

23.8.1 Treatment

23.8.1.1 Antiretrovirals

The FDA-approved antiretrovirals for the treatment of HBV are as follows: lamivudine, adefovir, entecavir, telbivudine, emtricitabine, and tenofovir. Most of the safety data on HBV medications during pregnancy are derived from the Antiretroviral Pregnancy Registry. Data from this registry have not detected an increased risk for congenital malformations with maternal antiviral use [89]. Of note, most of the included women were treated with lamivudine or tenofovir, thus extensive data on safety with the other antiretrovirals are lacking. Choice of antiretroviral should be based not only on safety profile, but also on efficacy, tendency to create resistance, and proposed length of treatment [90].

Lamivudine was the first oral drug approved for treatment of HBV. In a recent metaanalysis and systematic review, Shi et al. reported that women with high viral loads who were treated with lamivudine late in pregnancy had lower rates of perinatal HBV transmission [91]. Tenofovir and entecavir, however, are now favored as first-line therapy as they are less likely to lead to resistant viral strains [92]. Greater safety data exist for tenofovir than entecavir in pregnancy. Similar rates of HBV infection have been found in breast-fed and formula-fed babies; thus at this time, breastfeeding is not contraindicated for HBV-infected mothers [93]. However, if the mother is on antiviral therapy, breastfeeding is not recommended [85].

23.8.1.2 Interferon-α

Use of interferon-α is contraindicated during pregnancy due to abortifacient effects seen in animal studies [94].

23.9 Hepatitis C

The prevalence of hepatitis C virus (HCV) infection in pregnant women in Europe and North America is estimated to be between 0.2% and 4.3% [95]. Vertical transmission is the major cause of HCV infection among infants and children [96]. Several factors such as maternal HCV RNA levels, HIV coinfection, HCV genotype, prolonged membrane rupture, and intrapartum maternal blood exposure may influence the risk of transmission.

23.9.1 Treatment

The safety of direct acting antiviral therapy, now widely used for the treatment of hepatitis C, has not been studied in pregnancy, and thus these agents should not be used until after delivery [97]. Previous therapies commonly used to treat hepatitis C included ribavirin and interferon. Both of these are not recommended for use in pregnancy. Ribavirin, in particular, is a known teratogen and should be avoided for at least 6 months prior to conception.

23.10 Wilson disease

Wilson disease is an autosomal recessive disorder caused by the accumulation of copper, primarily in the liver and brain, which can lead to cirrhosis. Successful conception and pregnancies have been reported in patients with Wilson disease on or off treatment; however, fertility is commonly reduced and miscarriage rates may be higher [96].

23.10.1 Treatment

It is currently recommended that women with Wilson disease on stable treatment continue their medication during pregnancy as stopping therapy may lead to significant disease reactivation [98].

23.10.1.1 Penicillamine

Penicillamine is a copper chelator which, in nonpregnant patients, is first-line therapy for the treatment of Wilson disease. Cutis laxa syndrome, micrognathia, low-set ears, and congenital goitrous hypothyroidism have been reported in infants with in utero exposure to penicillamine [99,100]. Patients in these studies were generally treated with higher doses than are used for maintenance therapy in Wilson disease. Furthermore, other studies have reported good pregnancy outcomes [101]. For women on maintenance therapy, American Association for the Study of Liver disease (AASLD) recommends a 25%−50% dose reduction with close monitoring [102].

Patients should be given supplemental pyridoxine (vitamin B_6) as penicillamine inactivates pyridoxine.

23.10.1.2 Trientine

Trientine is also a chelating agent. Animal studies suggest it is teratogenic. Nevertheless, given the limited options in the treatment of Wilson disease, the benefit of trientine is believed to outweigh the risk, and can be used at reduced doses (i.e., 500−750 mg daily) with close monitoring [102].

23.10.1.3 Zinc

Zinc blocks intestinal cell absorption of copper and is associated with producing more steady serum copper levels than the chelating agents. It has not been found to be teratogenic in animal studies and is considered safe in pregnancy. The most notable side effect of zinc therapy in pregnancy is occasional gastric discomfort in the mother.

23.11 Autoimmune hepatitis

Autoimmune hepatitis is an idiopathic disorder that occurs more commonly in women than men. Flares during pregnancy are relatively common; thus, it is advisable for women to continue with immunosuppression during pregnancy. Furthermore, as postpartum flares are very common, immunosuppression should be continued and perhaps escalated after delivery [103].

The most commonly used agents for the treatment of autoimmune hepatitis are azathioprine and corticosteroids. Both of these agents are discussed in Section 23.7.

23.12 Intrahepatic cholestasis of pregnancy

Intrahepatic cholestasis of pregnancy (ICP) is the most common pregnancy-related liver disorder. Although it is typically a benign cholestatic disorder in the mother, it is associated with several fetal complications including meconium staining, preterm delivery, intrapartum fetal distress, and even intrauterine fetal demise [104]. Thus, aggressive treatment to lower bile acids is warranted. To decrease the incidence of intrauterine fetal demise, delivery as early as 36 weeks has been advised [105].

23.12.1 Ursodeoxycholic acid

Ursodeoxycholic acid (UDCA) modifies the bile acid pool and displaces toxic bile acids from hepatocyte cell membranes. A randomized trial found UDCA to be superior to cholestyramine for the treatment of pruritus in women with ICP [106]. More recently, however, it has not been shown to improve fetal outcomes [107].

23.12.1.1 Cholestyramine

Treatment with cholestyramine results in limited improvement in pruritus in ICP. It does not improve fetal prognosis. Cholestyramine is discussed further in Section 23.2.1.3.

23.12.1.2 Antihistamines

Antihistamines such as hydroxyzine or chlorpheniramine may be used to relieve itching but may be limited by their sedating properties.

23.12.1.3 Other agents

Dexamethasone also has been used but in a randomized controlled trial did not normalize transaminases or improve pruritis in ICP [108]. No adverse effects have been seen in long-term follow-up evaluations in children exposed to dexamethasone in utero [109].

Rifampin and phenobarbital have been used after first-line agents have failed to relieve pruritus. Rifampin eliminates bile acids through conjugation. In animal models, it has been found to be teratogenic when administered at high doses. Studies in humans have not found it to be teratogenic; however, it has been associated with hemorrhagic disease of the newborn [110]. Small studies have shown rifampin can be safely used with UDCA with good outcomes [111,112]. Phenobarbital works similarly to rifampin. Third trimester exposure did not find it to be associated with fetal complications in two observational studies [113].

23.13 Primary biliary cirrhosis and primary sclerosing cholangitis

Primary biliary cirrhosis (PBC) and primary sclerosing cholangitis (PSC) are chronic cholestatic disorders that destroy the bile ducts. There are limited data on either disease in pregnancy. Patients with PBC should be treated with UDCA [109]. Conversely, 2010 AASLD guidelines recommend against UDCA in PSC [114]. UDCA is discussed in Section 23.12.

The drugs used to treat the liver diseases discussed above are summarized in Table 23.5.

Table 23.5 Medications used to treat liver disease.

Drug	FDA category	Recommendations for pregnancy	Recommendations for breast feeding
Antiretrovirals			
Adefovir	C	Limited human data; probably safe	Not recommended
Entecavir	C	Limited human data; probably safe	Not recommended
Tenofovir	B	Probably safe	Not recommended
Telbivudine	B	Limited human data	Not recommended
Lamivudine	C	Probably safe	Not recommended
Interferon α	C	Not recommended	Not recommended
Ribavirin	X	Contraindicated due to fetal neurotoxicity	Not recommended
Penicillamine	D	May cause fetal toxicity at high doses; reduce dose 25%−50%. Give supplemental pyridoxine	Probably compatible
Trientine	C	Possible fetal toxicity	Probably compatible
Ursodiol		Low risk	Probably compatible

Direct acting antiretrovirals used for Hepatitis C should be avoided in pregnancy as there is currently no safety data available.

References

[1] Ali RA, Egan LJ. Gastroesophageal reflux disease in pregnancy. Best Pract Res Clin Gastroenterol 2007;21(5):793−806.

[2] Marrero JM, Goggin PM, de Caestecker JS, Pearce JM, Maxwell JD. Determinants of pregnancy heartburn. Br J Obstet Gynaecol 1992;99:731−4.

[3] Wesdorp IC. Reflux oesophagitis: a review. Postgrad Med 1986;62(Suppl. 2):43−55.

[4] Fisher RS, Robert GS, Grabowowski CJ, et al. Altered lower esophageal sphincter function during early pregnancy. Gastroenterology 1978;74:1233−7.

[5] Cappell MS. Clinical presentation, diagnosis and management of gastroesophageal reflux disease. Med Clin 2005;89:243−91.

[6] Richter JE. Review article: the management of heartburn in pregnancy. Aliment Pharmacol Ther 2005;23:749−57.

[7] Katz PO, Castell DO. Gastroesophageal reflux disease during pregnancy. Gastroenterol Clin N Am 1998;27:153−67.

[8] Christopher LA. The role of proton pump inhibitors in the treatment of heartburn during pregnancy. J Am Acad Nurse Pract 2005;17:4−8.

[9] Lewis JH, Weingold AB. The use of gastrointestinal drugs during pregnancy and lactation. Am J Gastroenterol 1985;80:912−23.

[10] Lindow SW, Regnell P, Sykes J, Little S. An open-label multi-center study to assess the safety and efficacy of a novel reflux supplement (Gaviscon advance) in the treatment of heartburn of pregnancy. Int J Clin Pract 2003;57:175−9.

[11] Ranchet G, Gangemi O, Petrone M. Sucralfate in the treatment of gravid pyrosis. G Ital Ostet Ginecol 1990;12:1−6.

[12] Rao AS, Camilleri M. Review article: metoclopramide and tardive dyskinesia. Aliment Pharmacol Therapeut 2010;31(1):11−9 (25.1.4).

[13] Gill SK, O'Brien L, Koren G. The safety of histamine 2 (H2) blockers in pregnancy: a meta-analysis. Dig Dis Sci 2009;154:1835−8.

[14] Larson JD, Patatanian E, Miner PB, Rayburn WF, Robinson MG. Double-blind, placebo controlled study of ranitidine for gastroesophageal reflux symptoms during pregnancy. Am J Obstet Gynecol 1997;90(1):83−7.

[15] U.S. Food and Drug Administration. FDA requests removal of all ranitidine products (Zantac) from the market. https://www.fda.gov/news-events/press-announcements/fda-requests-removal-all-ranitidne-products-zantac-market. Accessed May 26, 2020.

[16] Finkelstein W, Isselbacker KJ. Cimetidine. N Engl J Med 1978;229:992−6.

[17] Smallwood RA, Berlin RG, Castagnoli N, Festen HP, Hawkey CJ, Lam SK, et al. Safety of acid suppressing drugs. Dig Dis Sci 1995;40(Suppl. l):63S−80S.

[18] Broussard CN, Richter JE. Treating gastro-oesophageal reflux disease during pregnancy and lactation: what are the safest therapy options? Drug Saf 1998;19:325−37.

[19] U.S. Food and Drug Administration. Amneal Pharmaceuticals, LLC. Issues Voluntary Nationwide Recall of Nizatidine Oral Solution, 15 mg/mL, Due to Potential Levels of N-nitrosodimethylamine (NDMA) Impurity Amounts Above the Levels Established by FDA. https://www.fda.gov/safety/recalls-market-withdrawals-safety-alerts/amneal-pharmaceuticals-llc-issues-voluntary-nationwide-recall-nizatidine-oral-solution-15-mgml-due. Accessed May 26, 2020.

[20] Morton DM. Pharmacology and toxicity of nizatidine. Scand J Gastroenterol 1987;22(Suppl. 136):1−8.

[21] Richter JE. Gastroesophageal reflux disease during pregnancy. Gastroenterol Clin N Am 2003;32:235−61.

[22] Gill SK, O'Brien L, Einarson TR, Koren G. The safety of proton pump inhibitors (PPIs) in pregnancy: a meta-analysis. Am J Gastroenterol 2009;104(6):1541−5.

[23] Pasternak B, Hviid A. Use of proton-pump inhibitors in early pregnancy and the risk of birth defects. N Engl J Med 2010;363:2114−23.

[24] Cappell MS. Gastric and duodenal ulcers during pregnancy. Gastroenterol Clin N Am 2003;32:263−8.

[25] Othman MO, Stone E, Hashimi M, Parasher G. Conservative management of cholelithiasis and its complications in pregnancy is associated with recurrent symptoms and more emergency department visits. Gastrointest Endosc 2012;76:564−9.

[26] Pitchumoni CS, Yegneswaran B. Acute pancreatitis in pregnancy. World J Gastroenterol 2009;15(45):5641.

[27] Tsynman DN, Thor S, Kroser JA. Treatment of irritable bowel syndrome in women. Gastroenterol Clin N Am 2011;40(2):265−90.

[28] American College of Gastroenterology Functional Gastrointestinal Disorders Task Force. Evidence-based position statement on the management of irritable bowel syndrome in North America. Am J Gastroenterol 2002;97(Suppl. 11):S1−5.

[29] Thukral C, Wolf JL. Therapy insight: drugs for gastrointestinal disorders in pregnant women. Nat Clin Pract Gastroenterol Hepatol 2006;3(5):256−66.

[30] Khashan AS, Quigley EM, McNamee R, McCarthy FP, Shanahan F, Kenny LC. Increased risk of miscarriage and ectopic pregnancy among women with irritable bowel syndrome. Clin Gastroenterol Hepatol 2012;10(8):902−9.

[31] Saha S, Manlolo J, McGowan C, Reinert S, Degli Esposti S. Gastroenterology consultations in pregnancy. J Womens Health 2011;20(3):359−63.

[32] Anderson AS. Constipation during pregnancy: incidence and methods used in treatment in a group of Cambridgeshire women. Health Visit 1984;57:363−4.

[33] Cullen G, O'Donoghue D. Constipation and pregnancy. Best Pract Res Clin Gastroenterol 2007;21(5):807−18.

[34] Body C, Christie JA. Gastrointestinal diseases in pregnancy: nausea, vomiting, hyperemesis gravidarum, gastroesophageal reflux disease, constipation, and diarrhea. Gastroenterol Clin N Am 2016;45(2):267−83.

[35] Bonapace ES, Fisher RS. Constipation and diarrhea in pregnancy. Gastroenterol Clin N Am 1998;27:197−211.

[36] Rungsiprakarn P, Laopaiboon M, Sangkomkamhang US, Lumbiganon P, Pratt JJ. Interventions for treating constipation in pregnancy. Cochrane Database Syst Rev 2015;(9).

[37] Mahadevan U, Kane S. American Gastroenterological Association Institute technical review on the use of gastrointestinal medications in pregnancy. Gastroenterology 2006;131(1):283−311.

[38] Xing JH, Soffer EE. Adverse effects of laxatives. Dis Colon Rectum 2001;44:1201−9.

[39] Mahadevan U, Kane S. American Gastroenterological Association Institute medical position statement on the use of gastrointestinal medications in pregnancy. Gastroenterology 2006;131:278−82.

[40] Heinonen OP, Slone D, Shapiro S. Drugs taken for gastrointestinal disturbances. Birth defects and drugs in pregnancy. Littleton, MA: Publishing Sciences Group; 1997. p. 384−7.

[41] Acs N, Bánhidy F, Puhó EH, Czeizel AE. Senna treatment in pregnant women and congenital abnormalities in their offspring − a population-based case− control study. Reprod Toxicol 2009;28(1):100−4.

[42] Nelson MM, Forfar JO. Association between drugs administered during pregnancy and congenital abnormalities of the fetus. Br Med J 1971;1:523−7.

[43] Gatusso JM, Kamm MA. Adverse effects of drugs used in the management of constipation and diarrhea. Drug Saf 1994;10:47−65.

[44] Linaclotide data sheet. http://www.allergan.com/assets/pdf/linzess_pi.

[45] Vijayvargiya P, Camilleri M. Use of prucalopride in adults with chronic idiopathic constipation. Expet Rev Clin Pharmacol 2019;12(7):579−89.

[46] Levy N, Lemberg E, Sharf M. Bowel habits in pregnancy. Digestion 1977;4:216.

[47] Wolf J. Acute diarrhea. In: Branch WT, editor. Office Practice of medicine. 3rd ed. Philadelphia: WB Saunders; 1994.

[48] Einarson A, Mastroiacovo P, Arnon J, Ornoy A, Addis A, Malm H, et al. Prospective, controlled, multicentre study of loperamide in pregnancy. Can J Gastroenterol 2000; 14:185−7.

[49] Wald A. Constipation, diarrhea, and symptomatic hemorrhoids during pregnancy. Gastroenterol Clin N Am 2003;32:309−22.

[50] Lotronex Information. Center for drug evaluation and research. 2002. http://www.fda.gov/cder/drug/infopage/lotronex/lotronex.htm.

[51] Misri S, Sivertz K. Tricyclic drugs in pregnancy and lactation: a preliminary report. Int J Psychiatr Med 1991;21:157−71.

[52] McElhatton PR, Garbis HM, Elefant E, et al. The outcome of pregnancy in 689 women exposed to therapeutic doses of antidepressants. A collaborative study of the European Network of Teratology Information Services (ENTIS). Reprod Toxicol 1996;10:285−94.

[53] Hasler WL. The irritable bowel syndrome during pregnancy. Gastroenterol Clin N Am 2003;32(1):385−90.

[54] Ericson A, Kallen B, Wiholm B. Delivery outcome after the use of antidepressants in early pregnancy. Eur J Clin Pharmacol 1999;55(7):503−8.

[55] Study EPIP083. GSK medicine GlaxoSmithKline. Bupropion and paroxetine. Epidemiology study: preliminary report on bupropion in pregnancy and the occurrence of cardiovascular and major congenital malformation. 2005. http://ctr.gsk.co.uk/summary/paroxetine/epip083.pdf.

[56] McCredie J, Kricker A, Elliott J, et al. The innocent bystander: doxylamine/dicyclomine/pyridoxine and congenital limb defects. Med J Aust 1984;140(9):525−7.

[57] Jepsen P, Skriver MV, Floyd A, et al. A population-based study of maternal use of amoxicillin and pregnancy outcome in Denmark. Br J Clin Pharmacol 2003;55(2):216−21.

[58] Einarson A, Phillips E, Mawji F, D'Alimonte D, Schick B, Addis A, et al. A prospective controlled multicentre study of clarithromycin in pregnancy. Am J Perinatol 1998;15(9):523−5.

[59] Drinkard CR, Shatin D, Clouse J. Postmarketing surveillance of medications and pregnancy outcomes: clarithromycin and birth malformations. Pharmacoepidemiol Drug Saf 2009;9(7):549−56.

[60] Genot MT, Golan HP, Porter PJ, Kass EH. Effect of administration of tetracycline in pregnancy on the primary dentition of the offspring. J Oral Med 1970;25:75−9.

[61] Wenk RE, Gebhardt FC, Bhagavan BS, Lustgarten JA, McCarthy EF. Tetracycline-associated fatty liver of pregnancy, including possible pregnancy risk after chronic dermatologic use of tetracycline. J Reprod Med 1981;26:135−41.

[62] Burtin P, Taddio A, Ariburnu O, Einarson TR, Koren G. Safety of metronidazole in pregnancy: a meta-analysis. Am J Obstet Gynecol 1995;172:525−9.

[63] Caro-Paton T, Carvajal A, Martin de Diego I, Martin-Arias LH, Alvarez Requejo A, Rodríguez Pinilla E. Is metronidazole teratogenic? A meta-analysis. Br J Clin Pharmacol 1997;44:179−82.

[64] Piper JM, Mitchel EF, Ray WA. Prenatal use of metronidazole and birth defects: no association. Obstet Gynecol 1993;82:348−52.

[65] Loebstein R, Addis A, Ho E, Andreou R, Sage S, Donnenfeld AE, et al. Pregnancy outcome following gestational exposure to fluoroquinolones: a multicenter prospective controlled study. Antimicrob Agents Chemother 1998;42:1336−9.

[66] Schwethelm B, Margolis LH, Miller C, Smith S. Risk status and pregnancy outcome among medicaid recipients. Am J Prev Med 1989;5:157−63.

[67] Czeizel AE, Rockenbauer M, Sorensen HT, Olsen J. The teratogenic risk of trimethoprim-sulfonamides: a population based case−control study. Reprod Toxicol 2001;15:637−46.

[68] Norgard B, Hundborg HH, Jacobsen BA, Nielsen GL, Fonager K. Disease activity in pregnant women with Crohn's disease and birth outcomes: a regional Danish cohort study. Am J Gastroenterol 2007;102:1947−54.

[69] Mahadevan U, Sandborn WJ, Li DK, Hakimian S, Kane S, Corley DA. Pregnancy outcomes in women with inflammatory bowel disease: a large community-based study from northern California. Gastroenterology 2007;133:1106—12.

[70] Norgard B, Czeizel AE, Rockenbauer M, Olsen J, Sørensen HT. Population-based case control study of the safety of sulfasalazine use during pregnancy. Aliment Pharmacol Ther 2001;15:483—6.

[71] Diav-Citrin O, Park YH, Veerasuntharam G, Polachek H, Bologa M, Pastuszak A, et al. The safety of mesalamine in human pregnancy: a prospective controlled cohort study. Gastroenterology 1998;114:23—8.

[72] Rodriguez-Pinella E, Martinez-Frias ML. Corticosteroids during pregnancy and oral clefts: a case—control study. Teratology 1998;58:2—5.

[73] Mogadam M, Dobbins WO, Korelitz BI, Ahmed SW. Pregnancy in inflammatory bowel disease: effect of sulfasalazine and corticosteroids on fetal outcome. Obstet Gynecol Surv 1981;36:385—6.

[74] Bealieu DB, Ananthakrishnan AN, Issa M, Rosenbaum L, Skaros S, Newcomer JR, et al. Budesonide induction and maintenance therapy for Crohn's disease during pregnancy. Inflamm Bowel Dis 2009;15:25—8.

[75] McKay DB, Josephson MA. Pregnancy in recipients of solid organs — effects on mother and child. N Engl J Med 2006;354:1281—93.

[76] Francella A, Dyan A, Bodian C, Rubin P, Chapman M, Present DH. The safety of 6-mercaptopurine for childbearing patients with inflammatory bowel disease: a retrospective cohort study. Gastroenterology 2003;124:9—17.

[77] Mahadevan U, Robinson C, Bernasko N, et al. Inflammatory bowel disease in pregnancy clinical care pathway: a report from the American Gastroenterological Association IBD Parenthood Project Working Group. Inflamm Bowel Dis 2019;25(4):627—41.

[78] Bröms G, Granath F, Linder M, et al. Birth outcomes in women with inflammatory bowel disease: effects of disease activity and drug exposure. Inflamm Bowel Dis 2014;20:1091—8.

[79] Cleary BJ, Källén B. Early pregnancy azathioprine use and pregnancy outcomes. Birth Defects Res A Clin Mol Teratol 2009;85:647—54.

[80] Lichtenstein G, Cohen RD, Feagan BG, et al. Safety of infliximab in Crohn's disease: data from the 5000-patient TREAT registry. Gastroenterology 2004;126(Suppl. l):A54.

[81] Vesga L, Terdiman JP, Mahadevan U. Adalimumab use in pregnancy. Gut 2005;54:890.

[82] Luu M, Benzenine E, Doret M, et al. Continuous anti-TNFα use throughout pregnancy: possible complications for the mother but not for the fetus. A retrospective cohort on the French national health insurance database (EVASION). Am J Gastroenterol 2018;113(11):1669—77.

[83] Mahadevan U. PIANO: a 1000 patient prospective registry of pregnancy outcomes in women with IBD exposed to immunomodulators and biologic therapy. Gastroenterology 2012;142(Suppl. 1):Se149.

[84] Dowty ME, Lin J, Ryder TF, et al. The pharmacokinetics, metabolism, and clearance mechanisms of tofacitinib, a janus kinase inhibitor, in humans. Drug Metab Dispos 2014;42:759—73.

[85] Degli Esposti S, Shah D. Hepatitis B in pregnancy. Gastroenterol Clin N Am 2011;40(2):355—72.

[86] Hou J, Cui F, Ding Y, et al. Management algorithm for interrupting mother-to-child transmission of hepatitis B virus. Clin Gastroenterol Hepatol 2019;17(10):1929–36.

[87] Dionne-Odom J, Tita AT, Silverman NS, Society for Maternal-Fetal Medicine (SMFM). #38: Hepatitis B in pregnancy screening, treatment, and prevention of vertical transmission. Am J Obstet Gynecol 2016;214(1):6–14.

[88] Núñez M, Soriano V. Hepatotoxicity of antiretrovirals: incidence, mechanisms and management. Drug Saf 2005;28(1):53–66.

[89] Antiretroviral Pregnancy Registry. http://www.apregistry.com.

[90] Bzowej NH. Hepatitis B therapy in pregnancy. Curr Hepat Rep 2010;9:197–204.

[91] Shi Z, Yang Y, Ma L, Li X, Schreiber A. Lamivudine in late pregnancy to interrupt in utero transmission of hepatitis B virus: a systematic review and meta-analysis. Obstet Gynecol 2010;116:147–59.

[92] Lok AS, McMahon BJ. Chronic hepatitis B: update 2009. Hepatology 2009;50:661–2.

[93] Lok AS, McMahon BM. Chronic hepatitis B: update 2009. Hepatology 2009;50:1–36.

[94] Trotter JF, Zygmunt AJ. Conception and pregnancy during interferon-alpha therapy for chronic hepatitis C. J Clin Gastroenterol 2001;32(1):76–8.

[95] Silverman NS, Jenkin BK, Wu C, McGillen P, Knee G. Hepatitis C virus in pregnancy: seroprevalence and risk factors for infection. Am J Obstet Gynecol 1993;169(3): 583–7.

[96] Kumar S, Balki M, Williamson C, Castillo E, Money D. Disorders of the liver, biliary system and exocrine pancreas in pregnancy. In: Powrie RO, Greene MF, Camann W, editors. DeSwiet's medical disorders in obstetric Practice. 5th ed. Wiley-Blackwell; 2010. p. 223–55.

[97] Hughes BL, Page CM, Kuller JA. Society for Maternal-Fetal Medicine (SMFM). Hepatitis C in pregnancy: screening, treatment, and management. Am J Obstet Gynecol 2017;217(5):B2–12.

[98] Shimono N, Ishihashi H, Ikematsu H, Kudo J, Shirahama M, Inaba S, et al. Fulminant hepatic failure during perinatal period in a pregnant woman with Wilson's disease. Gastroenterol Jpn 1991;26:69–73.

[99] Sinha S, Taly AB, Prashanth LK, Arunodaya GR, Swamy HS. Successful pregnancies and abortions in symptomatic and asymptomatic Wilson's disease. J Neurol Sci 2004; 217:37–40.

[100] Hanukoglu A, Curiel B, Berkowitz D, Levine A, Sack J, Lorberboym M. Hypothyroidism and dyshormonogenesis induced by D-penicillamine in children with Wilson's disease and healthy infants born to a mother with Wilson's disease. J Pediatr 2008; 153:864–6.

[101] Sternlieb I. Wilson's disease and pregnancy. Hepatology 2000;31(2):531–2.

[102] Roberts EA, Schilsky ML, American Association for Study of Liver Diseases (AASLD). Diagnosis and treatment of Wilson disease: an update. Hepatology 2008; 47:2089.

[103] Buchel E, Van Steenbergen W, Nevens F, Fevery J. Improvement of auto-immune hepatitis during pregnancy followed by flare-up after delivery. Am J Gastroenterol 2002; 97(12):3160–5.

[104] Riely C, Bacq Y. Intrahepatic cholestasis of pregnancy. Clin Liver Dis 2004;8:167–76.

[105] Lo JO, Shaffer BL, Allen AJ, Little SE, Cheng YW, Caughey AB. Intrahepatic cholestasis of pregnancy and timing of delivery. J Matern Fetal Neonatal Med 2015;28(18): 2254–8.

[106] Kondrackiene J, Beuers U, Kupcinskas L. Efficacy and safety of ursodeoxycholic acid versus cholestyramine in intrahepatic cholestasis of pregnancy. Gastroenterology 2005;129:894−901.

[107] Chappell LC, Bell JL, Smith A, et al. Ursodeoxycholic acid versus placebo in women with intrahepatic cholestasis of pregnancy (PITCHES): a randomised controlled trial. Lancet 2019;394:849.

[108] Glantz A, Marschall HU, Lammert F, Mattsson LA. Intrahepatic cholestasis of pregnancy: a randomized controlled trial comparing dexamethasone and ursodeoxycholic acid. Hepatology 2005;42:1399.

[109] Matin A, Sass DA. Liver disease in pregnancy. Gastroenterol Clin N Am 2011;40(2): 335−53.

[110] Bothamley G. Drug treatment for tuberculosis during pregnancy; safety considerations. Drug Saf 2001;24:553−65.

[111] Liu J, Murray AM, Mankus EB, et al. Adjuvant use of rifampin for refractory intrahepatic cholestasis of pregnancy. Obstet Gynecol 2018;132:678.

[112] Geenes V, Chambers J, Khurana R, et al. Rifampicin in the treatment of severe intrahepatic cholestasis of pregnancy. Eur J Obstet Gynecol Reprod Biol 2015;189:59.

[113] Briggs GG, Freeman RK, Yaffe SJ. Drugs in pregnancy and lactation. A reference guide to fetal and neonatal risk. 6th ed. Baltimore: Williams and Wilkins; 2002. p. 1222−5.

[114] Chapman R, Fevery J, Kalloo A, et al. Diagnosis and management of primary sclerosing cholangitis. Hepatology 2010;51:660.

Further reading

[1] James LF, Lazar VA, Binns W. Effects of sublethal doses of certain minerals on pregnant ewes and fetal development. Am J Vet Res 1966;27:132−5.

[2] Shapiro S, Siskind V, Monson RR, Heinonen OP, Kaufman DW, Slone D. Perinatal mortality and birth-weight in relation to aspirin taken during pregnancy. Lancet 1976;1: 1375−6.

[3] Hernandez A, Petrov MS, Brooks DC, Banks PA, Ashley SW, Tavakkolizadeh A. Acute pancreatitis and pregnancy: a 10-year single center experience. J Gastrointest Surg 2007; 11:1623−7.

[4] Han G, Cao MK, Zhao W. A prospective and open-label study for the efficacy and safety of telbivudine in pregnancy for the prevention of perinatal transmission of hepatitis B virus infection. J Hepatol 2011;55:1215−21.

Challenges in predicting the pharmacokinetics of drugs in premature and mature newborns: example with piperacillin and tazobactam*

24

Jeffrey W. Fisher[1,3], Darshan Mehta[1], Miao Li[1], Xiaoxia Yang[2]

[1]*Division of Biochemical Toxicology, National Center for Toxicological Research, Food and Drug Administration, Jefferson, AR, United States;* [2]*Division of Infectious Disease Pharmacology, Center for Drug Evaluation and Research, Food and Drug Administration, Silver Spring, MD, United States;* [3]*ScitoVation, LLC, Durham, NC, United States*

24.1 Introduction

Using pharmacokinetic models to predict drug plasma time courses after drug or chemical administration to newborns is an active field of research and application [2–32]. Physiologically based pharmacokinetic (PBPK) modeling is one of the more sophisticated computational tools. This type of mathematical modeling has its foundational methodology based on physiology and biochemistry, which is important when considering maternal physiology changes that occur during pregnancy and lactation, and for the growth of the fetus and neonate. Human PBPK models have been constructed for drugs [33–37] and chemicals [33,38–41] during pregnancy and lactation, and in infants and children [33,42–46].

For pediatrics, PBPK models submitted to the FDA for drug registration were judged to be inadequate in a 2016 publication [47]. In a 2017 review [5] of published pediatric PBPK models, the authors discussed the challenges and needs for this field to advance. While limited pharmacokinetic plasma time course data are available for newborns, opportunistic data sets are more common. Variability in drug pharmacokinetic data for newborns, preterm, and term is a recognized challenge [48].

This chapter reviews the recent research effort to develop a neonate PBPK model, which was described in three manuscripts [49–51]. Many of the recent pediatric PBPK models are constructed using scripted commercial software. To

---

* Disclaimer: The views expressed in this book chapter do not necessarily reflect those of the US Food and Drug Administration.

Clinical Pharmacology During Pregnancy. https://doi.org/10.1016/B978-0-12-818902-3.00019-1

carefully evaluate the model code assumptions, we scripted (constructed) our neonate PBPK model using acslX simulation software [24]. Writing code to create a PBPK model is a common practice in chemical toxicology. In our case, we constructed a fit-for-purpose PBPK model to describe the pharmacokinetics of the combination drug piperacillin (PIP) and tazobactam (TAZ) in preterm and term neonates. The research goal was to determine if the variability associated with neonate maturation (physiology and renal excretion) accounted for the variability observed in plasma concentrations for PIP and TAZ in newborns [49], both preterm and term neonates. A careful evaluation of the neonate PBPK model that we constructed allowed us to better understand model failures and successes in predicting PIP and TAZ plasma concentrations.

24.2 What is a PBPK model?

PBPK modeling is a cross-disciplinary approach that leverages physiological and biochemical knowledge for estimating the disposition of drugs and chemicals and their metabolites in humans and other animal species. These models are useful in predicting the internal doses of drugs or chemicals at target tissues of concern and in understanding their absorption, distribution, metabolism, and excretion (ADME) profiles in different species of interest. In this approach, the body is conceptually divided into several compartments or tissue groupings consisting of different organs such as the liver, kidney, heart, and brain that are interconnected by arterial and venous blood flows. This framework is then described mathematically using a system of ordinary differential equations that govern the rate of transfer, formation, and accumulation of a drug or chemical and its metabolites in different body tissues. Knowledge about physiological parameters such as organ weights and blood flow rates as well as biochemical parameters such as partition coefficients in body tissues is essential for adequate description of the disposition and fate of a drug or chemical in the body. Equally important is knowledge about clearance mechanisms by which a drug or chemical is eliminated from the body, especially metabolism rates in the liver and glomerular filtration rate (GFR) for the kidneys. A recent review article examines the influence of birth on GFR maturation [52]. Data from in vitro and animal studies are used when clinical data are not available and suitable approaches such as IVIVE (in vitro to in vivo extrapolation) and allometric scaling are used for extrapolating parameter values across species. Allometric scaling is an empirical approach for extrapolating the pharmacokinetics of an administered chemical or drug across species [27]. The default application of allometric scaling relies on multiplying model parameters by body surface area or body weight (BW) using a power function of less than 1.0, usually 0.75. Scaled model parameters include biochemical reactions (e.g., metabolism), physiological parameters (e.g., cardiac output), or permeability constants for describing trans-membrane movement of drugs or chemicals in organs. Default allometric scaling methods do not usually describe systemic clearance of drugs in children [13] because during development these simple scaling methods do not reflect the impact of maturation processes. PBPK models allow for simulating "what if" scenarios to better understand the ADME processes. PBPK models can be used for route-to-route extrapolation and provide optimum dosing design for targeted therapeutic levels. For susceptible subpopulations with gaps in data and knowledge, PBPK models provide important in silico pharmacokinetic projections, such as in pregnancy (mother and fetus) and in lactation (mother and nursing neonate or infant).

24.3 Neonates are not just "little adults"

The FDA [53] defines "the neonatal period for term and postterm newborns as the day of birth plus 27 days, and for the preterm newborn, as the day of birth, through the expected date of delivery, plus 27 days". Generally, children grow rapidly from birth to about 1 or 2 years during the neonate and infant periods. The dynamic and nonlinear development of children makes them not just "little adults" [54]. Similarly, neonates are not just "little children." Compared to children, the differences in physiology of neonates and infants have impacts on the ADME of drugs. For instance, the GFR is at a much lower level in the term infant, increases rapidly, and approaches adult levels by the first year of age [55]. In addition, important phase 1 drug metabolism enzymes, including CYP1A2, CYP2C9, CYP2D6, and CYP3A4, are substantially lower in neonates, but increase significantly to the adult levels within weeks to 1 or 2 years after birth [56]. In another study, the age-specific plasma half-lives of 40 substrates in premature and term neonates and in infants up to 2 months of age were greater than corresponding plasma half-lives for adults [57]. Simply scaling drug doses from adults to children or neonates per BW may lead to overdosing or underdosing of neonates and infants. Also, administration of drug combinations in neonates may indicate that drug—drug interactions (DDIs) are of concern, in addition to differences in physiology. Among hospitalized neonates and infants in US children's hospitals in 2011, over 37% of them were reported to have potential DDIs [58]. PBPK modeling has been intensively applied for new drug approvals in FDA. Based on 254 Investigational New Drug and New Drug Applications submissions reviewed by FDA's Office of Clinical Pharmacology from 2008 to 2017, 15% included PBPK modeling and simulations for pediatrics and 67% for DDIs [59]. PBPK modeling is a powerful tool for dose adjustment of neonatal drug treatment based on our current knowledge of ontogeny for physiological developments in neonates. Besides maturation of PK-relevant physiologies in neonates, neonatal diseases may not be the same as those in children or adults, which leads to additional considerations in the dose selection for neonatal drugs [60].

24.4 PIP and TAZ PBPK model for preterm and term neonates [49—51]

24.4.1 Overview

One seven-compartment PBPK neonate model was developed for PIP and another for TAZ (Fig. 24.1). This PBPK model is called fit for purpose, meaning that the

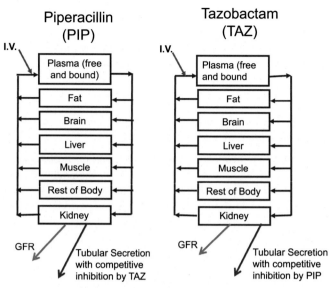

FIGURE 24.1

A static schematic of a dynamic seven-compartment PBPK model for intravenous administration of the combination drugs PIP and TAZ in neonates. Preterm and term neonate growth and urinary excretion of PIP and TAZ are described for birth ages ranging from 25 weeks to term to postnatal ages of 3–4 months.

Credit: Fisher JW, Wu H, Cohen-Wolkowiez M, Watt K, Wang J, Burckart GJ, et al. Predicting the pharmacokinetics of piperacillin and tazobactam in preterm and term neonates using physiologically based pharmacokinetic modeling. Comput Toxicol 2019;12:100104.

construct of the model is limited in its use and is not considered a generic PBPK model. Additional coding is required to consider drugs that are metabolized or administered by routes other than intravenous dosing. Special features for each PBPK model included maturation of the organs or lumped compartments, cardiac output, blood flows, and BW gain. The BW gain was described for five categories of birth age; four groups were preterm (gestation age (GA) 25 (24−26), 28 (27−29), 31 (30−32), and 34 (33−36) weeks) and one group was term (GA ≥37 weeks). The maturation of blood flows and tissue weights was directly or indirectly linked to BW. Renal excretion of PIP and TAZ was described by glomerular filtration and active transport (tubular secretion). In addition, the variability of each model parameter was accounted for using 90% distribution intervals obtained by Monte Carlo simulations. Readers are referred to Yang et al. 2019 [51] and Fisher et al. 2019 [49] to find details about model parameters.

PIP and TAZ have a long history of use in adults, children, and newborns to treat infections [61]. The ADME for drugs and chemicals, in general, are not well studied in detail for neonates because of experimental and clinical limitations and ethical concerns. In this case study of 31 neonates [1], 3 or 4 blood samples were taken from several neonates after an intravenous dose of PIP and TAZ, which provided important clearance information for these drugs. Here, armed with pharmacokinetic information in older children and adults combined with the neonatal clearance information [1], we were able to create a PBPK model for the neonate. An inactive minor metabolite of TAZ, called M1, has been reported in adults and was reported intermittently in children with an average age of 3.4 years [62]. In healthy adults, approximately 20% of the administered TAZ is excreted in urine [63−65]. Because of this uncertainty associated with the metabolic pathway in newborn neonates, metabolism was not considered as a clearance pathway for TAZ. Biliary excretion of PIP is another nonrenal clearance process that was not included in the model but has been reported in adult patients [66].

24.4.2 Neonate physiology

Describing growth in BW is a fundamental requirement for PBPK models because several PBPK model parameters are expressed as a function of BW, and in a few cases height (Ht). Deterministic (central tendency) longitudinal BW and Ht growth curves were constructed for preterm and term newborns [50], and then the equations were expanded to describe the 90% distribution intervals [49] for BW and Ht. BW gain in premature neonates is usually represented as intrauterine growth (at birth) and not by collecting longitudinal BW gain. Age-specific polynomial growth equations were developed for male and female neonates grouped into gestational birth ages of 25, 28, 31, 34, and term weeks. This resulted in 10 polynomial equations describing BW and Ht. Data sets to create these equations included anonymized longitudinal BW and Ht data for preterm neonates provided by Dr. Mary Sullivan [67], several publications containing cross-sectional and limited longitudinal neonate data for BW and Ht, and NHANES 2007−10 cross-sectional survey data [68]. Newborns from a PIP and TAZ study [1] were assigned to the closest age group. Gestational births less than 25 weeks were not included.

An important observation was that BW gain lagged for all premature groups compared to term births. Catch-up for the median BW ranged from 1 year for GA 25 neonates to a few months for older premature neonates. Variabilities in BW and Ht maturation were computed for each GA group with Monte Caro methods and were reported in Yang et al. 2019 [51].

Data for other neonate physiological model parameters were less abundant. These model parameters were organ weight, cardiac output, blood flows to organs, GFR, and tubular secretion. Limited longitudinal data for a few physiological measurements were reported for neonates. By no means could 10 separate maturation profiles (based on BW) for each model parameter be created. Longitudinal data were reported for GFR for GA (weeks) 28, 29, 30, and 31 age groups over a postnatal period of 4 weeks [69]. To overcome the gaps in data and knowledge about neonatal maturation, model interpolation and extrapolation methods were used to estimate maturation rates for each physiological parameter within a GA grouping (GA 25, 28, 31, 34, and term). This was accomplished by first creating a model parameter maturation equation based on the reported GA and BW or postmenstrual age (PMA) projections described above. PMA is the gestational age (weeks) plus the postnatal age (weeks). Each equation, developed using cross-sectional data and/or very limited longitudinal data, was then computed using the assigned BW or PMA growth equation depending on GA at birth. Monte Carlo simulations were implemented to describe the interindividual variability for each physiological model parameter value. Data for some physiological parameters were more robust than others. The variability for model parameters was described using a normally distributed random variable with a default standard deviation (SD, corresponding to the coefficient of variation) value of 0.3 when empirical data were not available (refer to Yang et al. 2019 [51] for equations). Most data-driven SD estimates were less than 0.3 except for preterm body fat weight, which had an SD value of 0.4. Equations for each model parameter, their 90% distribution intervals, and the data associated with each model parameter can be found in Yang et al. 2019 [51].

24.4.3 Drug-specific model parameters

Tubular secretion of PIP was suspected in older children because renal excretion of PIP exceeded GFR [62]. We described the competitive inhibition of PIP on TAZ and vice versa for tubular secretion by human renal transporters hOAT1 and hOAT3. This was accomplished using IVIVE methods [49]. Km, the affinity constants for PIP and TAZ for the two renal transporter proteins, were assigned an SD estimate of 0.3 and for Vmax, 0.7, for the normally distributed random variable, based on reported variability in tubular secretion of the anion, para-aminohippuric acid (PAH) in term neonates. Vmax values for PIP and TAZ (nmol/h) for each transporter were scaled per gram kidney weight. Thus, the estimated Vmax value increased during maturation as a function of kidney weight gain. Serum protein binding equations for PIP and TAZ were each assigned an SD of 0.25 for this normally distributed random variable. Weak serum protein binding was assumed in neonates based on adults (20%–30%) [70]. This was accounted for in neonates by adjusting the fraction of protein binding based on calculated albumin levels in the neonate. Tissue to plasma partition coefficients for the PBPK model compartments (liver, fat, muscle, brain, and rest of body) were derived from data (fat and muscle) or calculated using PK-Sim 7.2 simulation software, Rogers and Rowland algorithm. The corresponding SD values for the normally distributed random variables ranged from 0.29 to 0.56. The solubility (partition coefficients) values of PIP and TAZ were lowest in fat and highest in the kidney with all values of less than one, indicating hydrophilicity.

24.4.4 PBPK model sensitivity analyses

A restricted local sensitivity analysis of the neonate PBPK model was completed to determine which model parameters are most sensitive for predicting plasma levels of PIP and TAZ in preterm and term neonates. Of the approximately 35–40 model parameters, the most sensitive model parameters for preterm and term neonates are listed in Table 24.1. A complete listing can be found in Fisher et al. 2019 [49].

Table 24.1 The most sensitive model parameters with normalized sensitivity coefficient values.

Model parameter	PIP Preterm	PIP Term	TAZ Preterm	TAZ Term
GFR[a]	−2.88	−2.15	−2.78	−2.11
Volume of kidney[a]	−1.89	−1.19	−1.71	−1.11
Km hOAT3 renal transporter[b]	0.95	0.48	1.15	0.72
Vmax hOAT3 renal transporter[c]	−1.43	−0.94	−1.2	−0.77
BW[a]	−	0.76	−	0.77
Rest of body/plasma partition coefficient[b]	1.41	1.21	1.21	0.64

The larger the absolute value of the normalized sensitivity coefficient, the more sensitive the model parameter [49].
[a] *Described with a maturation equation.*
[b] *Fixed value.*
[c] *Described by scaling to kidney weight.*
Adapted from Fisher JW, Wu H, Cohen-Wolkowiez M, Watt K, Wang J, Burckart GJ, et al. Predicting the pharmacokinetics of piperacillin and tazobactam in preterm and term neonates using physiologically based pharmacokinetic modeling. Comput Toxicol 2019;12:100104.

One interesting assessment is to reexamine the availability of data for the sensitive model parameters and determine if the data were adequately described by the model-predicted 90% distribution intervals. Below is an evaluation of the sensitive model parameters (Table 24.1). Not unexpectedly, several of the model parameters associated with renal clearance of the drugs were found to be sensitive to predicting PIP and TAZ plasma concentrations.

24.4.4.1 Renal GFR
As reported in Yang et al. 2019 [51], the GFR for term neonates (mL/min) was predicted by creating an equation from data provided in Claassen et al. 2015 [4] (Fig. 24.2A). While the 50th percentile GFR is well predicted, the variability in GFR slightly exceeded the model predictions (5 and 95 percentiles) for the term neonate (GA ≥ 37 weeks). For preterm neonates, longitudinal data were used to create five equations (mL/min/1.73 m^2) for GA 27, 28, 29, 30, and 31 weeks based on data reported in Vieux et al. 2010 [69] (Fig. 24.2B−F). Body surface area of neonates was estimated using the Boyd equation as reported in Rhodin et al. 2009 [71], where BSA (cm^2) $= 4.688 \times BW^{0.8168 - 0.0154 \times \log(BW)}$. BW is in grams. The 50th percentile predictions for preterm neonates were adequately represented by each equation. There was a trend to slightly overpredict the 95th percentiles 3−4 weeks after birth. Urine is required to measure the rates of renal elimination of PIP and TAZ and compare to GFR and tubular secretion predictions. No urine was collected in this neonate study population.

24.4.4.2 Volume of kidney
Equations were developed based on cross-sectional measurements of the right and left kidneys from individual mixed sex autopsy measurements (solid circle) and

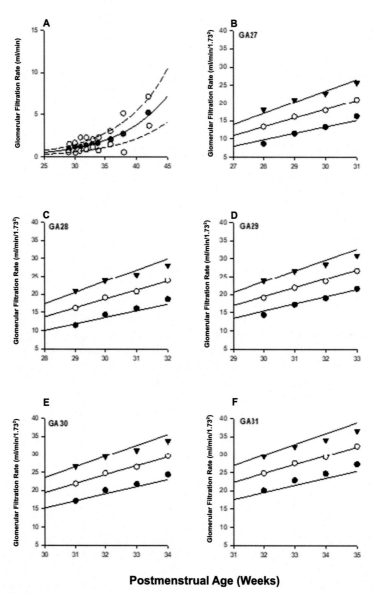

Postmenstrual Age (Weeks)

FIGURE 24.2

GFR. (A) Data representing mean (*solid circle*) and 5th and 95th percentiles (*open circle*) from Claassen et al. 2015 [4] with the 50th percentile predicted GFR (mL/min) represented by a *solid line* and the 5th and 95th percentiles represented by *dashed lines*. This equation [49] was used to predict GFR for term neonates only. (B—F) Observed and predicted GFR (mL/min/1.73 m²) for gestation ages 27, 28, 29, 30, and 31 weeks, respectively. The *solid lines* represent the equation-predicted 5th, 50th, and 95th percentiles and the *open circle* represents the mean observed GFR, the *solid circle* the 5th percentile, and the *upside-down solid triangle* the 95th percentile.

Credit: Yang X, Wu H, Mehta D, Sullivan MC, Wang J, Burckart GJ, et al. Ontogeny equations with probability distributions for anthropomorphic measurements in preterm and term neonates and infants for use in a PBPK model. Comput Toxicol 2019;11:101—17.

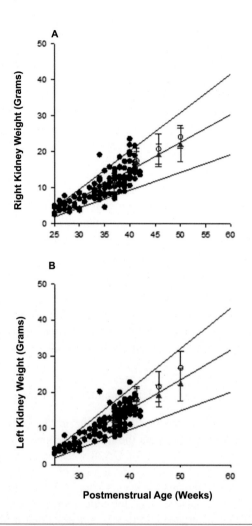

FIGURE 24.3

Kidney. Predicted 5th, 50th, and 95th percentiles (*solid lines*) for kidney weight (g) for right (A) and left (B) kidneys. Neonates of mixed sex born from GA25 to GA42 [72] are depicted as individual measurements (*solid circles*), and for older term neonates, males (open circle ± SD) and females (solid triangle ± SD) are shown [73]. Over 90% of the individual measures of kidney weight are within the 90% distribution intervals.

Credit: Yang X, Wu H, Mehta D, Sullivan MC, Wang J, Burckart GJ, et al. Ontogeny equations with probability distributions for anthropomorphic measurements in preterm and term neonates and infants for use in a PBPK model. Comput Toxicol 2019;11:101−17.

for older infants, male and female autopsy measurements [51] reported as mean values ± SD (Fig. 24.3). Many measurements represent intrauterine measurements. The equation-predicted 5th, 50th, and 95th percentiles are shown as solid lines. 90% of the individual data were within the model-predicted 90% distribution interval. The weights of right and left kidneys were summed for use as one compartment in the neonate PBPK model.

24.4.4.3 Renal tubular secretion (active transport)

Tubular secretions of PIP and TAZ were described as active transport using Michaelis—Menten equations based on in vitro studies with a common cell line, human embryonic kidney (HEK293) cells [74]. Competitive inhibition of each drug for the hOAT1 and hOAT3 transporters was apparent using HEK293 cells [74]. The methods to perform IVIVE were described in Fisher et al. 2019 [49]. Km (μM), the affinity constant, was assumed to not change throughout maturation. Vmax was scaled based on kidney weight (nmol/hr/g kidney). Michaelis—Menten model parameters, Vmax, and Km, describing the active transport of PIP and TAZ by hOAT3 were found to be more sensitive in the PBPK model than Vmax and Km values for hOAT1. Again, without collecting urine in neonates, the urinary excretion rates of PIP and TAZ are unknown, thus the evaluation of tubular secretion cannot be accomplished. Furthermore, information is needed about the abundance and the maturation rates of the hOAT1/3 protein transporters in the proximal renal tubule for this age group.

24.4.4.4 Body weight of term neonates

BW was a sensitive model parameter for term neonates in describing PIP and TAZ concentrations in plasma. When evaluating the observed BW data versus predictions [51], the variability in the data did exceed model predictions (Fig. 24.4A—C). However, using the World Health Organization (WHO) data set, a systematic over-prediction occurred during the first 30 days after birth for the WHO data for males and females (Fig. 24.4D and E). In this case, a reevaluation of the equations used to describe BW gain is needed to consider demographics for term neonates.

24.4.4.5 Partition coefficients for PIP and TAZ in the lumped compartment

The fraction of the BW that represents the lumped compartment (rest of body) is substantial, over 50% of BW at birth for GA28 week neonates, and decreases to near 25% by PMA 60. Fig. 24.5 shows maturation of organs and lumped tissues as a fraction of BW. Assigning a partition coefficient value for the lumped compartment/plasma equal to the muscle may introduce some error since the lumped compartment represents all organs and tissues not described in the PBPK model. The range of estimated partition coefficient values was about threefold for PIP and TAZ across tissue groups. Partition coefficient values influence the distribution phase of the drug in organs and tissues. The use of higher or lower tissue or organ/plasma partition coefficient values will result in lower and higher predicted plasma levels at steady state.

24.5 Ability of the neonate PBPK model to predict plasma levels of PIP and TAZ

For each of the 31 neonates, the reported intravenous dosing schedule in the hospital was simulated. Blood samples taken for each neonate ranged from minimal episodic

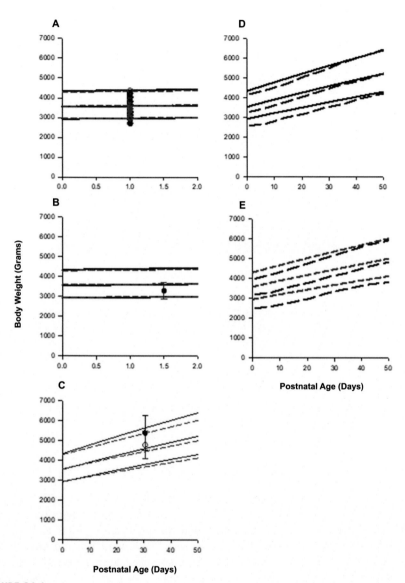

FIGURE 24.4

Term neonates, GA ≥ 37. Predicted BW growth for males (*sold lines*) and females (*dotted lines*) for medians and the ranges representing the 5th and 95th percentiles. (A) Postnatal age (PNA) 1 day with individual BW measurements for males (*solid circle*) and females (*empty circle*) [67]. (B) Mean and SD BW on PNA 1.5 days for male (*solid circle*) and female (*empty circle*) [75]. (C) Mean and SD BW on PNA 30 for male (*sold circle*) and female (*empty circle*) term birthed infants [68]. WHO reported 5th, 50th and 95th percentiles (*long-dashed lines*) for BW growth for males (D) and females (E) [76].

Credit: Yang X, Wu H, Mehta D, Sullivan MC, Wang J, Burckart GJ, et al. Ontogeny equations with probability distributions for anthropomorphic measurements in preterm and term neonates and infants for use in a PBPK model. Comput Toxicol 2019;11:101–17.

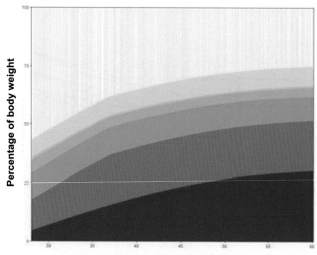

FIGURE 24.5

Predicted mean organ weight changes as a percent of body weight for GA28 weeks (PMA 28) to PMA 60 weeks for fat, muscle, brain, liver, kidney, blood, and the rest of the body. Less than 50% of the body was accounted for by organs at birth (GA28) in the neonate PBPK model and nearly 75% of the body was accounted for by organs at PMA 60, suggesting that more organs or tissue groups are needed for the preterm neonate PBPK model to reduce the size of the lumped compartment called "rest of body."

Credit: Yang X, Wu H, Mehta D, Sullivan MC, Wang J, Burckart GJ, et al. Ontogeny equations with probability distributions for anthropomorphic measurements in preterm and term neonates and infants for use in a PBPK model. Comput Toxicol 2019;11:101–17.

samples (2–3 samples) to one- or two-timed blood draws after dosing (3 or 4 samples). Treatment of neonates with PIP and TAZ was started soon after birth to days and weeks after birth. Details about the dosing schedules can be found in Fisher et al. (2019) [49]. The neonate PBPK model was constructed as briefly described above. Clearance of PIP and TAZ by renal excretion was predicted by GFR and tubular secretion. The expectation was that the neonate PBPK model would predict the PIP and TAZ concentrations measured in neonate plasma after dosing with this combination drug. Using a probability-based approach, if the PBPK model was successful, the measured PIP and TAZ plasma concentrations would be within the model-predicted 5th and 95th percentiles. No adjustments to model parameter values were undertaken to obtain better fits for neonates except for poor fits to data. In the case of poor fits to data or model failure (see below), model parameters in a deterministic form of the PBPK model were adjusted (not shown) in attempts to obtain better model fits with data.

For each neonate, the measured plasma PIP and TAZ concentrations were compared to model-predicted 90% distribution intervals and placed into bin categories of Satisfactory, Mixed, or Poor. Satisfactory was defined as all or all but one measured concentrations of PIP and TAZ falling within the 90% distribution interval. Poor was defined as all or all but perhaps one measured concentrations of PIP and TAZ falling outside the 90% distribution interval. The remainder of neonates were described as Mixed, where the PIP and TAZ measurements fell both inside and slightly outside of the 90% distribution interval.

In summary, model predictions were found to be Satisfactory (Fig. 24.6A and B) or Mixed (Table 24.2) for PIP and TAZ in 83% of the preterm neonates and 88% of the term neonates. 35% of the preterm neonates and 63% of term neonates were placed in the Mixed category. To clearly show the comparisons of observed and model-predicted PIP and TAZ plasma concentrations for the category "Mixed," a table is provided for one patient (Table 24.2). An evaluation of the most sensitive model parameters (discussed above) revealed that the data for the model parameters were more variable than first estimated, which may be responsible for this outcome. If greater variability was incorporated into the Monte Carlo procedures to better represent the distribution of sensitive model parameters, more of the observed PIP and TAZ plasma concentrations would fall within the 90% prediction intervals (Table 24.2). Of equal importance to model success is model failure. Model failure

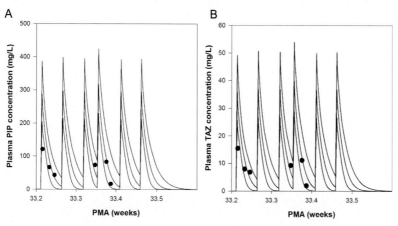

FIGURE 24.6

Example of a "Satisfactory" neonate PBPK model prediction for PIP and TAZ concentrations. Model-predicted (*solid lines*) 5th, 50th, and 95th percentiles for PIP (A) and TAZ (B) concentrations for a male neonate born at GA25 weeks and treated over PNA 60–62 days with 6 intravenous doses of PIP and TAZ. The *solid circles* represent measured concentrations of PIP (A) and TAZ (B). Of the 6 measurements of PIP and TAZ concentrations, only one time point resides slightly outside the model-predicted 90% distribution intervals.

Credit: Fisher JW, Wu H, Cohen-Wolkowiez M, Watt K, Wang J, Burckart GJ, et al. Predicting the pharmacokinetics of piperacillin and tazobactam in preterm and term neonates using physiologically based pharmacokinetic modeling. Comput Toxicol 2019;12:100104.

Table 24.2 Example of neonate PBPK model prediction and observation labeled as "Mixed."

Measured PIP in plasma (mg/L)	Model-predicted PIP 5th and 95th percentiles (mg/L)	Measured TAZ in plasma (mg/L)	Model-predicted TAZ 5th and 95th percentiles (mg/L)
335	121–248	23	15–31
179	29–132	17	4–17
25	4–84	4	0.8–11
108	1–93	20	0.3–12
381	142–311	36	18–39
245	21–170	23	3–22

The neonate was born at GA28 weeks and sampling of blood (n = 3) occurred twice after multiple intravenous doses with PIP and TAZ. Several measurements were outside the 90% distribution intervals, but within a factor of 2.

is very important for revealing gaps in knowledge about the biological system that is described by the PBPK model. 17% of preterm neonates and 12% of term neonates were labeled Poor (Fig. 24.7A and B) or model failure. A deterministic version of the model was exercised unsuccessfully to improve the fits to the entire dataset

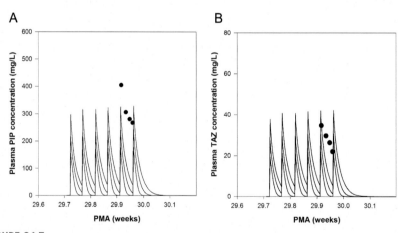

FIGURE 24.7

Example of "Poor" (model failure) neonate PBPK model predictions for PIP and TAZ concentrations. Model-predicted (*solid lines*) 5th, 50th, and 95th percentiles for PIP (A) and TAZ (B) concentrations for a male neonate born at GA30 weeks and small for gestational age. The neonate was treated over PNA 1–2 days with 6 intravenous doses of PIP and TAZ. All measured PIP (A) and TAZ (B) concentrations (*solid circles*) were not within the predicted 90% distribution intervals.

Credit: Fisher JW, Wu H, Cohen-Wolkowiez M, Watt K, Wang J, Burckart GJ, et al. Predicting the pharmacokinetics of piperacillin and tazobactam in preterm and term neonates using physiologically based pharmacokinetic modeling. Comput Toxicol 2019;12:100104.

for each neonate by making biologically plausible modest changes in model parameters. This suggests that other important factors (gaps in knowledge) need to be considered in the neonate PBPK model such as illness and organ function deficiency.

24.6 Conclusions

The outcome of this computational research using PIP and TAZ as an example is informative because it highlights the importance of the reported variability in maturation profiles for organ growth and function. As drug data sets become available for newborn neonates, a PBPK modeling metaanalysis would provide useful insights into the benefits and drawbacks of this in silico technology.

Depending on the drug-specific safety considerations and efficacy requirements, the ability to reliably predict the plasma pharmacokinetics in newborns with a PBPK model may require more information to reduce uncertainties. For example, biomarkers to evaluate renal function for renally cleared drugs would be useful, or if metabolism is expected to be the major clearance pathway, biomarkers of metabolic functionality. Monitoring urine excretion in neonates for renally excreted drugs would provide critically important data for renally excreted drugs. Obtaining noninvasive longitudinal data via imaging may be useful for monitoring physiologic maturation processes. Of course, the availability of drug plasma time course data is critical for the construction or evaluation of PBPK model performance.

References

[1] Cohen-Wolkowiez M, Watt KM, Zhou C, Bloom BT, Poindexter B, Castro L, et al. Developmental pharmacokinetics of piperacillin and tazobactam using plasma and dried blood spots from infants. Antimicrob Agents Chemother 2014;58(5):2856—65.
[2] Emoto C, Johnson TN, Neuhoff S, Hahn D, Vinks AA, Fukuda T. PBPK model of morphine incorporating developmental changes in hepatic OCT1 and UGT2B7 proteins to explain the variability in clearances in neonates and small infants. CPT Pharmacometrics Syst Pharmacol 2018;7(7):464—73.
[3] Donovan MD, Abduljalil K, Cryan JF, Boylan GB, Griffin BT. Application of a physiologically-based pharmacokinetic model for the prediction of bumetanide plasma and brain concentrations in the neonate. Biopharm Drug Dispos 2018;39(3):125—34.
[4] Claassen K, Thelen K, Coboeken K, Gaub T, Lippert J, Allegaert K, et al. Development of a physiologically-based pharmacokinetic model for preterm neonates: evaluation with in vivo data. Curr Pharmaceut Des 2015;21(39):5688—98.
[5] Michelet R, Bocxlaer JV, Vermeulen A. PBPK in preterm and term neonates: a review. Curr Pharmaceut Des 2017;23(38):5943—54.
[6] Smits A, De Cock P, Vermeulen A, Allegaert K. Physiologically based pharmacokinetic (PBPK) modeling and simulation in neonatal drug development: how clinicians can contribute. Expert Opin Drug Metabol Toxicol 2019;15(1):25—34.

[7] Salerno SN, Edginton A, Gerhart JG, Laughon MM, Ambalavanan N, Sokol GM, et al. Physiologically-based pharmacokinetic modeling characterizes the CYP3A-mediated drug-drug interaction between fluconazole and sildenafil in infants. Clin Pharmacol Therapeut 2021;109(1):253−62. online ahead of print.

[8] Willmann S, Frei M, Sutter G, Coboeken K, Wendl T, Eissing T, et al. Application of physiologically-based and population pharmacokinetic modeling for dose finding and confirmation during the pediatric development of moxifloxacin. CPT Pharmacometrics Syst Pharmacol 2019;8(9):654−63.

[9] Gerhart JG, Watt KM, Edginton A, Wade KC, Salerno SN, Benjamin Jr DK, et al. Physiologically-based pharmacokinetic modeling of fluconazole using plasma and cerebrospinal fluid samples from preterm and term infants. CPT Pharmacometrics Syst Pharmacol 2019;8(7):500−10.

[10] Lee CM, Zane NR, Veal G, Thakker DR. Physiologically based pharmacokinetic models for adults and children reveal a role of intracellular tubulin binding in vincristine disposition. CPT Pharmacometrics Syst Pharmacol 2019;8(10):759−68.

[11] Verscheijden LFM, van der Zanden TM, van Bussel LPM, de Hoop-Sommen M, Russel FGM, Johnson TN, et al. Chloroquine dosing recommendations for pediatric COVID-19 supported by modeling and simulation. Clin Pharmacol Ther 2020; 108(2):248−52.

[12] Duan P, Wu F, Moore JN, Fisher J, Crentsil V, Gonzalez D, et al. Assessing CYP2C19 ontogeny in neonates and infants using physiologically based pharmacokinetic models: impact of enzyme maturation versus inhibition. CPT Pharmacometrics Syst Pharmacol 2019;8(3):158−66.

[13] Mahmood I, Tegenge MA. A comparative study between allometric scaling and physiologically based pharmacokinetic modeling for the prediction of drug clearance from neonates to adolescents. J Clin Pharmacol 2019;59(2):189−97.

[14] Yamamoto K, Fukushima S, Mishima Y, Hashimoto M, Yamakawa K, Fujioka K, et al. Pharmacokinetic assessment of alprazolam-induced neonatal abstinence syndrome using physiologically based pharmacokinetic model. Drug Metabol Pharmacokinet 2019;34(6):400−2.

[15] Yun YE, Edginton AN. Model qualification of the PK-Sim® pediatric module for pediatric exposure assessment of CYP450 metabolized compounds. J Toxicol Environ Health 2019;82(14):789−814.

[16] Yoon M, Ring C, Van Landingham CB, Suh M, Song G, Antonijevic T, et al. Assessing children's exposure to manganese in drinking water using a PBPK model. Toxicol Appl Pharmacol 2019;380:114695.

[17] Wei L, Mansoor N, Khan RA, Czejka M, Ahmad T, Ahmed M, et al. WB-PBPK approach in predicting zidovudine pharmacokinetics in preterm neonates. Biopharm Drug Dispos 2019;40(9):341−9.

[18] Ota M, Shimizu M, Kamiya Y, Emoto C, Fukuda T, Yamazaki H. Adult and infant pharmacokinetic profiling of dihydrocodeine using physiologically based pharmacokinetic modeling. Biopharm Drug Dispos 2019;40(9):350−7.

[19] Ke AB, Milad MA. Evaluation of maternal drug exposure following the administration of antenatal corticosteroids during late pregnancy using physiologically-based pharmacokinetic modeling. Clin Pharmacol Ther 2019;106(1):164−73.

[20] Krekels EHJ, Calvier EAM, van der Graaf PH, Knibbe CAJ. Children are not small adults, but can we treat them as such? CPT Pharmacometrics Syst Pharmacol 2019; 8(1):34−8.

[21] Russo FM, De Bie F, Hodges R, Flake A, Deprest J. Sildenafil for antenatal treatment of congenital diaphragmatic hernia: from bench to bedside. Curr Pharmaceut Des 2019; 25(5):601—8.

[22] Kenyon EM, Lipscomb JC, Pegram RA, George BJ, Hines RN. The impact of scaling factor variability on risk-relevant pharmacokinetic outcomes in children: a case study using bromodichloromethane (BDCM). Toxicol Sci 2019;167(2):347—59.

[23] Hahn D, Emoto C, Euteneuer JC, Mizuno T, Vinks AA, Fukuda T. Influence of OCT1 ontogeny and genetic variation on morphine disposition in critically ill neonates: lessons from PBPK modeling and clinical study. Clin Pharmacol Ther 2019;105(3): 761—8.

[24] Zheng L, Xu M, Tang SW, Song HX, Jiang XH, Wang L. Physiologically based pharmacokinetic modeling of oxycodone in children to support pediatric dosing optimization. Pharm Res 2019;36(12):171.

[25] Mansoor N, Ahmad T, Alam Khan R, Sharib SM, Mahmood I. Prediction of clearance and dose of midazolam in preterm and term neonates: a comparative study between allometric scaling and physiologically based pharmacokinetic modeling. Am J Therapeut 2019;26(1):e32—7.

[26] T'Jollyn H, Vermeulen A, Van Bocxlaer J. PBPK and its virtual populations: the impact of physiology on pediatric pharmacokinetic predictions of tramadol. AAPS J 2018; 21(1):8.

[27] Michelet R, Van Bocxlaer J, Allegaert K, Vermeulen A. The use of PBPK modeling across the pediatric age range using propofol as a case. J Pharmacokinet Pharmacodyn 2018;45(6):765—85.

[28] Myhre O, Låg M, Villanger GD, Oftedal B, Øvrevik J, Holme JA, et al. Early life exposure to air pollution particulate matter (PM) as risk factor for attention deficit/ hyperactivity disorder (ADHD): need for novel strategies for mechanisms and causalities. Toxicol Appl Pharmacol 2018;354:196—214.

[29] Emoto C, Johnson TN, McPhail BT, Vinks AA, Fukuda T. Using a vancomycin PBPK model in special populations to elucidate case-based clinical PK observations. CPT Pharmacometrics Syst Pharmacol 2018;7(4):237—50.

[30] Johnson TN, Bonner JJ, Tucker GT, Turner DB, Jamei M. Development and applications of a physiologically-based model of paediatric oral drug absorption. Eur J Pharmaceut Sci 2018;115:57—67.

[31] Shin MY, Kim S, Lee S, Kim HJ, Lee JJ, Choi G, et al. Prenatal contribution of 2, 2', 4, 4'-tetrabromodiphenyl ether (BDE-47) to total body burden in young children. Sci Total Environ 2018;616—617:510—6.

[32] Zhou W, Johnson TN, Bui KH, Cheung SYA, Li J, Xu H, et al. Predictive performance of physiologically based pharmacokinetic (PBPK) modeling of drugs extensively metabolized by major cytochrome P450s in children. Clin Pharmacol Ther 2018; 104(1):188—200.

[33] Fisher J, Wang J, Duan P, Yang X. Pharmacokinetics and PBPK models. In: McQueen C, editor. Comprehensive toxicology. Elsevier Science; 2018.

[34] Ventrella D, Forni M, Bacci ML, Annaert P. Non-clinical models to determine drug passage into human breast milk. Curr Pharmaceut Des 2019;25(5):534—48.

[35] Dallmann A, Pfister M, van den Anker J, Eissing T. Physiologically based pharmacokinetic modeling in pregnancy: a systematic review of published models. Clin Pharmacol Ther 2018;104(6):1110—24.

[36] De Sousa Mendes M, Hirt D, Urien S, Valade E, Bouazza N, Foissac F, et al. Physiologically-based pharmacokinetic modeling of renally excreted antiretroviral drugs in pregnant women. Br J Clin Pharmacol 2015;80(5):1031–41.

[37] Colbers A, Greupink R, Litjens C, Burger D, Russel FG. Physiologically based modelling of darunavir/ritonavir pharmacokinetics during pregnancy. Clin Pharmacokinet 2016;55(3):381–96.

[38] Haddad S, Ayotte P, Verner M-A. Derivation of exposure factors for infant lactational exposure to persistent organic pollutants (POPs). Regul Toxicol Pharmacol 2015; 71(2):135–40.

[39] McLanahan ED, White P, Flowers L, Schlosser PM. The use of PBPK models to inform human Health risk assessment: case study on perchlorate and radioiodide human life-stage models. Risk Anal 2014;34(2):356–66.

[40] Lumen A, Mattie DR, Fisher JW. Evaluation of perturbations in serum thyroid hormones during human pregnancy due to dietary iodide and perchlorate exposure using a biologically based dose-response model. Toxicol Sci 2013;133(2):320–41.

[41] Loccisano AE, Longnecker MP, Campbell Jr JL, Andersen ME, Clewell 3rd HJ. Development of PBPK models for PFOA and PFOS for human pregnancy and lactation life stages. J Toxicol Environ Health 2013;76(1):25–57.

[42] Hornik CP, Wu H, Edginton AN, Watt K, Cohen-Wolkowiez M, Gonzalez D. Development of a pediatric physiologically-based pharmacokinetic model of clindamycin using opportunistic pharmacokinetic data. Clin Pharmacokinet 2017;56(11):1343–53.

[43] Verscheijden LFM, Koenderink JB, Johnson TN, de Wildt SN, Russel FGM. Physiologically-based pharmacokinetic models for children: starting to reach maturation? Pharmacol Ther 2020;211:107541.

[44] Duan P, Fisher JW, Yoshida K, Zhang L, Burckart GJ, Wang J. Physiologically based pharmacokinetic prediction of linezolid and emtricitabine in neonates and infants. Clin Pharmacokinet 2017;56(4):383–94.

[45] Yellepeddi V, Rower J, Liu X, Kumar S, Rashid J, Sherwin CMT. State-of-the-Art review on physiologically based pharmacokinetic modeling in pediatric drug development. Clin Pharmacokinet 2019;58(1):1–13.

[46] Maharaj AR, Wu H, Hornik CP, Balevic SJ, Hornik CD, Smith PB, et al. Simulated assessment of pharmacokinetically guided dosing for investigational treatments of pediatric patients with coronavirus disease 2019. JAMA Pediatr 2020:e202422.

[47] Mehrotra N, Bhattaram A, Earp JC, Florian J, Krudys K, Lee JE, et al. Role of quantitative clinical pharmacology in pediatric approval and labeling. Drug Metabol Dispos 2016;44(7):924.

[48] Allegaert K, Peeters MY, Verbesselt R, Tibboel D, Naulaers G, de Hoon JN, et al. Inter-individual variability in propofol pharmacokinetics in preterm and term neonates. Br J Anaesth 2007;99(6):864–70.

[49] Fisher JW, Wu H, Cohen-Wolkowiez M, Watt K, Wang J, Burckart GJ, et al. Predicting the pharmacokinetics of piperacillin and tazobactam in preterm and term neonates using physiologically based pharmacokinetic modeling. Comput Toxicol 2019;12:100104.

[50] Troutman JA, Sullivan MC, Carr GJ, Fisher J. Development of growth equations from longitudinal studies of body weight and height in the full term and preterm neonate: from birth to four years postnatal age. Birth Defects Res 2018;110(11):916–32.

[51] Yang X, Wu H, Mehta D, Sullivan MC, Wang J, Burckart GJ, et al. Ontogeny equations with probability distributions for anthropomorphic measurements in preterm and term neonates and infants for use in a PBPK model. Comput Toxicol 2019;11:101–17.

[52] Salem F, Johnson TN, Hodgkinson ABJ, Ogungbenro K, Rostami-Hodjegan A. Does "birth" as an event impact maturation trajectory of renal clearance via glomerular filtration? Reexamining data in preterm and full-term neonates by avoiding the creatinine bias. J Clin Pharmacol 2020;61(2):159−71.

[53] U.S. Food Drug Administration. General clinical pharmacology considerations for neonatal studies for drugs and biological products guidance for industry. 2019.

[54] Ferro A. Paediatric prescribing: why children are not small adults. Br J Clin Pharmacol 2015;79(3):351−3.

[55] Hines RN. The ontogeny of drug metabolism enzymes and implications for adverse drug events. Pharmacol Ther 2008;118(2):250−67.

[56] Hines RN. Developmental expression of drug metabolizing enzymes: impact on disposition in neonates and young children. Int J Pharm 2013;452(1):3−7.

[57] Ginsberg G, Hattis D, Sonawane B, Russ A, Banati P, Kozlak M, et al. Evaluation of child/adult pharmacokinetic differences from a database derived from the therapeutic drug literature. Toxicol Sci 2002;66(2):185−200.

[58] Feinstein J, Dai D, Zhong W, Freedman J, Feudtner C. Potential Drug−Drug interactions in infant, child, and adolescent patients in children's hospitals. Pediatrics 2015; 135(1):e99−108.

[59] Grimstein M, Yang Y, Zhang X, Grillo J, Huang SM, Zineh I, et al. Physiologically based pharmacokinetic modeling in regulatory science: an update from the U.S. Food and Drug Administration's Office of clinical pharmacology. J Pharm Sci 2019; 108(1):21−5.

[60] Van den Anker JN, McCune S, Annaert P, Baer GR, Mulugeta Y, Abdelrahman R, et al. Approaches to dose finding in neonates, illustrating the variability between neonatal drug development programs. Pharmaceutics 2020;12(7).

[61] Wolf MF, Simon A. The use of piperacillin−tazobactam in neonatal and paediatric patients. Expert Opin Drug Metab Toxicol 2009;5(1):57−69.

[62] Reed MD, Goldfarb J, Yamashita TS, Lemon E, Blumer JL. Single-dose pharmacokinetics of piperacillin and tazobactam in infants and children. Antimicrob Agents Chemother 1994;38(12):2817−26.

[63] Derendorf H, Dalla Costa T. Pharmacokinetics of piperacillin, tazobactam and its metabolite in renal impairment. Int J Clin Pharmacol Ther 1996;34(11):482−8.

[64] Halstenson CE, Wong MO, Johnson CA, Zimmerman SW, Onorato JJ, Keane WF, et al. Pharmacokinetics of tazobactam M1 metabolite after administration of piperacillin/ tazobactam in subjects with renal impairment. J Clin Pharmacol 1994;34(12):1208−17.

[65] Chandorkar G, Xiao A, Mouksassi MS, Hershberger E, Krishna G. Population pharmacokinetics of ceftolozane/tazobactam in healthy volunteers, subjects with varying degrees of renal function and patients with bacterial infections. J Clin Pharmacol 2015;55(2):230−9.

[66] Giron JA, Meyers BR, Hirschman SZ. Biliary concentrations of piperacillin in patients undergoing cholecystectomy. Antimicrob Agents Chemother 1981;19(2):309−11.

[67] Sullivan MC, McGrath MM, Hawes K, Lester BM. Growth trajectories of preterm infants: birth to 12 years. J Pediatr Health Care 2008;22(2):83−93.

[68] Fryar CD, Gu Q, Ogden CL, Flegal KM. Anthropometric reference data for children and adults; United States, 2011−2014. National Center for Health Statistics. Vital Health Stat 2016;3(39).

[69] Vieux R, Hascoet JM, Merdariu D, Fresson J, Guillemin F. Glomerular filtration rate reference values in very preterm infants. Pediatrics 2010;125(5):e1186−92.

[70] Sörgel F, Kinzig M. The chemistry, pharmacokinetics and tissue distribution of piper-acillin/tazobactam. J Antimicrob Chemother 1993;31(Suppl. 1A):39−60.

[71] Rhodin MM, Anderson BJ, Peters AM, Coulthard MG, Wilkins B, Cole M, et al. Human renal function maturation: a quantitative description using weight and postmenstrual age. Pediatr Nephrol 2009;24(1):67−76.

[72] Phillips JB, Billson VR, Forbes AB. Autopsy standards for fetal lengths and organ weights of an Australian perinatal population. Pathology 2009;41(6):515−26.

[73] Ogiu N, Nakamura Y, Ijiri I, Hiraiwa K, Ogiu T. A statistical analysis of the internal organ weights of normal Japanese people. Health Phys 1997;72(3):368−83.

[74] Wen S, Wang C, Duan Y, Huo X, Meng Q, Liu Z, et al. OAT1 and OAT3 also mediate the drug-drug interaction between piperacillin and tazobactam. Int J Pharm 2018; 537(1−2):172−82.

[75] Cruise MO. A longitudinal study of the growth of low birth weight infants. I. Velocity and distance growth, birth to 3 years. Pediatrics 1973;51(4):620−8.

[76] WHO Multicentre Growth Reference Study Group. WHO child growth standards: length/height-for-age, weight-for-age, weight-for-length, weight-for-height and body mass index-for-age: methods and development. Geneva: World Health Organization; 2006.

Index

Note: 'Page numbers followed by *f* indicate figures and *t* indicate tables.'

Printed in the United States
by Baker & Taylor Publisher Services